Introduction to Vascular Ultrasonography

Introduction to Vascular Ultrasonography

Fifth Edition

William J. Zwiebel, MD

Professor of Radiology
University of Utah School of Medicine
Staff Radiologist
University of Utah Medical Center
and VA Medical Center
Salt Lake City, UT

John S. Pellerito, MD

Chief, Division of Ultrasound, CT, and MRI
Director, Peripheral Vascular Laboratory
North Shore University Hospital
Manhasset, NY
Assistant Professor of Radiology
New York University School of Medicine
New York, NY

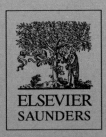

ELSEVIER
SAUNDERS

ELSEVIER
SAUNDERS
An Imprint of Elsevier

The Curtis Center
170 S Independence Mall W 300E
Philadelphia, Pennsylvania 19106

INTRODUCTION TO VASCULAR ULTRASONOGRAPHY
Copyright © 2005, Elsevier Inc. All rights reserved.

Notice

Ultrasonography is an ever-changing field. Standard safety precautions must be followed, but as new research and clinical experience broaden our knowledge, changes in treatment and drug therapy may become necessary or appropriate. Readers are advised to check the most current product information provided by the manufacturer of each drug to be administered to verify the recommended dose, the method and duration of administration, and contraindications. It is the responsibility of the licensed physician, relying on experience and knowledge of the patient, to determine dosages and the best treatment for each individual patient. Neither the Publisher nor the author assumes any liability for any injury and/or damage to persons or property arising from this publication.

The Publisher

Previous editions copyrighted 2000, 1992, 1986, 1983.

Library of Congress Cataloging-in-Publication Data
Introduction to vascular ultrasonography.–5th ed. / [edited by] William J. Zwiebel,
    John S. Pellerito.
        p. ; cm.
    Rev. ed. of: Indtroduction to vascular ultrasonography / William J. Zwiebel. 4th ed. c2000.
    Includes bibliographical references and index.
    ISBN-13: 978–0–7216–0631–6   ISBN-10: 0–7216–0631–8
        1. Blood-vessels–Ultrasonic imaging. I. Zwiebel, William J. II. Pellerito, John S.
    III. Zwiebel, William J. Introduction to vascular ultrasonography.
        [DNLM: 1. Vascular Diseases–ultrasonography. 2. Blood Vessels–ultrasonography.
    WG 500 I637 2004]
    RC691.6.U47I57 2004
    616.1`307543–dc22

                                                                                            2003069337

ISBN-13: 978–0–7216–0631–6
ISBN-10: 0–7216–0631–8

Acquisitions Editor: Allan Ross
Developmental Editor: Jennifer Shreiner
Project Manager: Mary Stermel
Book Designer: Steven Stave

Printed in China.
Last digit is the print number: 9   8   7   6   5

*To Margaret K. Batson, CNM, my wife, for her caring
and her support of my academic projects, and to my sons,
Colin and Aaron, for being such wonderful children.*
—W.J.Z.

*To my wife, Elizabeth Maltin Pellerito, MD, and my children,
John, Alana, and Daniel, for their patience, encouragement,
and support throughout this endeavor.*
—J.S.P.

Acknowledgments

With sincere gratitude, I acknowledge the contributions of the following individuals:

The authors, whose combined expertise is the foundation of this publication. They have provided their knowledge and experience with great willingness and generosity, and they have graciously tolerated our rigorous (some might say tedious) editing of their material.

John Pellerito, MD, for sharing his great knowledge of vascular sonography with so many people and for taking on the task of editor.

Ms. Jennifer Shreiner, Developmental Editor for Elsevier, Inc., Publishers, who shepherded the book through the production process. The timely publication of this work is the result of her excellent sense of organization, her attention to detail, and her patient prodding of the authors and editors.

Mr. Allan Ross, Executive Editor for Elsevier, Inc., Publishers, for supporting this publication and for his administrative advice.

Ms. Linnea Hermanson, project editor for P. M. Gordon Associates, Inc., for her diligent and expert assemblage of the text.

Nancy Cottrell, RDMS; Shelley Smith, RDMS; and Janice McChesney, RVT, our excellent general ultrasound/vascular technologists at the Salt Lake City VA Medical Center, for their assistance with securing clinical illustrations.

Finally, to my family, for tolerating disappearances of many hours while I was writing and editing this text.

—W.J.Z.

I gratefully acknowledge the following persons who have directly or indirectly contributed to the publication of this work:

My administrative assistants, Barbara Stanco, Carole Magid-Green, Doreen Magri, and Patricia McMahon, for their support and good humor.

My chairman, Mitchell A. Goldman, MD, for his encouragement and leadership.

My colleagues and friends, Robin Warshawsky, MD; Gwen Harris, MD; Brian Burke, MD; Eran Ben Levi, MD; Rakesh D. Shah, MD; and James Naidich, MD, for their understanding and commitment to excellence.

My chief technologist, Amalia Pose, and all the sonographers in the Ultrasound section and the Vascular Laboratory at North Shore University Hospital, for their dedication and assistance.

My fellow educators and partners in crime, Irwin Kuperberg; Joseph Polak, MD, MPH; Marsha Neumyer; BS, RVT; Larry Needleman, MD; and Faye Laing, MD, for making learning fun.

My mentor, Kenneth J. W. Taylor, for his unique contributions to ultrasound and for his passion for innovation.

Saiedeh "Nanaz" Maghoul; Adam Cooper, RBP; and James Cooper, MD, for their images, photos, and illustrations.

All the authors of this book, for their outstanding contributions.

Jennifer Shreiner, Allan Ross, and everyone at Elsevier for their help and expertise.

My co-editor, William J. Zwiebel, MD, for his guidance and trust with this project.

Last but not least, my wife, Elizabeth; children, John, Alana, and Daniel; brother, Peter; and parents, Marie and Peter, for their endless consideration and love.

—J.S.P.

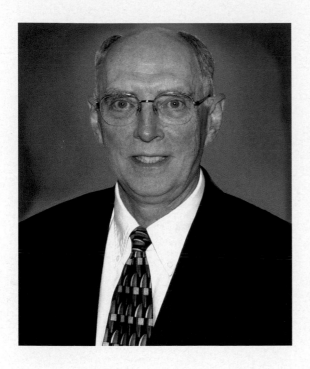

William J. Zwiebel, MD, is Professor of Radiology at the University of Utah in Salt Lake City, and he practices radiology at both the University of Utah Medical Center and the Salt Lake City VA Medical Center. He graduated from the Hahnemann Medical College (now Drexel University School of Medicine), Philadelphia, in 1969. Following an internship at Mercy Hospital, Pittsburgh, he completed a diagnostic radiology residency at the University of Wisconsin, Madison, in 1976, and joined the faculty of that institution the same year. He remained at the University of Wisconsin until 1984, when he joined the Department of Radiology at the University of Utah. Dr. Zwiebel's involvement with vascular sonography dates from 1977. He is the editor of four editions of this text, and he authored two additional textbooks concerned with ultrasound and vascular imaging. For 25 years he has been co-editor of the bimonthly review journal *Seminars in Ultrasound, CT and MRI.* He is a member of the editorial board of *Ultrasound in Medicine and Biology* and holds fellowships in the Society of Radiologist in Ultrasound and the American College of Radiology. He was a founding board member of the Intersocietal Commission for the Accreditation of Vascular Laboratories.

John S. Pellerito, MD, is the Chief of the Division of Ultrasound, CT, and MRI and Director of the Peripheral Vascular Laboratory in the Department of Radiology at North Shore University Hospital in Manhasset, New York. He is also the Director of the Body Imaging Fellowship Program at North Shore University Hospital and Assistant Professor of Radiology at New York University School of Medicine. Dr. Pellerito graduated from New York University before receiving his MD from Albany Medical College. He served as a radiologist at Yale-New Haven Hospital before his current positions at North Shore University Hospital. He is the author of multiple original articles and book chapters and his current research interests include developing new imaging strategies for OB/GYN and cardiovascular diseases. Dr. Pellerito is in great demand as a speaker both nationally and internationally and currently holds multiple editorial appointments including *Radiology, RadioGraphics,* and *Journal of Ultrasound in Medicine.* He is a board examiner for the American Board of Radiology and he currently serves on the Board of Governors of the American Institute of Ultrasound in Medicine (AIUM) and the Board of Directors of the Intersocietal Commission for the Accreditation of Vascular Laboratories (ICAVL).

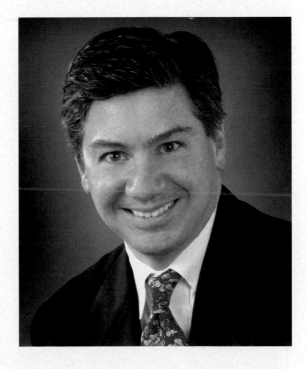

Preface to the Fifth Edition

This edition of *Introduction to Vascular Ultrasonography* is organized along the same lines as the preceding edition but is different in several important ways, most notably the addition of a second editor. One objective of co-editorship is to add new perspectives on the authorship and content of the text. Our success in this regard is verified by the expanded scope of this edition, as outlined below. The second goal of co-editorship is to ensure continued publication of this popular text after the original editor, Dr. Zwiebel, retires in the next few years.

A variety of new chapters has been added throughout the text, substantially expanding the content. These chapters cover various subjects such as hemodialysis access, aortic stent grafts, and Doppler assessment of the female pelvis. With the inclusion of this new material, we feel that all major applications of Doppler sonography are represented, literally from head to toe. The addition of new chapters also has broadened the authorship of the text, providing a wider view of technical and clinical matters than in the previous edition. The authors were chosen for their recognized expertise in the field of vascular ultrasound, and their contributions have enriched this new edition.

Another significant change is the printing of this edition in full color, allowing color illustrations to be shown throughout the text. Color figures were confined to "wells" in previous editions, which diminished their educational value, as they often were located several pages from related text. In this edition, the color illustrations and text are in proximity. Full color publication also enlivens the text, as color artwork and page borders are included throughout. Hopefully this enhances the educational value of the book by holding the reader's attention. The downside of full color publication is added production cost, but the publisher has accomplished this change while keeping the price of the text sufficiently low for access by all potential readers.

Although many changes and additions are apparent in this edition, we have not substantially altered the format of the book because it previously served well to introduce readers to the principles and practice of vascular sonography. Although new chapters have been added, the basic-knowledge chapters have been retained—in updated forms, of course. As with previous editions, we have included material that is sufficiently deep to meet the needs of our readers without delving into esoteric subjects. We also have attempted to meet the educational needs of readers with varying backgrounds. The strength of previous editions has resided in achieving these objectives, and we hope this edition succeeds in a like manner.

William J. Zwiebel, MD
John S. Pellerito, MD

Contributors

Andrei V. Alexandrov, MD
Assistant Professor, Departments of Neurology and Radiology, Director, Cerebrovascular Ultrasound, University of Texas Stroke Treatment Team, The University of Texas Medical School, Houston, TX

J. Dennis Baker, MD
Professor of Surgery, Division of Vascular Surgery, David Geffen School of Medicine at UCLA; Chief, Vascular Surgery Service, VA West Los Angeles Healthcare Center, Los Angeles, CA

Dennis Bandyk, MD
Professor of Surgery, University of South Florida College of Medicine, Tampa, FL

Phillip J. Bendick, PhD
Director of Surgical Research, Director, Peripheral Vascular Diagnostic Center, William Beaumont Hospital, Royal Oak, MI

Carol B. Benson, MD
Professor of Radiology, Harvard Medical School; Director of Ultrasound and Co-Director of High-Risk Obstetrical Ultrasound, Brigham and Women's Hospital, Boston, MA

George L. Berdejo, BA, RVT
Director, Vascular Diagnostic Laboratories, Montefiore Medical Center and Jack D. Weiler Hospital, Bronx, NY

Brian J. Burke, MD, RVT
Assistant Professor of Radiology, New York University School of Medicine, New York, NY; Attending Radiologist, Section of Body Imaging, North Shore University Hospital, Manhasset, NY

Stefan A. Carter, MD, MSc, FRCP(C)
Professor of Physiology and Medicine, University of Manitoba, Winnipeg, Manitoba, Canada

John J. Cronan, MD
Professor, Chairman of Diagnostic Imaging, Brown Medical School; Radiologist-in-Chief, Rhode Island Hospital, Providence, RI

Edward B. Diethrich, MD
Medical Director, Arizona Heart Institute, Arizona Heart Hospital, Phoenix, AZ

Peter M. Doubilet, MD, PhD
Professor of Radiology, Harvard Medical School; Senior Vice-Chair of Radiology, Brigham and Women's Hospital, Boston, MA

Steven G. Friedman, MD
Associate Professor of Surgery, New York University Medical School, New York, NY

Spencer W. Galt, MD
Associate in Vascular Surgery, Geisinger Medical Center, Danville, PA

Gregory Keck, MD
Interventional Radiologist, Southwest Medical Imaging Associates, Department of Radiology, Midland Memorial Hospital, Midland, TX

Evan C. Lipsitz, MD
Assistant Professor of Surgery, Albert Einstein College of Medicine; Attending Surgeon and Medical Director, Vascular Diagnostic Laboratory, Montefiore Medical Center, New York, NY

Mark E. Lockhart, MD, MPH
Assistant Professor, Director, Medical Student Education, Director, Fellowship Program, University of Alabama at Birmingham, Birmingham, AL

Erica L. Mitchell, MD
Vascular Fellow, Oregon Health & Science University, Portland, OR

Gregory L. Moneta, MD
Professor of Surgery, Chief of Vascular
Surgery, Oregon Health & Science
University, Portland, OR

Darius G. Nabavi, MD
Assistant Professor of Neurology, Head of
Neurological Ultrasound Laboratory and
Stroke/Intensive Care Unit, University
Hospital of Münster, Wilhelms
University, Münster, Germany

Laurence Needleman, MD
Jefferson Medical College; Attending
Radiologist, Thomas Jefferson University
Hospital, Philadelphia, PA

Marsha M. Neumyer, RVT, FSVU, FAIUM
International Director, Vascular Diagnostic
Educational Service, Vascular Resource
Associates, Harrisburg, PA

Shirley M. Otis, MD
Professor, Scripps Clinic; Assistant
Professor, University of California, San
Diego; Senior Neurologist, Green
Hospital Scripps Clinic, La Jolla, CA

John S. Pellerito, MD
Chief, Division of Ultrasound, CT, and
MRI, Director, Peripheral Vascular
Laboratory, North Shore University
Hospital, Manhasset, NY; Assistant
Professor of Radiology, New York
University School of Medicine, New
York, NY

E. Bernd Ringelstein, MD
Professor of Neurology, Chairman and
Head, Department of Neurology,
University Hospital of Münster,
Wilhelms University, Münster, Germany

Michelle L. Robbin, MS, MD
Professor of Radiology, Professor of
Biomedical Engineering, Chief of
Ultrasound, University of Alabama at
Birmingham, Birmingham, AL

Robert S. Singh, MD
Vascular Fellow, Geisinger Medical Center,
Danville, PA

Steven R. Talbot, RVT, FSVU
Supervising Technologist, Vascular
Laboratory, University of Utah Hospitals
and Clinics, Salt Lake City, UT

James A. Zagzebski, PhD
Professor and Chairman, Department of
Medical Physics, University of
Wisconsin, Madison, WI

R. Eugene Zierler, MD
Professor of Surgery, University of
Washington School of Medicine;
Medical Director, Vascular Diagnostic
Service, University of Washington
Medical Center, Seattle, WA

William J. Zwiebel, MD
Professor of Radiology, University of Utah
School of Medicine; Staff Radiologist,
University of Utah Medical Center and
VA Medical Center, Salt Lake City, UT

Contents

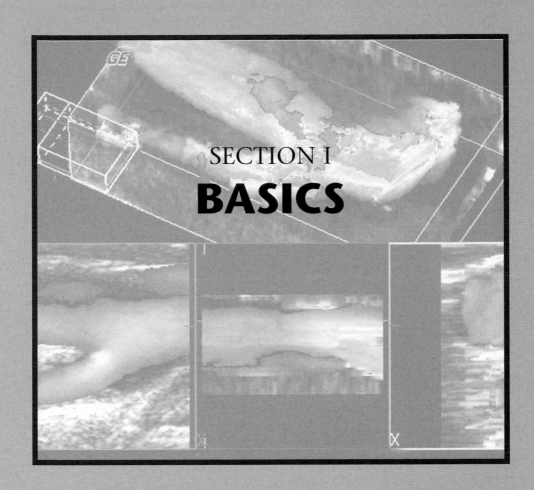

SECTION I
BASICS

Hemodynamic Considerations in Peripheral Vascular and Cerebrovascular Disease

Stefan A. Carter, MD, MSc, FRCP(C)

The circulatory system is extremely complex in both structure and function, and blood flow is influenced by many factors, including cardiac function; elasticity of the vessel walls (compliance); the tone of vascular smooth muscle; and the various patterns, dimensions, and interconnections of millions of branching vessels. Some of these factors can be measured and described in reasonably simple terms, but many others cannot be described succinctly because they are difficult to quantify and generally are not well understood.

With these limitations in mind, this chapter presents the basic principles of the dynamics of blood circulation, the many factors that influence blood flow, and the hemodynamic consequences of occlusive disease. These considerations are helpful in understanding the normal physiology of blood circulation and the abnormalities that can occur in the presence of vascular obstruction.

PHYSIOLOGIC FACTORS GOVERNING BLOOD FLOW AND ITS CHARACTERISTICS

Energy and Pressure

For blood flow to occur between any two points in the circulatory system, there must be a difference in the energy level between these two points. Usually, the difference in energy level is reflected by a difference in pressure, and the circulatory system generally consists of a high-pressure, high-energy arterial reservoir and a venous pool of low pressure and energy. These reservoirs are connected by a system of distributing vessels (smaller arteries) and by the resistance vessels of the microcirculation, which consist of arterioles, capillaries, and venules.

During flow, energy is continuously lost from the blood because of the friction between its layers and particles. Both pressure and energy levels therefore decrease from the arterial to the venous ends. The energy necessary for flow is continuously restored by the pumping action of the heart, which forces blood to move from the venous system into the arterial system, and thus maintains the arterial pressure and the energy difference needed for flow to occur.

The high arterial energy level is a result of the large volume of blood in the arterial reservoir. The function of the heart and blood vessels is normally regulated to maintain volume and pressure in the arteries within the limits required for smooth function. This is achieved by maintaining a balance between the amounts of blood that enter and leave the arterial reservoir. The amount that enters the arteries is the cardiac output. The amount that leaves depends on the arterial pressure and on the total peripheral resistance, which is controlled in turn by the amount of vasoconstriction in the microcirculation.

Under normal conditions, flow to all the body tissues is adjusted according to the tissues' particular needs at a given time. This adjustment is accomplished by alterations in the level of vasoconstriction of the arterioles within the organs supplied. Maintenance of normal volume and pressure in the arteries thus allows for both adjustment of blood flow to all parts of the body and regulation of cardiac output (which equals the sum of blood flow to all the vascular beds).

Forms of Energy in the Blood and Its Dissipation During Flow

This section considers the forms in which energy exists in the circulation and the important factors that govern the dissipation of energy during flow, including friction, resistance, and the influence of laminar and turbulent flow. Poiseuille's law and the equation that summarizes the basic relationships among flow, pressure, and resistance are discussed, as well as the effects of connecting vascular resistances in parallel and in series.

Forms of Energy

Potential and Kinetic Energy

The main form of energy present in flowing blood is the pressure distending the vessels (a form of potential energy), which is created by the pumping action of the heart. However, some of the energy of the blood is kinetic; namely, the ability of flowing blood to do work as a result of its velocity. Usually, the kinetic energy component is small compared with the pressure energy, and under normal resting conditions, it is equivalent to only a few millimeters of mercury or less. The kinetic energy of blood is proportional to its density (which is stable in normal circumstances) and to the square of its velocity. Therefore, important increases in kinetic energy occur in the systemic circulation when flow is high (e.g., during exercise) and in stenotic lesions, in which luminal narrowing leads to high velocities. Kinetic energy is converted back into pressure (potential energy) when velocity is decreased (e.g., in a normal segment of the artery distal to a stenosis).

Energy Differences Related to Differences in the Levels of Body Parts

There is also variation in the energy of the blood associated with differences in the levels of body parts. For example, the pressure in the vessels in the dependent parts of the body, such as the lower portions of the legs, increases by an amount that depends on the weight of the column of blood resting on the blood in the legs. This hydrostatic pressure increases the transmural pressure and the distention of the vessels. Gravitational potential energy (potential for doing work related to the effect of gravity on a free-falling body), however, is reduced in the dependent parts of the body by the same amount as the increase resulting from hydrostatic pressure. Therefore, differences in the level of the body parts usually do not lead to changes in the driving pressure along the vascular tree unless the column of blood is interrupted, as may be the case when the venous valves close. Changes in energy and pressure associated with differences in level are important under certain conditions, such as with changes in posture or when the venous pump is activated because of muscular action during walking.

Dissipation of Energy

During Laminar Flow

In most vessels, blood moves in concentric layers, or laminae; hence, the flow is said to be laminar. Each infinitesimal layer flows with a different velocity. In theory, a thin layer of blood is held stationary next to the vessel wall at zero velocity because of an adhesive force between the blood and the inner surface of the vessel. The next layer flows with a certain velocity, but its movement is delayed by the stationary layer because of friction between the layers, generated by the viscous properties of the fluid. The second layer, in turn, delays the next layer, which flows at a greater velocity. The layers in the middle of the vessel flow with the highest velocity, and the *mean velocity across the vessel is half of the maximal velocity*. Because the rate of change of velocity is greatest near the walls and decreases toward the center of the vessel, a velocity profile in the shape of a parabola exists along the vessel diameter (Fig. 1–1A).

Loss of energy during blood flow occurs because of friction, and the amount of friction and energy loss is determined in large part by the dimensions of the vessels. In small vessels, especially in the microcirculation, even the layers in the middle of the lumen are relatively close to the wall and are thus delayed considerably, resulting in a significant opposition or resistance to flow. In large vessels, by contrast, a large central core of blood is far from the walls, and the frictional energy losses are minimal. As indicated later, friction and energy losses increase if laminar flow is disturbed.

Poiseuille's Law and Equation. In a cylindric tube model, the mean linear velocity of laminar flow is directly proportional to the energy difference between the ends of the tube and the square of the radius and is inversely proportional to the length of the tube and the viscosity of the fluid. In the circulatory system, however, volume flow is of more interest than velocity. Volume flow is proportional to the fourth power of the vessel radius, because it is equal to the product of the mean linear velocity and the cross-sectional area of the tube. These important considerations are helpful in understanding Poiseuille's law, as expressed in Poiseuille's equation:

$$Q = \frac{\pi(P_1 - P_2)r^4}{8L\eta} \qquad (1-1)$$

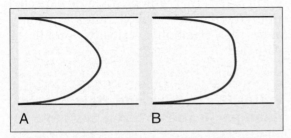

FIGURE 1–1. Flow velocity profiles across a normal arterial lumen. A, Parabolic profile of laminar flow. B, Flattened profile with a central core of relatively uniform velocity encountered in the proximal portion (inlet length) of arterial branches or with turbulent flow.

where Q is the volume flow; P_1 and P_2 are the pressures at the proximal and distal ends of the tube, respectively; r and L are the radius and length of the tube, respectively; and η is the viscosity of the fluid.

Because volume flow is proportional to the fourth power of the radius, even small changes in radius can result in large changes in flow. For example, a decrease in radius of 10% would decrease flow in a tube model by about 35%, and a decrease of 50% would lead to a 95% decrease in flow. *Because the length of the vessels and the viscosity of blood do not change much in the cardiovascular system, alterations in blood flow occur mainly as a result of changes in the radius of the vessels and in the difference in the pressure energy level available for flow.*

Poiseuille's equation can be rewritten, therefore, as follows:

$$\frac{8L\eta}{\pi r^4} = \frac{P_1 - P_2}{Q} \qquad (1-2)$$

$$R = \frac{8L\eta}{\pi r^4} \qquad (1-3)$$

$$R = \frac{P_1 - P_2}{Q} \qquad (1-4)$$

The resistance term (R) depends on the viscous properties of the blood and on the dimensions of the vessels. Although these parameters cannot be measured in a complex system, the pressure difference $(P_1 - P_2)$ and the blood flow (Q) can be measured, and the resistance can thus be calculated. Because resistance is equal to the pressure difference divided by the volume flow (the pressure difference per unit flow), it can be thought of as the pressure difference needed to produce one unit of flow and, therefore, can be considered as an index of the difficulty in forcing blood through the vessels.

Vessel Interconnection and Energy Dissipation. Poiseuille's law applies with precision only to constant laminar flow of a simple fluid (such as water) in a rigid tube of a uniform bore. In the blood circulation, these conditions are not met. Instead, the resistance is influenced by the presence of numerous interconnected vessels with a combined effect similar to that observed in electrical resistances. In the case of vessels in series, the overall resistance is equal to the sum of the resistances of the individual vessels, whereas in the case of parallel vessels, the reciprocal of the total resistance equals the sum of the reciprocals of the individual vessel resistances. Thus, *the contribution of any single vessel to the total resistance of a vascular bed, or the effect of a change in the dimension of a vessel, depends on the presence and relative size of the other vessels linked in series or in parallel.*

Deviations from the conditions to which Poiseuille's law applies also occur in relation to changes in blood viscosity, which is affected by hematocrit, temperature, vessel diameter, and rate of flow.

During Nonlaminar Flow

Various degrees of deviation from orderly laminar flow occur in the circulation under both normal and abnormal conditions. Factors responsible for these deviations include the following: (1) the flow velocity, which changes throughout the cardiac cycle as a result of acceleration during systole and deceleration in diastole; (2) alteration of the lines of flow, which occurs whenever a vessel changes dimensions, including variations in diameter associated with each pulse; and (3) the lines of flow, which are distorted at curves, at bifurcations, and in branches that take off at various angles. For example, the parabolic velocity profile is often not re-established in branches for a considerable distance beyond their origin. Instead, the parabola is flattened so that there is a relatively large central core of blood that flows with a relatively uniform speed (Fig. 1–1*B*).

Because of these and other factors, laminar flow may be disturbed or fully turbulent, even in a uniform tube. The factors that affect the development of turbulence are expressed by the dimensionless Reynold's number (Re):

$$\text{Re} = \frac{vq2r}{\eta} \qquad (1\text{--}5)$$

where v is the velocity, q is the density of the fluid, r is the radius of the tube, and η is the viscosity of the fluid. Because the density (q) and viscosity (η) of the blood are relatively constant, *the development of turbulence depends mainly on the size of the vessels and on the velocity of flow.* In a tube model, laminar flow tends to be disturbed if Reynold's number exceeds 2000. However, in the circulatory system, disturbances and various degrees of turbulence are likely to occur at lower values because of body movements, the pulsatile nature of blood flow, changes in vessel dimensions, roughness of the endothelial surface, and other factors. Turbulence develops more readily in large vessels under conditions of high flow and can be detected clinically by the finding of bruits or thrills. Bruits may sometimes be heard over the ascending aorta during systolic acceleration in normal individuals at rest and are frequently heard in states of high cardiac output and blood flow, even in more distal arteries, such as the femoral artery.[1] Distortion of laminar flow velocity profiles can be assessed using ultrasound flow detectors, and such assessments can be applied for diagnostic purposes. For example, in arteries with severe stenosis, pronounced turbulence is a diagnostic feature observed in the poststenotic zone. Turbulence occurs because a jet of blood with high velocity and high kinetic energy suddenly encounters a normal diameter lumen or a lumen of increased diameter (because of poststenotic dilatation), where both the velocity and energy level are lower than in the stenotic region.

During turbulent flow, the loss of pressure energy between two points in a vessel is greater than that which would be expected from the factors in Poiseuille's equation, and the parabolic velocity profile is flattened.[2]

Pulsatile Pressure and Flow Changes in the Arterial System

With each heartbeat, a stroke volume of blood is ejected into the arterial system, resulting in a pressure wave that travels throughout the arterial tree. The speed of propagation, amplitude (strength), and shape of the pressure wave change as it traverses the arterial system. These alterations are influenced by the varying characteristics of the vessels traversed by the pressure wave. The velocity and, in some parts of the circulation, the direction of flow, also vary with each heartbeat. Correct interpretation of noninvasive tests based on recordings of arterial pressure and velocity, as well as pressure and velocity waveforms, requires knowledge of the factors that influence these variables. This section considers these factors as they occur in various portions of the circulatory system.

Pressure Changes from Cardiac Activity

As indicated previously, the pumping action of the heart maintains a high volume of blood in the arterial end of the circulation and thus provides the high pressure difference between the arterial and venous ends necessary to maintain flow. Because of the intermittent pumping action of the heart, pressure and flow vary in a pulsatile manner. During the rapid phase of ventricular ejection, the volume of blood at the arterial end increases, raising the pressure to a systolic peak. During the latter part of systole, when cardiac ejection decreases, the outflow through the peripheral resistance vessels exceeds the volume being ejected by the heart, and the pressure begins to decline. This decline continues throughout diastole as blood continues to flow from the arteries into the microcirculation. Part of the work of the heart leads directly to forward flow, but a large portion of the energy of each cardiac contraction results in distention of the arteries that serve as reservoirs for storing the blood volume and the energy supplied to the system. This storage of energy and blood volume provides for continuous flow to the tissues during diastole.

Arterial Pressure Wave

The pulsatile variations in blood volume and energy occurring with each cardiac cycle are manifested as a pressure wave that can be detected throughout the arterial system. The amplitude and shape of the arterial pressure wave depend on a complex interplay of factors, which include the stroke volume and time course of ventricular ejection, the peripheral resistance, and the stiffness of the arterial walls. In general, an increase in any of these factors results in an increase in the pulse amplitude (i.e., pulse pressure, difference between systolic and diastolic pressures) and frequently in a concomitant increase in systolic pressure. For example, increased stiffness of the arteries with age tends to increase both the systolic and pulse pressures.

The arterial pressure wave is propagated along the arterial tree distally from the heart. The speed of propagation, or pulse wave velocity, increases with stiffness of the arterial walls (the elastic modulus of the material of which the walls are composed) and with the ratio of the wall thickness to diameter. In the mammalian circulation, arteries become progressively stiffer from the aorta toward the periphery. Therefore, the speed of propagation of the wave increases as it moves peripherally. Also, the gradual increase in stiffness tends to decrease wave reflection (discussed later) and has a beneficial effect in that the pulse and systolic pressures in the aorta and proximal arteries are relatively lower than in peripheral vessels. The pressure against which the heart ejects the stroke volume and the associated cardiac work are accordingly reduced.[3]

Pressure Changes Throughout the Circulation

Figure 1–2 illustrates changes in pressure in the systemic circulation from large arteries through the resistance vessels to the veins. Because there is little loss of pressure energy from friction in large and distributing arteries, they offer relatively little resistance to flow, and the mean pressure decreases only slightly between the aorta and the small arteries of the limbs, such as the radial or the dorsalis pedis.[4,5] The diastolic pressure also shows only minor changes. The

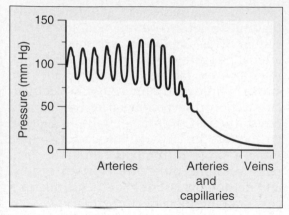

FIGURE 1–2. Schematic representation of normal pressure changes in the systemic circulation. (From Carter SA: Peripheral artery disease: Pressure measurements ease evaluation. Consultant 19[9]:102–115, 1979.)

amplitude of the pressure wave and the systolic pressure actually increase, however, as the wave travels distally (systolic amplification), because of increasing stiffness of the walls toward the periphery and the presence of reflected waves. These waves arise where the vessels change diameter and stiffness, divide, or branch and are superadded to the oncoming primary pulse wave.[3,4] The reflected waves, at least in the extremities, are strongly enhanced by increased peripheral resistance.[4] Direct measurements of pressure in small arteries in experimental animals and humans, and indirect measurements of systolic pressure in human digits, have shown that the pulse amplitude and systolic pressure decrease in smaller vessels, such as the digital vessels of the human extremities.[6–9] However, some pulsatile changes in pressure and flow may remain evident even in minute arteries and capillaries, at least under conditions of peripheral vasodilatation, and can be recorded by various methods, including plethysmography. The effect of peripheral vasoconstriction on pulsatility in the microcirculation is opposite to that seen in the proximal small or medium arteries of the extremities. *Pulsatile changes in minute arteries, arterioles, and capillaries are reduced by vasoconstriction and enhanced by vasodilatation. In small and medium arteries of the limbs, however, pulsatile changes are increased by vasoconstriction, as a result of enhanced wave reflection, and are decreased by vasodilatation.* Figure 1–3 shows arterial pressure pulses recorded directly from the femoral and dorsalis pedis arteries during peripheral vasoconstriction and vasodilatation induced, respectively, by body cooling and heating.

There is almost a complete disappearance of amplification in the dorsalis pedis artery in response to vasodilatation induced by body heating. Similar changes in the distal pressure waves result from other factors that alter peripheral resistance; for example, reactive hyperemia and exercise. Exercise, by decreasing resistance in the working muscle, would be expected to decrease reflection in the exercising extremity. Because of vasoconstriction in other parts of the body during exercise (the result of cardiovascular reflexes that regulate blood pressure and circulation), however, the reflection may be increased and lead to a high degree of amplification. For example, it has been shown that during walking, the pulse pressure in the radial arteries can exceed that in the aorta by perhaps 100%.[10]

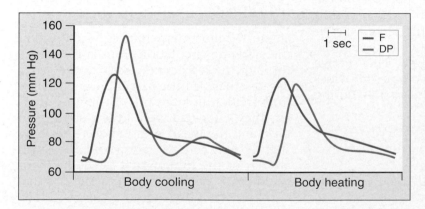

FIGURE 1–3. Pressure waves from the femoral (F) and dorsalis pedis (DP) arteries during heating and cooling. Note that the pulse pressure of the dorsalis pedis artery is greater with vasoconstriction (body cooling) and falls dramatically with vasodilatation (body heating). (From Carter SA: Effect of age, cardiovascular disease, and vasomotor changes on transmission of arterial pressure waves through the lower extremities. Angiology 29:601–616, 1978.)

These considerations are important for correct interpretation of pressure measurements in peripheral arterial obstruction. For example, brachial systolic pressure corresponds well to aortic or femoral systolic pressure and is used as a standard against which ankle pressure can be compared. The systolic pressure at the ankle usually exceeds brachial pressure in normal subjects; therefore, the finding of ankle systolic pressure that is even slightly lower than brachial systolic pressure indicates a high likelihood of a proximal stenotic lesion. However, systolic pressure in human digits is usually lower than systolic pressure proximal to the wrist or the ankle. This observation has to be taken into account when measurements of digital systolic pressures are used as an index of distal arterial obstruction. In such cases, the appropriate norms for the differences between the proximal and digital systolic pressures have to be applied.[11]

Pulsatile Flow Patterns

Pulsatile changes in pressure are associated with corresponding acceleration of blood flow with systole and deceleration in diastole. Although the energy stored in the arterial walls maintains a positive arteriovenous pressure gradient and overall forward flow in the microcirculation during diastole, temporary cessation of forward flow or even diastolic reversal occurs frequently in portions of the human arterial system. How these phenomena occur may be clarified by considering pulsatile pressure changes at two points along the arterial tree. Figure 1–3

shows arterial pressure pulses in the femoral and dorsalis pedis arteries. The corresponding pressure gradient between the two arteries (Fig. 1–4) varies during the cardiac cycle, not only because of differences in the shape and magnitude of the original pressure waves but also, more importantly, because the wave arrives later at the dorsalis pedis. The pressure gradient is greatest during the first half of systole, at which time the peak of the wave arrives at the femoral site. Thereafter, the gradient decreases, and by the time the peak arrives at the dorsalis pedis, the femoral pressure has fallen and a negative pressure gradient appears. Such negative gradients, related to different arrival times of the pressure wave at various sites in the arterial system, are commonly observed along human arteries and are conducive to the reversal of blood flow. Despite the reversal of the pressure gradient, however, the direction of flow may not be reversed if there is a large forward mean flow component.[12]

The presence of reversed flow during diastole can also be understood if one imagines a major arterial segment, with a certain diastolic pressure, that has several branch vessels leading to areas with different levels of resistance. If one of the proximal branches leads to an area with low peripheral resistance, flow during diastole in the main vessel will occur toward this branch, and flow will reverse in the distal portion of the main vessel if distal branches supply areas with higher peripheral resistance. Such situations of transient flow reversal may exist in the limb during cooling (see Fig. 1–4), but during body heating, when

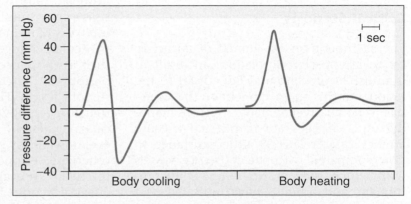

FIGURE 1–4. Pressure differences between the femoral and dorsalis pedis arteries obtained from the waves shown in Figure 1–3. Note the effect of vasodilatation (body heating) on the negative (reverse flow) component.

peripheral resistance in the distal cutaneous circulation is reduced to a low level, reversed flow is decreased or may be abolished. Diastolic flow reversal is generally present in vessels that supply vascular beds with high peripheral resistance. It tends to be absent in low-resistance vascular beds or when peripheral resistance is reduced by peripheral dilatation, such as that which occurs in the skin with body heating, or in the working muscle during exercise or reactive hyperemia. These principles are important in assessing blood flow in arteries that supply various regions, including the cranial circulation. For example, flow reversal can be observed in the external carotid because extracranial resistance is relatively high, but it is absent in the internal carotid because the cerebrovascular resistance is low.

EFFECTS OF ARTERIAL OBSTRUCTION

Arterial obstruction can result in reduced pressure and flow distal to the site of blockage, but the effects on pressure and flow are greatly influenced by a number of factors proximal and especially distal to the lesion. One must be familiar with these factors when interpreting noninvasive studies, because they affect the pressure and velocity waveforms observed both proximal and distal to the obstructive lesion. In this section of the chapter, the concept of the critical stenosis is considered, as well as the pressure, velocity, and flow manifestations of arterial obstructive disease.

Critical Stenosis

Encroachment on the lumen of an artery by an arteriosclerotic plaque can result in diminished pressure and flow distal to the lesion, but this encroachment on the lumen has to be relatively extensive before hemodynamic changes are manifested because arteries offer relatively little resistance to flow compared with the resistance vessels with which they are in series. Studies in humans and animals have indicated that about 90% of the cross-sectional area of the aorta must be encroached upon before there is a change in the distal pressure and flow, whereas in smaller vessels, such as the iliac, carotid, renal, and femoral arteries, the critical stenosis level varies from 70% to 90%.[13,14] It is important to differentiate between percentage decrease in cross-sectional area and diameter. For example, a decrease in diameter of 50% corresponds to a 75% decrease in cross-sectional area, and a diameter narrowing of 66% is equivalent to about a 90% reduction in area.

Whether a hemodynamic abnormality results from a stenosis and how severe it may be depend on several factors, including (1) the length and diameter of the narrowed segment; (2) the roughness of the endothelial surface; (3) the degree of irregularity of the narrowing and its shape (i.e., whether the narrowing is abrupt or gradual); (4) the ratio of the cross-sectional area of the narrowed segment to that of the normal vessel; (5) the rate of flow; (6) the arteriovenous pressure gradient; and (7) the peripheral resistance beyond the stenosis.

The concept of critical stenosis (i.e., a stenosis that causes a reduction in flow and pressure) has been treated extensively in the literature. This concept has been accepted because there is generally little or no change in hemodynamics when an artery is first narrowed by disease, but a relatively rapid decrease in pressure and flow occurs with greater degrees of narrowing. The critical stenosis concept is of practical significance, because lesser degrees of narrowing of human arteries often do not produce significant changes in hemodynamics or clinical manifestations. It must be recognized, however, that the concept of critical stenosis is a gross simplification of a very complex interplay of numerous circulatory factors. In particular, changes in peripheral resistance, such as those occurring with exercise, may profoundly alter the effect of a given stenotic lesion. These considerations dictate that the hemodynamic and clinical significance of stenotic lesions be assessed, whenever possible, by physiologic measurements; otherwise, erroneous conclusions may be reached.[12] In evaluating the hemodynamic effect of stenotic lesions, it is also important to recognize that two or more stenotic lesions that occur in series have a more pronounced effect on distal pressure and flow than does a single lesion of equal total length. This difference is a result of large losses of energy at the entrance, and particularly at the exit, of the lesion resulting from grossly disturbed flow patterns, including jet effects, turbulence, and eddy formation. Thus, the energy losses in tandem lesions far exceed those that result from frictional resistance in a solitary stenosis, as represented in Poiseuille's equation.

Pressure Changes

Experiments with graded stenoses in animals have indicated that, whereas the diastolic pressure does not fall until the stenosis is quite severe, a decrease in systolic pressure is a sensitive index of reduction in both the mean pressure and the amplitude of the pressure wave distal to a relatively minor stenosis (Fig. 1–5).[15,16] Also, damping of the waveform, increased time to peak, and greater width of the wave at half-amplitude can be detected distal to an arterial stenosis or occlusion.[17,18]

These abnormal features of the pulse wave correlate well with the results of measurement of systolic pressure and can be demonstrated by noninvasive techniques

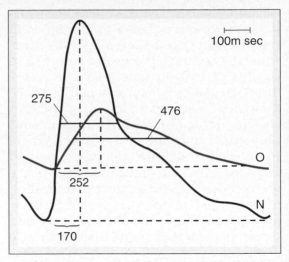

FIGURE 1–6. Dorsalis pedis pulse waves from a normal limb (N) and a limb with a proximal occlusion (O). The wave from the limb with occlusion shows a prolonged time to peak (252 msec) and increased width at half of the amplitude (476 msec). (From Carter SA: Investigation and treatment of arterial occlusive disease of the extremities. Clin Med 79[5]:13–24, 1972 [Part I]; Clin Med 79[6]:15–22, 1972 [Part II].)

employing pulse waveforms recorded using various types of plethysmography (Fig. 1–6). In the case of very mild stenotic lesions, however, little or no pressure or pulse abnormality may be evident distal to the lesion when the patient is at rest. The presence of such lesions may be demonstrated if blood flow is increased with exercise or through the induction of hyperemia. Enhanced flow through the stenosis results in increased loss of energy, which can be detected by a decrease in pressure distal to the lesion.[15,19]

Flow Changes

At rest, the total blood flow to an extremity may be normal in the presence of a severe stenosis or even a complete obstruction of the main artery because of the development of collateral circulation, as well as a compensatory decrease in the peripheral resistance. In such circumstances, measurement of systolic pressure, as discussed earlier, is a better method of assessing the presence and severity of the occlusive or stenotic process than measurement of blood flow.[12,17] Resting blood flow is reduced only when the

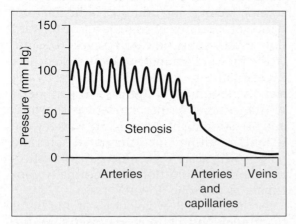

FIGURE 1–5. Decrease in pulse amplitude and systolic and mean pressures distal to a stenosis. In minimal stenosis, alterations in pulse pressure such as this may be evident only during high-volume flow induced by exercise or hyperemia. (From Carter SA: Peripheral artery disease: Pressure measurements ease evaluation. Consultant 19[9]:102–115, 1979.)

occlusion is acute and the collateral circulation has not had a chance to develop or, in the case of a chronic arterial obstruction, when the occlusive process is extensive and consists of two or more lesions in series. Although single lesions might not be associated with symptoms or significant changes in blood flow at rest, such lesions can significantly affect the blood supply when need is increased during exercise. In such cases, the sum of the resistances of the obstructions (stenosis, collateral resistance, or both) and of the peripheral resistance may prevent a normal increase in flow, and symptoms of intermittent claudication may develop.

Arterial obstruction can lead to changes in the distribution of the available blood flow to neighboring regions or vascular beds, depending on the relative resistance and anatomic arrangement of these areas. For example, flow during exercise can increase in the skeletal muscle of the extremity distal to an arterial obstruction, but because the distal pressure is reduced during exercise, the muscle "steals" blood from the skin and the blood supply to the skin of the foot is diminished. Such reduction in flow to the skin may be manifested clinically by numbness of the foot, a common symptom in patients with claudication. In lower extremities with extensive large vessel occlusion and additional obstruction in small distal branches, vasodilator drugs or sympathectomy may divert flow from the critically ischemic distal areas by decreasing resistance in less ischemic regions.[20] Obstruction of the subclavian artery is known to cause cerebral symptoms in some patients because of reversal of flow in the vertebral arteries (the subclavian steal syndrome); similarly, obstructive lesions of the internal carotid artery may lead to reversal of flow in the ophthalmic vessels, which communicate with external carotid branches on the face and scalp.

Velocity Changes

In normal arteries, flow velocity increases rapidly to a peak during early systole and decreases during diastole, when flow reversal can occur. The shape of the resulting pulse velocity wave resembles the pressure gradient shown in Figure 1–4. The character of this velocity profile can be quantified from analogue velocity recordings by calculating various indices of pulsatility and damping.[12,21] The characteristics of the waveform can also be appreciated by listening to the arterial flow sounds emitted by Doppler flow detectors.[12] Over normal peripheral arteries, double or triple sounds are heard; the second sound represents the diastolic flow reversal, and the third sound represents the second forward component. Whether the sounds are double or triple is probably not of practical clinical significance and may be related to a complex interplay of several factors. These factors include the basal heart rate and the shape of the pressure and flow waves. As discussed earlier, the latter factors depend on the degree of peripheral vasoconstriction and elastic properties of the arteries.

Distal to an arterial stenosis the pulse velocity wave is more damped than normal and is similar in pattern to the pressure wave seen in Figure 1–6. Also, flow reversal disappears distal to an arterial stenosis. The calculated wave indices are thus altered, and the audible Doppler signals have a single component rather than the double or triple components usually heard.[12,21] The disappearance of reversed flow distal to a stenosis probably results from a combination of several factors, including (1) the maintenance of a relatively high level of forward flow throughout the cardiac cycle (because of the pressure gradient across the stenosis); (2) resistance to reverse flow created by the stenotic lesion; (3) a decrease in peripheral resistance as a result of relative ischemia; and (4) damping of the pressure wave by the lesion, resulting in attenuated pressure pulses, which are less subject to the reflections and amplification that normally contribute to diastolic flow reversal.

Recordings of flow velocities at and distal to arterial obstructions are useful in the assessment of occlusive processes. The introduction of online frequency spectrum analysis allows better detection and quantification of flow abnormalities resulting from stenotic lesions. This subject is considered in further detail in Chapters 2 and 3, but it is of interest to comment on the physiologic principles illustrated by frequency spectra in normal and abnormal vessels. As noted previously, the velocity pattern across a vessel is flattened by such factors as the effect of branching (see Fig. 1–1B). As a result, the particles in the central core of normal arteries flow with relatively uniform and high velocities during systole. This can be demonstrated by spectrum analysis of the arterial velocity Doppler signals, which reveals a narrow band of velocities near the maximum velocity.[22] Stenotic lesions result in marked disturbance of flow with the occurrence of abnormally high velocities, jet effects, irregular travel of particles in various directions and at different velocities, and eddy formation. The change in the direction of particle movement with respect to the axis of the vessel alters the observed Doppler shifts and also contributes to the occurrence of a large range of flow velocities registered with frequency spectral analysis. These effects of arterial stenosis are manifest as widening or dispersal of the band of systolic velocity (spectral broadening) or complete filling in of the spectral tracing, as discussed in Chapter 3.

VENOUS HEMODYNAMICS

As shown in Figure 1–2, the pressure remaining in the veins after the blood has traversed the arterioles and capillaries is low when the subject is in the supine position. Because of their relatively large diameters, medium and large veins offer little resistance to flow, and blood moves readily from the small veins to the right atrium, where the pressure is close to atmospheric pressure. Although the effects of arterial pressure and flow waves are rarely transmitted to the systemic veins, phasic changes in venous pressure and flow do occur in response to cardiac activity and because of alterations of intrathoracic pressure with respiration. Knowledge of these changes is necessary for correct assessment of peripheral veins by noninvasive laboratory studies.

The final section of this chapter discusses changes in pressure and flow in various portions of the venous system that are associated with cardiac and respiratory cycles. Also considered are alterations in lower extremity veins that occur with changes in posture, the important consequences of competence or incompetence of venous valves, and the effects of venous obstruction.

Flow and Pressure Changes During the Cardiac Cycle

Figure 1–7 shows changes in pressure and flow in large veins such as the venae cavae that occur during phases of the cardiac cycle. Such oscillations in pressure and flow may, at times, be transmitted to more peripheral vessels. Characteristically, three positive pressure waves (a, c, v) can be distinguished in central venous pressure and reflect corresponding changes in pressure in the atria. The *a wave* is caused by atrial contraction and relaxation. The upstroke of the *c wave* is related to the increase in pressure when the atrioventricular valves are closed and bulge during isovolumetric ventricular

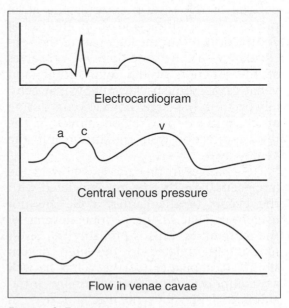

FIGURE 1–7. Schematic representation of normal changes in pressure and flow in the central veins associated with the cardiac cycle. a, a wave; c, c wave; v, v wave.

contraction. The subsequent downstroke results from the fall in pressure caused by pulling the atrioventricular valve rings toward the apex of the heart during ventricular contraction, thus tending to increase the atrial volume. The upstroke of the *v wave* results from a passive rise in atrial pressure during ventricular systole when the atrioventricular valves are closed and the atria fill with blood from the peripheral veins. The v wave downstroke is caused by the fall in pressure that occurs when the blood leaves the atria rapidly and fills the ventricles, soon after the opening of the atrioventricular valves, early in ventricular diastole.

The venous pressure waves are associated with changes in flow. There are two periods of increased venous flow during each cardiac cycle. The first occurs during ventricular systole, when shortening of the ventricular muscle pulls the atrioventricular valve rings toward the apex of the heart. This movement of the valve ring tends to increase atrial volume and decrease atrial pressure, thus increasing flow from the extracardiac veins into the atria. The second phase of increased venous flow occurs after the atrioventricular valves open and blood rushes into the ventricles from the atria. Venous flow is reduced in the intervening periods of the cardiac cycle as the atrial pressure rises during and soon after atrial contraction and in the later part of the ventricular systole. Because there are no valves at the junction of the right atrium and venae cavae, some backward flow may actually occur in the large thoracic veins during atrial contraction as blood moves in the reverse direction from the atrium into the venae cavae.

The changes in pressure and flow in the large central veins that are associated with the events of the cardiac cycle are not usually evident in the peripheral veins of the extremities. This is probably the result of damping related to the high distensibility (compliance) of the veins, as well as compression of the veins by intra-abdominal pressure and mechanical compression in the thoracic inlet. Because the effects of right-sided heart contractions are more readily transmitted to the large veins of the arms, the pulsatile changes in venous velocity associated with the events of the cardiac cycle tend to be more obvious in the upper extremities than in the veins of the legs.

In abnormal conditions, such as congestive heart failure or tricuspid insufficiency, venous pressure is increased. This elevation of venous pressure may lead to the transmission of cardiac phasic changes in pressure and flow to the peripheral veins of the upper and lower limbs. Such phasic changes may occasionally be found in healthy, well-hydrated individuals, probably because a large blood volume distends the venous system.

Venous Effects of Respiration

Respiration has profound effects on venous pressure and flow. During inspiration, the volume in the veins of the thorax increases and the pressure decreases in response to reduced intrathoracic pressure. Expiration leads to the opposite effect, with decreased venous volume and increased pressure. The venous response to respiration is reversed in the abdomen, where the pressure increases during inspiration because of the descent of the diaphragm and decreases during expiration as the diaphragm ascends. Increased abdominal pressure during inspiration decreases pressure gradients between peripheral veins in the lower extremities and the abdomen, thus reducing flow in the peripheral vessels. During expiration, when intra-abdominal pressure is reduced, the pressure gradient from the lower limbs to the abdomen is increased and flow in the peripheral veins rises correspondingly.

In the veins of the upper limbs, the changes in flow with respiration are opposite to those in the lower extremities. Because of reduced intrathoracic pressure during inspiration, the pressure gradient from the veins of the upper limbs to the right atrium increases and flow increases. During expiration, flow decreases because of the resulting increase in intrathoracic pressure and the corresponding rise of the right atrial pressure. The respiratory changes in flow in the upper limbs may be influenced by changes in posture. With the upper parts of the body elevated, venous flow tends to stop at the height of inspiration and resumes with expiration, probably because of the compression of the subclavian vein at the level of the first rib during contraction of the accessory muscles of respiration.

The respiratory effects are usually associated with clear phasic changes in venous flow in the extremities; these can be detected by various instruments, including many forms of plethysmographs and Doppler flow detectors. The respiratory changes in venous velocity may be exaggerated by respiratory maneuvers such as the Valsalva maneuver, which increases intrathoracic and abdominal pressures and decreases, abolishes, or even reverses flow in some peripheral veins. Also, the respiratory effects on venous flow may be diminished in the lower limbs in individuals who are chest or shallow breathers and whose diaphragm may not descend sufficiently to elevate intra-abdominal pressure. Venous flow then tends to be more continuous.

Venous Flow and Peripheral Resistance

Blood flow and flow velocity in the peripheral veins, particularly in the extremities, are profoundly influenced by local blood flow, which is in turn largely determined by the peripheral resistance or the state of vasoconstriction or vasodilatation. When limb blood flow is markedly increased as a result of peripheral vasodilatation (e.g., secondary to infection or inflammation), the flow tends to be more continuous, and the respiratory changes in flow are less evident. When there is increased vasoconstriction in the extremities (e.g., when there is a need to conserve body heat and blood flow through the skin is decreased), venous flow is also markedly decreased and there may be no audible Doppler flow signals over a peripheral vein, such as the posterior tibial vein. Also, severe arterial obstruction may decrease overall blood flow and velocity in the vessels of the extremities and lead to decreased velocity signals over the venous channels.

Effect of Posture

In the upright position, the hydrostatic pressure is greatly increased in the dependent part of the body, particularly in the lower portions of the lower extremities. This increase in hydrostatic pressure, as indicated earlier, is associated with high transmural pressures in the blood vessels and, in turn, leads to greater vascular distention. In the veins, which have low pressure to start with and are distensible, considerable pooling of the blood occurs in the lower parts of the legs. The resulting decrease in venous return to the right atrium is associated with diminished cardiac output. When the normal compensatory reflexes that increase peripheral resistance are impaired, decreased cardiac output can lead to hypotension and fainting.

The movement of the skeletal muscles of the legs, such as that which occurs during walking, leads to decreased venous pressure because of the presence of one-way valves in the peripheral veins. Contraction of the voluntary muscle squeezes the veins and propels the blood toward the heart. Muscular contraction not only increases venous return and cardiac output but also interrupts the hydrostatic column of venous blood from the heart and thus decreases pressure in the peripheral veins (e.g., in the veins at the ankle). Activity of the skeletal muscles of the legs in the presence of competent venous valves therefore results in the lowering of pressure in the veins of the extremity, leading to decreased venous pooling, decreased capillary pressure, reduced filtration of fluid into the extracellular space than would otherwise occur, and increased blood flow because of increased arteriovenous pressure difference.

Effect of External Compression

Sudden pressure on the veins of the extremities, whether caused by an active muscular contraction or external manual compression of the limb, increases venous flow and velocity toward the heart and stops the flow distal to the site of the compression in the presence of competent venous valves.

The responses to sudden pressure changes are affected by venous obstruction and damage to the venous valves. The detection of such changes is important when assessing patients for the presence of venous disease. (This is discussed further in Chapter 22.)

Venous Obstruction

Venous obstruction can be acute or chronic. In the case of severe chronic obstruction, edema may occur. Also, the nutrition of the skin in the affected region may be impaired, and characteristic trophic changes in the skin and venous stasis ulcers may result. Acute obstruction, usually associated with thrombosis, may lead to potentially fatal pulmonary embolism. Because the clinical diagnosis of acute deep vein thrombosis is unreliable, noninvasive procedures have been developed to enhance the accuracy of this diagnosis.[12] Various forms of plethysmographs, Doppler flow detectors, and duplex ultrasound scanners may be used for this purpose.

An audible Doppler signal should be present over peripheral veins; it can be easily distinguished from an arterial flow signal because of the absence of pulsatility synchronous with the heart. As indicated earlier, a signal may be absent in low-flow states, especially when the limb is cold and auscultation is carried out over small peripheral veins. Squeezing of the limb distal to the site of examination should temporarily increase flow and result in an audible signal if the vein is patent. Spontaneous venous flow signals normally possess clear respiratory phases. However, if there is an obstruction between the heart and the examination site, the respiratory changes in venous velocity are absent or attenuated. Over larger, more proximal veins, such as the popliteal and more proximal vessels, the absence of audible signals after an adequate search is indicative of an obstructed venous segment.

The presence or absence of obstruction is also gauged by increasing flow toward the examination site by squeezing the limb distally or by activating the *distal* muscle groups and thus increasing venous blood flow toward the flow-detecting probe. Absence of increased flow sounds or attenuation of increased flow is associated with obstruction between the probe location and the site from which the enhancement of venous flow is attempted.

Increase in flow is also elicited when manual compression of the limb proximal to the flow-detecting probe is released, because of low filling and pressure in the proximal veins that have been emptied by the compression. If the proximal veins at or near the point of compression are occluded, the augmentation of flow after release of the compression is attenuated.

Venous Valvular Incompetence

When the valves are competent, flow in the peripheral veins is toward the heart. However, flow may be temporarily diminished or stopped soon after assumption of the upright posture, at the height of inspiration, or during the Valsalva maneuver. The peripheral veins normally fill from the capillaries, and the rate at which they fill depends on the peripheral resistance and blood flow, as determined by the degree of peripheral vasoconstriction. When there are incompetent veins proximally, there may be retrograde filling of the peripheral veins, such as those in the ankle region, from the more proximal veins, in addition to normal filling from the capillary beds.[12] This retrograde filling may have serious consequences because of a resulting increase in hydrostatic pressure and filtration of fluid into the extravascular spaces in the upright position.

The presence or absence of the retrograde flow may be detected by listening with a Doppler flow detector and squeezing the limb proximally. Also, various plethysmographic methods can detect the rate of filling through measurement of venous volume, which changes with pressure, after the volume and pressure have been reduced by muscular action such as flexion-extension of the ankle in the upright position. After such exercise, the venous volume and pressure increase more rapidly when the valves are incompetent, because the peripheral veins fill as a result of retrograde flow from the more proximal parts of the limbs. The application of a tourniquet or cuff with appropriate pressure compresses the superficial veins and allows localization of incompetent veins, not only to the various segments of the limbs, but also to the superficial veins as opposed to the perforating or deep veins.

Acknowledgments. The author held grants-in-aid of research from the Manitoba Heart and the St. Boniface Hospital Research Foundations, which supported the studies whose results are discussed in this chapter. He is also grateful to Dr. William J. Zwiebel for the valuable exchange of ideas and assistance and the excellent secretarial work of Mrs. Constance Twomey.

References

1. Carter SA: Arterial auscultation in peripheral vascular disease. JAMA 246:1682–1686, 1981.
2. Kaufman W: Fluid Mechanics, 2nd ed. New York, McGraw-Hill, 1963.
3. Taylor MG: Wave travel in arteries and the design of the cardiovascular system. In Attinger EO (ed): Pulsatile Blood Flow. New York, McGraw-Hill, 1964, pp 343–372.
4. Carter SA: Effect of age, cardiovascular disease, and vasomotor changes on transmission of arterial pressure waves through the lower extremities. Angiology 29:601–616, 1978.
5. Kroeker EJ, Wood EH: Comparison of simultaneously recorded central and peripheral arterial pressure pulses during rest, exercise and tilted position in man. Circ Res 3:623–632, 1955.
6. Gaskell P, Krisman A: The brachial to digital blood pressure gradient in normal subjects and in patients with high blood pressure. Can J Biochem Physiol 36:889–893, 1958.
7. Lezack JD, Carter SA: Systolic pressures in the extremities of man with special reference to the toes. Can J Physiol Pharmacol 48:469–474, 1970.
8. Nielsen PE, Barras J-P, Holstein P: Systolic pressure amplification in the arteries of normal subjects. Scand J Clin Lab Invest 33:371–377, 1974.
9. Sugiura T, Freis ED: Pressure pulse in small arteries. Circ Res 11:838–842, 1962.
10. Rowell LB, Brengelmann GL, Blackmon JR, et al: Disparities between aortic and peripheral pulse pressure induced by upright exercise and vasomotor changes in man. Circulation 37:954–964, 1968.
11. Carter SA: Role of pressure measurements in vascular disease. In Bernstein EF (ed): Noninvasive Diagnostic Techniques in Vascular Disease. St. Louis, CV Mosby, 1985, pp 513–544.
12. Strandness DE Jr, Sumner DS: Hemodynamics for Surgeons. New York, Grune & Stratton, 1975, pp 3–20; 73–120; 209–289; 396–511.
13. May AG, Van de Berg L, DeWeese JA, et al: Critical arterial stenosis. Surgery 54:250–259, 1963.
14. Schultz RD, Hokanson DE, Strandness DE Jr: Pressure-flow and stress-strain measurements of normal and diseased aortoiliac segments. Surg Gynecol Obstet 124:1267–1276, 1967.
15. Carter SA: Peripheral artery disease: Pressure measurements ease evaluation. Consultant 19(9):102–115, 1979.
16. Widmer LK, Staub H: Blutdruck in stenosierten Arterien. Z Kreislaufforsch 51:975–979, 1962.
17. Carter SA: Indirect systolic pressures and pulse waves in arterial occlusive disease of the lower extremities. Circulation 37:624–637, 1968.
18. Carter SA: Investigation and treatment of arterial occlusive disease of the extremities. Clin Med 79(5):13–24, 1972 (Part I); Clin Med 79(6):15–22, 1972 (Part II).
19. Carter SA: Response of ankle systolic pressure to leg exercise in mild or questionable arterial disease. N Engl J Med 287:578–582, 1972.
20. Uhrenholdt A, Dam WH, Larsen OA, et al: Paradoxical effect on peripheral blood flow after sympathetic blockades in patients with gangrene due to arteriosclerosis obliterans. Vasc Surg 5:154–163, 1971.
21. Johnston KW, Taraschuk I: Validation of the role of pulsatility index in quantitation of the severity of peripheral arterial occlusive disease. Am J Surg 131:295–297, 1976.
22. Reneman RS, Hoeks A, Spencer MP: Doppler ultrasound in the evaluation of the peripheral arterial circulation. Angiology 30:526–538, 1979.

Chapter 2

Physics and Instrumentation in Doppler and B-Mode Ultrasonography

James A. Zagzebski, PhD

This chapter presents an overview of the physical and technical aspects of vascular sonography, including the following: (1) a brief review of relevant ultrasound–soft-tissue interactions, (2) pulse-echo principles and display techniques, (3) harmonic and chirp imaging, (4) the Doppler effect as it applies to vascular sonography, (5) continuous-wave (CW) and pulsed Doppler instrumentation, (6) the common techniques used for displaying Doppler signal spectral information, and (7) extended field-of-view and three-dimensional (3D) techniques.

SOUND PROPAGATION IN TISSUE

Sound waves are produced by vibrating sources, which cause particles in the medium to oscillate, setting up the wave. As sound energy propagates, it is attenuated, scattered, and reflected, producing echoes from various interfaces. In medical ultrasonography, *piezoelectric elements* inside an ultrasound transducer serve as the source and detector of sound waves. The design of the transducer is such that the waves travel in a beam with a well-defined direction. The reception of reflected and scattered echo signals by the transducer makes possible the production of ultrasound images and allows detection of motion using the Doppler effect. This section inspects factors that are important in the transmission and reflection of ultrasound in tissue.

Speed of Sound

Most ultrasound applications involve transmitting short bursts, or pulses, of sound into the body and receiving echoes from tissue interfaces. The time between transmitting a pulse and receiving an echo is used to determine the depth of the interface. The speed of sound in tissue must be known to apply pulse-echo methods.

Sound propagation speeds depend on the properties of the transmitting medium and not significantly on frequency or wave amplitude. As a general rule, gasses, including air, exhibit the lowest sound speed; liquids have an intermediate speed; and firm solids such as glass have very high speeds of sound. Speeds of sound in common media and tissues are listed in Table 2–1. For soft tissues, the average speed of sound has been found to be 1540 m/sec.[1] Most diagnostic ultrasound instruments are calibrated with the assumption that the sound beam propagates at this average speed. Slight variations exist in the speed of sound from one tissue to another, but as Table 2–1 indicates, speeds of sound in specific soft tissues deviate only slightly from the assumed average. Adipose tissues have sound speeds that are lower than the average, whereas muscle tissue exhibits a speed of sound that is slightly greater than 1540 m/sec.

Table 2–1. Speed of Sound for Biologic Tissue

Tissue	Speed of Sound (m/sec)	Change from 1540 m/sec (%)
Fat	1450	−5.8
Vitreous humor	1520	−1.3
Liver	1550	+0.6
Blood	1570	+1.9
Muscle	1580	+2.6
Lens of eye	1620	+5.2

From Wells PNT: Propagation of ultrasonic waves through tissues. In Fullerton G, Zagzebski J (eds): Medical Physics of CT and Ultrasound. New York, American Institute of Physics, 1980, p 381.

Table 2–2. Wavelengths for Various Ultrasound Frequencies

Frequency (MHz)	Wavelength* (mm)
1	1.54
2.25	0.68
5	0.31
10	0.15
15	0.103

*Assuming a speed of sound of 1540 m/sec.

Frequency and Wavelength

The number of oscillations per second of the piezoelectric element in the transducer establishes the frequency of the ultrasound wave. Frequency is expressed in cycles per second, or hertz (Hz). Audible sounds are in the range of 30 Hz to 20 kHz. *Ultrasound* refers to any sound whose frequency is above the audible range (i.e., above 20 kHz). Diagnostic ultrasound applications use frequencies in the 1-MHz to 30-MHz (1 million to 30 million Hz) frequency range. Manufacturers of ultrasound equipment and clinical users strive to use as high a frequency as practical that still allows adequate visualization depth into tissue (see section on attenuation). Higher frequencies are associated with improved spatial detail, or better resolution.

Figure 2–1 shows what might be called a snapshot of a sound wave, captured at an instant of time. It illustrates accompanying compressions and rarefactions in the medium that result from the particle oscillations. The wavelength λ is the distance over which a property of a wave repeats itself. It is defined by the equation

$$\lambda = \frac{c}{f} \qquad (2\text{–}1)$$

where c is the speed of sound and f is the frequency. Table 2–2 presents values for the wavelength in soft tissue, where the speed of sound is taken to be 1540 m/sec, for several frequencies. A good rule of thumb for tissues is the wavelength $\lambda_t = 1.5$ mm/F, where F is the frequency expressed in MHz. For example, if the frequency is 5 MHz, the wavelength in soft tissue is approximately 0.3 mm. Higher frequencies have shorter wavelengths and vice versa.

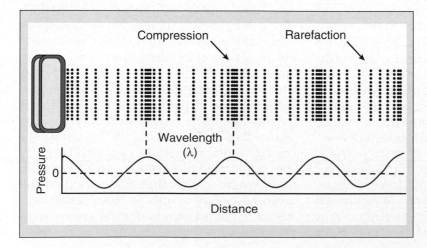

FIGURE 2–1. Sound waves produced by an ultrasound transducer. Vibrations of the transducer are coupled into the medium, producing local fluctuations in pressure. The fluctuations propagate through the medium in waves. The pressure amplitude is the maximum pressure swing, positive or negative. The diagram schematically illustrates compressions and rarefactions at an instant of time. The symbol λ is the acoustic wavelength.

Wavelength has relevance when describing dimensions of objects, such as reflectors and scatterers in the body. The size of an object is most meaningfully expressed if given relative to the ultrasonic wavelength for the frequency of the sound beam. Similarly, the width of the ultrasound beam from a transducer depends in part on the wavelength. Higher-frequency beams have shorter wavelengths and are narrower than lower-frequency beams.

Amplitude, Intensity, and Power

A sound wave is accompanied by pressure fluctuations in the medium. The pressure profile that could occur for the wave in Figure 2–1 might appear as in the graph in the lower part of this figure. The pressure *amplitude* is the maximal increase (or decrease) in the pressure caused by the sound wave. The unit for pressure is the pascal (Pa). Pulsed ultrasound scanners can produce peak pressure amplitudes of several million pascals in water when power controls on the machine are adjusted for maximal levels. As a benchmark for comparison, atmospheric pressure is approximately 0.1 MPa, so it is clear that ultrasound fields from medical devices significantly exceed this mark. The high-pressure amplitudes of an ultrasound pulse can easily burst contrast agent bubbles (see later) that are sometimes injected into the blood stream to enhance echo signals. Diagnostic levels, however, are not believed to create biologic effects in tissues if such gas bodies are not present.

The intensity (I) of a sound wave at a point in the medium is estimated by squaring the pressure amplitude (P) and using $I = P^2/2\rho c$, where ρ is the density and c is the speed of sound. Units for ultrasound intensity are watts per meter squared (W/m^2) or multiples thereof, such as mW/cm^2. In water, a 2-MPa amplitude during the pulse corresponds to a pulse average intensity of 133 W/cm^2! This is a high intensity, but, fortunately, it is not sustained by a diagnostic ultrasound device because the duty factor (i.e., the fraction of time the transducer

actually emits ultrasound) typically is less than 0.005. Therefore, the time-averaged acoustic intensity from an ultrasound machine, found by averaging over a time that includes transmit pulses as well as the time between pulses, is much lower than the intensity during the pulse. Typical time-averaged intensities at the location in the ultrasound beam where the maximal values are found are on the order of 10 to 20 mW/cm^2 for B-mode imaging. Doppler and color flow imaging modes have higher duty factors. Moreover, these modes tend to concentrate the acoustic energy into smaller areas. Time-averaged intensities for Doppler modes may be a few hundred mW/cm^2 for color flow imaging and as high as 1000 to 2000 mW/cm^2 for pulsed Doppler![2,3]

The acoustic *power* produced by a scanner is the rate at which energy is emitted by the transducer. Average acoustic power levels in diagnostic ultrasonography are low because of the small duty factors used in most equipment. Typical power levels are on the order of 10 to 20 mW for black and white imaging, but may be three to times this value for color flow modes of operation.

Acoustic Output Labels on Machines

The transmit level, or the output power, on most scanners may be adjusted by the operator. Increasing the power applies a more energetic signal to the transducer, thereby increasing the pressure amplitude and increasing the power and the intensity of the waves produced. Higher power levels are advantageous because they enable detection of echoes from more weakly reflecting interfaces in the body. The disadvantage of high power levels is that they expose the tissue to greater amounts of acoustic energy, increasing the potential for biologic effects. Although there are no confirmed effects of ultrasound on patients during diagnostic ultrasound exposures, most operators attempt to follow the ALARA principal (as low as reasonably achievable) when adjusting the power level and other instrument controls that affect output levels.

It would be difficult to follow ALARA without labels on the machine to inform the operator "how much" ultrasound energy is being applied. Although some ultrasound machines display relative output indications, such as a transmit level percentage, a relative level in decibels, or simply the setting of a power control knob, such labels do not provide users sufficient information to help them understand the likelihood that the sound levels produced might be in an undesirable zone.

To help operators implement the ALARA principle, output labels are used that are related to the biologic effects of ultrasound.[4] One of the potential effects is "cavitation," which describes activity of small gas bodies under the action of an ultrasound field. When gas bodies are present, such as when there are contrast agents in the ultrasound field, cavitation increases the local stresses on tissue that are associated with the ultrasound waves. If the wave amplitude is high enough, collapse of the gas body occurs, and this is accompanied by localized energy depositions that significantly exceed depositions that might occur without cavitation. Cavitation is believed to be most closely associated with the peak negative pressure in the ultrasound wave. Scientists have developed a "mechanical index" (MI) that is derived from the peak negative pressure in the medium. For most ultrasound machines, the current maximum MI in the field is displayed in a prominent position on the display (Fig. 2–2).

Another way that ultrasound energy may affect tissue is by heating through absorption of the waves. Absorption is one of the mechanisms that result in attenuation of a sound beam as it propagates through tissue. A corresponding index, the "thermal index" (TI) is displayed to indicate the likelihood of heating (see Fig. 2–2). This is estimated using the time average acoustic power or the time average intensity, along with detailed mathematical models for the sound beam pattern and assumptions on the ultrasonic and thermal properties of the tissue. Depending on the application, a machine will exhibit either a soft tissue thermal index value (TI_s) or a thermal index for the case in which absorbing bone is at the beam focus (TI_b). Another value that sometimes is used is TI_c, a thermal index that is appropriate for transcranial Doppler, (TI_c), where heating could occur in bone.

The acoustic output labeling standard calls for a clear display of MI and TI.[4] The standard is followed by most ultrasound equipment manufacturers, and it provides ultrasound system operators values of acoustic output quantities that are relevant to the possibility of biologic effects from the ultrasound exposures.

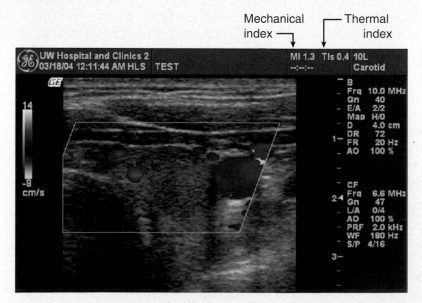

FIGURE 2–2. Ultrasound image showing display of the mechanical index (MI) and thermal index (TI).

Decibel Notation

Decibels are used frequently to indicate relative power, intensity, and amplitude levels. Their use is a way to express the ratio of two signal amplitudes or two intensities. Suppose one wishes to express how much greater (or smaller) intensity (I_1) is relative to another (I_2). Their relative value in decibels is given by

$$dB = 10\log\frac{I_1}{I_2} \qquad (2\text{--}2)$$

Thus, the decibel relation between two intensities is just the log of their ratio multiplied by 10. The same equation holds for expressing the ratio of two power levels. The difference in decibels between two powers is found by taking the log of their ratio and multiplying by 10.

Sometimes amplitudes rather than the intensities of two signals are used to express decibels. For a given decibel level, one must account for the fact that the intensity is proportional to the square of the amplitude. Substituting the corresponding amplitudes (A_1 and A_2) into equation 2–2, squaring them, and taking into account that $\log (x^2)$ is $2(\log x)$, we have the relationship

$$dB = 20\log\frac{A_1}{A_2}$$

Notice, the multiplicative factor is 20 rather than 10 when converting amplitude ratios to decibels.

Table 2–3 lists decibel values for various intensity and amplitude ratios. Notice that a 3-dB increase in the intensity is the same as doubling the quantity. A 10-dB increase corresponds to a 10-fold increase, and a 20-dB increase means that the intensity is multiplied by 100. The lower half of the table shows decibel changes corresponding to reductions of the intensity. A 3-dB decrease is the same as halving the intensity, and so forth.

Frequently, decibels are used to describe the loudness of audible sounds. Here, the level of one sound often is expressed with no explicit comparison to another, such as

Table 2–3. Decibel Differences Corresponding to Various Intensity and Amplitude Ratios*

Amplitude Ratio (A_1/A_2)	Intensity Ratio (I_1/I_2)	Decibel Difference (dB)
1	1	0
1.41	2	+3
2	4	+6
2.828	8	+9
3.16	10	+10
4.47	20	+13
10	100	+20
100	10,000	+40
1	1	0
0.707	0.5	−3
0.5	0.25	−6

*For example, if I_1 is 10 times I_2, it is 10 dB greater than I_2. A 20-dB difference between two signals corresponds to both a ratio of 10 for their amplitude or a ratio of 100 for their intensities, and so forth.

"the sound intensity of the jet at takeoff was 110 dB." However, with airborne sounds, a reference intensity is implied when not stated explicitly. This reference is $I_2 = 10^{-12}\ W/m^2$, the accepted threshold for human hearing.

Attenuation

As a sound beam propagates through tissue, its intensity decreases with increasing distance. This decrease with path length is called *attenuation*. Attenuation of medical ultrasound beams is caused by reflection and scatter of the waves at boundaries between media having different densities or speeds of sound and absorption of ultrasonic energy by tissues. As mentioned previously, absorption may lead to heating if beam power levels are sufficiently high.

The rate of attenuation in relation to distance is called the *attenuation coefficient*, expressed in decibels per centimeter. The attenuation coefficient depends on both the medium and the ultrasound frequency. Figure 2–3 illustrates attenuation coefficients for a few tissues, plotted versus the frequency. Attenuation is quite high for

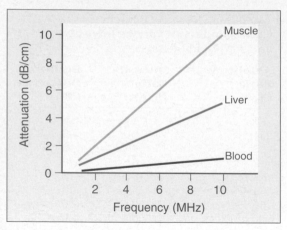

FIGURE 2–3. Variation of attenuation with tissue type and frequency.

muscle and skin, has an intermediate value for large organs such as the liver, and is very low for fluid-filled structures. For the liver, it is approximately 0.5 dB/cm at 1 MHz, whereas for blood, it is about 0.17 dB/cm at 1 MHz. An important characteristic of attenuation is its frequency dependence. For most soft tissues, the attenuation coefficient is nearly proportional to the frequency.[1] The attenuation expressed in

decibels would roughly double if the frequency were doubled. Thus, higher-frequency sound waves are more severely attenuated than lower-frequency waves, and the high-frequency beams cannot penetrate as far as low-frequency beams. Diagnostic studies with higher-frequency sound beams (7 MHz and above) are usually limited to superficial regions of the body. Lower frequencies (5 MHz and below) must be used for imaging large organs, such as the liver.

Reflection

Figure 2–4 shows an ultrasound image of the carotid artery of a normal adult. The walls of the vessel can be seen because of reflection of sound waves. Echoes from muscle and other tissues are also produced by reflections and by ultrasonic scatter. Both reflection and scatter contribute to the detail seen on clinical ultrasound scans.

Partial reflection of ultrasound waves occurs when they are incident on interfaces separating tissues having different acoustic

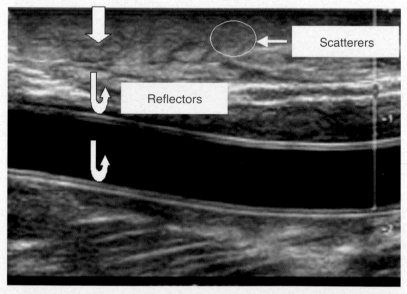

FIGURE 2–4. B-mode image of an arterial graft. Such images are constructed from echoes detected from large interfaces (*arrows*) and from small scatterers (*smooth echo region*). Bright dots on ultrasound B-mode images indicate high amplitude echoes, and dim dots indicate low amplitudes. Notice how the echoes from the vessel wall vary as the orientation changes slightly, characteristic of a specular reflector. The highest-amplitude echoes occur when the interface is perpendicular to the ultrasound beam. The interior of the vessel appears anechoic because blood has a lower backscatter level (lower echogenicity) than surrounding tissues. Scattering from small interfaces produces the vast majority of echoes visualized throughout the image.

properties. The fraction of the incident energy that is reflected depends on the acoustic impedances of the tissues forming the interface. The acoustic impedance (Z) is the speed of sound (c) multiplied by the density (ρ) of a tissue. The amplitude or strength of the reflected wave is proportional to the difference between the acoustic impedances of tissues forming the interface.

The *reflection coefficient* quantifies the relative amplitude of a wave reflected at an interface. It is the ratio of the reflected amplitude to the incident amplitude. For perpendicular incidence of the ultrasound beam on a large, flat interface (Fig. 2–5), reflection coefficient (R) is given by

$$R = \frac{Z_2 - Z_1}{Z_2 + Z_1} \qquad (2\text{–}3)$$

where the impedances Z_1 and Z_2 are identified in Figure 2–5.

Equation 2–3 shows that the larger the difference between impedances Z_2 and Z_1, the greater will be the amplitude of the echo from an interface, and hence, the less will be the transmitted signal. Large impedance differences are found at tissue-to-air and tissue-to-bone interfaces. In fact, such interfaces are nearly impenetrable to an ultrasound beam. In contrast, significantly weaker echoes originate at interfaces formed by two soft tissues because, generally, there is not a large difference in impedance between soft tissues.[6]

Large, smooth interfaces, such as those indicated in Figure 2–5, are called *specular reflectors*. The direction in which the reflected wave travels after striking a specular reflector is highly dependent on the orientation of the interface with respect to the sound beam. The wave is reflected back toward the source only when the incident beam is perpendicular or nearly perpendicular to the reflector. The amplitude of an echo detected from a specular reflector thus also depends on the orientation of the reflector with respect to the sound beam direction. The ultrasound image in Figure 2–4 was obtained using a linear array probe, which sends individual ultrasound beams into the scanned region in a vertical direction as viewed on the image. Sections of the vessel wall that are nearly horizontal yield the highest amplitude echoes and hence appear brightest because they were closest to being perpendicular to the ultrasound beams during imaging. Sections where the vessel is slightly inclined are seen as less bright.

Some soft-tissue interfaces are better classified as *diffuse reflectors*. The reflected waves from a diffuse reflector propagate in various directions with respect to the incident beam. Therefore, the amplitude of an echo from a diffuse interface is less dependent on the orientation of the interface with respect to the sound beam than the amplitude detected from a specular reflector.

Scattering

For interfaces whose dimensions are small, reflections are classified as "scattering." Much of the background information viewed in Figure 2–4 results from scattered echoes, where no one interface can be identified but usually echoes from many small interfaces are picked up simultaneously. The scattered waves spread in all directions, as suggested in Figure 2–6. Consequently, there is little angular dependence on the strength of echoes detected from scatterers. Unlike the vessel wall, which is best visualized when the ultrasound beam is perpendicular to it, the scatterers are detected with relatively uniform average amplitude from all directions. Echoes resulting from scattering within organ parenchyma are

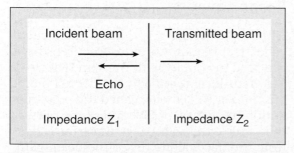

FIGURE 2–5. Reflection at a specular interface. The echo amplitude depends on the difference between the acoustic impedances Z_1 and Z_2 of the materials forming the interface.

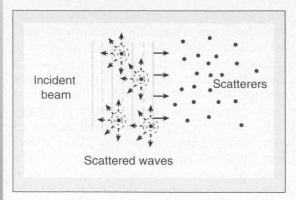

FIGURE 2–6. Scattering of ultrasound by small in-homogeneities.

clinically important because they provide much of the diagnostic detail seen on ultrasound scans.

In Doppler ultrasound, blood flow is detected by processing signals resulting from scattering by red blood cells. At diagnostic ultrasound frequencies, the size of a red blood cell is very small compared with the ultrasonic wavelength. Scatterers of this size range are called *Rayleigh scatterers*. The scattered intensity from a distribution of Rayleigh scatterers depends on several factors: (1) the dimensions of the scatterer, with a sharply increasing scattered intensity as the size increases; (2) the number of scatterers present in the beam (e.g., Shung has demonstrated that when the hematocrit is low, scattering from blood is proportional to the hematocrit[7]); (3) the extent to which the density or elastic properties of the scatterer differ from those of the surrounding material; and (4) the ultrasonic frequency. (For Rayleigh scatterers, the scattered intensity is proportional to the frequency to the fourth power.)

Nonlinear Propagation

A sound wave traveling through tissue will also undergo gradual distortion with distance if the amplitude is high enough. This is a manifestation of *nonlinear* sound propagation, and it leads to creation of harmonic waves, or waves that have frequencies that are multiples of that of the original transmitted wave. When partial reflection of the distorted beam occurs at an interface, the reflected echo consists of both the original, "fundamental frequency signals" and harmonic components. A 3-MHz fundamental echo is accompanied by a 6-MHz second harmonic echo and so on. Higher-order harmonics are possible, but attenuation in tissue usually limits the ability to detect them. Although the second harmonic echoes themselves are of lower amplitude than the fundamental, it is possible to distinguish them from the fundamental in the processor of an ultrasound machine and to use them to construct an image, called a tissue harmonic image.[8]

A noteworthy character of tissue harmonic images is that they appear less noisy and have fewer reverberation artifacts than images made with the fundamental. This is believed to be related to the way the harmonic component of the beam forms; i.e., the harmonics gradually grow in amplitude with increasing depth. The harmonic is not present at the skin surface but gradually develops as the beam propagates deeper and deeper into tissue. The second harmonic reaches a peak at some intermediate depth in the patient, then reduces with further increases in depth. Any reverberations or other sources of acoustic noise generated when the transmitted pulse is near the skin surface preferentially contains fundamental frequencies because the harmonics have not built up to any appreciable level at that point. Examples of harmonic images are presented later in this chapter.

B-MODE IMAGING

Range Equation

Ultrasound imaging is done using "pulse-echo" techniques. An ultrasonic transducer is placed in contact with the skin (Fig. 2–7). The transducer repeatedly emits brief pulses of sound at a fixed rate, called the pulse repetition frequency, or PRF. After transmitting each pulse, the transducer waits for echoes from interfaces along the sound beam path. Echo signals picked up by the transducer are amplified and processed into a format suitable for display.

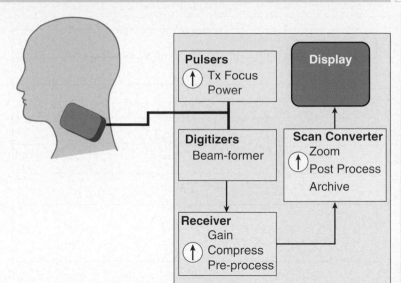

FIGURE 2–7. Simple block diagram of a pulse-echo ultrasound instrument.

The distance to a reflector is determined from the arrival time of its echo. Thus,

$$d = \frac{cT}{2} \qquad (2\text{–}5)$$

where d is the depth of the interface, T is the echo arrival time, and c is the speed of sound in the tissue. The factor 2 accounts for the roundtrip journey of the sound pulse and echo. Equation 2–5 is called the *range equation* in ultrasound imaging.[9] A speed of sound of 1540 m/sec is assumed in most scanners when calculating and displaying reflector depths from echo arrival times. The corresponding echo arrival time is 13 μs/cm of distance to the reflector.

Signal Processing

To create images, pulses of sound are transmitted along various beam lines, each followed by reception and processing of resultant echo signals. Imaging is done with transducer arrays, where echo signals are acquired by individual elements and are combined within a beam former into a single signal for each beam line. The role of the beam former will be discussed in more detail later. Following the beam former, echo signal processing for imaging consists of amplifying the signals; applying time gain compensation to offset effects of beam attenuation; applying nonlinear, logarithmic amplification to compress the wide range of echo signal amplitudes (called the displayed echo dynamic range) into a range that can be displayed effectively on a monitor; demodulation, which forms a single spike-like signal for each echo; and B-mode (for brightness mode) processing. The B-mode display is used in imaging. Signal processing steps are shown in Figure 2–8.

Forming the Image

Two well-known echo display techniques are also illustrated in the lower two panels of Figure 2–8. The amplitude (A)-mode display is a presentation of the echo signal amplitude versus the echo return time, or the reflector depth. This is a one-dimensional display portraying echo signals and their amplitudes along a single beam line; i.e., along one direction. In contrast, the more versatile B-mode display is used for gray-scale imaging. The display is formed by converting echo signals to dots on a monitor, with the brightness indicating echo amplitudes.

In B-mode scanning, sound beams are swept over a region (Fig. 2–9), and echo signals are registered on a two-dimensional (2D) matrix in a position that corresponds to their anatomic origin. Registration is done by placing the B-mode dots along a

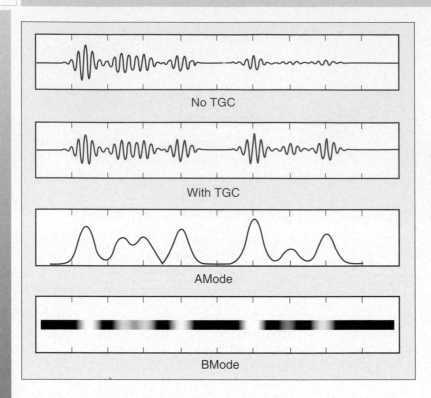

No TGC

With TGC

AMode

BMode

Figure 2–8. Signal processing for imaging. From *top to bottom*, the diagram illustrates the radio frequency signal versus depth for a single beam line; the same signal after application of time gain compensation (TGC); the demodulated, or A-mode waveform; and the B-mode display of the echoes for this line.

line that corresponds to the axis of the ultrasound beam as it sweeps across the scanned field; the proper depth of each echo is determined from the arrival time. In Figure 2–9, the sound beam is swept by electronic switching between groups of elements in a linear array transducer. The B-mode display on the monitor follows the axis of the ultrasound beam as it is swept across the imaged region. Usually, 100 to 200 or more separate ultrasound beam lines are used to construct each image. Most ultrasound systems have controls that allow the operator to vary the beam line density, either directly or indirectly when some other image processing control is manipulated.

Image Memory

An image memory, or *scan converter*, temporarily retains images for review and

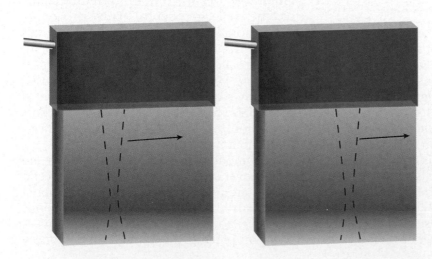

Figure 2–9. Ultrasound B-mode scanning using a linear array. Each sketch shows the position of an ultrasound beam line interrogating the scanned field. The resultant B-mode echo display trace changes with the position of the beam line.

photography and converts the image format into one that can be viewed on a video monitor or that can be recorded on videotape. The scan converter is a digital device and may be thought of as a matrix of pixels (image elements); typically, 500 or more pixels are arranged vertically, and about 500, horizontally. The more pixels horizontally and vertically, the better the detail that is represented in the memory, which is particularly important if a post-processing digital zoom is applied.

Image attributes such as the echo amplitude at each pixel location are represented using a sequence of 1s and 0s, as is the practice for digital devices. The fundamental unit of storage in a digital device is a singular entity called a bit. A single bit can take on a value of either 1 or 0, but by grouping bits into multi-bit storage cells, each multi-bit word can represent a large range of values because of the different combinations of 1 and 0 that can be accommodated. For example, "8-bit" memories divide the echo signal into 255 (2^8) different amplitude levels and store an appropriate level at each pixel location. Twelve-bit memories represent the echo amplitudes using 4096 (2^{12}) levels, and so forth. The more bits (amplitude levels), the more different shades of gray are possible from the stored image, especially during post-processing (see later). Modern scanners also allow storage of cine loops, using a memory that can retain many separate images.

A variety of types of storage media are used in ultrasound. Some laboratories continue their use of hard copy, such as film or other print media. For studies where flow or other dynamic information must be viewed, video tape recorders can store significant quantities of information and facilitate archiving.

Today's ultrasound machines are equipped with digital storage devices, including fixed computer disks, removable magnetic media such as ZIP disks, and CD-ROMs, and these devices are used to archive study results. Software on the machine can be invoked to recall specific studies and display the image or cine loop sequence. In addition, the majority of installations now utilize computer networks for transferring images, making it possible to view study results on workstations and archive information in centrally organized digital collections. PACS (Picture Archiving and Storing) software is available to do these tasks, either on the ultrasound machine itself or off line. A standard file organization system, the Digital Imaging and Communications in Medicine (DICOM) standard, was created by the National Electrical Manufacturers Association and other standards bodies to aid in the distribution and viewing of ultrasound and other medical images created by equipment from different manufacturers. Each DICOM file contains a "header section" that has information including the patient's name, the type of scan, image dimensions, and more, as well as the image data itself. Some scanners require a converter box to accept the image data from the scanner, convert it to a DICOM file, and then transfer the file to the PACS network. More commonly, scanning machines themselves have software to convert files to DICOM format and communicate with the external PACS network. When files are in DICOM format, users with access either to the archived data on the scanning machine or from the network itself can employ DICOM readers available for workstations and personal computers to view, archive externally, print, and manipulate the image data.

Frame Rate

In most applications, B-mode imaging is performed with "real-time" scanning machines. These machines automatically sweep ultrasound beams over the imaged region at a rapid rate, say 30 sweeps per second or higher. The *image frame rate* is the number of complete scans per second carried out by the system. Fundamentally, image frame rates are limited by the sound propagation speed in tissue. An image is produced in the machine by sending ultrasound pulses along 100 to 200 different beam directions (beam lines) into the body. For each beam line, the scanner transmits a pulse and waits for echoes along that beam line, all the way down to the maximum depth setting. Then it transmits a pulse along a new beam direction and repeats the process. Beam lines are addressed serially, meaning the scanner does not transmit a pulse along a new beam line until echoes have been picked up from the maximum depth in the previous line. The speed with which the pulse propagates through tissue, the depth setting of the scanner, the number of transmit focal zones, and the number of beam lines used to form a single image frame all intermix to establish the maximal possible image frame rate.

Using the range equation, if the maximum depth setting is D, it takes a time ($T = 2D/c$) to receive echoes from the entire beam line. The amount of time for a complete image frame constructed with data from N beam lines is simply $N \times T$, or $2ND/c$. If the maximum frame rate is FR_{max}, FR_{max} will be equal to the inverse of the time needed for a complete image. This may be written as

$$FR_{max} = \frac{1}{NT} = \frac{c}{2ND} \qquad (2\text{–}6)$$

For soft tissue in which the speed of sound is about 1540 m/sec, or 154,000 cm/sec, if the depth setting (D) is expressed in centimeters, Equation 2–6 also works out to

$$FR_{max} = \frac{77,000}{ND(\text{cm})} \text{ Hz}$$

For example, with $N = 200$ beam lines and an image depth of 15.4 cm, FR_{max} is 25 Hz.

Operators can easily verify that reducing the depth setting on the machine will increase the frame rate, and vice versa. Often, the machine is programmed to provide as high a frame rate as is practical for the operator settings. Some machines allow the operator to change N, the number of beam lines used to form the image, for example, by increasing the angular separation between beam lines. This, in turn, also affects the frame rate, as does changing the horizontal size of the image and changing the number of transmit focal zones.

TRANSDUCER PROPERTIES

An ultrasound transducer provides the communicating link between the imaging system and the patient. Medical ultrasound transducers use piezoelectric ceramic elements to generate and detect sound waves. Piezoelectric materials convert electric signals into mechanical vibrations and pressure waves into electric signals. The elements, therefore, serve a dual role of pulse transmission and echo detection.

Internal components of an array transducer are shown in Figure 2–10. In the figure, the elements are seen from the side, and the ultrasound waves would be projected upward. The thickness of the piezoelectric element governs the resonance frequency of the transducer. Quarter-wave matching layers between the piezoelectric elements and a protective outer faceplate are used on most transducers. Analogous to special optical coatings on lenses and on picture frame glass, the matching layers improve sound transmission between the transducer and the patient. This improves the transducer's sensitivity to weak echoes. Backing material is often used in pulse-echo

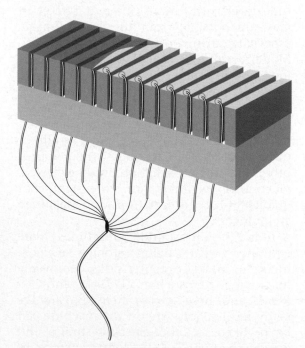

FIGURE 2–10. Drawing of an array transducer. A number of rectangular-shaped piezoelectric elements are mounted side by side within the array housing.

applications to dampen the element vibrations after the transducer is excited with an electric impulse. Dampening shortens the duration of the transmitted pulse, improving the axial (or range) resolution. With optimized designs of the matching and backing layers, transducers can be made to operate over a range of frequencies. Hence, ultrasound machines provide a frequency control switch that the operator manipulates to select the frequency from a menu of choices available for each probe. Some transducers have sufficient frequency range that harmonic imaging can be done, where a low-frequency transmit pulse is sent out, and echoes whose frequency is twice that transmitted are detected and used in imaging.

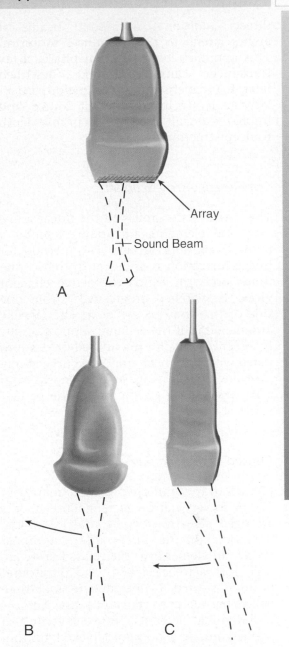

FIGURE 2–11. Transducer types. *A*, Linear array transducer. *B*, Curvilinear array scanner. *C*, Phased array scanner.

Types of Transducers

The operation of three principal types of array transducers is presented in Figure 2–11. The most important transducer for peripheral vascular applications is the "linear array." "Curvilinear arrays" and "phased arrays" also are used in the clinic but mainly for imaging deeper structures in the body. Their use in imaging superficial vessels is rather limited.

Linear (Sequential) Array Scanner

An array of perhaps 200 separate rectangularly shaped transducer elements is arranged side by side in the transducer housing. Conceptually, groups of perhaps 15 to 20 elements are activated simultaneously to produce each ultrasound beam. The beam line would be centered over the central element in the group, except when beam lines are near the lateral margins of the image and an asymmetric element arrangement would be used. An image frame is initiated by a group of elements on one end of the array. The group transmits a pulsed beam and collects the echo signals for this beam line. The active element group is shifted (translated) by one element, forming a new element group, and the pulse-echo process is repeated along a second, parallel beam line. The active element group progresses from one end of the array to the other by switching among the elements. Beam lines are parallel to one another, and the resultant image format is rectangular.

The linear array image format may be expanded by applying "beam steering" that directs additional ultrasound beams at angles lateral to the transducer footprint. This approach borrows from phased-array transducer scanning methods, described later. It broadens the imaged field, particularly at depths away from the source, and improves overall visualization of mid-depth to deep structures.

Curvilinear Array Scanner

These arrays are similar to the linear array, only the elements are arranged along a convex scanning surface. The method for image formation is identical to that of the linear array, in which the active element group is switched progressively from one side of the array to the next. The fan-like arrangement of the element support results in a sector shape for the imaged field. Compared with the linear array, the curved array provides a wider image at large depths from a narrow scanning window on the patient surface.

Phased-Array Scanner

Phased-array scanners consist of an array of 120 or so very narrow rectangular elements arranged side by side. In contrast to the operation of the linear and curvilinear arrays, all elements in the phased array are used for each beam line. The ultrasound beam is "steered" by introducing small-time delays between the transmit pulses applied to individual elements. Time delays are also applied among echo signals picked up from individual elements during reception, steering the received directionality as well. An image is formed using perhaps 100 beams steered in different directions. The advantage of the phased array is that it provides a very broad imaged field at large depths, and this is done with a narrow transducer footprint. The transducer readily fits between the ribs or underneath the rib cage for cardiac scanning. It also makes easy the search for scanning windows in the abdomen, where wound dressings or gas bodies may be present to impede ultrasound beam transmission.

Axial Resolution, Lateral Resolution, and Slice Thickness

Spatial resolution describes the minimum spacing between two reflectors for which they can be distinguished on the display. Important factors are the axial resolution, the lateral resolution, and the slice thickness. These define a "resolution cell," as illustrated in Figure 2–12. Like the size of a paintbrush affecting the detail on a painting, the dimensions of the resolution cell ultimately limit the tissue detail that can be resolved on an ultrasound image.

Axial resolution is the ability to resolve reflectors that are closely spaced along a sound beam axis. It is determined by the pulse duration, the length of time the transducer oscillates for each transmit pulse. Short-duration pulses enable the axial resolution to be 1 mm or less in imaging applications. Damping material attached to the back of the elements helps reduce the pulse duration and improve axial resolution. Axial resolution is considerably better at higher frequencies (Fig. 2–13) because pulse durations can be made much shorter than at low frequencies. A measurement of the intima-media thickness of a blood vessel requires excellent axial resolution to visualize the interfaces and enable the operator to position the distance measuring cursors for an accurate result (Fig. 2–14).

Lateral resolution refers to the closest possible reflector spacing perpendicular to the beam that allows them to be distinguished. It is determined by the width of the ultrasound beam at the location of the reflectors. Beam forming with array imaging systems is a two-step process, first involving shaping a transmitted field and then focusing the sensitivity pattern during echo reception.[5]

The transmitted field from an individual element would spread quickly with distance if it were driven in isolation because the element is narrow. However, when a group of elements is excited, a directional beam can be formed. This beam can be focused by applying infinitesimal time delays to the transmit pulses applied to individual elements, exciting the outer elements of the group a little earlier than the neighboring inner ones, and so on, as in Figure 2–15.

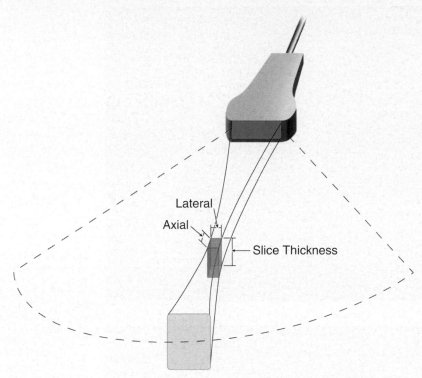

FIGURE 2–12. Typical pulse dimensions emerging from an ultrasound transducer along a single beam line. The pulse duration affects the axial resolution. The width of the beam in the scanning plane determines lateral resolution, whereas the dimensions of the beam perpendicular to the scanning plane determine the slice thickness.

When the operator adjusts the "focus" of a machine, he or she is changing the focal distance of the transmitted beam. The machine responds by adjusting the precise arrangement of the time delays applied to the individual elements producing the beam. Focusing narrows the ultrasound beam at the focal depth. Multiple transmit focal depths are also possible. Usually, this is done by sending several different transmit pulses along each beam line, each transmit pulse focused at a slightly different depth. Because the system must wait for echoes from the focal zone of the previous transmit pulse before a subsequent transmit can be initiated, image frame rate suffers when multiple transmit foci are applied.

Focusing also is done on the received echoes. After a transmit pulse, echoes are picked up by each element of the active aperture. These are digitized and sent to the digital "beam former." The beam former combines the digital signals from each of the array elements and adds them together, forming one extended signal for each trans-mit pulse. However, the echo from any reflector will need to travel slightly different distances to be picked up by the different array elements. This will create phase differences between the signals from the individual elements. This is corrected by "receive focusing," where precisely programmed focusing time delays are applied to the individual signals before summation. The required delay pattern for focusing must change as echoes arrive from progressively greater depths following the transmit pulse. Therefore, the receive beam former is designed to adjust the time delays in real-time. So-called "dynamic receive focusing" enables the receive focus of the array to track the depth of the reflector as echoes arrive from deeper and deeper structures. Dynamic receive focusing is not affected directly by the transmit focus adjustment done by the operator, but rather it is internal to the machine. Some machines even run parallel beam formers during reception, creating several dynamically focused received echo beam lines for each transmit pulse.

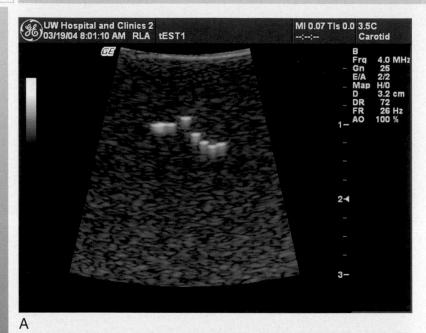

A

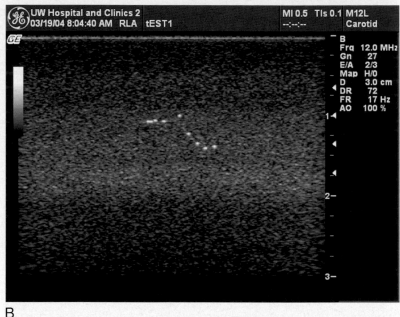

B

FIGURE 2–13. Images of a test object for determining resolution. The reflectors are spaced axially by 2 mm, 1 mm, 0.5 mm, and 0.2 mm. The horizontal row also has reflectors spaced at 2 mm, 1 mm, 0.5 mm, and 0.2 mm. *Part A* was obtained using a transducer running at 4 MHz. *Part B* was obtained using a 11-MHz setting on a different probe.

Focusing reduces the beam width and improves the lateral resolution over a volume called the *focal region*. The beam width (W) in the focal region is approximated by

$$W = \frac{1.2\lambda F}{A} \qquad (2\text{–}8)$$

where F is the focal distance, A is the aperture (i.e., the length of the active part of

the transducer when signals are picked up), and λ is the wavelength. Higher-frequency transducers, for which the wavelength is smaller, provide narrower sound beams and better lateral resolution than lower-frequency transducers. For a given focal depth, the larger the aperture, the narrower is the beam. Often, a system will employ a dynamically changing aperture, increasing A as the echoes arrive from progressively deeper structures, which maintains approximately the same pulse-echo beam width at

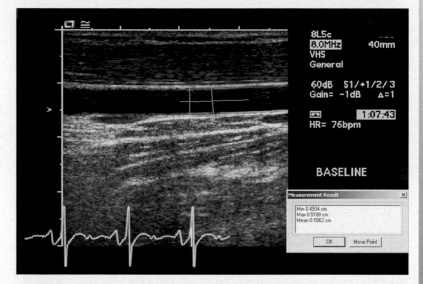

FIGURE 2–14. Intima-media thickness measurements in a brachial artery. Axial resolution is important in being able to make these measurements with high precision.

all depths. In Figure 2–13, the images at both frequencies also include a horizontal row of reflectors, where the separation is from 2 mm to 0.25 mm. As is clearly seen, the detail is much better in the image obtained at a higher ultrasound frequency.

The *slice thickness* is the thickness of the scanned section of tissue that contributes to the image. It depends on the width of the ultrasound beam perpendicular to the image plane (see Fig. 2–12), often called the elevational beam width. Many phased, linear, and curvilinear array transducers still use a one dimensional array (Fig. 2–16) along with a mechanical lens to provide focusing in this direction. While the in-plane beam width and, hence, the lateral

resolution is exquisitely controlled by electronic focusing, the slice thickness for these units is not. The elevational focusing mechanical lens provides good detail near the focal zone but poor detail at depths proximal and distal to this zone (see Fig. 2–16B). Not surprising, therefore, slice thickness is the worst aspect of the resolution of array transducers. Manufacturers are rapidly developing "multi-D," such as "one-and-a-half–dimensional" arrays that will enable electronic focusing in the slice thickness as well as in the lateral direction (Fig. 2–17). These arrays, though more complex and expensive, significantly improve the resolution of small spherical objects, as illustrated in Figure 2–17B.

FIGURE 2–15. Electronic focusing of an array during pulse transmission. By exciting the outer elements of an array group slightly before the inner elements in the sequence shown, the waves from individual elements converge, forming a focused beam. The transmit focal distance is user selectable.

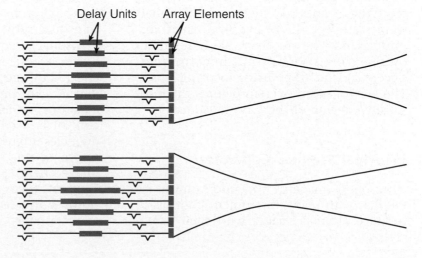

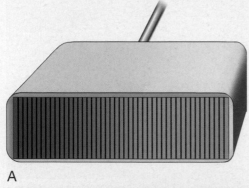

A

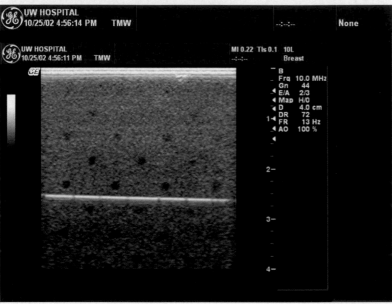

B

FIGURE 2–16. A, View looking towards a linear array of typical element cuts. B, Image of a test phantom containing 2.4-mm diameter spherical targets. Only targets in the mid-range for this transducer are visualized.

Transducers that are used with standalone CW Doppler units are not intended for imaging and therefore are much simpler. Most employ two elements, one for continuously transmitting and the other for receiving echoes. To detect echo signals from scatterers, the beams from the transmitter and the receiver are caused to overlap. This is done by inclining the transducer elements or by using focusing lenses. The area of beam overlap defines the most sensitive region of the CW transducer.

Principal Scanner Controls

Ultrasound machine operators must be familiar with many instrument controls to produce optimal images with their equipment. Details and examples of different control settings can be found in standard textbooks.[5] The major controls found on scanners include these:

- Transducer select, to activate one of two to four probes physically attached to transducer ports on the machine.
- Transducer frequency select, to select the center frequency of ultrasound pulses emitted by the transducer. Modern transducers can produce ultrasound beams covering a range of frequencies. This control is used to determine which frequencies are used in the image.
- Depth setting, to select the size of the imaged field.
- Transmit focus, to enable users to set the number and depth of transmit beam focal zones.

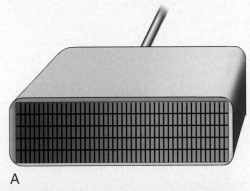

A

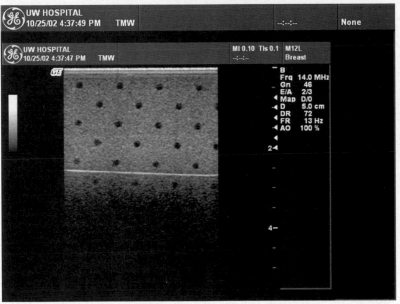

B

FIGURE 2–17. *A*, 1½ Dimensional array. *B*, Image of the same test phantom as in Figure 2–16, using a one-and-a-half-dimensional array.

- Output power control, to vary the scanner sensitivity. Increasing the transmit power allows the operator to view weaker echo signals from the body. (Higher transmit power levels also increase the acoustical exposure to the patient.)
- Overall receiver gain, also to vary the scanner sensitivity. Gain describes the amount of amplification of echoes in the receiver. Higher gains apply more amplification than lower gains; overall gain adjusts the gain throughout the imaged field.
- Time gain compensation, to compensate for attenuation of the ultrasound beam in tissue. With time gain compensation, the receiver amplification increases automatically with the depth of origin of the echoes, so echo signals from deep struc-

tures, which have undergone significant attenuation, are amplified more than signals from shallow structures that have undergone less attenuation. Time gain compensation is controlled in most machines using a set of six to eight gain knobs, each adjusting the receiver gain at a different depth.
- Compression, to vary the amplitude range (dynamic range) of echoes displayed as shades of gray on the image. Most machines apply logarithmic compression to the echo signals emerging from the receiver; the amount of compression is under user control.
- Other preprocessing, to alter the echo signals before they are sent to the scan converter. Some machines, for example, apply edge-enhancing filters to the

signals. Others allow the operator to vary the "beam line density," packing more beam lines into the image in hopes of improving image quality but trading off image frame rate.

- Post-processing, to change the appearance of echo signals, already stored in memory, on the image. Various post-processing curves are available, each emphasizing different portions of the echo amplitudes stored in the image memory.
- Persistence, to include the images from several successive sweeps of the transducer with the current image. High persistence has the effect of smoothing out the image but at the expense of losing some temporal detail.

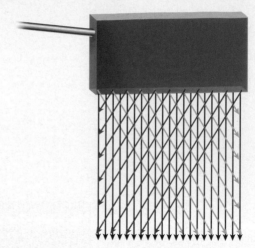

FIGURE 2–18. Compound scanning with a linear array transducer. Echo data resulting from scans done at several beam angles are superimposed on the same image.

SPECIAL PROCESSING TECHNIQUES

Compound Imaging

B-mode images produced using conventional linear or curvilinear arrays appear "granular" or noisy, and this can contribute to uncertainties when interpreting scan results. The granular pattern originates from two sources. First, ultrasound images are subject to a process called speckle, which leads to the random arrangement of B-mode dots on images of organs. The speckle pattern originates from the presence of many unresolvable scatterers that contribute to the echo signal at each location in the image. Once the number of scatterers gets so dense that the imaging machine cannot resolve them, a distribution of dots occurs, whose origin is the underlying, random arrangement of scatterers. The second reason images appear noisy is that small surface reflectors, such as tissue boundaries, muscle facia, and vessel walls, often are at an unfavorable angle to the incident ultrasound beam. Echoes are difficult to pick up, or are even lost, when the surface is at a steep angle (not perpendicular) to the ultrasound beam.

Compound imaging[5,9] addresses both of these issues by sweeping ultrasound beams that are oriented at different angles across the imaged region (Fig. 2–18). The speckle pattern from any location will vary with the direction of the incident beam, because the positions of the individual scatterers relative to the ultrasound beam axis will differ. Therefore, by averaging the angled image data at each location, a smoother pattern can be produced. This improvement in image quality results in greater ability to visualize regions that exhibit subtle changes in echogenicity compared with the background tissue. Additionally, with interrogating beams incident at various angles, surfaces that may not be favorably inclined to the ultrasound beam for one beam direction may turn out to be so for other angles in the compound acquisition. Thus, there usually is more complete outlining of structural boundaries.

The sketch in Figure 2–18 shows only three acquisition angles, but as many as 9 to 10 are available in some imaging systems. In these systems, operators can choose between different levels of compounding when scanning. A greater degree of compounding requires longer scanning times and, hence, lower image frame rates.

Harmonic Imaging

We mentioned earlier that sound pulses undergo nonlinear distortion as they propagate through tissue (Fig. 2–19). The distor-

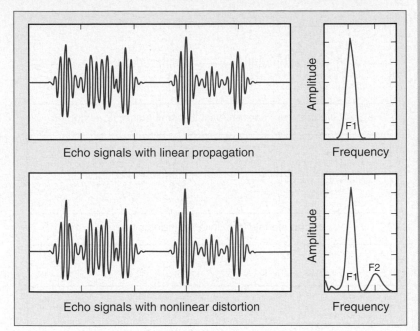

FIGURE 2–19. Echo signal waveforms with their frequency spectra for (*top*) linear propagation and (*bottom*) nonlinear propagation through tissues, with generation of harmonic signals.

Echo signals with linear propagation

Echo signals with nonlinear distortion

tion is accompanied by the production of harmonic frequencies; i.e., added components to the pulse that are integral multiples of the fundamental transmitted pulse frequency. A 2-MHz incident pulse has harmonic components of 4-MHz, 6-MHz, and so on, and echoes will contain mixtures of fundamental and harmonic components. These components, while not present in the transmit pulse emitted by the transducer, build gradually as the pulse makes its way deeper into the tissue. Because this is a nonlinear phenomenon, higher-amplitude pulses undergo much more distortion than lower-amplitude pulses, and the central portion of the ultrasound beam, where the beam intensity is highest, undergoes greater harmonic conversion than the weak edges of the beam.

Although the existence of harmonic distortion in ultrasound has been known for some time, the means to exploit this phenomenon has been only recently incorporated into ultrasound instruments. "Tissue harmonic imaging" is done by filtering out the low-frequency, fundamental components of the ultrasound echoes and using the second harmonic components to form B-mode images. Two signal processing approaches are common.[8] The first applies frequency filtering to isolate the second harmonic frequency component of echo signals from the fundamental. The second method applies "pulse inversion" techniques, explained later.

The frequency filtering methods require special pulse shaping applied to the transmit pulse to ensure there is no overlap between echoes within the fundamental frequency band and those in the harmonic spectrum. A short-duration pulse, optimized for achieving high axial resolution by its nature, contains a spectrum of frequencies; the shorter the pulse, the wider the range of frequencies. The filtering method sometimes is referred to as "narrow-band harmonics" because of the need to restrict the frequencies in the transmit pulse to be sure the higher-frequency components in the much stronger fundamental frequency echoes do not overlap with the low-frequency components of the harmonic echoes. Harmonics tend to be of much lower amplitude than the fundamental, so a significant overlap would offset the benefits to be gained in employing the harmonic mode.

The pulse inversion approach requires two transmit pulses along the same beam line (Fig. 2–20). The first is a conventional imaging pulse of short duration and

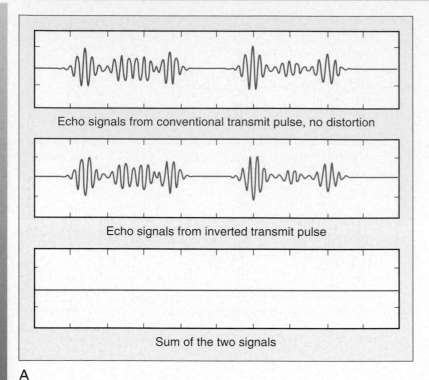

Echo signals from conventional transmit pulse, no distortion

Echo signals from inverted transmit pulse

Sum of the two signals

A

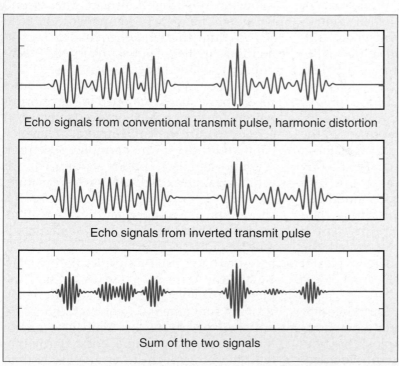

Echo signals from conventional transmit pulse, harmonic distortion

Echo signals from inverted transmit pulse

Sum of the two signals

B

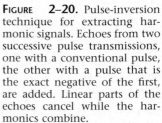

FIGURE 2–20. Pulse-inversion technique for extracting harmonic signals. Echoes from two successive pulse transmissions, one with a conventional pulse, the other with a pulse that is the exact negative of the first, are added. Linear parts of the echoes cancel while the harmonics combine.

wide-frequency bandwidth. After echoes are collected for this transmit pulse, a second pulse is launched that is 180 degrees out of phase; i.e., the exact negative of the first pulse. The resultant echo signals from the two pulse-echo sequences are then added. For linear propagation, the two echoes should cancel each other, and no signal would be displayed along that beam line. However, when significant nonlinear propagation occurs, the echo signals from the different-shaped transmit pulses will not cancel, because the nonlinear distortion occurs more for the positive-going, compressional half cycles of the wave than for the negative, rarefactional half cycles. The noncancelling part is the harmonic signal (see Fig. 2–20B). The apparent advantage of pulse or phase inversion over narrow band harmonics is the use of shorter-duration pulses with their inherently better axial resolution. A disadvantage of pulse inversion is the need to employ two transmit pulse-echo sequences for each beam line, decreasing the image frame rate.

Either method is supposed to help reduce reverberation noise in images and thus improve image quality. An example is presented in Figure 2–21. The echoes within this cystic mass in the breast are caused by reverberation of parts of the incident pulse as it progresses through the tissue layers proximal to the mass. Harmonic echoes are not as strongly affected by the reverberations taking place in the overlying tissues, because the harmonic components have not yet built up to an appreciable degree when the incident pulse is near the skin surface.

Imaging with Contrast Agents

It is possible to enhance the echo signals from a region if small gas bubbles are present. This is exactly how contrast agents may be used to enhance the echo signals from blood. Ultrasound contrast agents consist of tiny gas bubbles, either air of a heavy molecular weight gas, stabilized with a type of shell. One of the earliest contrast agents available was Albunex (Mallinckrodt Medical, St. Louis, MO), manufactured by sonicating human serum albumin in the presence of air. A number of similar agents have evolved and are available commercially, each having a particular shell material or gas. The bubble sizes commonly are in the 1- to 5-μm range. Even though bubbles are small, they can produce large-amplitude echoes and so are used to intensify echoes from small blood vessels and sometimes from the chambers of the heart.

Special properties of gas bubbles can be exploited to help distinguish between echoes from contrast agents and echoes from tissues that have no agent present.[10] The first property is the ease to which the bubbles reflect nonlinearly, producing echoes not only of the frequency transmitted by the transducer but also at harmonics of the transmitted frequency. For example, when 3-MHz waves are reflected by contrast agent bubbles, fundamental (3-MHz), second harmonic (6-MHz), and higher, as well as subharmonic (1.5-MHz) echoes result. Tuning the scanner to pick out the harmonic frequencies helps isolate the echo signals from the contrast agent. Ultrasound machines set up for contrast agent imag-

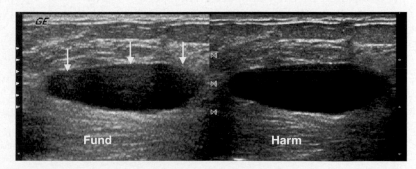

FIGURE 2–21. Image of a breast cyst with conventional processing (*left*) and with harmonic processing (*right*).

ing sometimes apply complex pulse-echo sequences, where the resultant echoes can be combined in a way that draws out the echoes resulting from nonlinear reflections from the bubbles and cancels the echoes from other reflectors.

Another property that can be exploited in their detection is that contrast agent bubbles are easily destroyed by high-amplitude ultrasound pulses. Thus, bubbles are detected by transmitting a high-amplitude destructive pulse, collecting the echoes, then transmitting a second pulse and comparing the echoes from the two. Echoes from the contrast agent bubbles would be present for the first pulse but absent for the second because of the destructive effects of the first pulse. Manipulation of the echo signals is done to isolate signals from the agent only, which is sometimes useful to detect flow in small vessels. Ultrasound machines with contrast agent imaging modes may thus implement special pulse sequences to draw out the echo signal from the agent itself.

Codes and Chirps

To achieve the best spatial resolution, equipment operators attempt to use as high an ultrasound frequency as possible when scanning. Unfortunately, high ultrasound frequencies are severely attenuated, so the need for adequate beam penetration usually limits the frequency that can be effectively used. If it were possible to increase the transmit power, sending more energetic pulses into the tissues, this might improve penetration of these high frequencies somewhat. The transmit power can be increased by increasing the amplitude of the ultrasound pulse emitted by the transducer. This works only up to a point, however, because non-linear distortion, equipment limitations, and regulations on ultrasound equipment for safety purposes result in limitations on the amplitude of the transmitted pulses from the transducer. Related to the question of potential biologic effects, current practice by the U.S. Food and Drug Administration requires manufacturers of ultrasound equipment to limit the amplitude of the

transmitted pulse to levels that have MI values of 1.9 or less.

Another way to provide a more energetic transmit pulse without exceeding the amplitude limits or equipment capabilities is to make the pulse duration longer. However, it is first necessary to encode the pulse in a special way that would enable recovery of a short-duration pulse with its accompanying good axial resolution after echoes are received. Use of "coded excitation" is one means of achieving this.

Coded excitation applies a unique signature to the transmitted ultrasound pulse. The pulse itself has a very long duration compared with conventional pulses applied in ultrasound. However, it is modulated by a specific pattern of 1s and 0s before being applied to the transducer. An example of a waveform detected from one manufacturer's coded transmit by a detector in water is presented in Figure 2–22. This long-duration transmit pulse undergoes

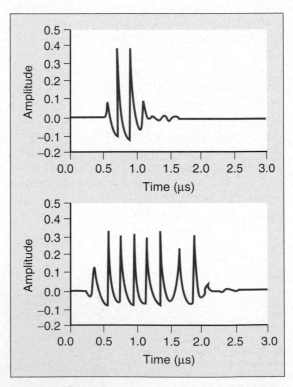

FIGURE 2–22. Comparison of transmitted waveforms using conventional pulsing (*top*) and coded excitation (*bottom*). The short-duration nature of the system response is recovered following coded excitation by applying special decoding, or matched filter schemes.

reflections at interfaces, and echoes are detected once again by the transducer. After amplification and beam forming, the echo signals are sent to a special decoding process, often referred to as a matched filter, to recover signals exhibiting short-duration pulse properties. Certain codes require two pulse-echo sequences, each transmit pulse having slightly different timing features but the two together having complimentary properties. When echo signals are combined, the process eliminates artifacts known as range side-lobes that sometimes are present when codes are used. Nevertheless, with coded excitation methods, it is possible to recover both the effects of having a short-duration pulse and a pulse of much higher amplitude.

Another type of code is a "chirp pulse."[11] A chirp is a brief transmit burst, or pulse, whose frequency varies over the pulse duration. Again, special decoding schemes allow the original short pulse duration to be recovered while providing much better beam penetration than would be provided with conventional, short-duration pulse transmission.

DOPPLER ULTRASOUND

The Doppler effect is a change in the frequency of a detected wave when the source or the detector is moving. In medical ultrasonography, a Doppler shift occurs when reflectors move relative to the transducer. The frequency of echo signals from moving reflectors is higher or lower than the frequency transmitted by the transducer, depending on whether the motion is toward or away from the transducer. The Doppler shift frequency, or simply the Doppler frequency, is the difference between the received and transmitted frequencies.

Doppler Equation

Ultrasonic Doppler equipment is for detecting and evaluating blood flow. A typical arrangement is illustrated in Figure 2–23. An ultrasonic transducer is placed in contact

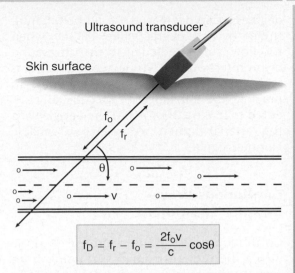

$$f_D = f_r - f_o = \frac{2f_o v}{c} \cos\theta$$

FIGURE 2–23. Arrangement for detecting Doppler signals from blood. The angle θ is the Doppler angle, which is the angle between the direction of motion and the beam axis, looking toward the transducer.

with the skin surface; it transmits a beam whose frequency is f_o. The received frequency f_R will differ from f_o when echoes are picked up from moving scatterers, such as the red blood cells. The Doppler frequency (f_D) is defined as the difference between the received and transmitted frequencies. The f_D is calculated by the following:

$$f_D = f_R = f_o = \frac{2f_o V \cos\theta}{c} \qquad (2\text{--}7)$$

where c is the speed of sound, V is the flow velocity, and θ is the angle between the direction of flow and the axis of the ultrasound beam, looking toward the transducer.

The symbol θ is called the *Doppler angle* and strongly influences the detected Doppler frequency for a given reflector velocity. When flow is directly toward the transducer, θ is 0 degrees and cos θ is 1. The Doppler frequency detected for this orientation would be the maximum one could obtain for the flow conditions. More typically, the ultrasound beam will be incident at an angle other than 0 degrees, and the detected Doppler frequency will be reduced according to the cos θ term. For example, at 30 degrees, the Doppler frequency would be 0.87 multiplied by what it is at 0 degrees; at 60 degrees, it would be 0.5 multiplied by its 0-degree value. Finally, when the flow is perpendicular to the ultrasound beam direction, θ is 90 degrees and cos θ is 0; there is no detected Doppler shift! In practice, the transducer beam is usually oriented to make a 30- to 60-degree angle with the arterial lumen to receive a reliable Doppler signal.

Continuous-Wave Doppler Equipment

Continuous-wave (CW) Doppler is done in a variety of instruments, ranging from simple, inexpensive hand-held Doppler units, to "high-end" duplex scanners in which CW Doppler is one of several operating modes. A simplified block diagram of the necessary components of a CW Doppler unit is presented in Figure 2–24. The transmitter continuously excites a transmit section of the ultrasonic transducer, sending a continuous beam whose frequency is f_o. Echoes returning to the transducer have frequency f_R. These signals are amplified in the receiver and then sent to a demodulator to extract the Doppler signal. Here, the signals are multiplied by a reference signal from the transmitter, producing a mixture of signals, part having a frequency equal to $(f_R + f_o)$ and part having a frequency $(f_R - f_o)$. The sum frequency $(f_R + f_o)$ is very high—about twice the ultrasound frequency—and is easily removed by electronic filtering. This leaves signals with frequency $(f_R - f_o)$ at the output, which is the Doppler signal!

What are typical Doppler frequencies for blood flow? Suppose V = 20 cm/sec; the ultrasound frequency (f_o) is 5 MHz (5 × 10^6 cycles/sec); and the speed of sound (c) is 1540 m/sec. Let θ equal 0 degrees, so that cos θ is 1. Using Equation 2–7, we find

$$f_D = \frac{2 \times (5 \times 10^6 \, \text{cycles/sec}) \times 0.2 \, \text{m/sec}}{1540 \, \text{m/sec}}$$

$$= 1299 \, \text{cycles/sec}$$

or about 1.3 kHz, which is within the audible frequency range. The filtered output Doppler signal can be applied to a loudspeaker or headphones for interpretation by the operator. The signals can also be recorded on audiotape or applied to any of several spectral analysis systems (see later).

It is possible to eliminate signals of certain frequency ranges from the output. This is done in instruments that have additional electric filters in their circuitry. For example, when studying blood flow, relatively low-frequency Doppler signals originating from movement of vessel walls may be eliminated from the output by applying a high-pass filter. The lower cutoff frequency of such "wall filters" is usually operator selectable.

Continuous-Wave Doppler Controls

Basic CW Doppler units usually have only a few controls, but operators should be familiar with those on their own equipment. Examples include the following:

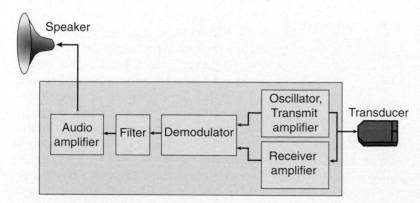

Figure 2–24. A continuous-wave Doppler instrument. The Doppler signal is obtained by demodulating the amplified echo signals and then applying a low-pass filter. Because the signals are generally in the audible range, a loudspeaker may be used to display the Doppler signals.

- Transmit power, to vary the amplitude of the signal from the transmitter to the transducer, thus changing the sensitivity to weak echoes. Some simple units omit this control, keeping the transmit level constant.
- Gain, to vary the sensitivity of the unit.
- Audio gain, to vary the loudness of Doppler signals applied to loudspeakers.
- Wall filter, to vary the low-frequency cutoff frequency of the wall filter.

Directional Doppler

A basic CW Doppler instrument allows detection of the magnitude of the Doppler frequency, but it provides no indication of whether flow is toward or away from the transducer; i.e., whether the Doppler shift is positive or negative. A common technique for determining flow direction is to use quadrature detection in the Doppler device. After the received echo signals are amplified, they are split into two identical channels for demodulation. The channels differ only in that the reference signals from the transmitter sent to the two demodulators are 90 degrees out of phase. Two separate Doppler signals are produced. They are identical except for a small phase difference between them, and this phase difference can be used to determine whether the Doppler shift is positive or negative.[12] Various schemes are used that combine the two quadrature signals to enable presentation of positive and negative flow in stereo speakers.[13]

Pulsed Doppler

With CW Doppler instruments, reflectors and scatterers anywhere within the beam of the transducer can contribute to the instantaneous Doppler signal. A pulsed Doppler instrument provides for discrimination of Doppler signals from different depths, allowing for the detection of moving interfaces and scatterers only from within a well-defined sample volume (Fig. 2–25). The sample volume can be posi-

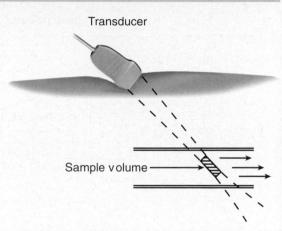

FIGURE 2–25. Sample volume in pulsed Doppler. Echo signals from a fixed depth are selected by a range gate. The size of the sample volume depends on the beam width, the duration of the gate, and the pulse duration from the transducer.

tioned anywhere along the axis of the ultrasound beam.

The principal components of a pulsed Doppler instrument are shown in Figure 2–26. The ultrasonic transducer is excited with a short-duration burst, rather than continuously as in the CW instrument. Scattered and reflected echo signals are detected by the same transducer, amplified in the receiver, and applied to the demodulator. The output of the demodulator is then applied to a sample-and-hold circuit, which integrates (or averages) a portion of the signal, selected by a range gate. The gate position and duration are controlled by the operator. The gated signal, taken over a series of pulse-echo sequences, forms the Doppler signal heard over the loudspeaker of the device. In Figure 2–26, quadrature detectors are used to form two output channels, enabling the flow direction to be determined.

The Doppler signal produced by a pulsed Doppler instrument is generated from the changes in phase of the echo signals from moving targets from one pulse-echo sequence to the next. Thus, the PRF of the instrument must be high enough so that important details of the Doppler signal are not lost between transmit pulses. (See section on aliasing in pulsed doppler.) After each transmit pulse, only a brief portion of the Doppler signal is available within the

Pulsed Doppler

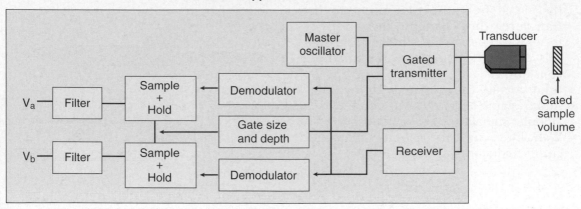

FIGURE 2–26. Principal components of a pulsed Doppler instrument. The transducer is excited by a brief pulse; echo signals are amplified in the receiver and sent to the quadrature demodulators. A portion of the demodulated waveform is held in the sample and hold unit, which forms the Doppler signal by using several pulse-echo sequences. V_a and V_b are quadrature signals that can be processed to indicate flow toward and away from the transducer.

demodulated echo signals selected by the gated region. Multiple pulse-echo sequences are required to construct the Doppler signal heard over the loudspeakers. By filtering the sample-and-hold output from one pulse-echo sequence to the next, a smooth Doppler signal is formed.

Duplex Instruments

A real-time B-mode imager and a Doppler instrument provide complementary information because the scanner can best outline anatomic structures, whereas a Doppler instrument yields information regarding flow and movement patterns. *Duplex ultrasound instruments* are real-time B-mode scanners with built-in Doppler capabilities. In typical applications, the pulse-echo B-mode image obtained with a duplex scanner is used to localize areas where flow is to be examined using Doppler.

The region of interest for Doppler studies may be selected on the B-mode image by placement of a sample volume indicator, or cursor (Fig. 2–27). Most duplex instruments allow the operator to indicate the Doppler angle or the direction of blood flow with respect to the ultrasound beam. The Doppler angle must be known to estimate flow velocity from the Doppler signal.

Choice of Ultrasound Frequency

Competing physical interactions govern the choice of the operating frequency employed in an ultrasound instrument. For Doppler work, the choice is usually dictated by the need to obtain adequate signal strength for reliable interpretation of Doppler signals. It was mentioned previously that the intensity of ultrasonic waves scattered from small

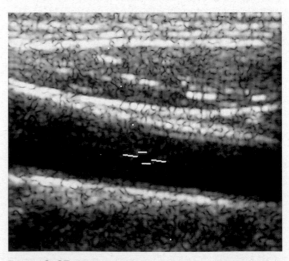

FIGURE 2–27. Image of a carotid artery obtained with a duplex ultrasound machine. A sample volume cursor is positioned to detect Doppler signals from within the artery, and a Doppler angle cursor is oriented to "angle correct" the Doppler signals for displaying the velocity.

scatterers such as red blood cells increases rapidly with increasing frequency, being proportional to the frequency raised to the fourth power. It thus would seem reasonable to use a high ultrasonic frequency to increase the intensity of scattered signals from blood. As the frequency increases, however, the rate of beam attenuation also increases (see Fig. 2–3). In selecting the optimal frequency for detecting blood flow, these competing processes must be balanced, and the choice of operating frequency is often determined by the tissue depth of the vessel of interest. For small, superficial vessels, in which attenuation from overlying tissues is not significant, B-mode and Doppler probes operating at 7 to 10 MHz are commonly used. Doppler applications in the carotid artery usually employ somewhat lower frequencies to avoid significant attenuation losses, and frequencies of 4 to 5 MHz are typical. Frequencies as low as 2 MHz are used for detecting flow in deeper arteries and veins.

Doppler Spectral Analysis

For many structures of interest, the Doppler signal is in the audible frequency range. For some applications, adequate clinical interpretations can be made simply by listening to the signals. The listener then characterizes the flow according to the qualities of the audible signal.

In the case of blood flow, the Doppler signal is fairly complex because of the complicated blood velocity patterns found in most vessels. In a large blood vessel, the blood velocity is not the same at all points but follows some type of flow profile. If the ultrasound beam and the sample volume are large compared with the lumen diameter, scattered ultrasound signals are received simultaneously from blood that is moving at different velocities. The resultant Doppler signal, therefore, is complex.

A complex signal such as that shown in Figure 2–28A may be shown to be composed of many single-frequency signals (see Fig. 2–28B). Each of these has a particular amplitude and phase so that, when added together, they form the original signal. *Spectral analysis* is a way to separate a complicated signal into its individual frequency components so that the relative contribution of each frequency component to the original signal can be determined (see Fig. 2–28C). Often, the relative contribution is denoted by the signal power in a given frequency interval, and the spectrum is referred to as the *power spectrum*.

Most instruments use a Fast Fourier Transform to do spectral analysis of Doppler signals. The Doppler signal is fed into the spectral analyzer in small time segments (e.g., 5 msec). The power spectrum is computed and is displayed along a vertical line, where the height represents a frequency bin and the brightness represents the signal power or intensity for that bin (Fig. 2–29). The relative intensity of Doppler signals depends on the amount of blood generating that signal, so the brightness of each frequency bin indicates the amount of flow at the velocity corresponding to that Doppler frequency. As the spectral signals from one segment are being displayed, a subsequent segment is being analyzed, producing a continuous display.

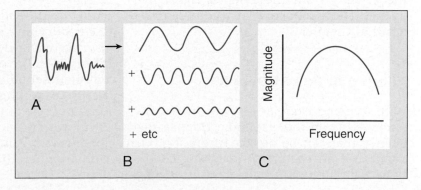

FIGURE 2–28. A complex signal waveform (*A*) can be generated by a combination of single-frequency signals (*B*). *C*, Spectral analysis involves the separation of the complex signal into its frequency components and the display of the magnitude of each frequency component that contributes to the signal.

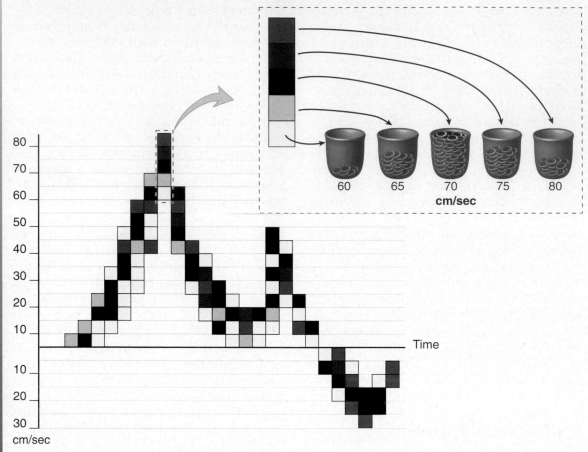

FIGURE 2–29. Information on a spectral Doppler display. Doppler frequency (or reflector velocity) is plotted vertically and time, horizontally. For each time segment, the amount of signal within specific frequency bins is indicated by a shade of gray. The amount of signal corresponds to the amount of blood flowing at the corresponding velocity.

Duplex instruments display a B-mode image along with a Doppler spectral display. An example is presented in Figure 2–30. The vertical scale on the spectral display can be either Doppler frequency (in hertz) or velocity (in centimeters per second or meters per second). To display the velocity, the analyzer solves the Doppler equation to derive the velocity from the Doppler signal frequency. The spectral display is considered in detail in Chapter 3.

Aliasing in Pulsed Doppler

With a pulsed Doppler instrument, a limitation exists on the maximum Doppler frequency that can be detected from a given depth and on the set of operating conditions. The limitation referred to is *aliasing*

and, if present, can lead to anomalies on Doppler signal spectral waveforms.

Consider the situation illustrated in Figure 2–31. As mentioned earlier, a pulsed Doppler instrument forms the Doppler signal using multiple pulse-echo sequences. The Doppler signal is said to be sampled, and the sampling frequency is the PRF of the instrument. In Figure 2–31, the Doppler signal is represented by the *solid line*, and the *arrows* represent successive samples of this signal. The *lower waveform* depicts the sampled signal. In this case, the sampled signal is an excellent representation of the original signal because sampling occurred multiple times for each cycle of the original waveform.

Unfortunately, with pulsed Doppler, it is not always possible to have the PRF significantly higher than the frequency of the Doppler signal. As discussed in the next

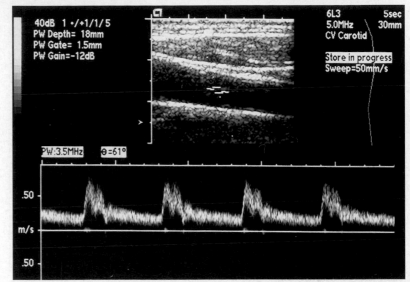

FIGURE 2–30. Spectral display from a carotid artery.

section, we must limit the PRF, so sufficient time is available to collect all signals from one pulsing of the transducer before a subsequent pulsing. This restriction on the PRF depends on the depth of the sample volume. The greater the distance to the sample volume, the longer it takes to pick up echoes from that region and the lower the PRF must be.

At a minimum, the PRF must be at least twice the frequency of the Doppler signal to construct the signal successfully. When the PRF equals twice the F_D, this is known as the *Nyquist sampling rate*. The Nyquist rate is the minimum sampling rate that can be used for a signal of a given frequency. If the sampling rate is lower than the Nyquist

rate, aliasing occurs. Aliasing is a production of artifactual, lower-frequency signals when the sampling rate (the PRF) is less than twice the Doppler signal frequency.

Aliasing is illustrated schematically in Figure 2–32. The actual Doppler signal (*top*) is sampled (*arrows*) at a rate less than twice each cycle of the signal. The resulting sampled waveform (see *lower part* of Fig. 2–32) is one whose frequency is less than that of the actual signal.

A common way that aliasing is manifested on a Doppler spectral display is illustrated in Figure 2–33. The Doppler spectrum wraps around the display, with high

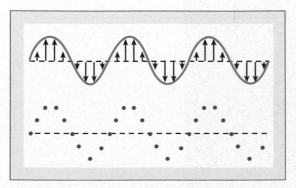

FIGURE 2–31. Sampling a Doppler signal. The *solid line* on top is a sine wave, and *arrows* represent the times when discrete samples of the signal are taken. The *dotted line* on the bottom is the sampled signal.

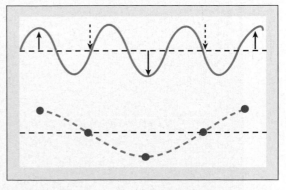

FIGURE 2–32. Production of aliasing when the sampling rate is less than 2 times the frequency of the signal. The upper curve is the signal, which is being sampled at the discrete times indicated by *arrows*. The lower curve is a lower frequency alias of the signal resulting from the inadequate sampling.

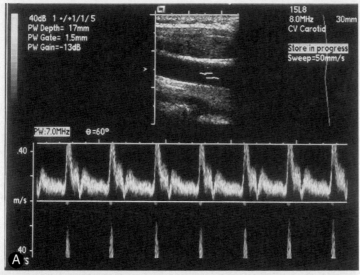

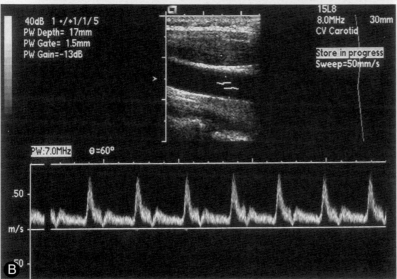

FIGURE 2–33. Manifestation of aliasing on a spectral display. *A*, The spectrum warps around. *B*, Correction of aliasing by increasing the velocity scale on the machine. *C*, Elimination of aliasing by adjusting the baseline.

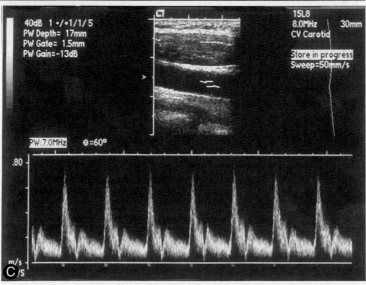

velocities being converted to reversed flow immediately at the point of aliasing and still higher velocities in the flow signal appearing as progressively lower velocities.

Several methods are used to eliminate aliasing. It can often be eliminated by increasing the velocity/frequency scale limits of the spectral display (see Fig. 2–33B). When the scale is increased, the Doppler instrument increases the PRF, keeping it at the Nyquist limit for the maximum Doppler frequency shown on the spectral scale. The operator can also adjust the spectral baseline, the line representing 0 velocity, assigning the entire spectral display to flow moving in just one direction (see Fig. 2–33C). This is successful when flow is in one direction only. Yet another way to eliminate aliasing may be to use a lower-frequency transducer. The Doppler frequency is proportional to both the reflector velocity and the ultrasound frequency (f_o), so a lower ultrasound frequency results in a lower-frequency Doppler signal for a given velocity.

Maximum Velocity Detectable with Pulsed Doppler

As mentioned earlier, to detect a Doppler signal without aliasing, the PRF of the instrument must be at least twice the Doppler frequency. An upper limit on the PRF is established, however, by the time interval required for ultrasound pulses to propagate to the range of interest and return. If the time between pulses is insufficient, "range ambiguities" arise because of overlap of echoes from successive pulses. With the sample volume set at depth d, the minimum time needed between pulses (T_d) is $2d/c$ (from the range equation). The maximum PRF possible, PRF_{max}, is just the inverse of T_d. Thus,

$$PRF_{max} = 1/T_d = c/2d \qquad (2–9)$$

What is the highest flow velocity that can be detected, given the limitation expressed in Equation 2–9? The maximum Doppler frequency we can detect without aliasing will now be $PRF_{max}/2 = c/4d$. Using the

Doppler equation and substituting for f_D, we get

$$\frac{2f_o V_{max}}{c} = \frac{c}{4d}$$

where V_{max} is the maximum velocity detectable without aliasing. Solving for V_{max},

$$V_{max} = \frac{c^2}{8f_o d} \qquad (2–10)$$

Assuming a speed of sound of 1540 m/sec, the plots in Figure 2–34 were generated using Equation 2–10, relating the maximum reflector velocity that can be detected to reflector depth for three different ultrasound frequencies. As the sample volume depth increases, the maximum detectable Doppler signal frequency, and hence the maximum reflector velocity that can be detected, decreases. At any depth, lower ultrasound frequencies permit detection of greater velocities than higher frequencies.

In some instruments, higher velocities than those shown in Figure 2–34 can be obtained using a "high PRF" selection. In this mode, the PRF of the instrument is allowed to be increased beyond the limit set by Equation 2–9. Now, range ambiguity is present because the echo data from successive transmit pulses overlap. This is

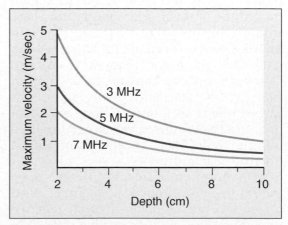

FIGURE 2–34. Maximum velocity detectable with pulsed Doppler versus sample volume depth for three different ultrasound frequencies.

indicated on the display by the presence of multiple sample volumes displayed on the image. In general, however, the range ambiguities are not a problem, because the operator already has the area of flow sampling isolated before activating high PRF, and the exact origin of the Doppler signals is still known.

COLOR FLOW IMAGING

Forming Color Images

Color flow imaging (or color-velocity imaging) is done by estimating and displaying the mean velocity relative to the ultrasound beam direction of scatterers and reflectors in a scanned region. Echo signals from moving reflectors are generally displayed so that the color hue, saturation, or brightness indicates the relative velocity. Color flow image data are superimposed on B-mode data from stationary structures to obtain a composite image.

Several methods for processing echo signals to produce color flow images have been described. Some of these operate on the signals produced after Doppler signal processing,[5,14,15] whereas a few process echo signals directly.[16] (Specific mathematical details of the methods are given in the references, especially references 13 and 16.) For each method, a series of pulse-echo sequences are produced along a single-beam axis. Echo signals from each succeeding transmit pulse are compared with signals from those of the previous pulse, and phase shifts in the succeeding signals are then estimated. Once this is done for all pulse-echo sequences along the beam line, a mean Doppler frequency shift and, hence, a mean velocity are calculated. This process is carried out at all locations along the beam line, and the estimated velocity is displayed using a color. Then, another beam line is interrogated, and so on.

With most instruments, 10 or more transmit-receive sequences might be used to produce an estimate of mean reflector velocities along each beam line. The term *pulse packets* has been adopted to designate the transmit-receive pulse-echo sequences, with *packet size* designating the number of such sequences along each beam line.[17] Some instruments allow the operator to vary the packet size directly; most vary the packet size when the operator changes other control settings, such as color preprocessing.

Because data for each acoustic line that forms a color-velocity image are acquired using multiple pulse-echo sequences, frame rates in color flow imaging tend to be lower than frame rates in standard B-mode imaging. In color flow imaging, noticeable tradeoffs are evident among factors affecting color-image quality and scanning speed or frame rate. Most instruments provide signal processing controls that allow the user to optimize imaging parameters for specific applications. Higher frame rates are often accompanied by reduced image quality, because fewer acoustic lines are used to form the image. In contrast, very detailed color images, sensitive to low-flow states, are frequently obtained at the expense of lower frame rates.

The direction of blood flow is indicated by the display color; for example, red might encode flow toward the transducer, and blue, away from the transducer. It should be kept in mind that the color processor displays motion relative to the ultrasound beam direction for each beam line forming the flow image. Different parts of a vessel are often interrogated from different beam directions, either because of the orientation of the vessel or as a result of the transducer scan format. The latter problem is illustrated in Figure 2–35, in which continuous flow through a horizontal vessel appears both blue (away) and red (toward) because of the different beam angles that interrogate the vessel when a sector scanner is used.

Aliasing on Color Displays

The color-velocity image is produced with pulsed Doppler techniques; therefore, the image is subject to aliasing, as discussed previously. A common manifestation of aliasing is a wraparound of the display, resulting in an apparent reversal of the flow direction (Fig. 2–36A). For example, aliased flow

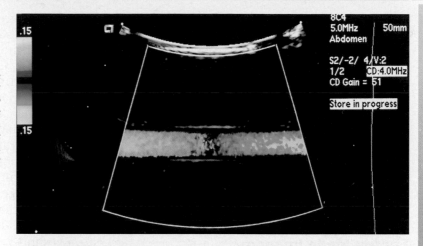

FIGURE 2–35. Color flow image of a horizontal vessel in a flow phantom. Flow is from left to right on the image, so for the sector transducer, it is directed toward the transducer on the left-hand side of the image and away from the transducer on the right-hand side.

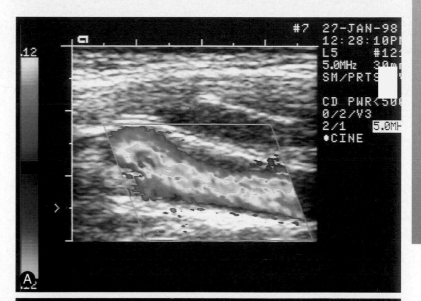

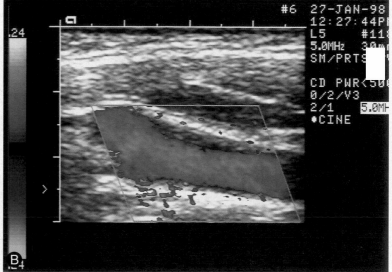

FIGURE 2–36. Aliasing in color flow imaging. A, Color flow image of a carotid artery, with aliasing. B, Same as in part A, only the velocity scale has been adjusted to eliminate aliasing.

toward the probe is interpreted as flow moving away. Increasing the color flow velocity scale essentially increases the PRF of the processor and eliminates the aliasing problem if flow velocities remain within the allowable range of velocities on the instrument (see Fig. 2–36*B*). Also, changing the color baseline (the zero-flow position on the spectral display) can shift the allowable Doppler frequency range; this method is effective when flow signals are only in one direction.

Energy Mode Imaging

Color flow imaging displays scatterer velocities relative to the interrogating ultrasound beam direction at positions throughout the scanned field. An alternative processing method ignores the velocity and simply estimates the strength (or power or energy) of the Doppler signal detected from each location. So-called power or energy mode imaging[18] has both advantages and limitations.

An energy mode image of the horizontal vessel in the flow phantom depicted in Figure 2–35 is presented in Figure 2–37. The energy mode image is continuous rather than divided into segments because of the different beam directions. In other words,

the energy image is not sensitive to relative flow direction, as is the color velocity image. Another advantage of the energy mode image is that it is not affected by aliasing. Figure 2–30 contrasts color velocity images with energy-mode images of a flow phantom when aliasing is present. The energy mode image does not depict velocities but only a value related to the strength of the Doppler signal, so the effects of aliasing are not manifested.

The advantages of this modality over color velocity imaging are, therefore

1. Energy mode seems to be more sensitive to low- and weak-flow states than color velocity.
2. Angle effects on the Doppler frequency are ignored, unless the angle becomes so close to perpendicular that the Doppler signals are below the flow detectability threshold of the color processor.
3. Aliasing does not affect the energy mode display. Thus, a more continuous display of flow, especially in difficult to scan regions, is provided.

Disadvantages of energy mode imaging are also clear:

1. Information on reflector velocity and flow direction relative to the transducer is not displayed. Sometimes these features are important to a diagnosis.

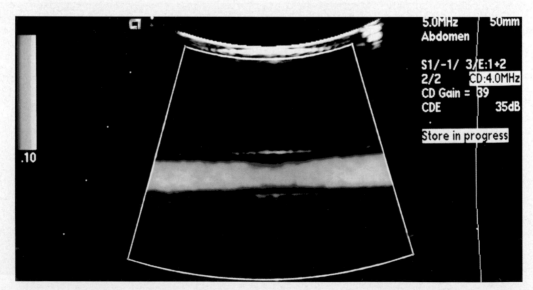

FIGURE 2–37. Power-mode image of the same vessel as in Figure 2–27. The energy-mode image is almost insensitive to the Doppler angle.

2. Image build-up tends to be slower, and image frame rates lower, because of the use of more signal averaging in energy mode than in velocity mode. Consequently, problems with flash artifact caused by Doppler signals from slowly moving soft tissues are more severe in energy mode than in velocity mode.

BEYOND TWO-DIMENSIONAL IMAGING

Extended Field of View Imaging

Sometimes it is desirable to display a larger imaged region than that provided simply by the format of the ultrasound transducer. To some extent, this has already been addressed in technology that widens the image format of linear array transducers. It might be possible to produce images whose view is much larger than that provided by the transducer alone if the probe were attached to a mechanical translation system and the transducer were moved in a direction parallel to the image plane as image data are acquired. However, the idea of mechanically linking the transducer for the purpose of providing an image that has a wider format might not appeal to operators, who need extensive freedom to manipulate the probe to desired image planes. An alternative and effective method for extending the image field is one in which the operator freely translates the probe parallel to the image plane, and probe motion is tracked by changes in the image itself. As the transducer is translated manually, image processing software identifies the amount of lateral motion from one frame to the next. This enables the software to register new image information in a location that correctly corresponds to its anatomic position with respect to structures appearing in the original image.

An image of a femoral-tibial artery graft shown in Figure 2–38 illustrates one result of this process. Although the original image from the linear array transducer used in creating the image would be only about 4 cm wide, careful translation of the probe along

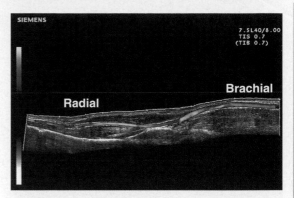

FIGURE 2–38. Extended field of view imaging. This image of a femoral tibeal graft extends over 20 cm. It is constructed by tracking motion of the transducer during the scan using correlation processing applied to the B-mode image data. (Courtesy of Siemens Medical.)

with the image registration software provides a view of the artery that extends for nearly its entire length.

Three-Dimensional Ultrasound

The real-time nature of ultrasound imaging and the need to view structures through scanning windows that sometimes provide poor acoustic access has limited the use of 3D volume acquisition and display techniques. However, transducers that are comparable in size to conventional probes but with 3D capabilities are leading to a renewed interest in 3D imaging in ultrasound. Some applications appear to benefit greatly from using 3D, especially imaging the fetus and certain vascular structures (Fig. 2–39). Three-dimensional scanning acquires ultrasound B-mode or color images over an entire volume. Besides the more extensive data set than is obtained using large numbers of 2D images, a 3D set enables new views that sometimes can save time during interpretation and analysis. Moreover, 3D images often are more intuitive than sets of conventional, 2D images for those who are not specialists in medical imaging, making communication with patients and referring physicians more easily done.

Typically, to acquire 3D data, the ultrasound transducer is translated perpendicular to the plane of the acquired image (Fig. 2–40), and images are stored at predeter-

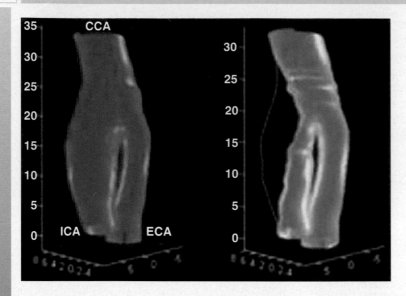

FIGURE 2–39. Surface-rendered three-dimensional image of the carotid bifurcation. CCA, common carotid artery; ECA, external carotid artery; ICA, internal carotid artery.

mined spatial intervals. The stack of images so acquired may be thought of as a volume scan. We think of "acquired image planes" (i.e, images generated by the real-time beam sweeping methods discussed earlier) and "reconstructed planes," or new images gen-

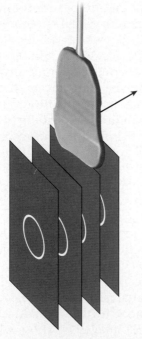

FIGURE 2–40. Arrangement for acquiring three-dimensional images by freehand translation of a transducer. Probe tracking methods vary from no tracking, where the assumption is made that the translation is at a uniform speed, to detecting changes in the image texture pattern when the changes can be associated with scan plane translation, to attaching sensors to the transducer so that the position and orientation of each recorded image plane are known precisely.

erated using the entire 3D image data set. The shorter the distance between acquired planes, the better will be the resolution, particularly of reconstructed planes from the set, but the greater will also be the storage and image handling requirements. "Freehand" scanning, mechanical movement within a specialized 3D probe housing, and 2D transducer arrays have all been implemented to translate the acquisition plane across the volume.

In the simplest freehand scanning method, the operator translates the probe over the scanned volume and a loop of image data is stored during a preset time interval. 3D image reconstruction is then done by assuming that all image planes are equidistant from one another, with the interval between planes essentially being controlled subjectively by the operator. Rough 3D data sets are thus acquired and can be displayed with this method, but the distance between image planes is not known precisely. The spatial relationship between any two structures that are not in one of the acquired image planes can be erroneous because it depends on the operator providing perfectly spaced scans, which is unlikely for this type of system.

More accurate tracking of the transducer position can be done by systems that process the image data to sense changes in the image texture patterns from one frame to the next while the operator does a freehand sweep. The texture changes are measured as reductions in the degree of information correlation within a region from one acquired image to the next. Once the rate of reduction with translation distance is calibrated, the system can use the image data to estimate distances between successive image planes and reconstruct 3D data sets.

A third freehand tracking scheme uses sensors attached to the transducer or otherwise placed in the scanning room and measures the position and orientation of the probe directly.[19] For example, one method uses video cameras to record the positions of small reflectors affixed to the transducer, while a more common tracking system uses an electromagnetic coil attached to the probe with transmitters distributed around the scanning room. These methods place each acquired image in a properly registered location and orientation in the 3D ultrasound data set. Reconstruction and display methods then can be used quite reliably for producing 3D images.

More precise acquisitions of volumetric data are done using mechanically translated transducer arrays within special-purpose 3D probes. Mechanical systems for 3D vascular imaging have been pioneered by Fenster and colleagues.[20] Commercial versions of the mechanically scanned arrays operate with special array transducers that are slightly larger than conventional one dimensional arrays. With these, the image plane is manipulated by an internal motor system, such as the pivoting system shown in Figure 2–41, that translates the acquired image plane. Thus, a series of 2D images is acquired at volumetric scanning rates that are high enough to track slow movements, such as fetal limbs. However, blood flow in vascular studies usually requires electrocardiogram gating, particularly when precise measurements of vessel sizes are being made.

Progress is being made gradually in the development of full 2D ultrasound transducer arrays.[21] These enable acquisition of volumetric data sets without the need for mechanical manipulations inside the transducer housing or translations of the probe by the operator. One such system is rapid enough to provide live images of the adult

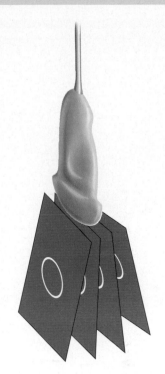

FIGURE 2–41. Commonly used three-dimensional transducer assembly. In this arrangement, the image plane is translated by mechanical movement, within the transducer housing, of a curvilinear array probe.

heart. Two-dimensional arrays require large channel counts to enable individual elements to be driven. For example, a typical high-quality one-dimensional array operates with a channel count of 128 or more elements. If one were to repeat the same channel density in two dimensions, it would require more than 10,000 channels, which currently is prohibitive, given the status of miniaturization of circuits and other factors. Thus, the usual strategy is to get by on fewer elements. The Duke system, for example, uses randomly positioned elements.

There are various ways to display the volumetric data during acquisition and for analysis. The preferred methods depend on the nature of the data and their potential uses. For example, in echocardiology, a simultaneous display of two orthogonal image planes that represent traditional ultrasound acquisition planes, along with one or more reconstructed "C-planes" (constant-depth planes) depicting structures in a plane at a selected distance from the transducer, has been found extremely useful.[21]

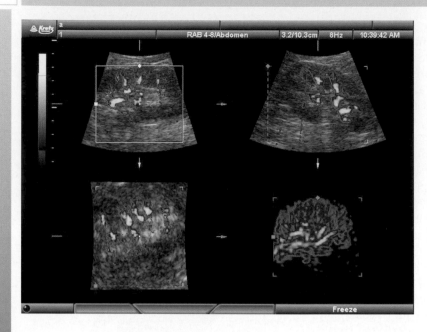

FIGURE 2–42. Display of three-dimensional ultrasound information from a kidney. *Top left,* One of multiple acquisition planes. *Top right,* Constructed plane orthogonal to the acquisition planes. *Lower left,* reconstructed c-plane (constant depth) representing a coronal view. *Lower right,* volume-rendered image depicting the blood vessels derived using color flow imaging. (Courtesy of General Electric.)

Volumetric acquisition and display techniques often support multi-view displays, as shown in Figure 2–42. The *image in the lower right* represents the entire color data volume acquired from a kidney. The gray-scale echo data have been suppressed in this view. The other three images depict single image planes. The *top left* is the normal acquisition plane, representing one of the planes used as input to the data set volume. An orthogonal, reconstructed plane is presented in the *top right image.* Although this image could have been generated simply by rotating the original scanning plane 90 degrees, here it is computed from the 3D data set. The *lower left image* is another reconstructed plane, this one at a fixed depth from the transducer. One of the very useful aspects of this type of 3D scanning is the ability to generate new image planes, such as that shown here, which are not accessible with conventional, 2D imaging.

Besides multiview displays, various volume rendering and surface rendering techniques have been found useful for 3D ultrasound data. The fetal image in Figure 2–43 is one that uses thresholding and surface rendering to portray a view similar to a visual image of the structures. This method works in cases where the image contrast is sufficiently high that the surface

can be detected by automated methods. Contrast with color flow imaging is also very good, so surface rendered images of major vessels (see Fig. 2–39) can portray information on the lumen shape and diameter, the course of the vessel, and the relationship between flow features in adjacent vessels. Volume rendered images, such as the kidney in Figure 2–42 can also be useful, particularly when the image includes vascular information displayed in color. The complex relationship among vessels of different diameters and locations can be readily appreciated with such methods.

As computational and image processing techniques become more powerful and processor speeds intensify, we can anticipate that there will be increasing uses of 3D ultrasound. The tremendous data overhead that is required for these techniques used to be a burden, even for powerful workstations, but this is no longer the case. Furthermore, it is likely that the data-handling capabilities of tomorrow's processors will hardly be challenged by present-day approaches to acquisition, image processing, and display. Hopefully, diagnostic capabilities of ultrasound machines will also continue to increase, benefiting greater numbers of patients.

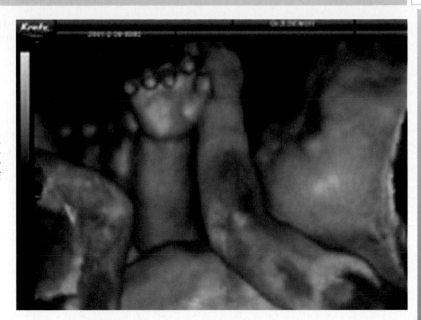

FIGURE 2–43. Surface-rendered image of a fetus, clearly depicting facial features and other anatomic details. (Courtesy of General Electric.)

EQUIPMENT SAFETY

In an ultrasound examination, acoustic energy must be transmitted into the tissue. The possibility that the energy could produce a detrimental biologic effect has been considered extensively by bioacoustics researchers; it continues to be studied to this day. At this time, most workers conclude that diagnostic ultrasound equipment is safe and that it is unlikely that bioeffects could result from prudent use of this modality, at least with current scanners. The American Institute of Ultrasound in Medicine's official statement on the clinical safety of diagnostic ultrasound instrumentation reads as follows:

. . . There are no confirmed biological effects on patients or instrument operators caused by exposures from present diagnostic ultrasound instruments. Although the possibility exists that such biological effects may be identified in the future, current data indicate that the benefits to patients of the prudent use of diagnostic ultrasound outweigh the risks, if any, that may be present.[22]

Readers should consult more detailed reports[23] on postulated mechanisms for bioeffects; acoustic exposure parameters of concern; reports of the nature of biologic effects, especially high-power and intensity levels; and acoustic output data from current scanners.[4]

The responsibility for safety of medical diagnostic ultrasound equipment falls on everyone involved in manufacturing, regulating, and using this equipment.[24] Until recently, manufacturers in the United States were required to adhere to "application-specific limits" on the intensity, peak pressure levels, and acoustic power levels of scanners. When a new scanner or a new transducer was planned for marketing, the U.S. Food and Drug Administration considered acoustic output data submitted by the manufacturer of the device. If the intensities were lower than these limits, the product was considered satisfactory as far as acoustic output was concerned.

Most equipment manufacturers in the United States and Canada now follow the acoustic output labeling standard described earlier in this chapter (see Fig. 2–2).[4] It requires manufacturers to provide output indicators on their scanners to inform users of levels as they relate to potential biologic effects. These quantities enable users to implement the ALARA principle. Although regulators continue to impose a 720-mW/cm^2 limit on the time-average intensity and a limit of 1.9 on the MI value, it is feasible that such upper limits could be relaxed at some future date. Presumably, this would open up the potential of still further diagnostic capabilities with medical ultrasonography. It would, of course, also place greater responsibility for clinical safety on the operator and physician responsible for the ultrasound examination.

Some individuals are concerned that the removal of application-specific intensity limits will not be recognized by ultrasound equipment users and they may operate a scanner at an unnecessarily high output setting. As the new labels become more familiar to ultrasonographers, the likelihood of this occurring will diminish.

References

1. Wells PT: Biomedical Ultrasonics. New York, Academic Press, 1977, pp 120–123.
2. 1993 Acoustical Data for Diagnostic Ultrasound Equipment: Laurel, MD, American Institute of Ultrasound in Medicine, 1993.
3. Duck FA: Output data from European studies. Ultrasound Med Biol 15(Suppl 1):61–64, 1989.
4. Standard for real-time display of thermal and mechanical acoustic output indices on diagnostic ultrasound equipment. Laurel, MD, American Institute of Ultrasound in Medicine, 1991.
5. Zagzebski JA: Essentials of Ultrasound Physics. St. Louis, CV Mosby, 1996.
6. Shung KK: In vitro experimental results on ultrasonic scattering in biological tissues. In Shung KK, Thieme GA (Eds): Ultrasonic Scattering in Biological Tissues. Boca Raton, FL, CRC Press, 1993, pp 219–312.
7. Desser T, Jaffrey B: Tissue harmonic imaging techniques: Physical principles and clinical applications. Semin Ultrasound CT MR 22: 1–10, 2001.
8. Kremkau F: Diagnostic Ultrasound Principles, Instrumentation and Exercises, 5th ed. Orlando, FL, Grune & Stratton, 1993.
9. Entrekin R, Porter B, Sillesen H, et al: Real-time spatial compound imaging: Application to breast, vascular, and musculoskeletal ultrasound. Semin Ultrasound CT MR 22:50–64, 2001.
10. Burns P: Instrumentation for contrast echocardiography. Echocardiography J CV Ultrasound Allied Technol 19:241–259, 2002.
11. Pedersen MH, Misaridis TX, Jensen JA: Clinical evaluation of chirp-coded excitation in medical ultrasound. Ultrasound Med Biol 29(6):895–905, 2003.
12. Taylor KJW, Wells PNT, Burns PN: Clinical Applications of Doppler Ultrasound. New York, Raven Press, 1995.
13. Beach K, Philips D: Doppler instrumentation for the evaluation of arterial and venous disease. In Jaffe C (Ed): Vascular and Doppler Ultrasound. Clinics in Diagnostic Ultrasound Series. New York, Churchill Livingstone, 1984.
14. Omoto R, Kasai C: Basic principles of Doppler color flow imaging. Echocardiography 3:463, 1986.
15. Evans D: Doppler ultrasound physics instrumentation and clinical applications. New York, John Wiley & Sons, 1989.
16. Embree P, O'Brien W: Volumetric blood flow via time-domain correlation: Experimental verification. IEEE Trans Ultrasonics Ferroelec Frequency Con 37:176–185, 1990.
17. Kisslo J, Adams AB, Belkin RN: Doppler Color Flow Imaging. New York, Churchill Livingstone, 1988.
18. Rubin JM, Bude RO, Carson PL, et al: Power Doppler US: A potentially useful alternative to mean frequency-based color Doppler US. Radiology 190:853–856, 1994.
19. Nelson TR, Pretorius DH: Three-dimensional ultrasound imaging. Ultrasound Med Biol 24:1243–1270, 1998.
20. Fenster A, Downey DB, Cardinal HN: Three-dimensional ultrasound imaging. Phys Med Biol 46(5):R67–99, 2001.
21. Kisslo J, Firek B, Ota T, et al: Real-time volumetric echocardiography: The technology and the possibilities Echocardiography J Cardiol 17(8):773–779, 2000.
22. 1997 Statement on Clinical Ultrasound Safety. Laurel, MD, American Institute of Ultrasound in Medicine, 1997.
23. Exposure Criteria For Medical Diagnostic Ultrasound: II. Criteria Based On All Known Mechanisms. NCRP Report 140. National Council on Radiation Protection and Measurements, Bethesda MD, 2002.
24. Medical Ultrasound Safety: Bioeffects and Biophysics; Prudent Use; Implementing ALARA. Laurel, MD, American Institute of Ultrasound in Medicine, 1994.

Basic Concepts of Doppler Frequency Spectrum Analysis and Ultrasound Blood Flow Imaging

WILLIAM J. ZWIEBEL, MD, AND JOHN S. PELLERITO, MD

SPECTRUM ANALYSIS

If blood flow were continuous rather than pulsatile, if blood vessels followed straight lines and were uniform in caliber, if blood flowed at the same velocity at the periphery and in the center of the lumen, and if vessels were disease free, then each blood vessel would produce a single Doppler ultrasound frequency. However, blood flow *is* pulsatile, vessels are not always straight or uniform in size, flow is slower at the periphery than in the center of the vessel, and the vessel lumen may be distorted by atherosclerosis and other pathology. For these reasons, blood flow produces a mixture of Doppler frequency shifts that changes from moment to moment and from place to place within the vessel lumen. Spectrum analysis is needed to sort out the jumble of Doppler frequencies generated by blood flow and to provide quantitative information that is critical for diagnosis of vascular pathology.

The Doppler Spectrum

The word *spectrum,* as derived from Latin, means *image.* You may think of the Doppler spectrum as an image of the Doppler frequencies generated by moving blood.[1-8] In fact, this image is a graph showing the mixture of Doppler frequencies present in a small area of a vessel over a short period of time.[1-3] The key elements of the Doppler spectrum are *time, frequency, velocity,* and Doppler signal *power.* These elements are best described in pictorial form; therefore, this information is provided in Figure 3–1, rather than in the text. Please review this figure now, directing particular attention to the four key elements cited previously.

The Power Spectrum

The Doppler frequency spectrum that you have just reviewed in Figure 3–1 is sometimes called a *power spectrum,*[1-3] because the power, or strength, of each frequency is shown by the *brightness* of the pixels. The power of a given frequency shift, in turn, is proportionate to the *number* of red blood cells producing that frequency shift. If a large number of blood cells are moving at a certain velocity, the corresponding Doppler frequency shift is powerful, and the pixels assigned to that frequency are bright. Conversely, if only a small number of cells are causing a certain frequency shift, the pixels assigned to that frequency are dim. The power spectrum concept is important for understanding power Doppler flow imaging, which is discussed later in this chapter. The concept of the power Doppler spectrum is nicely illustrated in Figure 2–29.

Frequency versus Velocity

The echoes that return to the transducer from a blood vessel contain only Doppler frequency shift information; yet the Doppler spectrum often displays both velocity (cm/sec or m/sec) and frequency (kHz) information. How does the instrument

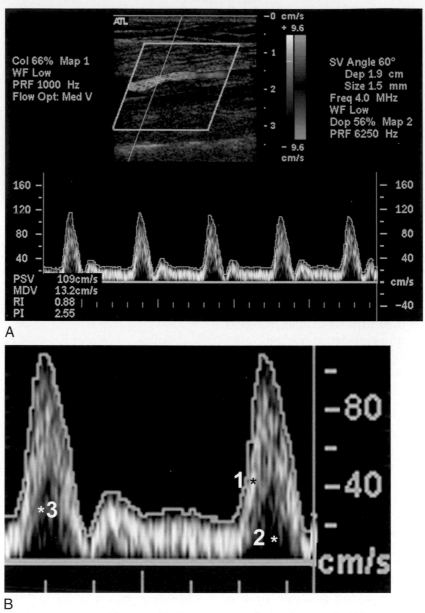

Figure 3–1. The Doppler spectrum display. The following information is presented on the display screen (*A,* Entire display; *B,* Magnified Doppler spectrum).

Color flow image: The vessel, the sample volume, and the Doppler line of sight are shown in the color flow image at the top of the display screen.

Color flow information: The "color bar" to the right of the image shows the relationship between the direction of blood flow and the colors in the flow image. By convention, the upper half of the bar shows flow *toward* the transducer. This is logical, as this part of the bar is nearest to the transducer in the image. The lower half represents flow *away* from the transducer. In this case, red/orange colors correspond to flow toward the transducers, and blue/green colors indicate flow in the opposite direction. A shift in color from red to orange or from blue to green represents increasing flow velocity.

Doppler angle: The Doppler angle for the spectral Doppler appears at the upper right of the display screen, in this case 60 degrees.

FIGURE 3–1, cont'd. *Time:* The time is represented on the horizontal (x) axis of the Doppler spectrum, at the base of the display. The lines represent divisions of a second, but typically a scale is not provided.

Velocity: Blood flow velocity (cm/sec) is shown on the vertical (y) axis of the spectrum. In this case, velocity is shown on both vertical axes. On some instruments, the velocity is shown on one vertical axis and the Doppler-shifted frequency (KHz) on the other.

The distribution of velocities within the sample volume is illustrated by the brightness of the spectral display (the z-axis). To better understand the z-axis concept, examine the magnified spectrum shown in *B* and imagine that the spectral display is made of tiny squares called *pixels* (for picture elements). You cannot see the pixels in this image because they are purposely blurred to smooth the picture. The pixels are there, however, and each corresponds to a specific moment in time and a specific frequency shift or velocity. *The brightness of a pixel (its z-axis) is proportionate to the number of blood cells causing that frequency shift at that specific point in time.* In this example, the pixels at *asterisk 1* are bright white, meaning that a large number of blood cells have the corresponding velocity (about 41 cm/sec) at that moment in time. The pixels at *asterisk 2* are black, meaning that no (or very few) blood cells have the corresponding velocity (about 12 cm/sec) at that moment. The pixels at *asterisk 3* are gray, meaning that a moderate number of blood cells have the corresponding velocity (about 35 cm/sec) at that moment. Got it? If not, read this again and remember that the brightness of each pixel is proportionate to the *relative* number of blood cells with a specific velocity at a specific moment in time. Since the brightness of the pixels also shows the distribution of flow energy, or power, at each moment in time, the spectrum display is also called a *power* spectrum.

Flow direction: The direction of flow is shown in relation to the spectrum baseline. In this case, flow toward the transducer is shown above the baseline, and flow away from the transducer is shown below the baseline. Note that the number 40 in the lower right corner is preceded by a minus sign. This is because the area below the baseline corresponds to flow away from the transducer, which would generate a negative Doppler shift. The relationship between the flow direction and the Doppler baseline may be reversed by the operator, but flow toward the transducer will always be represented by positive velocity or frequency values.

Peak velocity envelope: The peak velocity throughout the cardiac cycle is shown by the *green line* outlining the Doppler spectrum. Based on this envelope, a numeric output is provided at the bottom left, showing the peak systolic velocity (PSV) and the minimum diastolic velocity (MDV). In this case, the MDV also corresponds to the end diastolic velocity, but this is not necessarily the case. The instrument also automatically calculates the resistivity index (RI) and the pulsatility index (PI), as shown below the velocity values.

Pulse repetition frequency: A noteworthy number shown on the display is the pulse repetition frequency (PRF). The PRF for the color flow image is shown at the left of the image (1000 Hz, or cycles, or pulses per second). The PRF for the spectral Doppler is much higher (6250 Hz), as shown to the right of the color flow image. This difference illustrates the fact that the color flow image is based on the average Doppler frequency shift or velocity, while the spectral Doppler values are shown as absolutes, without averaging. A higher PRF is needed for the spectral Doppler to ensure that systolic velocities are shown accurately, without aliasing.

convert the Doppler frequency shift to velocity? This conversion occurs when the sonographer "informs" the duplex instrument of the Doppler angle,[1,2,9] which is shown in Figure 3–2. If the instrument "knows" the Doppler angle, it can then compute the blood flow velocity via the Doppler formula (see Chapter 2). You may note in this formula that the frequency shift is proportional to the cosine of the Doppler angle, theta. When the operator informs the ultrasound machine of this angle, the frequency shift is proportional to blood flow velocity. Voila! The frequency spectrum becomes a velocity spectrum. A Doppler angle of *60 degrees or less* is required to derive accurate frequency and velocity measurements. If the angle is greater than 60 degrees, velocity measurements are unreliable. Some ultrasound instruments will not calculate velocity if the angle is much greater than 60 degrees. Measurement variability also occurs when the Doppler angle approaches zero, and it is generally recom-

mended that the Doppler angle should be between 45 and 60 degrees for greatest accuracy.

In spite of potential measurement inaccuracy described in the previous paragraphs, it is desirable to operate the duplex instrument in the velocity mode rather than the frequency mode for two reasons.[1,2,9] First, velocity measurements compensate for variations in vessel alignment relative to the skin surface. For instance, the Doppler frequency shift observed in a tortuous internal carotid artery might be radically different from one point to another, but angle-corrected velocity measurements will be similar throughout the vessel, in spite of dramatic changes in vessel orientation relative to the skin. Second, the Doppler frequency shift is inherently linked to the output frequency of the transducer, but velocity measurement is independent of the transducer frequency. For instance, if the output frequency goes from 5 to 10 MHz, the frequency shift is doubled. Imagine the clinical consequences of such frequency changes. For instance, to determine stenosis severity, different diagnostic parameters would be needed for different ultrasound transducers (e.g., 3.5, 5, or 7.5 MHz). This problem is eliminated when the instrument converts the "raw" frequency information to velocity data.

Auditory Spectrum Analysis

The human ear was the spectrum analysis instrument used initially for Doppler blood flow studies. The ear is a highly capable spectrum analysis instrument, which is evident in its ability to distinguish one person's voice from another. Even though duplex ultrasound instruments are equipped with electronic spectrum analysis devices, an audible Doppler output is provided as well, to take advantage of the human ear's capabilities. Certain features of the Doppler flow signal can be appreciated aurally that are difficult or impossible to display electronically, and as a result, the audible Doppler signal remains important in ultrasound vascular diagnosis. For instance, in very high–grade carotid

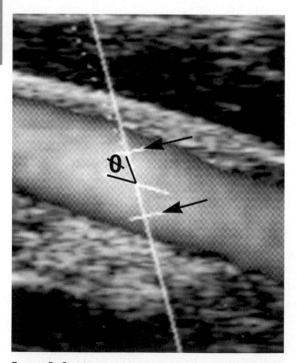

FIGURE 3–2. The Doppler angle and sample volume. The *nearly vertical line* is the Doppler line of sight. The *line in the center of the blood vessel* indicates the axis of blood flow. The angle formed by these two lines is the Doppler angle (θ). The parallel lines (*arrows*) indicate the length of the Doppler sample volume.

stenoses, a distinctive whining or whistling sound is heard. In spite of its abilities, however, the human ear has three major drawbacks. First, the ear is a purely qualitative device; second, it is not equipped with a hard copy output for permanent storage; and third, some ears work better than others—some cannot hear very high frequencies. Electronic spectrum analysis overcomes these obstacles.

The Sample Volume

The frequency spectrum shows blood flow information from a specific location called the *Doppler sample volume,* which is illustrated in Figure 3–2. You should be familiar with the following three characteristics of the Doppler sample volume: First, it is, in fact, a volume (three dimensions), even though only two of its dimensions are shown on the duplex image. The "thickness" of the sample volume cannot be shown on the two-dimensional spectrum display, and this can sometimes lead to errors of localization. Doppler signals may be obtained from vessels that are marginally within the sample volume but are not shown on the two-dimensional display. For instance, the ultrasound image may show the internal carotid artery, but you may actually be receiving flow signals from an adjacent external carotid branch. Second, the actual shape and size of the sample volume may be somewhat different from the linear representation shown on the duplex image. Third, and most important, the Doppler spectrum displays flow information only within the sample volume and does not provide information about flow in other portions of the blood vessel that are visible on the ultrasound image. Therefore, if the sample volume is positioned incorrectly, key diagnostic information may be overlooked.

Flow Direction

The frequency spectrum shows blood flow *relative to the transducer.* Flow in one direction, with respect to the transducer, is displayed above the spectrum baseline, and flow in the opposite direction is shown below the baseline. One must always remember that the flow direction is *relative* to the transducer and is not absolute. The apparent direction of flow can be reversed by turning the transducer around or by pressing a button on the instrument that inverts the spectrum! The arbitrary nature of this arrangement can lead to significant diagnostic error. When accurate determination of flow direction is necessary, a comparison should be made with a reference vessel in which the flow direction is known (e.g., when working in the abdomen, the aorta is a handy reference vessel).

Waveforms and Pulsatility

In arteries, each cycle of cardiac activity produces a distinct "wave" on the Doppler frequency spectrum that begins with systole and terminates at the end of diastole. The term *waveform* refers to the shape of each of these waves, and this shape, in turn, defines a very important flow property called *pulsatility.*[1,2,10–28] In general terms, Doppler waveforms have low, moderate, or high pulsatility features, as illustrated in Figure 3–3. Please review this figure before proceeding to the material that follows.

Low-pulsatility Doppler waveforms have broad systolic peaks and forward flow throughout diastole (see Fig. 3–3A). The carotid, vertebral, renal, and celiac arteries all have low-pulsatility waveforms in normal individuals because these vessels feed circulatory systems with low resistance to flow (low peripheral resistance). Low-pulsatility waveforms are also *monophasic,* meaning that flow is always forward, and the entire waveform is either above or below the Doppler spectrum baseline (depending on the orientation of the ultrasound transducer).

Moderate-pulsatility Doppler waveforms have an appearance somewhere between the low- and high-resistance patterns (see Fig. 3–3B). With moderate flow resistance, the systolic peak is tall and sharp, but

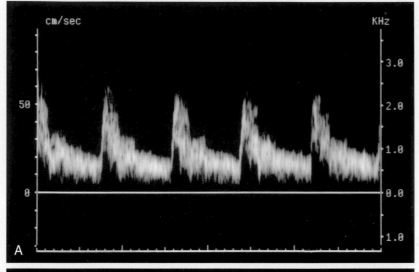

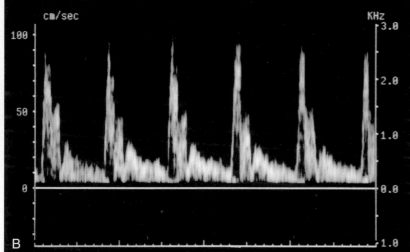

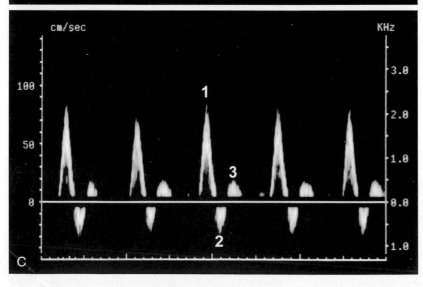

FIGURE 3–3. Pulsatility. *A,* Low pulsatility is indicated by broad systolic peaks and persistent forward flow throughout diastole (e.g., the internal carotid artery). *B,* Moderate pulsatility is indicated by tall, sharp, and narrow systolic peaks and relatively little diastolic flow (e.g., the external carotid artery). *C,* High pulsatility is characterized by narrow systolic peaks, flow reversal early in diastole, and absence of flow late in diastole. In this classic triphasic example, the first phase (1) is systole, the second phase (2) is brief diastolic flow reversal, and the third phase (3) is diastolic forward flow. Triphasic flow is seen in normal extremity arteries at rest.

forward flow is present throughout diastole (perhaps interrupted by early-diastolic flow reversal). Examples of moderate pulsatility are found in the external carotid artery and the superior mesenteric artery (during fasting).

High-pulsatility Doppler waveforms have tall, narrow, sharp systolic peaks and reversed or absent diastolic flow. The classic example of high pulsatility is the triphasic flow pattern seen in an extremity artery of a resting individual (see Fig. 3–3C). A sharp systolic peak (first phase) is followed by brief flow reversal (second phase) and then by brief forward flow (third phase). High-pulsatility waveforms are a feature of circulatory systems with high resistance to blood flow (high peripheral resistance).

Pulsatility and flow resistance may be gauged qualitatively, either by visual inspection of the Doppler spectrum waveforms or by listening to the auditory output of a Doppler instrument. Qualitative assessment of pulsatility is often sufficient for clinical vascular diagnosis, but in some situations (e.g., assessment of renal transplant rejection), quantitative assessment is desirable. A variety of mathematical formulae can be used for this purpose, but the most popular measurements are the pulsatility index (of Gosling), the resistivity index (of Pourcelot), and the systolic/diastolic ratio,[24,26,28,29] all of which are illustrated in Figure 3–4.

Normal values for pulsatility measurements vary from one location in the body to another. Furthermore, both physiology and pathology may alter arterial pulsatility. For example, the normal high-pulsatility pattern seen in extremity arteries during rest converts to a low-resistance, monophasic pattern after vigorous exercise (because the capillary beds open and flow resistance decreases). Although this monophasic pattern is *normal* after exercise, it is distinctly *abnormal* in a resting patient and, in that circumstance, indicates arterial insufficiency resulting from obstruction of more proximal arteries. The point to be made here is that proper interpretation of pulsatility requires knowledge of the normal waveform characteristics of a given vessel *and* the physiologic status of the circulation

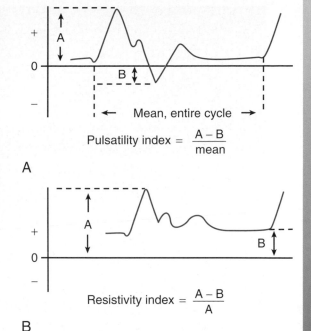

$$\text{Pulsatility index} = \frac{A - B}{\text{mean}}$$

A

$$\text{Resistivity index} = \frac{A - B}{A}$$

B

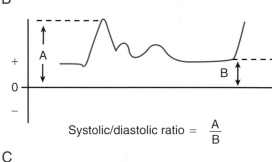

$$\text{Systolic/diastolic ratio} = \frac{A}{B}$$

C

FIGURE 3–4. Pulsatility measurements. *A,* The pulsatility index (Gosling). *B,* The resistivity index (Pourcelot). *C,* The systolic/diastolic ratio.

at the time of examination. The status of cardiac function is also important; slowed ventricular emptying, valvular reflux, valvular stenosis, and other factors may significantly affect arterial pulsatility.

Acceleration

Acceleration is another important flow feature evident in Doppler spectral waveforms.[24,25] In most normal situations, flow velocity in an artery accelerates very rapidly in systole, and the peak velocity is reached within a few hundreds of a second after ventricular contraction begins. Rapid flow acceleration produces an almost vertical

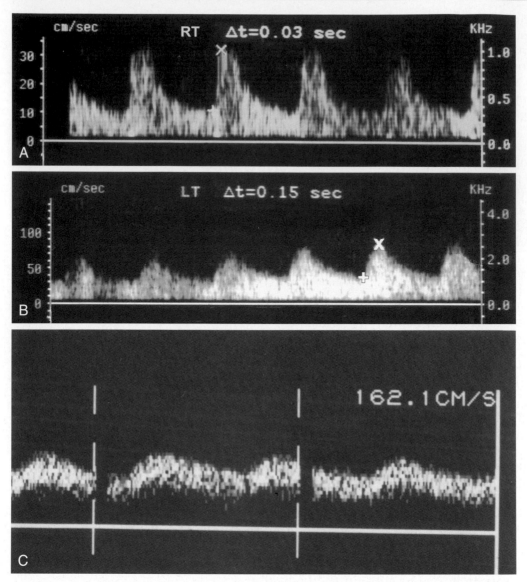

FIGURE 3–5. Acceleration and damping. *A,* The acceleration time (0.03 sec) is normal in the right kidney. *B,* The acceleration time is prolonged (0.15 sec) in the left kidney due to severe proximal renal artery stenosis. (*A* and *B* are from the same patient.) *C,* Severely damped dorsalis pedis artery waveform distal to common iliac and superficial femoral artery occlusion. Normally, this waveform should look like Figure 3–3*C.* Acceleration is severely delayed, and a large amount of flow is present throughout diastole, consistent with severe ischemia.

deflection of the Doppler waveform at the start of systole (Fig. 3–5*A*). If, however, severe arterial obstruction is present proximal (upstream) to the point of Doppler examination, systolic flow acceleration may be slowed substantially, as shown in Figure 3–5*B* and *C.* Quantitative measurement of acceleration is achieved by measuring the acceleration time and the acceleration index, as illustrated in Figure 3–6. These measurements are used, for example, in evaluating renal artery stenosis.

Vessel Identity

As you may have already surmised, vessels can be identified by their waveform pulsatility features.[1,2,14,21–23,26] For example, Doppler waveforms readily differentiate between lower extremity arteries, which are distinctly pulsatile, and veins, which have gently undulant flow features. Doppler waveforms are particularly helpful in identifying the internal and external carotid arteries, which have low and moderate

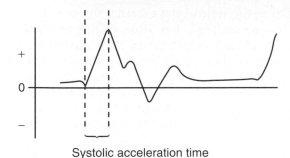

Systolic acceleration time

A

Systolic acceleration rate $= \dfrac{\Delta V}{\Delta T}$

B

FIGURE 3–6. Acceleration measurements: acceleration time (A) and acceleration rate (B).

pulsatility, respectively. Pulsatility is also of value within the liver for differentiating among the portal veins, hepatic veins, and hepatic arteries, as discussed in Chapter 31.

Laminar and Disturbed Flow

Blood generally flows through arteries in an orderly way, with blood in the center of the vessel moving faster than the blood at the periphery. This flow pattern is described as *laminar,* because the movement of blood is in parallel lines.[1,2,4,14,15] When flow is laminar, the great majority of blood cells are moving at a uniform speed, and the Doppler spectrum shows a thin line that outlines a clear space called the *spectral window* (Fig. 3–7).*

*The term *plug flow* is actually more precise for this spectral pattern, as discussed in Chapter 1, but the term *laminar* is used throughout this text, in keeping with common convention.

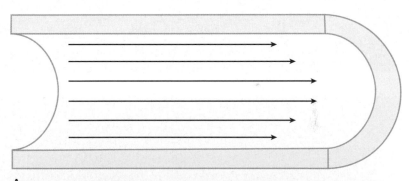

FIGURE 3–7. Laminar flow. A, Illustration of parallel lines of blood cell movement. B, Doppler spectrum during laminar flow. At all times, the blood cells are moving at similar velocities. As a result, the spectrum is a thin line that encloses a well-defined black "window" (W).

A

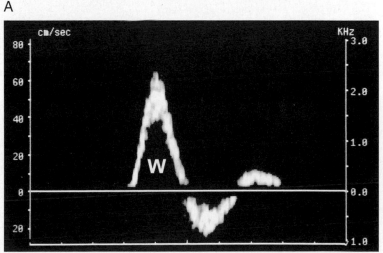

B

In *disturbed flow,* the movement of blood cells is less uniform and orderly than in laminar flow. Disturbed flow is manifested as spectral broadening or widening of the spectral waveform.[1,2,4,15–19] The *degree* of spectral broadening is proportionate to the *severity* of the flow disturbance, as illustrated in Figure 3–8. Although disturbed blood flow often indicates vascular disease, it must be recognized that flow disturbances also occur in normal vessels. Kinks, curves, and arterial branching may produce normal flow disturbances, as illustrated quite vividly in the carotid bulb, where a prominent area of reversed flow is a normal occurrence[11,20,21] (Fig. 3–9). In addition, a spurious

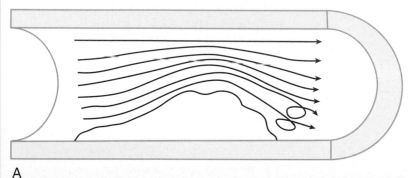

A

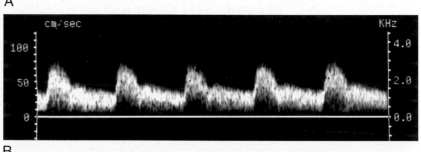

B

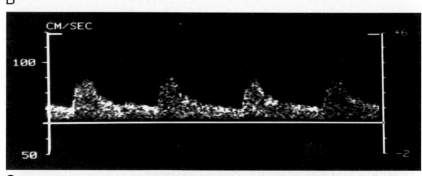

C

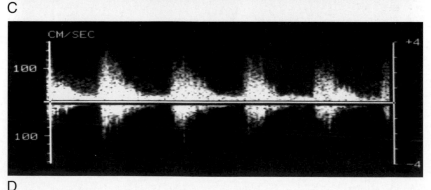

D

FIGURE 3–8. Disturbed flow. *A,* Disturbed flow illustration. *B,* Minor flow disturbance is indicated by spectral broadening at peak systole and through diastole. *C,* Moderate flow disturbance causes fill-in of the spectral window. *D,* Severe flow disturbance is characterized by spectral fill-in, poor definition of spectral borders, and simultaneous forward and reversed flow. The audible Doppler signal has a loud, gruff character when flow is severely disturbed.

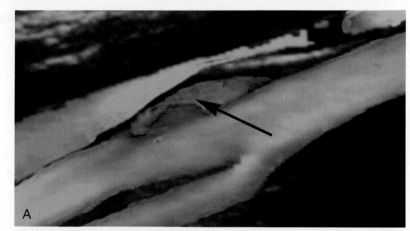

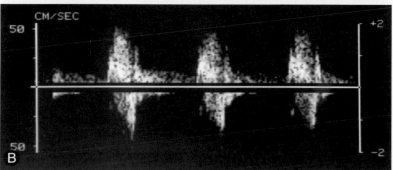

FIGURE 3–9. Normal bifurcation flow disturbance. *A,* Flow reversal in the bulbous portion of the common and internal carotid arteries causes localized color changes (*arrow,* blue color). *B,* Simultaneous forward and reverse flow is evident in the bulbous region on the Doppler spectrum.

disturbed flow appearance may be created in normal arteries through the use of a large sample volume that encompasses both the slow flow area near the vessel wall and more rapid flow at the vessel center.[16–19] The Doppler spectrum, in such cases, appears broadened because both the high-velocity flow at the vessel center and the slow flow at the periphery of the vessel are encompassed by the wide sample volume.

Volume Flow

Modern duplex instruments are capable of measuring the volume of blood flowing through a vessel (volume flow).[1,2,30–32] This is done by measuring the average flow velocity across the entire lumen (slow peripheral flow and high central flow) through several cardiac cycles while simultaneously measuring the vessel diameter, which is converted mathematically into cross-sectional area. Knowing the average velocity and the vessel area, it is an easy matter for the Doppler instrument to calculate the blood flow (in mL/min), and this is done automatically by the ultrasound instrument. Although the ability to calculate volume flow has been available on duplex instruments for more than 20 years and measurement accuracy appears satisfactory, volume flow measurements have found surprisingly little use in a clinical setting.[4–9,14–16,30,31,33,34]

DIAGNOSIS OF ARTERIAL OBSTRUCTION

Now that we have covered the basic concepts of Doppler spectral analysis, we can turn to the "heart of the matter," namely, how to use Doppler spectral analysis to diagnose arterial obstruction. Five main categories of information are used in this process: (1) increased stenotic zone velocity, (2) disturbed flow in the poststenotic zone, (3) proximal pulsatility changes, (4) distal pulsatility changes, and (5) indirect effects of obstruction, such as collateralization.* These categories are summarized in Table 3–1, and each is discussed in the following sections.

*See references 2, 4–10, 13, 15–19, 22–27, 29, 33, 35

Table 3–1. Spectral Features of Arterial Obstruction

Local effects
  Elevated flow velocity in the stenotic lumen
  Poststenotic flow disturbance
Proximal (upstream) pulsatility changes
  Increased pulsatility
  Decreased velocity overall, due to decreased flow
Distal (downstream) pulsatility changes
  Slowed systolic acceleration
  Broad systolic peak
  Increased diastolic flow (reduced peripheral resistance)
  Decreased velocity overall
Secondary (collateral) effects
  Increased size, velocity, and volume flow in collateral vessels
  Reversed flow in collateral vessels
  Decreased pulsatility (flow resistance) in collateral vessels

Increased Stenotic Zone Velocity

The term *stenotic zone* refers to the narrowed portion of the arterial lumen. For determining the severity of arterial stenosis, the single most valuable Doppler finding is increased velocity in the stenotic zone. Flow velocity is increased in the stenotic zone because blood must move more quickly if the same volume is to flow through the narrowed lumen as through the larger, normal lumen. The increase in stenotic zone velocity is directly proportional to the severity of luminal narrowing.

Three stenotic zone velocity measurements are commonly used to determine the severity of arterial stenoses (Fig. 3–10): (1) *peak systolic velocity* (also called peak systole), which is the highest systolic veloc-

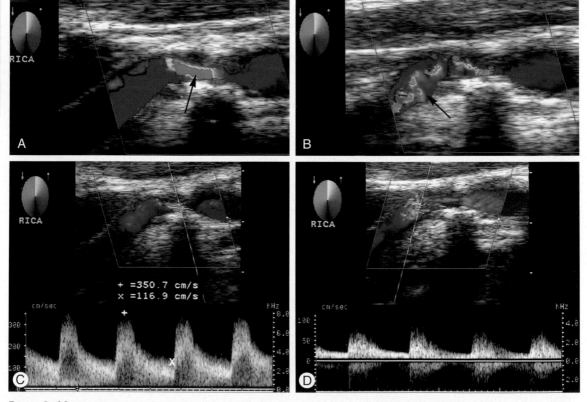

FIGURE 3–10. Local effects of arterial stenosis. *A,* The high velocities present in the narrowed portion of the arterial lumen generate an area of color aliasing (*arrow*) within the stenotic lumen. (The color Doppler pulse repetition frequency is not high enough to accurately record the average velocity, and flow is shown in reverse-flow colors.) *B,* Disturbed flow in the poststenotic area generates a mixture of colors (*arrow*). *C,* Doppler spectrum analysis shows markedly elevated flow velocity, with a peak systolic velocity of 350.7 cm/sec and end diastolic velocity of 116.9 cm/sec. *D,* Severe flow disturbance is evident in the poststenotic region, as indicated by simultaneous forward and reverse flow, spectrum fill-in, and poor definition of the spectrum margins.

ity within the stenosis; (2) *end-diastolic velocity* (also called end diastole), which is the highest end-diastolic velocity; and (3) the *systolic velocity ratio,* which compares peak systole in the stenosis with peak systole proximal to the stenosis (in a normal portion of the vessel).

Peak systole in the stenotic zone is the first Doppler parameter to become abnormal as an arterial lumen becomes narrowed. The region of maximum velocity within the stenotic zone may be quite small, and for that reason, the sonographer must "search" the stenotic lumen with the sample volume to locate the highest flow velocity. If the highest flow velocity is overlooked, the degree of stenosis may be underestimated. As shown in Figure 3–11, peak systole rises steadily with progressive narrowing, but ultimately the flow resistance becomes so high (at about 80% diameter reduction) that peak systole falls to normal or even subnor-

mal levels. This drop in velocity can cause the unwary to underestimate the severity of a high-grade stenosis. Low flow velocity in a very high–grade stenosis may also lead to false diagnosis of arterial occlusion, if the velocity is so low that Doppler signals cannot be detected with ultrasound.

The end-diastolic velocity (end diastole) in the stenotic zone, generally remains normal with less than 50% (diameter) narrowing, as there is no pressure gradient across the stenosis in diastole. With moderate stenosis (50%–70% diameter reduction), however, a pressure gradient exists throughout diastole, and end-diastolic velocity is elevated in proportion to stenosis severity. With severe stenosis (70%–90% diameter reduction), a substantial pressure gradient exists throughout diastole, and diastolic velocities are high. Furthermore, with progression of stenosis severity, end-diastolic velocity increases at a greater rate,

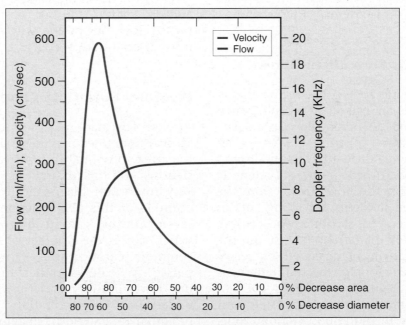

FIGURE 3–11. Relationship among velocity, flow, and lumen size. This graph refers specifically to internal carotid artery stenosis, but the principles illustrated apply to stenoses in other arteries throughout the body. Note that peak systolic velocity in the stenotic internal carotid lumen (labeled *velocity*) increases exponentially as the lumen diameter decreases (from right to left). The highest velocities correspond to approximately 70% diameter reduction. With greater stenosis severity, peak systolic velocity falls off rapidly to zero (because of rapidly increasing flow resistance). In contrast to velocity, volume flow (labeled *flow*) remains stable until the lumen diameter is reduced by about 50%. With further reduction in lumen size, volume flow falls off very rapidly to zero. Finally, note the relationship of percent diameter and area reduction, as shown at the base of the figure. Fifty percent diameter reduction equals about 70% area reduction, and 70% diameter reduction equals about 90% area reduction! (Modified from Spencer MP: Full capability Doppler diagnosis. In Spencer MP, Reed JM [eds]: Cerebrovascular Evaluation with Doppler Ultrasound. The Hague, Netherlands, Martinus Nijhoff, 1981, p 213, with kind permission from Kluwer Academic Publishers.)

proportionately, than the peak systolic velocity, and as a result, the *difference* between peak systolic and end-diastolic velocity decreases. End-diastolic velocity, therefore, is a particularly good marker for severe stenosis.[9]

The *systolic velocity ratio*, as defined previously, is an additional important parameter for the diagnosis of arterial stenosis. This parameter is used to compensate for patient-to-patient hemodynamic variables, such as cardiac function, heart rate, blood pressure, and arterial compliance. Tachycardia, for instance, tends to increase peak systole in the stenotic zone, whereas poor myocardial function may decrease peak systole. The systolic velocity ratio allows the patient to act as his or her own physiologic "standard," because peak systole in the stenotic zone is compared with peak systole in a normal arterial segment (e.g., the common carotid artery). The systolic velocity ratio is used clinically in a number of circumstances, including the measurement of internal carotid, renal, and extremity artery stenoses.

Post-stenotic Flow Disturbance

The post-stenotic zone is the region immediately beyond an arterial stenosis in which disorganized or "disturbed" flow occurs. The demonstration of disturbed flow is an important diagnostic feature. To understand why flow is disturbed in the post-stenotic region, envision the flow stream from the stenotic lumen suddenly spreading out" in the much larger, post-stenotic zone, causing the laminar flow pattern to be lost and the flow to become disorganized, which generates a disturbed Doppler spectral pattern, as illustrated in Figures 3–8 and 3–10D. In some cases, frank swirling movements (or turbulence) occur in the post-stenotic zone, producing simultaneous forward and reverse flow on the Doppler spectrum. The maximal flow disturbance occurs within 1 cm beyond the stenosis,[16] and in very severe stenoses, soft tissues adjacent to this portion of the artery may vibrate, causing a "visible bruit" on color Doppler images, as illustrated later in this chapter. Approximately 2 cm beyond the stenosis, the flow distur-

bance becomes less violent and spectral broadening diminishes. An orderly, laminar flow pattern may be reestablished within 3 cm beyond the stenosis,[4,16] but this distance is variable.

Post-stenotic flow disturbances can be visually graded,[2,4,6,9,15–19] as shown in Figure 3–8. In general, minimal and even moderate flow disturbances are of little diagnostic value, because they may occur in both normal and abnormal vessels. Severe flow disturbance, however, generally does not occur in normal vessels and is an important sign of high-grade arterial narrowing or other arterial pathology such as an intimal flap, dissection, or an arteriovenous fistula. Severe flow disturbances are "beacons" indicating the presence of arterial disease. Whenever a severe flow disturbance is detected, the sonographer should search carefully for an adjacent stenosis or other vascular lesion. In some cases, the stenosis may be obscured by plaque calcification (preventing direct ultrasound visualization), and in such instances, poststenotic disturbed flow may be the only sign of significant arterial narrowing.

Proximal Pulsatility Changes

Arterial obstruction causes increased pulsatility (as defined previously) in portions of the artery proximal to (upstream from) the stenosis, and this finding, therefore, may be very important diagnostically. The classic example of this phenomenon occurs with severe internal carotid artery obstruction, which causes the Doppler spectrum in the common carotid artery to have high-pulsatility features rather than the normal low-pulsatility pattern (Fig. 3–12). To understand why pulsatility is increased proximal to a stenosis, imagine that blood flowing in the common carotid artery is being propelled toward a "valve" in the internal carotid artery that is 90% or 100% closed rather than wide open. How do you think the velocity waveform will appear in the common carotid artery? First, you can imagine that in systole, flow will go forward for only a brief moment and will then slow abruptly; therefore, the systolic peak will be

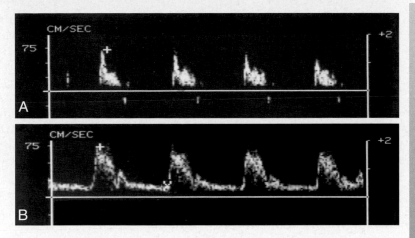

FIGURE 3–12. Increased common carotid artery pulsatility due to internal carotid artery occlusion. *A*, A high-resistance flow pattern is evident in this common carotid artery, consisting of sharp systolic peaks, diastolic flow reversal, and absence of flow throughout most of diastole. The ipsilateral internal carotid artery was occluded. *B*, The contralateral common carotid artery shows normal flow features.

sharp and narrow. Second, there will be relatively little flow in diastole, because intra-arterial pressure will be insufficient to force blood through the closed valve. Third, back-pressure from the blockage may cause a brief flow reversal early in diastole, equivalent to the reflected wave seen in normal extremity arteries. Finally, flow velocity in the common carotid artery will be low throughout the entire cardiac cycle because the closed valve will reduce blood flow overall. The increase in pulsatility proximal to a stenosis may be lessened in the presence of collateral flow. For instance, abnormal common carotid pulsatility may be absent, in spite of a high-grade internal carotid stenosis, if a large volume of collateral flow occurs via the external carotid artery. In such cases, collateral vessels provide an alternative, low-resistance pathway for blood flow and decrease the level of pulsatility.

Distal Pulsatility Changes

Doppler waveform abnormalities seen distal to a stenosis (downstream) also have considerable value in the diagnosis of arterial stenosis. As noted previously in the section on acceleration, the flow velocity in a normal, wide open, artery increases abruptly in systole, and the systolic peak is reached quickly (see Fig. 3–5A). In contrast, the Doppler waveform distal to a *severe* arterial obstruction has a "damped" appearance (see Fig. 3–5B and C), which means that the

systolic acceleration is slowed, the systolic peak is rounded, the maximum systolic velocity is lower than normal, and diastolic flow is increased. The terms *pulsus tardus* and *pulsus parvus* are also used to describe these damped, postobstructive waveforms. *Tardus* refers to delayed arrival of the systolic peak, and *parvus* refers to overall low velocity. There are three causes for the pulsus tardus and parvus appearance. First, it can be imagined that blood is being "squeezed" slowly through the obstructed lumen (or tiny collaterals), rather than "flying" along a broad tube. Therefore, it takes longer to reach peak velocity in systole, and systolic acceleration is reduced. Second, flow velocity is low, because less blood is moving through the obstructed vessel. This makes the Doppler waveform smaller than normal overall. Finally, ischemic distal tissues arc "begging" for blood, with capillary beds wide open. The resultant decrease in peripheral resistance allows blood to flow throughout diastole, even in vessels that normally would not have diastolic flow (e.g., extremity arteries). The net effect of all three factors is the damped (also called *dampened*) waveform appearance described previously. The importance of this waveform shape cannot be overstated, since it clearly indicates the presence of arterial obstruction proximal to the Doppler examination site.

Waveform damping due to proximal obstruction may be assessed visually, but it also is possible to quantify damping by measuring the acceleration time or acceleration index and with pulsatility indices described previously in this chapter.

Secondary (Collateral) Effects

The final diagnostic features of arterial obstruction of diagnostic importance are flow changes in collateral vessels. Arterial obstruction commonly alters flow in collateral channels that may be near to or distant from the site of obstruction. These flow alterations include increased velocity, increased volume flow, reversed flow direction, and pulsatility changes. For example, the external carotid artery may become an important collateral vessel in the event of ipsilateral or contralateral internal carotid stenosis or occlusion. Likewise, the vertebral artery may become a collateral source of arm perfusion in cases of subclavian artery obstruction. In such cases, blood flow may reverse in the ipsilateral vertebral artery and flow may be substantially increased in the contralateral vertebral artery, accompanied, in turn, by increased vessel size and flow velocity.

Secondary manifestations of arterial obstruction can be important diagnostically for the following reasons: (1) they may indicate that an obstructive lesion exists that would not be apparent otherwise, for example, when reversed vertebral flow calls attention to subclavian stenosis; (2) the location of collaterals roughly indicates the level of obstruction; and (3) secondary flow changes provide some data, albeit limited, about the adequacy of the collateral system circumventing an obstructive lesion. Such changes are of particular importance in transcranial Doppler applications, as considered in Chapter 12.

COLOR FLOW ULTRASOUND IMAGING

One of the more remarkable developments in ultrasound instrumentation is color flow ultrasound imaging, which superimposes a blood flow image on a standard gray-scale ultrasound image, permitting visual assessment of blood flow. Color flow imaging is an essential component of ultrasound vascular diagnosis, and for that reason, the proper use of this modality is very important. Color flow has certain idiosyncrasies and limitations that can cause significant diagnostic error if the sonographer has insufficient understanding of this modality and its applications. Therefore, it is worthwhile to review this subject.

Principles of Color Flow Imaging

There are three methods of generating color flow images, color Doppler, time domain imaging, and power Doppler. We generally lump these together under the general term *color flow*, but the more specific terms *color Doppler* and *power Doppler* also are commonly used. You will appreciate the differences among these color imaging methods after reading the following material.

Color Doppler Imaging

Gray-scale ultrasound instruments use only two pieces of information from each echo that returns from the patient's body: the distance from the echo to the transducer (determined by the time of flight of the ultrasound pulse) and the strength of the echo. The echo signal typically contains other information, such as a Doppler frequency shift, but this information is disregarded. Color Doppler instruments[36–40] utilize the Doppler shift information, in addition to time of flight and amplitude information, to illustrate blood flow in color, as shown in Figure 3–13. For each echo shown on the color Doppler image, the instrument makes five determinations:

1. *How long has it taken for the sound beam to travel to and from the site of the echo?* As is the case in all ultrasound machines, this "time of flight" of the ultrasound beam indicates the distance of the echo reflector from the transducer.
2. *How strong is the echo?* The strength or amplitude of the ultrasound signal

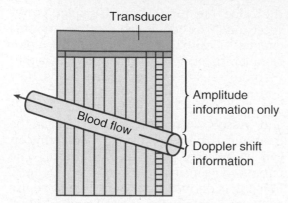

Transducer

Blood flow

Amplitude
information only

Doppler shift
information

FIGURE 3–13. Color Doppler instrumentation. Stationary reflectors generate only amplitude information and are represented in shades of gray. Moving reflectors generate a Doppler frequency shift and are shown in color. Different colors can be used to show flow toward the transducer (increased Doppler-shifted frequency) and away from the transducer (decreased Doppler-shifted frequency).

determines how brightly the echo is displayed on the image, both for the grayscale and the color Doppler components.

3. *Is a Doppler frequency shift present?* If so, the echo is represented in color; if not, it is represented in shades of gray.

4. *What is the magnitude of the Doppler frequency shift?* The magnitude of the Doppler shift is proportionate to the blood flow velocity and the Doppler angle (shown in Fig. 3–2). Different frequency levels are shown on the image as different color shades or hues.

5. *What is the direction of the Doppler shift?* The instrument determines whether flow is toward or away from the transducer by noting whether the echo has a higher or lower frequency than the ultrasound beam sent out from the transducer. A higher Doppler frequency means flow is (relatively) toward the transducer, and a lower Doppler frequency means flow is away from transducer. It is customary to show flow in one direction in blue and flow in the other direction in red. However, the operator can select other color schemes, if desired.

You should note that both the direction of flow and the velocity of flow (Doppler shift) are shown on the color Doppler image (Fig. 3–14). This can be done in two ways. With the shifting hue method, different colors are used to represent different frequency levels (e.g., with increasing frequency/velocity, the color shifts through

FIGURE 3–14. Color flow schemes. A variety of color schemes are used in color Doppler instruments. *A,* With this scheme, progressive increase in the frequency shift changes the image color from red to pink to white, or from dark blue to light blue to white, depending on the flow direction. *B,* With this scheme, the color changes from red to yellow or from blue to green.

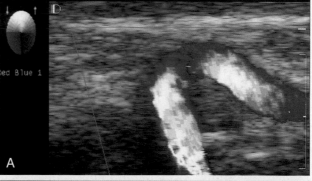

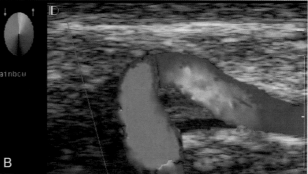

blue, green, yellow, and white). With the changing shade method, the same color is shown, but the color gets lighter as the frequency increases (e.g., through dark red, light red, pink, and, finally, white). Some sonologists prefer the shifting hue method, believing that it more clearly represents changes in the frequency shift and may demonstrate aliasing more clearly, as considered later.

Time-Domain Color Flow Imaging

The color flow images generated with the time-domain method[41] look like the flow images produced with the Doppler method previously described, but these color flow techniques are actually quite different. In the time-domain method, the ultrasound instrument identifies clusters of echoes (called *speckle*) within the ultrasound image and notes how far these clusters move on successive ultrasound pulses. By repeatedly "testing" echo clusters for movement, the instrument recognizes regions where flow is present. Flow direction and flow velocity are ascertained directly with the time-domain method, by noting which way and how fast the clusters move.[41] Time-domain flow imaging is not widely used by ultrasound equipment manufacturers. The most commonly used color flow methods are color Doppler and power Doppler.

Power Doppler Flow Imaging

The third method of color flow imaging is used widely in vascular diagnosis and is called *power Doppler flow imaging*, or *power Doppler*, for short. As its name implies, this is a Doppler method, but it differs from standard color Doppler imaging, previously described, in that the *power* or intensity of the Doppler signal is measured and mapped in color, rather than the Doppler frequency shift, per se.[42] Stated differently, the instrument determines how strong the Doppler shift is at all locations within the image field and displays locations where the strength of the Doppler signal exceeds a threshold level (Fig. 3–15). The term *power,* as used here, has

the same meaning as in "Doppler power spectrum," as described earlier in this chapter. Compared with standard color Doppler imaging, power Doppler[42] is said to be more sensitive in detecting blood flow and less dependent on the Doppler angle. These advantages mean that smaller vessels and vessels with slow flow rates can be imaged; furthermore, even tissue perfusion can be assessed, to a limited degree. The enhanced sensitivity of power Doppler imaging is derived from more extensive use of the dynamic range of the Doppler signal than is possible with standard color Doppler imaging. More of the dynamic range can be used, because noise that would overwhelm the standard color Doppler image can be assigned a uniform background color (e.g., light blue). Hence, anything that represents noise is blue (Fig. 3–15C), and anything that represents flow is another color (usually gold). Furthermore, power Doppler imaging is not affected by aliasing. Even the aliased (wrapped-around) portion of the signal (see Chapter 2) has power and can be displayed as flow.

Power Doppler imaging has one additional advantage that makes it especially valuable for use with ultrasound echo-enhancing agents (see Chapter 4). Power Doppler imaging is less subject to *blooming* than standard color Doppler imaging. Blooming is the spread of color outside of the blood vessel that occurs when the amplification of the Doppler signal is too great. Blooming is a particular problem when an echo-enhancing agent (ultrasound contrast agent) is used to improve the detection of blood flow. Intravenous injection of the echo-enhancing agent greatly increases the Doppler signal intensity, causing over-amplification and severe blooming. With power Doppler imaging, blooming does *not* occur, owing to the way that the flow–no flow determination is made.[42] Power Doppler imaging, therefore, may be the preferred method for ultrasound imaging with echo enhancement.

In spite of its potential advantages over color Doppler, power Doppler has two major limitations. First, the frame rate is agonizingly slow, which renders this imaging method useless for rapidly moving

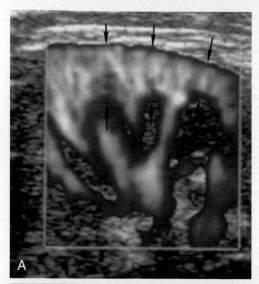

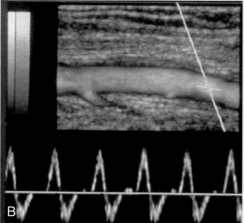

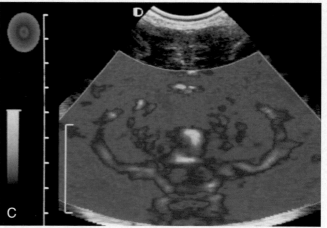

FIGURE 3–15. Power Doppler illustrations. *A*, Renal vessels are seen with striking detail, including small vessels in the renal cortex (*arrows*). Note the absence of flow direction information; all vessels are yellow even though flow in some vessels is toward the cortex (arteries) and in others is toward the renal hilum (veins). *B*, Quantitative spectral information can be obtained in the power Doppler mode. *C*, This power Doppler image of the cranial vasculature uses a blue background, which enhances flow detection because noise is converted to a uniform blue color. With color Doppler, noise would blur the margins of the vessels.

vessels, rapidly moving patients (especially children), and areas subject to respiratory or cardiac motion. Second, power Doppler does not provide flow direction information! (Remember, the power of the Doppler signal is imaged, not the Doppler shift, per se.) Without measuring the Doppler shift, the flow direction cannot be determined.

Advantages of Color Flow Imaging

Leaving the technical details behind, let us consider color flow imaging from a clinical perspective: Where does color flow help, and where does it have problems? Stated differently, what are the capabilities and limitations of color flow ultrasound?

Technical Efficiency

Perhaps the greatest advantage of color flow imaging is technical efficiency. When moving blood is encountered, the vessel "lights up," even if the vessel is too small to be resolved on the gray-scale image. Because vessels stand out in vivid color, they may be located and followed much more easily than with gray-scale instruments. Furthermore, basic judgments about blood flow can be made relatively easily with color flow imaging. The sonographer can quickly determine the presence of flow, the direction of flow, and the existence of focal flow disturbances. These capabilities have expanded the applications of duplex sonography. For example, with color flow imaging, it is possible to quickly examine long vascular segments, such as a vascular bypass graft, with relative ease. Furthermore, color flow imaging facilitates examination of vessels that are difficult to study with gray-scale imaging, such as the calf veins and the renal arteries.

Assistance in Sorting out Abdominal Anatomy

Another advantage of color flow imaging is simplified differentiation between vascular and nonvascular structures, which is particularly useful in the abdomen. From a radiologist's perspective, one of the most obvious applications is sorting out porta hepatis anatomy. The bile ducts, which do not exhibit flow, may be differentiated visually from the porta hepatis vessels; moreover, the hepatic artery and portal vein may be differentiated visually by their flow characteristics.

Flow Assessment in the Entire Lumen

A major advantage of color flow imaging is the depiction of blood flow throughout entire vascular segments, rather than only within the Doppler sample volume. Because flow features are visible over a large area, localized flow abnormalities are readily apparent and are less likely to be overlooked than with gray-scale duplex methods. The sonographer is immediately made aware of the location of any flow abnormality, which speeds up the examination and permits rapid assessment of long segments of vessels for obstruction and other pathology.

Visual Measurement of Stenoses

As compared with gray-scale ultrasound, color flow imaging makes it easier to define the residual lumen in stenotic vessels,[43,44] permitting visual (non-Doppler) measurement of arterial stenoses (Fig. 3–16). Direct, visual stenosis measurement remains problem prone, however, due to vessel tortuosity, color blooming, and acoustic shadows from calcified plaque.

Differentiation of Severe Stenosis and Occlusion

The ability of color flow imaging, and especially power Doppler, to detect low velocity flow in a tiny residual lumen facilitates the differentiation between occlusion of an artery and near occlusion with a "trickle" of residual flow (Fig. 3–17). Personal experience suggests that color flow imaging is of value in this regard, and studies of the carotid arteries have shown improved

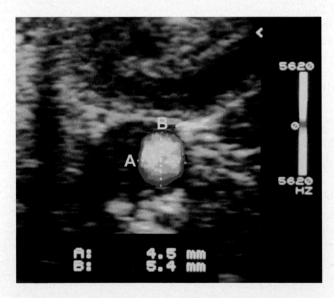

FIGURE 3–16. Enhanced visual stenosis measurement. The residual lumen (cursors *A* and *B*) is clearly visualized in this color flow image, potentially enhancing measurement accuracy.

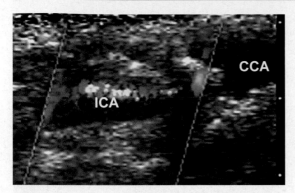

FIGURE 3–17. Small residual lumen. The tiny residual lumen in this internal carotid artery (ICA) would not be visible without color flow imaging. CCA, common carotid artery.

results for detecting flow in near-occluded internal carotid arteries.[45,46]

Limitations of Color Flow Imaging

So much for the advantages of color flow imaging, most of which quickly become obvious with use. Now to the limitations, which can have adverse diagnostic consequences if they are not understood by the sonographer. Many of the limitations listed here also occur with three-dimensional color flow imaging, which is discussed later in this chapter.

Flow Information Is Qualitative

It is most important to recognize that color flow information is *qualitative* and not quantitative.[36–41] There are three reasons for this.

First, *the color flow image is based on the average Doppler shift* within the vessel, rather than the *peak* Doppler shift. Recall that quantitative Doppler spectrum measurements are based on the peak Doppler shifts, not the average shift. The average Doppler shift is *not* helpful for actually putting a number on a stenosis; you need the peak values. Furthermore, the average Doppler shift is lowered by flow disturbances (turbulence).

The second reason that color flow information is qualitative is *the lack of Doppler angle correction*. We previously indicated the importance of Doppler angle correction for accurate spectral Doppler measurements. It is easy to understand, therefore, that lack of angle correction is a significant contribution to the qualitative nature of the color flow image. Colors coded for high velocity may be seen in a vessel that is diving steeply away from the transducer when the velocities in that vessel are not actually very high.

Finally, *color flow information shows only a few frequency levels*. Color flow imaging is, in essence, a visual form of Doppler spectrum analysis, but it is a very crude form in which only a few large frequency "steps" are visible. These few steps provide only a general sense of altered flow velocity.

Because color flow images are qualitative, Doppler spectrum analysis must still be used to derive quantitative flow data (Fig. 3–18). However, quantitative flow data can be derived from the color flow display with some time-domain color flow imaging systems, but these instruments are not widely used.*

Low Pulse Repetition Frequencies and Frame Rates

A tremendous amount of data must be processed by the color flow instrument to generate each pixel (picture element) and each television frame. Processing these data takes time, which may significantly degrade both the gray-scale and color Doppler images. This problem results principally from reduction of the pulse repetition frequency [PRF], the number of pulses sent out per second) and the frame rate (the number of times per second that the television image is renewed). B-flow imaging, discussed later, is not subject to these image-resolution limitations.

Image degradation during color flow operation occurs in the following forms: (1) loss of spatial resolution; (2) a greater tendency for Doppler aliasing, which can cause spurious representation of high-velocity

*Philips Medical Systems, Ultrasound Division, Santa Ana, CA.

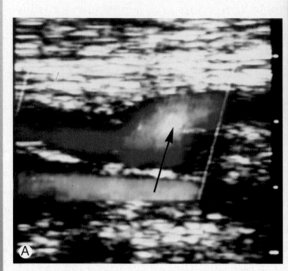
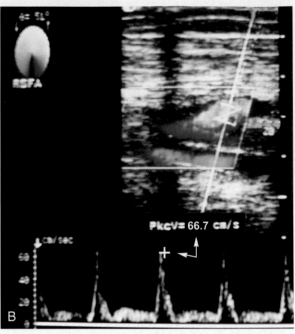

FIGURE 3–18. Color flow information is qualitative, not quantitative. *A,* It appears that the flow velocity is elevated at the origin of this arterial bypass graft (*arrow,* yellow color shift) because the color flow image is not angle corrected. *B,* Angle-corrected spectral Doppler measurement shows that the peak systolic velocity is not elevated (66.7 cm/sec).

flow; (3) diminished temporal resolution, limiting the ability to visualize rapidly moving cardiac or vascular events (for example, cardiac valve motion may be less clearly seen with color flow scanning than with gray-scale scanning); and (4) visible image flicker when the frame rate falls below 15 frames/sec. (At that point, the human eye no longer "blurs" the ultrasound images into a moving picture.)[47]

Blood Flow Detection Is Angle Dependent

Blood flow is not detected with color Doppler devices in vessels that are perpendicular to the ultrasound beam. (Color and spectral Doppler devices are similar in this respect.) A false-positive diagnosis of vascular occlusion may occur if a vessel is approximately perpendicular to the ultrasound beam, as shown in Figure 3–19. This is a particularly severe problem with curved array transducers. (Try imaging vessels with a curved array, and you will see what I mean.)

Flow Direction Is Arbitrary

It is crucial to remember that the color of the vessel on the color flow image is *not* an absolute indication of flow direction. The color is assigned relative to the transducer

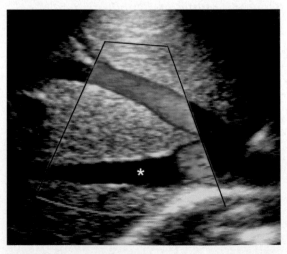

FIGURE 3–19. Spurious absence of flow. It appears that flow is absent in the right hepatic vein (*asterisk*) because this vessel is perpendicular to the color Doppler line of sight.

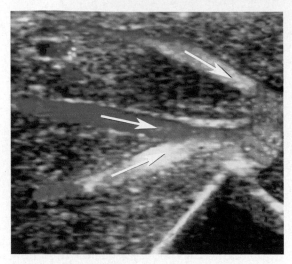

FIGURE 3–20. Color flow direction is relative to the transducer. Two of the hepatic veins are blue and one is red, implying that the flow direction in the red vessel is opposite that in the blue vessels. Flow actually is toward the inferior vena cava (*arrows*) in all of the vessels, but flow in the red vessel is *relatively* toward the transducer (top of image), while flow in the other vessels is *relatively* away from the transducer.

(Fig. 3–20; see Fig. 3–14). The operator may reverse the color scheme (e.g., arteries blue, veins red) simply by reversing the orientation of the transducer or by pushing a button. To determine the true direction of flow, the operator must closely observe the orientation of the vessel of interest relative to the transducer or refer to a vessel in which the flow direction is known (such as the aorta, if you are working in the abdomen).

Color May Obscure Vascular Pathology

If the instrument controls are improperly adjusted, the color flow information tends to "bloom" into the surrounding gray-scale image (Fig. 3–21). Important vascular pathology, including plaque and venous thrombus, may be obscured by blooming. The absence of blooming is a desirable feature of B-flow imaging, as mentioned later.

Color Flash

With color flow imaging, anything within the field of view that moves relative to the transducer is shown in color. In the abdomen, peristaltic motion, cardiac motion, or transmitted pulsations from great vessels may generate blotches of color on the ultrasound image called *color flash,* which can obscure large portions of the field of view, including structures of interest. The color flash problem is particularly apparent in the upper abdomen because of heart motion.

The Strange Case of the Visible Bruit

The *visible bruit* is a peculiar, but useful, flow phenomenon (Fig. 3–22) that can be seen with color flow imaging.[48] A montage of

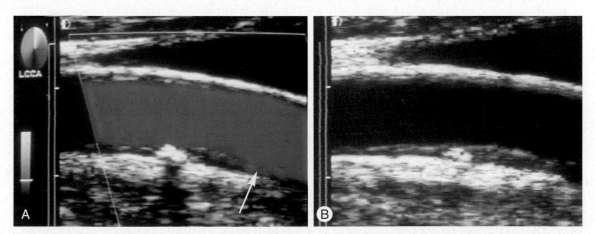

FIGURE 3–21. Color obscures plaque. *A,* Color blooming obscures part of the plaque (*arrow*). *B,* The plaque is seen optimally with color flow turned off.

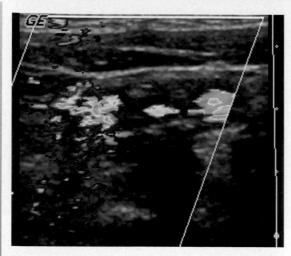

FIGURE 3–22. Visible bruit. Soft-tissue vibrations cause a montage of color adjacent to this stenotic internal carotid artery.

applicable to three-dimensional color flow imaging.

1. *Velocity range:* Consider whether the instrument is set for the proper velocity range. If the instrument is set to detect arterial velocities, it is not sensitive to venous velocities, or vice versa. Adjust the PRF or the velocity range to a level appropriate for the vessel of interest.

2. *Doppler angle:* Remember that the Doppler angle profoundly affects the color flow image. The strength of the color flow image diminishes as the Doppler angle approaches 90 degrees; that is, the ultrasound beam is perpendicular to the blood vessel. So, when flow is absent in a vessel, ask, "Do I have an appropriate Doppler angle?" If not, move the color flow box or the transducer to improve the Doppler angle.

3. *Field of view:* Consider the depth of field shown on the image. Use only as much depth as you need! Greater depth requires a longer round-trip time for the ultrasound pulses, decreasing the PRF and the number of pulses per square centimeter of tissue and increasing the signal-processing time. The net result is diminished ability to display flow (as well as gray-scale image degradation).

4. *Color box size:* Consider the size of the color box. For the same reasons that were stated previously for *field of view,* pulse-echo information becomes increasingly "diluted" as the color box is enlarged. It is best to use a small color box, especially when examining vessels deep within the body.

color is seen within the soft tissues adjacent to the blood vessel as a result of vibration of the vessel wall and surrounding soft tissues. The wall vibration, in turn, is caused by a severe flow disturbance within the vessel. The visible bruit is associated particularly with arteriovenous fistulae but is also encountered with arterial stenoses and pseudoaneurysms.

A visible bruit suggests severe arterial stenosis, but caution is advised in interpreting this finding, because severe flow disturbances may sometime occur in the absence of significant stenosis. The term *visible bruit* is a misnomer, because a bruit is a sound and is not visible. Nonetheless, we like this term because the tissue vibration seen with color flow imaging also causes the bruit to be heard with a stethoscope.

Optimizing Color Flow Image Quality

The color flow image is derived from relatively weak reflections from red blood cells. Because of the weakness of these echoes, the ability to demonstrate flow with ultrasound is particularly sensitive to instrument settings. The following technical tricks, summarized in Table 3–2, should be tried when it is difficult to obtain an adequate color flow image. The same procedures are

Table 3–2. What to Check When You Cannot Detect Blood Flow

Velocity range
Doppler angle
Field of view
Color box size
Power and gain
Color priority
Gray-scale priority
Thump control
Wall filter
Is flow too slow?

5. *Power and gain:* Determine if the output power of the instrument, the time compensated gain, and the color gain are optimal. Insufficient power or gain can result in inadequate color flow information.

6. *Color priority:* Consider whether the gray-scale versus color priority is adjusted correctly. Most (if not all) color flow instruments permit the operator to determine whether the gray-scale or color image is given more attention. If the gray-scale image is prioritized, then the color image suffers, and vice versa. If you are having trouble detecting flow, shift the image processing priority toward color.

7. *Thump control:* See if the thump control is eliminating too much color flow information. *Thump control* refers to electronic filtering that removes color artifacts generated by the heart or vascular pulsations. Thump control is not needed in smaller peripheral vessels and should be set as low as is practical.

8. *Wall filter:* Check the wall filter setting. If the wall filter is set too high, low-frequency signals generated by low velocity flow are eliminated. The wall filter is designed to eliminate low frequency noise, but if it is set too high, it also eliminates flow information. This is not a problem with high-velocity flow, but it may be a major problem for detection of venous flow or for evaluating small intrarenal arteries.

9. *Very slow flow:* Finally, remember that flow might be present that simply is too slow for color flow visualization. Power Doppler or spectral Doppler may be more sensitive to the presence of slow flow than standard color Doppler imaging, and it may be useful to switch to these modalities when a vessel appears occluded.

THREE-DIMENSIONAL VASCULAR IMAGING

Advances in computer technology and transducer design have made three-dimensional (3D) ultrasound imaging a reality[49-53] (Fig. 3–23). Although the reconstruction algorithms utilized with current 3D ultrasound units are not as sophisticated as those used for computed tomography or magnetic resonance imaging, they are adequate for clinical use, and the utilization of 3D ultrasound continues to grow. Most studies have concentrated on obstetric, cardiac, and gynecologic applications. There are few clinical studies that have evaluated vascular applications of 3D ultrasound. Areas of current investigation include the carotid bifurcation and carotid

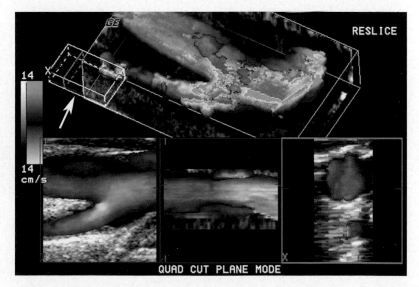

FIGURE 3–23. Three-dimensional ultrasound image. The large image at the top is shaded to display the three dimensionality inherent in this carotid bifurcation image. The three boxes at the bottom show different two-dimensional perspectives, based on the stored three-dimensional data. Orientation is provided by the navigator (*arrow*). The colored borders around the two-dimensional images correspond to the planes of section seen in the navigator.

stenosis, intracranial vascular disease, remodeling in bypass grafts, and abdominal aortic aneurysms.

Three-dimensional presentation of ultrasound data can be performed with commercially available ultrasound systems. Off-line graphics workstations can also be utilized to generate, view, and store 3D data sets. These data sets may be obtained by combining stacks of two-dimensional slices to generate a volume of tissue. More recently, 3D ultrasound information can be obtained directly, through the acquisition of a volume of data generated by sweeping, tilting, or rotating the transducer across the area of interest.

There are several options for review of 3D data. The images can be displayed as a set of sequential images that can be reviewed manually, with the use of a trackball or keyboard. Multiple planes, including axial, sagittal, and coronal images, can be displayed simultaneously for comparison. In addition, the information may be viewed as a volume-rendered data set, emphasizing different tissue or blood flow characteristics. Interactive review of the data allows the examiner to rotate the volume in any plane or section, scroll through individual slices, and subtract superficial or unwanted information. Real-time 3D examination (also known as four-dimensional imaging) is currently available on clinical ultrasound units. Future software modifications will allow virtual fly-through examination of blood vessels in real time.

The advantages of 3D ultrasound include the ability to obtain anatomic views not possible with two-dimensional imaging. The examiner can reformat the volume of image data in different imaging planes to extract information obscured by overlying tissue or artifacts. In addition, a surface (or transparent) display of the data can be obtained. Off-line review of patient data sets is also available. Recalculation of velocity measurements and assessment of different imaging planes for arterial stenosis, after the patient has left the ultrasound area, will be possible in the near future.

There are several limitations that have slowed widespread acceptance of 3D ultrasound. Reformatting and analysis of the 3D data is time consuming. Artifacts related to motion, scatter, attenuation, and color flash seriously degrade the quality of the 3D information. Current workstations that allow the analysis of 3D ultrasound data are expensive and do not readily interface with current picture archiving systems. Finally, it is also difficult to store and retrieve 3D ultrasound information with current picture archiving system technology.

B-MODE FLOW IMAGING

B-mode flow imaging[54-56] (B-flow for short) is one of the newest methods for flow imaging available on medical ultrasound instruments. As the name implies, B-flow shows blood flow with the gray-scale, or B-mode, image and is not a Doppler method. Both the flowing blood and the surrounding stationary structures are shown in shades of gray (Fig. 3–24). For B-flow

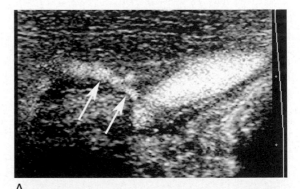

A

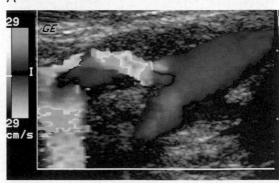

B

FIGURE 3–24. B-flow ultrasound. *A,* This long axis B-flow image accurately shows the size of the stenotic internal carotid artery lumen (*arrows*). *B,* The lumen size is greatly exaggerated by color flow imaging due to blooming and other artifacts.

imaging, digitally encoded wide-band pulses are transmitted and reflected from the moving blood cells. The returning echoes are decoded and filtered to increase sensitivity for the detection of moving scatterers and distinguish blood from tissue. Since this is not a Doppler technique, no velocity or frequency information is provided, and spectrum analysis does not apply. This is a purely visual, nonquantitative method of showing blood flow.

Probably the most useful aspect of B-flow is the precise definition of the boundary between flowing blood and the vessel wall. Because this is not a Doppler imaging method, the problems of blooming and overamplification of the flow signals, cited previously, do not apply. In addition, the B-flow technique does not degrade the spatial or temporal resolution of the B-mode image, as is the case with color flow imaging. Thus, the tendency of color Doppler to obscure the vessel wall and plaque is eliminated. In superficial arteries, such as the carotid arteries, the presence, extent, and severity of plaque in arteries is shown more clearly with B-flow than with color Doppler or even standard B-mode sonography. Potentially, B-flow may clarify the depiction of irregular plaque surfaces resulting from plaque ulceration, which would contribute significantly to its value for carotid artery imaging. In the venous system, small deep vein thrombi are well demonstrated with B-flow as filling defects that can be distinguished from flowing blood. Venous insufficiency and incompetent valves are also easily seen with this technique. Finally, B-flow is useful for demonstrating complex flow states, as seen with bypass grafts, arteriovenous fistulae, pseudoaneurysms, and dialysis grafts, where color Doppler artifacts may obscure flow information.

Because B-flow relies on the amplification of very weak echoes from red blood cells, it is limited by ultrasound attenuation, which restricts the depiction of deep vessels, especially those in which blood is moving rapidly. B-flow, therefore, is principally applicable for superficial vascular imaging. In the abdomen, it has been used to show blood flow in the portal and hepatic veins, but is less reliable for visualization of arterial flow.

References

1. Wells PNT, Skedmore R: Doppler developments in the last quinquennium. Ultrasound Med Biol 11:613–623, 1986.
2. Taylor KJW, Holland S: Doppler ultrasound: Part I. Basic principles, instrumentation, and pitfalls. Radiology 174:297–307, 1990.
3. Hutchison KJ, Oberle K, Scott JA, et al: A comparison of Doppler ultrasonic waveforms processed by zero crossing and spectrographic techniques in the diagnosis of peripheral arterial disease. Angiology 32:277–289, 1981.
4. Reneman RS, Spencer MP: Local Doppler audio spectra in normal and stenosed carotid arteries in man. Ultrasound Med Biol 5:1–11, 1979.
5. Johnston KW, deMorais D, Kassam M, et al: Cerebrovascular assessment using a Doppler carotid scanner and real-time frequency analysis. J Clin Ultrasound 9:443–449, 1981.
6. Brown PM, Johnston W, Kassam M, et al: A critical study of ultrasound Doppler spectral analysis for detecting carotid disease. Ultrasound Med Biol 8:515–523, 1982.
7. Zwiebel WJ: Color duplex imaging and Doppler spectrum analysis: Principles, capabilities, and limitations. Semin Ultrasound CT MR 11: 84–96, 1990.
8. Zwiebel WJ, Knighton R: Duplex examination of the carotid arteries. Semin Ultrasound CT MR 11:97–135, 1990.
9. Bluth EI, Wetzner SM, Stavros AT, et al: Carotid duplex sonography: A multicenter recommendation for standardized imaging and Doppler criteria. Radiographics 8:487–506, 1988.
10. Feigenbaum H: Doppler color flow imaging. Heart Dis Update 2:25–50, 1988.
11. Zierler RE, Phillips DJ, Beach KW, et al: Noninvasive assessment of normal carotid bifurcation hemodynamics with color flow ultrasound imaging. Ultrasound Med Biol 13:471–476, 1987.
12. Middleton WD, Foley WD, Lawson TL: Flow reversal in the normal carotid bifurcation: Color Doppler flow imaging analysis. Radiology 167:207–210, 1988.
13. Spencer MP: Frequency spectrum analysis in Doppler diagnosis. In Zwiebel WJ (ed): Introduction to Vascular Ultrasonography, 2nd ed. Philadelphia, WB Saunders, 1986, pp 53–80.
14. Smith JJ, Kampine JP: The peripheral circulation and its regulation. In Smith JJ, Kampine JP (eds): Circulatory Physiology: The Essentials. Baltimore, Williams & Wilkins, 1980.
15. Baker D: Application of pulsed Doppler techniques. Radiol Clin North Am 18:79–103, 1980.

16. Douville Y, Johnston KW, Kassam M: Determination of the hemodynamic factors which influence the carotid Doppler spectral broadening. Ultrasound Med Biol 11:417–423, 1985.

17. Campbell JD, Hutchison KJ, Karpinski E: Variation of Doppler ultrasound spectral width in the post-stenotic velocity field. Ultrasound Med Biol 15:611–619, 1989.

18. Merode TV, Hick P, Hoeks APG, et al: Limitations of Doppler spectral broadening in the early detection of carotid artery disease due to the size of the sample volume. Ultrasound Med Biol 9:581–586, 1983.

19. Knox RA, Phillips DJ, Breslau PJ, et al: Empirical findings relating sample volume size to diagnostic accuracy in pulsed Doppler cerebrovascular studies. J Clin Ultrasound 10:227–232, 1982.

20. Ku DN, Giddens DP, Phillips DJ, et al: Hemodynamics of the normal human carotid bifurcation: In vitro and in vivo studies. Ultrasound Med Biol 11:13–26, 1985.

21. Phillips DJ, Greene FM, Langlois Y, et al: Flow velocity patterns in the carotid bifurcations of young, presumed normal subjects. Ultrasound Med Biol 9:39–49, 1983.

22. Nimura Y, Matsuo H, Hayashi T, et al: Studies on arterial flow patterns: Instantaneous velocity spectrums and their phasic changes with directional ultrasonic Doppler technique. Br Heart J 36:899–907, 1974.

23. Rutherford RB, Kreutzer EW: Doppler ultrasound techniques in the assessment of extracranial arterial occlusive disease. In Nicolaides AN, Yao JST (eds): Investigation of Vascular Disorders. London, Churchill Livingstone, 1981.

24. Rutherford RB, Hiatt WR, Kreutzer EW: The use of velocity wave form analysis in the diagnosis of carotid artery occlusive disease. Surgery 82:695–702, 1977.

25. Nicolaides AN, Angelides NS: Waveform index and resistance factor using directional Doppler ultrasound and a zero crossing detector. In Nicolaides AN, Yao JST (eds): Investigation of Vascular Disorders. London, Churchill Livingstone, 1981.

26. Gosling RG: Doppler ultrasound assessment of occlusive arterial disease. Practitioner 220:599–609, 1978.

27. Kotval PS: Doppler waveform parvus and tardus. J Ultrasound Med 8:435–440, 1989.

28. Pourcelot L: Applications cliniques de l'examen Doppler transcutane. In Peronneau P (ed): Velocimetrie Ultrasonore Doppler, vol 34. Paris, INSERM 1974, pp 780–785.

29. Stuart B, Drumm J, Fitzgerald DE, Duignan NM: Foetal blood velocity waveforms in normal pregnancy. Br J Obstet Gynaecol 87:780–785, 1980.

30. Avasthi PS, Greene ER, Voyles WF, et al: A comparison of echo-Doppler and electromagnetic renal blood flow measurements. J Ultrasound Med 3:213–218, 1984.

31. Gill RW: Measurement of blood flow by ultrasound: Accuracy and sources of error. Ultrasound Med Biol 11:625–641, 1985.

32. Burns PN, Jaffe CC: Quantitative flow measurements with Doppler ultrasound: Techniques, accuracy, and limitations. Radiol Clin North Am 23:641–657, 1985.

33. Fei DY, Billian C, Rittgers SE: Flow dynamics in a stenosed carotid bifurcation model. Part I: Basic velocity measurements. Ultrasound Med Biol 14:21–31, 1988.

34. Chang BB, Leather RP, Kaufmann JL, et al: Hemodynamic characteristics of failing infrainguinal in situ vein bypass. J Vasc Surg 12:596–600, 1990.

35. Spencer MP: Full capability Doppler diagnosis. In Spencer MP, Reed JM (eds): Cerebrovascular Evaluation with Doppler Ultrasound. The Hague, Netherlands, Martinus Nijhoff, 1981, p 213.

36. Switzer DF, Nanda NC: Doppler color flow mapping. Ultrasound Med Biol 11:403–416, 1985.

37. Merritt CRB: Doppler blood flow imaging: Integrating flow with tissue data. Diagn Imaging 11:146–155, 1986.

38. Powis RL: Color flow imaging: Understanding its science and technology. J Diagn Med Sonograph 4:236–245, 1988.

39. Carroll BA: Carotid sonography: Pitfalls and color flow. Appl Radiol 10:15–21, 1988.

40. Nelson TR, Pretorius DH: The Doppler signal: Where does it come from and what does it mean? Am J Roentgenol 151:439–447, 1988.

41. Gardiner W, Fox MD: Color flow ultrasound imaging through the analysis of speckle motion. Radiology 172:866–868, 1989.

42. Murphy KJ, Rubin JM: Power Doppler: It's a good thing. Semin Ultrasound 18:13–21, 1997.

43. Erickson SJ, Mewissen MW, Foley WD, et al: Stenosis of the internal carotid artery: Assessment using color Doppler imaging compared with angiography. Am J Roentgenol 152:1299–1305, 1989.

44. Polak JF, Dobkin GR, O'Leary DH, et al: Internal carotid artery stenosis: Accuracy and reproducibility of color-Doppler assisted duplex imaging. Radiology 173:793–798, 1989.

45. Chang YJ, Lin SK, Ryu SJ, Wai YY: Common carotid artery occlusion: Evaluation with duplex sonography. Am J Neuroradiol 16:1099–1105, 1995.

46. Lee DH, Gao FQ, Rankin RN, et al: Duplex and color Doppler flow sonography of occlusion

and near occlusion of the carotid artery. Am J Neuroradiol 17:1267–1274, 1996.

47. Powis RL, Powis WD: A Thinker's Guide to Ultrasonic Imaging. Baltimore, Urban & Schwarzenberg, 1984, pp 345–364.

48. Middleton WD, Erickson S, Melson GL: Perivascular color artifact: Pathologic significance and appearance on color Doppler ultrasound images. Radiology 171:647–652, 1989.

49. Delcker A, Schurks M, Polz H: Development and applications of 4-D ultrasound (dynamic 3-D) in neurosonology. J Neuroimaging 9:229–234, 1999.

50. Delcker A, Diener HC: Quantification of atherosclerotic plaques in carotid arteries by 3-D ultrasound. Br J Radiol 67:672–678, 1994.

51. Leotta DF, Primozich JF, Beach KW, et al: Remodeling in peripheral vein graft revisions: Serial study with three-dimensional ultrasound imaging. J Vasc Surg 37:798–807, 2003.

52. Nelson TR, Pretorius DH, Lev-Toaff A, et al: Feasibility of performing a virtual patient examination using three-dimensional ultrasonographic data acquired at remote locations. J Ultrasound Med 20:941–952, 2001.

53. Pretorius DH, Borok NN, Coffler MS, et al: Three-dimensional ultrasound in obstetrics and gynecology. Radiol Clin North Am 39:499–521, 2001.

54. Umemura A, Yamada K: B-mode flow imaging of the carotid artery. Stroke 32:2055–2057, 2001.

55. Furuse J, Maru Y, Mera K, et al: Visualization of blood flow in hepatic vessels and hepatocellular carcinoma using B-flow sonography. J Clin Ultrasound 29:1–6, 2001.

56. Pellerito JS: Current approach to peripheral arterial sonography. Radiol Clin North Am 3:553–567, 2001.

Chapter 4

Contrast Agents in Arterial Sonography

Laurence Needleman, MD

INITIAL CONSIDERATIONS

The ability of ultrasound to generate spectral Doppler and color Doppler information is quite impressive. Nevertheless, using conventional ultrasound instruments, there are situations in which the reflected signals from vessels are weak and the accuracy of ultrasound becomes compromised. This is particularly true in deep-lying vessels, due to attenuation of the Doppler signal. In high-grade stenoses, the reduction in volume flow decreases the number of red blood cells that serve as reflectors, leading to a reduction of the Doppler signal. This problem can interfere with differentiation of occlusion and near-occlusion, which can be a critical issue in determining the most appropriate therapy for the patient.

Ultrasound contrast agents (UCAs) have been developed to increase the returning ultrasound echo signal.[1] Because most agents remain in the blood pool, they increase vascular signals. Although contrast agents are under development by several pharmaceutical firms, they share several general properties. They all consist of gas-filled microbubbles, which powerfully reflect sound, compared with soft tissue and blood. The microbubbles are small and nearly uniform, which allows the agent to cross capillaries. Therefore, an intravenous injection can pass through the lungs to enhance the arterial system. Most agents are also robust, so that the microbubbles persist in the circulation for minutes. Approved agents have undergone evaluation of their safety.

In the United States, some UCAs have been approved by the Food and Drug Administration for echocardiography. No agents have been approved for vascular ultrasound indications. Presently, UCA use in the United States requires understanding of the exclusion criteria for the agent (such as hypersensitivity to its components or a right-to-left shunt) and informed patient consent, either because the agent is part of a research study or it is used for a non-approved application. Some UCAs have been approved for use in countries other than the United States for a variety of indications, including vascular applications.

Outside of echocardiography, most of the clinical and research use of UCAs has been to investigate the microcirculation, particularly tumor vascularity (Fig. 4–1). There has been some research in the cerebrovascular, peripheral arterial, and abdominal arterial and venous systems, but there has been no dominant theme in the investigation of vascular UCAs. Aside from assessment of the characteristics and efficacy of diffcrent contrast agents under development, the spectral Doppler, color Doppler, and gray-scale applications (Fig. 4–2) are all being studied. Different doses of the same agent and the use of different intravenous administration schemes (bolus versus infusion) also have been reported.

There is no consensus on how peripheral vascular UCA should be used. Some investigators envision UCA as a problem-solver to be used following an unenhanced scan that is less than satisfactory. Others have introduced protocols under which the entire scan is performed with contrast enhancement. In this setting, the agent is expected to give more reliable information, speed up

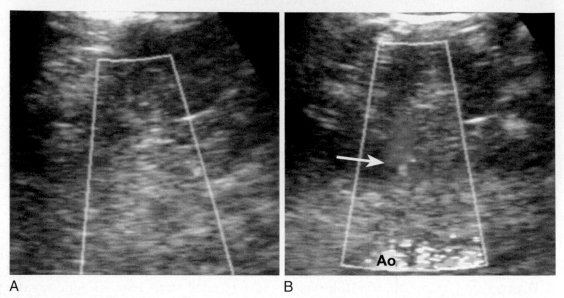

A   B

FIGURE 4–1. Normal renal artery. *A*, There is no detectable color Doppler signal in the renal artery. *B*, Following the administration of contrast, the aorta (Ao) and the entire length of the renal artery (*arrow*) can be identified into the renal hilum.

the examination, or both, and eliminate the need for an unenhanced scan.

Whereas earlier UCA research had been restricted to color, power, or spectral Doppler, newer agents demonstrate gray-scale enhancement, expanding potential applications. The gray-scale potential of UCAs has been further advanced by ultrasound instrument improvements, notably harmonic techniques.[2–5] In traditional ultrasound systems, ultrasound at a given frequency (the fundamental frequency) is sent into the patient, and echoes are received at the same frequency, altered only by the Doppler shift. Harmonic ultrasound utilizes an important property of microbubbles: They are powerful reflectors of the fundamental frequency, but they also generate strong signals at frequencies that are regular increments from the fundamental (i.e., the harmonic frequencies). Harmonic ultrasound filters out the fundamental frequency to collect information at a harmonic frequency, which is typically double the fundamental frequency. Because tissue gives off weak signals at harmonic frequencies, the harmonic technique suppresses tissue, making the UCA signals stand out.

Wideband harmonic imaging (also called pulse inversion technique)[3–6] capitalizes on another characteristic of a bubble, its non-linear response to the sound wave. A bubble expands more in low pressure than it is compressed in high pressure. This is a non-linear response. Typically, two inverted pulses of ultrasound are transmitted, causing the tissue signal to cancel itself out, while the microbubble signal persists. This technique improves the conspicuity of the UCA signal relative to the tissue background, allowing for better spatial resolution and better contrast–to-tissue differences while using lower power and causing less destruction of the agent microbubbles.

Each microbubble agent has a unique formulation. The type of gas used in the microbubbles is varied to improve longevity of the bubbles.[7] Most agents use air, SF_6, or fluorocarbons. The microbubbles used in different agents are stabilized by various means, including phospholipids, surfactants, and other compounds.[7] The composition of the agent affects its effectiveness, including its safety, length, and strength of enhancement, as well as its harmonic response.

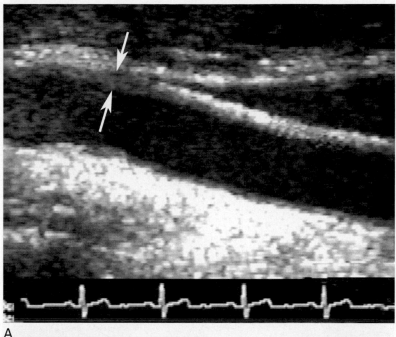

A

FIGURE 4-2. Harmonic gray-scale enhancement of the human carotid artery intima-media thickness measurements. *A*, Baseline unenhanced scan demonstrates slight thickening of the vessel. The near wall (*arrows*) is thicker than the far wall, which may be a real finding or an artifact due to reverberation. *B*, Following the administration of contrast, the blood is echogenic, compared with the now less echogenic wall, and the contrast-vessel interface is more conspicuous. Some of the thickening is real (*arrows*) and the slightly greater thickening in the distal vessel is easily seen, compared with the thinner proximal artery. (Case courtesy of Steven Feinstein, MD, Chicago, IL.)

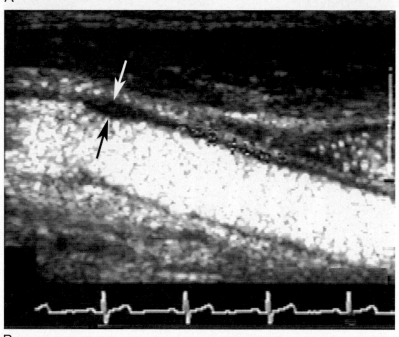

B

ARTIFACTS

An excessive amount of contrast enhancement can cause the color signal to "bloom," or spread beyond the borders of the vessel (Fig. 4–3).[8,9] This artifact is easily recognized and can be eliminated by allowing the contrast to dissipate or by reducing the gain of the color Doppler signal. The blooming arti-fact does not occur with gray-scale imaging, but desilhouetting of the gray-scale image may occur if the echogenicity of the contrast-enhanced blood equals that of the vessel wall, lessening the conspicuity of the vessel itself.

Spectral Doppler artifacts also exist.[8,9] Bubble destruction may cause spikes in the spectral Doppler waveforms, and

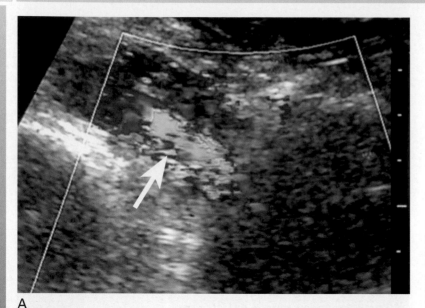

A

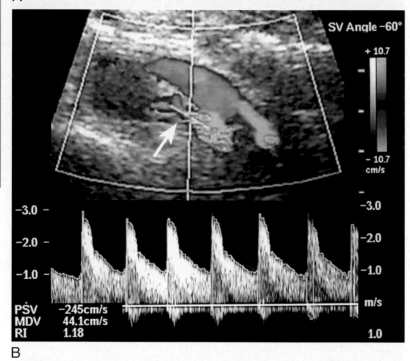

B

FIGURE 4–3. Color blooming in renal artery stenosis. *A,* In this patient with renal artery stenosis, the color extends over the artery obscuring the residual lumen. *B,* Scan-taking several minutes later demonstrates the blooming to resolve as the amount of contrast diminishes. The stenosis can now be optimally imaged as an area of color narrowing with mosaic color (representing aliasing). Spectral Doppler reveals a high-velocity stenotic jet with peak systolic velocity of 245 cm/sec. At baseline (not shown), the renal artery was not seen with color. (Case courtesy of Boris Brkljačić, MD, Zagreb, Croatia.)

contrast-enhanced spectral waveforms may demonstrate spectral broadening (Fig. 4–4). In some studies in animals, human breast tumors, and intracerebral vessels, enhancement of the spectral Doppler signal has increased the velocity detected with spectral Doppler.[8–11] This effect has been somewhat controversial, as it has not been observed by all investigators.[12] Basseau and associates[13] studied this artifact in rabbits and showed that it most likely is due to alteration of the power of the Doppler signal and the gain of the system. Artifactual elevation of Doppler velocity does not affect pulsatility indices or velocity ratios.[11,12,14] Larger trials are needed to determine if velocity elevation is a clinical problem.

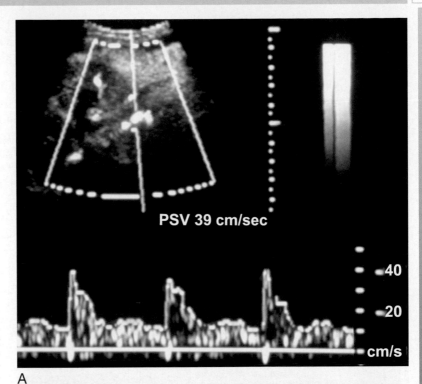

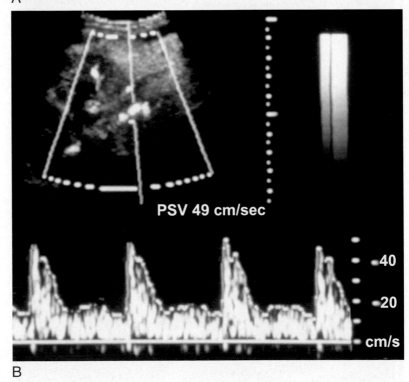

FIGURE 4–4. Spectral broadening and velocity increase after contrast administration. *A*, Unenhanced scan of a canine renal artery. Peak systolic velocity (PSV) is 39 cm/sec. *B*, Following contrast administration, spectral broadening is evident. The peak systolic velocity has increased to 49 cm/sec, an increase of 25%.

PERIPHERAL ARTERY APPLICATIONS

The majority of published peripheral arterial UCS studies have used Levovist (Schering AG, Germany), a so-called "first-generation" UCS primarily composed of galactose particles and air microbubbles. In most of the reported studies, this agent was used after a suboptimal initial ultrasound scan. The studies generally showed that difficult examinations can be improved by the introduction of contrast. The studies used both color and spectral Doppler.

In one of the Levovist studies, improved visualization of runoff vessels was seen in four of nine patients with peripheral arterial disease (two with occlusion and two with stenosis).[15] In another study of five arteries, the absence of detectable flow at baseline was proven to be a technical problem, as normal flow was identified after contrast enhancement. Collaterals were identified after contrast administration in patients with occlusion (Fig. 4–5). In this study, spectral Doppler was entirely adequate in only 19% of baseline examinations. Contrast enhancement significantly improved spectral Doppler signal adequacy, to 71%.

In a Phase III trial of Levovist, Schwarz and colleagues[16] reported on another group of patients studied after an inadequate baseline Doppler examination. One or two doses of 200-mg/mL Levovist were administered. The diagnostic confidence of the spectral Doppler examination improved from 35% unenhanced to 91% after contrast administration. In this multicenter study, there was no diagnostic standard, and the diagnostic accuracy of the contrast-enhanced examination was not assessed.

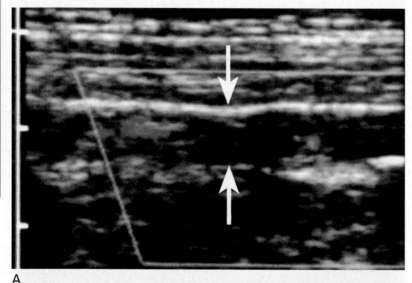

A

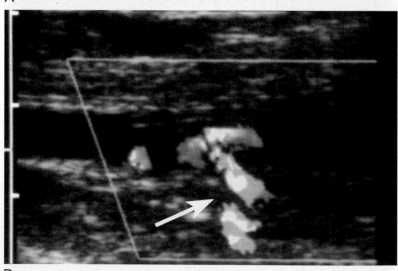

B

FIGURE 4–5. Peripheral artery occlusion. *A,* Baseline view of the femoral artery (*arrows*) shows abrupt termination of the vessel. *B,* Following administration of contrast, the occlusion is confirmed. Collateral flow reconstituting the vessel (*arrow*) is seen distal to the occluded vessel.

Langholz and associates[17] compared different concentrations of Levovist and found that a lower concentration (200 mg/mL) was adequate in the majority of patients, but 300 mg/mL was required in others. The concentration could be chosen based on the initial appearance of the vessel: In those with partial visualization, lower concentration could be attempted. An even higher concentration of 400 mg/mL was effective for patients in whom the lower concentration was not helpful. The iliac or thigh arteries were studied in 12 patients. The investigators remarked on improvement of visualization of blood flow in the iliac arteries, despite the presence of overlying bowel gas.

The study by Langholz and associates[17] also reported that contrast enhancement times increased with concentration. The mean arterial enhancement times in the upper extremity were 2.3, 5.2, and 6.1 minutes for concentrations of 200, 300, and 400 mg/mL, respectively. (Statistical significance was not reported.) In a different study, there was an increase in enhancement duration from 5.8 to 7.0 minutes when the dose was increased from 200 to 300 mg/mL, but this difference was not statistically significant.[15]

Albrecht and associates[18] reported on the effect of Levovist infusion on the enhancement of the femoral artery in six normal volunteers. The signal enhancement increased significantly as the infusion rate was increased from slow to standard to fast. The duration of enhancement was significantly longer lasting with a slow rate compared with faster rates. All infusions produced significantly longer enhancement than bolus administration. This study suggests a method to enhance the entire limb vasculature, although it has not been determined if SCA infusion would generate adequate enhancement for an entire arterial mapping examination (from the iliac artery to the runoff vessels).

A definitive protocol for Levovist administration has not been established. To evaluate a particular arterial segment, a 10-mL bolus at a concentration of 300 mg/mL is usually adequate for color and spectral Doppler. If there is partial visualization of the artery at baseline, a lower dose and concentration (16 mL of 200 mg/mL) can be tried. Correas and others[19] described a 1.5-mL bolus of 300 mg/mL, followed by an infusion of 1.0 mL/min. If there is color blooming, the infusion rate is reduced. If the enhancement is inadequate, the concentration can be increased to 400 mg/mL.

Spinazzi and Llull[20] reported on the use of SonoVue (Bracco, Italy), a second-generation agent, in various parts of the circulatory system. The anatomic areas studies were the peripheral arteries (58 patients), the extracranial carotid arteries (59 patients), the abdominal or renal arteries (55 patients), and the intracranial arteries (78 patients). The examinations of all patients were compared with reference ultrasound visualization standards. All subjects had baseline scans that were not fully diagnostic. The patients then underwent color or power Doppler examination, followed by spectral Doppler, utilizing one of four doses of Sonovue. For extracranial carotid and peripheral arteries, the percent agreement with the standard was significantly improved above baseline for the majority of readers. The best results were at the highest dose (2.4-mL bolus), where the agreement improved from 31% to 69%.

CEREBROVASCULAR APPLICATIONS

Several investigators have used contrast enhancement for the evaluation of the internal carotid artery. Most have evaluated the vexing problem of distinguishing carotid occlusion from pseudo-occlusion (near occlusion) (Fig. 4–6).[21–23]

Furst and associates[23] evaluated 20 patients with angiographically proven internal carotid artery pseudo-occlusion and compared the findings with those in a controlled group of 13 patients with occlusion. Sensitivity and specificity were 70% and 92%, respectively, for unenhanced color Doppler and 83% and 92%, respectively, for Levovist-enhanced color Doppler. The results for enhanced power Doppler were 94% and 100%, respectively. This did not represent a significant increase in accuracy,

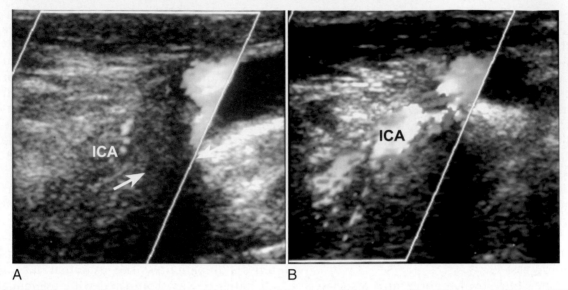

A   B

Figure 4–6. Carotid pseudo-occlusion. *A,* In a patient following endarterectomy, the internal carotid artery (ICA) ends abruptly. There is also shadowing (*arrow*) at the common carotid–internal carotid junction causing a break in the color column. *B,* Following contrast enhancement, color Doppler shows that the internal carotid is patent and there is a continuous color column from the common carotid throughout the internal carotid.

as unenhanced power Doppler was also quite accurate, being 95% sensitive and 92% specific.

Ferrer and associates[22] studied 88 patients with Doppler-diagnosed carotid occlusion who also underwent contrast-enhanced ultrasound. Levovist was injected at a concentration of 300 mg/mL in 79 patients, and in 9 patients, a second injection of 400 mg/mL was given because the first dose was inadequate. Three patients were excluded from the study. Of the 85 remaining patients, 7 were found to have a patent carotid artery by contrast-enhanced ultrasound, and all were subsequently confirmed to be patent angiographically.

Droste and associates[21] report that contrast enhancement can help clarify ultrasound assessment of the technically challenging vertebral artery. They report an improvement in differentiating vertebral occlusion from hypoplasia.

More recently, Kono and coinvestigators[24] used wide-band harmonic gray-scale to image carotid stenosis. In 20 patients, Optison (a suspension of a fluorocarbon in an albumin solution) (Amersham Health, Princeton, NJ) was injected in multiple boluses of 0.5 to 1.0 mL (up to the maximum allowable dose of 8.7 mL). Gray-scale images were obtained in long and short axis, and the degree of stenosis was measured using the technique described in the North American Symptomatic Carotid Endarterectomy Trial. In the 10 patients who underwent angiography, the correlation coefficient between contrast ultrasound angiography and conventional arteriography was 0.988 ($P < 0.001$). In two patients, calcifications obscured the lumen.

Currently, more research attention is being paid to the arterial wall itself, rather than the degree of lumenal narrowing, both to characterize atherosclerotic plaque and to study preclinical disease using intima-media thickness measurements and endothelial dysfunction. Contrast-enhanced ultrasound is being investigated for intima-media thickness measurement to better define the near wall of the carotid artery and to define the blood vessel interface with greater precision[25] (see Fig. 4–2). Endothelial injury and atherosclerotic lesions are being studied in experimental models.[26,27] The study by Kono and associates[28] also evaluated plaque appearance in human subjects. Plaque irregularities and a case of dissection not recognized by unenhanced gray-scale imaging were seen in several of their patients.

RENAL ARTERY APPLICATIONS

The use of ultrasound for detection of renal artery stenosis is a challenging but important duplex application. The renal arteries are deep seated within the abdomen, and in many individuals they also are tortuous, making ultrasound evaluation along the course of the vessel difficult. Accuracy in evaluating the main renal artery is directly related to the length of the vessel that can be insonated.

Missouris and coauthors[29] have investigated intrarenal waveforms following contrast administration. Levovist (10 mL at a 300-mg/mL concentration) was used in 21 subjects. Renal artery examination time was reduced from 25 to 14 minutes, the sensitivity for stenosis improved from 85% to 94%, and the specificity improved from 79% to 88% following contrast administration.

Most of the evaluation for renal artery stenosis has concerned the main renal artery (see Fig. 4–3). Melany and colleagues[30] reported improved visualization of the main renal artery and detected two additional stenoses of a total of eight after injection of perflenapent, a discontinued agent.

A Canadian multicenter trial utilized seven sites to assess renal artery stenosis in 78 patients.[31] Multiple boluses of Levovist at 300 mg/mL were utilized. Renal artery diagnosis was not possible in 18% of baseline studies, due to poor arterial visualization, whereas only 1% of studies remained inadequate after contrast enhancement. Complete visualization of the left and right main renal arteries was significantly increased after contrast (from 61% to 87% on the right and from 58% to 92% on the left). In 63 of 64 patients with an adequate noncontrast baseline scan, contrast ultrasound findings were the same as for the unenhanced scans. Sensitivity and specificity could not be determined, as only 14 patients underwent angiography. There was agreement between angiography and enhanced ultrasound in 12 patients (86%), compared to angiography in 11 patients with unenhanced ultrasound. Scintigraphy had only a 64% correlation. An economic evaluation revealed that the management costs were lower after contrast-enhanced ultrasound due to the higher success rate at reaching a conclusive diagnosis.[32]

A European trial of contrast-enhanced renal artery sonography consisted of 198 patients, all of whom underwent angiography.[33] Levovist dosage was determined by how well the renal artery was seen at baseline. It was possible to visualize a sufficient length of the renal artery to diagnose or exclude stenosis in 84% of 191 patients. This represented a significant improvment compared with 64% with unenhanced ultrasound. There was also significant improvement when visualization was compared on a per-kidney basis. Although different centers used different criteria for measuring renal artery stenosis, agreement with angiography improved significantly after contrast enhancement, from 52% unenhanced to 70% enhanced ($P = 0.001$) on an individual patient basis, and from 66% unenhanced to 78% enhanced on a per-kidney basis ($P = 0.001$). However, sensitivity and specificity for renal artery stenosis did not significantly improve after contrast enhancement. Sensitivity increased from 80% to 84% ($P = 0.248$) and specificity from 81% to 86% ($P = 0.665$). The significant agreement between baseline and contrast studies was due to relatively few inadequate noncontrast studies. The results show that the ability to visualize the renal arteries improves after contrast administration, but this does not necessarily result in a more accurate examination.

Frauscher and coworkers[34] used Levovist to detect crossing vessels in 29 patients with ureteropelvic junction obstruction. The detection of crossing vessels increased significantly ($P < 0.16$), from 65% to 96%, using Levovist. Vessels were detected in 22 of 23 laparoscopically confirmed cases. (Only a 2-mm–diameter posterior vein was missed.)

MESENTERIC AND HEPATIC ARTERY APPLICATIONS

Blebea and associates[35] investigated mesenteric vessels utilizing an infusion of Definity (perflutren) (Bristol Myers Squibb Medical Imaging, Billerica, MA) infusion.

Duplex Doppler without and with contrast enhancement was compared with angiography in 17 patients. The accuracy of the unenhanced study was 82% compared with 88% after contrast enhancement. The non-visualization rate went from 12 vessels to 3 after injection. Unenhanced celiac axis scans overcalled obstructive lesions in one vessel and did not detect obstruction in two others. After contrast administration, all celiac arteries were identified, but two vessels were falsely called stenotic (post-contrast velocities were higher than 300 cm/sec).The greatest improvement in this study concerned superior mesenteric artery diagnosis, where accuracy changed from 71% to 94%. After contrast administration, two occlusions and three stenoses were correctly identified, while baseline, non-contrast examinations missed one occlusion and one stenosis. Noncontrast accuracy for the inferior mesenteric artery was poor, at only 35%. The addition of contrast improved the accuracy to only 38%. For all vessels (aorta, superior mesenteric artery, celiac artery, and inferior mesenteric artery), stenosis or occlusion was correctly detected in 81% after contrast, compared with 55% at baseline. The specificity was similar—84% after contrast and 79% at baseline. The improvement was most evident in the celiac and superior mesenteric arteries, but the results did not reach statistical significance.

Hepatic transplants were studied using a UCA by Sidhu and colleagues[36] to detect the cause of a parvus tardus waveform in the hepatic artery. Although the agent allowed better delineation of the hepatic artery, postcontrast peak systolic velocities did not always accurately determine the degree of stenosis compared with arteriography. The agent permitted the confident diagnosis of an occluded vessel but could not eliminate the need for angiography to determine the number, grade, and lengths of hepatic artery stenoses.

ENDOVASCULAR GRAFT EVALUATION

Aortic endovascular stent graft placement requires postprocedural monitoring. Several investigators have reported on contrast-enhanced ultrasound for detection of graft complications, notably endoleaks. Ultrasound can evaluate the graft over several minutes, so that both fast-flowing and slow-flowing endoleaks can be detected, either by a color flow signal or an increase in echogenicity between the aneurysm sac and the graft (Fig. 4–7). This is a potential advantage over computed tomographic (CT) scanning, since the post-contrast CT scans may cover only one or a few time phases following contrast administration. Slow endoleaks may be overlooked if time delays are too short. Ultrasound may also determine the direction of flow in the leak, which may not be possible with CT. However, bowel gas may obscure part of the graft during ultrasound examination, and stent fractures may be missed by ultrasound as well.[37]

Early results with Levovist have shown endoleaks not visible prior to contrast administration.[38–40] In a follow-up to one of these studies, McWilliams and colleagues[41] evaluated 53 patients. Although they detected more leaks after contrast administration, contrast enhancement still failed to detect several type II endoleaks,* compared with biphasic (arterial and delayed phase) CT. In a more recent trial, Bendick and associates[42] reported excellent endoleak results using Optison. One cubic cm of the agent was injected with a 5-mL saline flush, and scans where obtained after 1 minute. The graft was scanned in gray-scale harmonic mode. Baseline ultrasound detected six endoleaks, and delayed-phase CT detected eight endoleaks. All eight were seen on the contrast-enhanced ultrasound, and it was possible to determine if they were type I or II endoleaks* using the UCA. Additionally, two proximal attachment leaks not seen with CT were visualized with contrast sonography and were subsequently shown at angiography. Nelms and colleagues[43] have also reported using Optison but in smaller doses (0.3 mL and up to three injections) than Bendick and associates[42] described. This group also detected four cases of extragraft flow not seen with CT,

*See Chapter 30.

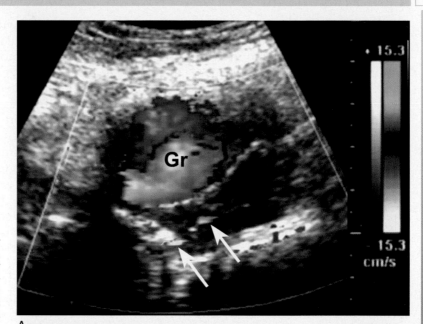

FIGURE 4–7. Endoleaks after aortic stent graft placement. *A*, Color Doppler obtained after injection of contrast demonstrates abnormal color (*arrows*) between the aortic wall and the stent graft (Gr). This could be traced to a lumbar artery. *B*, Pulse inversion harmonic imaging in a different patient demonstrates contrast (*arrow*) in the posterior aspect of the aneurysm sac distant from the enhanced graft seen more anteriorly. This was subsequently proven to be a type II endoleak. (Cases courtesy of Kathleen Carter, RN, FSVU, Richmond, VA.)

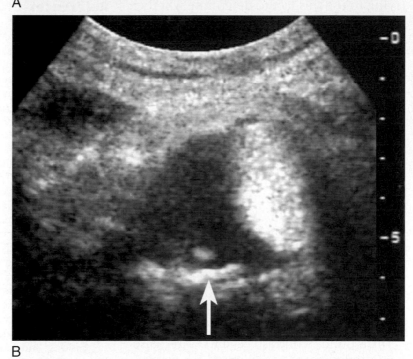

and at least one case was confirmed angiographically. For CT-confirmed endoleaks, ultrasound contrast improved visualization of the leak and facilitated detection of the source of leakage. These positive results concerning endograft assessment warrant further investigation with newer ultrasound contrast agents.

NEW TECHNIQUES

Intermittent pulses of ultrasound can destroy microbubbles in an insonated region, followed by replenishment of the agent by the blood pool. Therefore, the flow of blood into an organ can be investigated sonographically. The replenishment rate is related to the blood volume and the microbubble velocity, and these variables can be correlated with blood flow, as investigated in dogs using SonoVue.[44] In this study, the measurement of renal blood flow by the contrast-enhanced blood flow replenishment method correlated well with actual blood flow (R = 0.82; $P < 0.001$). In another study, renal transplant recipients were investigated using pulse inversion gray-scale ultrasound to generate time-intensity curves after bolus UCS injection. This work showed some differences between pathologic and normally functioning kidney transplants.[45]

Other novel uses of contrast agents are being investigated. The response of the bubble to ultrasound is related to the pressure around the bubble. Investigators are trying to use this fact to determine whether UCAs can be used to measure blood pressure noninvasively.[46]

Ultrasound contrast agents are generally thought of as blood pool agents that flow passively with the blood products; however, active, targeted contrast agents are being designed, and early research work in this area is ongoing.[47] UCAs have been targeted to atherosclerotic plaque and thrombus, both in vitro and in vivo.[48-50] The agent actively attaches to the designated target, increasing the echogenicity of the target surface relative to the unenhanced vessel. This approach might aid the detection of important findings, such as thrombus associated with plaque that might require a different type of therapy than the plaque itself. Investigators are also attempting to use targeted UCAs to identify different surface characteristics of the vessel wall.[27]

Ultrasound contrast agents are also being investigated as a method for accelerating thrombolysis.[47,48] Microbubble agents have also been proposed as a means for delivering therapeutic agents, such as chemotherapy or gene therapy, directly to a diseased vessel or organ.[47]

CONCLUSIONS

Contrast enhancement has been shown in many studies to improve visualization of blood vessels with ultrasound. In some cases, UCAs have improved the detection of pathology, but most studies have been small in scale and largely anecdotal. Larger trials are required to determine if the use of ultrasound contrast can be translated into more accurate or more cost-effective diagnoses. However, the lack of commercially available diagnostic contrast agents in the United States has restricted their more widespread investigation. Two important trends that may affect the future role of UCAs are ongoing improvements in ultrasound technology, which permit ultrasound instruments to better capitalize on the unique characteristics of microbubble agents, and the development of agents designed for therapeutic uses.

References

1. Goldberg BB, Liu JB, Forsberg F: Ultrasound contrast agents: A review. Ultrasound Med Biol 20:319–333, 1994.
2. Burns P, Powers JE, Fritzsch T: Harmonic imaging: A new imaging and Doppler method for contrast enhanced ultrasound. Radiology 185(P):142, 1992.
3. Simpson DH, Chin CT, Burns PN: Pulse inversion Doppler: A new method for detecting nonlinear echoes from microbubble contrast agents. IEEE Trans Ultrason Ferroelectr Freq Control 46:372–382, 1999.
4. de Jong N, Bouakaz A, Frinking PJA, et al: Contrast-specific imaging methods. In Goldberg BB, Raichlen JS, Forsberg F (eds): Ultrasound Contrast Agents: Basic Principles and Clinical Applications, 2nd ed. London: Martin Dunitz, 2001, pp 25–36.
5. Kono Y, Mattrey RF: Harmonic imaging with contrast microbubbles. In Goldberg BB, Raichlen JS, Forsberg F (eds): Ultrasound Contrast Agents: Basic Principles and Clinical Applications, 2nd ed. London: Martin Dunitz, 2001, pp 37–46.
6. Burns PN, Wilson SR, Simpson DH: Pulse inversion imaging of liver blood flow: Improved method for characterizing focal masses with microbubble contrast. Invest Radiol 35:58–71, 2000.
7. Wheatley MA, Schrope B, Shen P: Contrast agents for diagnostic ultrasound: Development and evaluation of polymer-coated microbubbles. Biomaterials 11:713–717, 1990.
8. Forsberg F, Liu JB, Burns PN, et al: Artifacts in ultrasonic contrast agent studies. J Ultrasound Med 13:357–365, 1994.

9. Forsberg F, Shi WT: Physics of contrast micro-bubbles. In Goldberg BB, Raichlen JS, Forsberg F (eds): Ultrasound Contrast Agents: Basic Principles and Clinical Applications, 2nd ed. London: Martin Dunitz, 2001, pp 15–24.

10. Khan HG, Gailloud P, Bude RO, et al: The effect of contrast material on transcranial Doppler evaluation of normal middle cerebral artery peak systolic velocity. Am J Neuroradiol 21: 386–390, 2000.

11. Needleman L, Forsberg F, Malguria NO, et al: US contrast does not change canine renal Doppler pulsatility indices. Radiology 209(P): 461, 1998.

12. Gutberlet M, Venz S, Zendel W, et al: Do ultrasonic contrast agents artificially increase maximum Doppler shift? In vivo study of human common carotid arteries. J Ultrasound Med 17:97–102, 1998.

13. Basseau F, Grenier N, Trillaud H, et al: Doppler frequency shift and time-domain velocity enhancement induced by an ultrasonographic contrast agent. J Ultrasound Med 19:171–176, 2000.

14. Kroger K, Massalha K, Rudofsky G: The use of the echo-enhancing agent Levovist does not influence the estimation of the degree of vascular stenosis calculated from peak systolic velocity ratio, diameter reduction and cross-section area reduction. Eur J Ultrasound 8:17–24, 1998.

15. Needleman L, Goldberg BB, Feld RI, et al: Evaluation of arterial diseases in humans using an ultrasound contrast agent. J Ultrasound Med 13:S48, 1994.

16. Schwarz KQ, Becher H, Schimpfky C, et al: Doppler enhancement with SH U 508A in multiple vascular regions. Radiology 193:195–201, 1994.

17. Langholz J, Schlief R, Schurmann R, et al: Contrast enhancement in leg vessels. Clin Radiol 1996:31–34, 1996.

18. Albrecht T, Urbank A, Mahler M, et al: Prolongation and optimization of Doppler enhancement with a microbubble US contrast agent by using continuous infusion: Preliminary experience. Radiology 207:339–347, 1998.

19. Correas JM, Boespflug O, Hamida K, et al: Doppler ultrasonography of peripheral vascular disease: The potential for ultrasound contrast agents. J Comp Assist Tomogr 23(Suppl 1): S119–S127, 1999.

20. Spinazzi A, Llull JB: Diagnostic performance of SonoVue-enhanced color duplex sonography of vascular structures. Acad Radiol 9(Suppl 1): S246–S250, 2002.

21. Droste DW, Kaps M, Navabi DG, et al: Ultrasound contrast enhancing agents in neurosonology: Principles, methods, future possibilities. Acta Neurol Scand 102:1–10, 2000.

22. Ferrer JM, Samso JJ, Serrando JR, et al: Use of ultrasound contrast in the diagnosis of carotid artery occlusion. J Vasc Surg 31:736–741, 2000.

23. Furst G, Saleh A, Wenserski F, et al: Reliability and validity of noninvasive imaging of internal carotid artery pseudo-occlusion. Stroke 30: 1444–1449, 1999.

24. Kono Y, Pinnell SP, Sirlin CB, et al: Carotid arteries: Contrast-enhanced US angiography—preliminary clinical experience. Radiology 230: 561–568, 2004.

25. Feinstein SB, Voci P, Pizzuto F: Noninvasive surrogate markers of atherosclerosis. Am J Cardiol 89:31C–43C; discussion, 43C–44C, 2002.

26. Sirlin CB, Lee YZ, Girard MS, et al: Contrast-enhanced B-mode US angiography in the assessment of experimental in vivo and in vitro atherosclerotic disease. Acad Radiol 8:162–172, 2001.

27. Villanueva FS, Wagner WR, Klibanov AL: Targeted ultrasound contrast agents: Identification of endothelial dysfunction. In Goldberg BB, Raichlen JS, Forsberg F (eds): Ultrasound Contrast Agents: Basic Principles and Clinical Applications, 2nd ed. London: Martin Dunitz, 2001, pp 353–365.

28. Kono Y, Moriyasu F, Nada T, et al: Gray scale second harmonic imaging of the liver: A preliminary animal study. Ultrasound Med Biol 23:719–726, 1997.

29. Missouris CG, Allen CM, Balen FG, et al: Noninvasive screening for renal artery stenosis with ultrasound contrast enhancement. J Hypertens 14:519–524, 1996.

30. Melany ML, Grant EG, Duerinckx AJ, et al: Ability of a phase shift US contrast agent to improve imaging of the main renal arteries. Radiology 205:147–152, 1997.

31. Lacourciere Y, Levesque J, Onrot JM, et al: Impact of Levovist ultrasonographic contrast agent on the diagnosis and management of hypertensive patients with suspected renal artery stenosis: A Canadian multicentre pilot study. Can Assoc Radiol J 53:219–227, 2002.

32. Levesque J, Lacourciere Y, Onrot JM, et al: Economic impact of an ultrasonographic contrast agent on the diagnosis and initial management of patients with suspected renal artery stenosis. Can Assoc Radiol J 53:228–236, 2002.

33. Claudon M, Plouin PF, Baxter GM, et al: Renal arteries in patients at risk of renal arterial stenosis: Multicenter evaluation of the echo-enhancer SH U 508A at color and spectral Doppler US. Levovist Renal Artery Stenosis Study Group. Radiology 214:739–746, 2000.

34. Frauscher F, Janetschek G, Helweg G, et al: Crossing vessels at the ureteropelvic junction: Detection with contrast-enhanced color Doppler imaging. Radiology 210:727–731, 1999.

35. Blebea J, Volteas N, Neumyer M, et al: Contrast enhanced duplex ultrasound imaging of the mesenteric arteries. Ann Vasc Surg 16:77–83, 2002.

36. Sidhu PS, Ellis SM, Karani JB, et al: Hepatic artery stenosis following liver transplantation: Significance of the tardus parvus waveform and the role of microbubble contrast media in the detection of a focal stenosis. Clin Radiol 57:789–799, 2002.

37. Heilberger P, Schunn C, Ritter W, et al: Postoperative color flow duplex scanning in aortic endografting. J Endovasc Surg 4:262–271, 1997.

38. McWilliams RG, Martin J, White D, et al: Use of contrast-enhanced ultrasound in follow-up after endovascular aortic aneurysm repair. J Vasc Interv Radiol 10:1107–1114, 1999.

39. Giannoni MF, Bilotta F, Fiorani L, et al: Ultrasound echo-enhancers in the evaluation of endovascular prostheses. Cardiovasc Surg 7: 532–538, 1999.

40. Giannoni MF, Palombo G, Sbarigia E, et al: Contrast-enhanced ultrasound imaging for aortic stent-graft surveillance. J Endovasc Ther 10: 208–217, 2003.

41. McWilliams RG, Martin J, White D, et al: Detection of endoleak with enhanced ultrasound imaging: Comparison with biphasic computed tomography. J Endovasc Ther 9:170–179, 2002.

42. Bendick PJ, Bove PG, Long GW, et al: Efficacy of ultrasound scan contrast agents in the noninvasive follow-up of aortic stent grafts. J Vasc Surg 37:381–385, 2003.

43. Nelms CR, Carter K, Meier G, et al: A technique to improve the confidence of color duplex ultrasound assessment of aortic endografts: The use of contrast agents. J Vasc Ultrasound (in press).

44. Wei K, Le E, Bin JP, et al: Quantification of renal blood flow with contrast-enhanced ultrasound. J Am Coll Cardiol 37:1135–1140, 2001.

45. Lefevre F, Correas JM, Briancon S, et al: Contrast-enhanced sonography of the renal transplant using triggered pulse-inversion imaging: Preliminary results. Ultrasound Med Biol 28:303–314, 2002.

46. Shi WT, Forsberg F, Raichlen JS, et al: Pressure dependence of subharmonic signals from contrast microbubbles. Ultrasound Med Biol 25:275–283, 1999.

47. Unger EC, Matsunaga TO, McCreery T, et al: Therapeutic applications of microbubbles. Eur J Radiol 42:160–168, 2002.

48. Unger E, Wu Q, McCreery T, et al: Thrombus-specific contrast agents for imaging and thrombolysis. In Goldberg BB, Raichlen JS, Forsberg F (eds): Ultrasound Contrast Agents: Basic Principles and Clinical Applications, 2nd ed. London, Martin Dunitz, 2001, pp 337–346.

49. Unger E, Metzger P 3rd, Krupinski E, et al: The use of a thrombus-specific ultrasound contrast agent to detect thrombus in arteriovenous fistulae. Invest Radiol 35:86–89, 2000.

50. Porter TR, Xie F: Targeted drug delivery using intravenous microbubbles. In Goldberg BB, Raichlen JS, Forsberg F (eds): Ultrasound Contrast Agents: Basic Principles and Clinical Applications, 2nd ed. London: Martin Dunitz, 2001, pp 347–352.

SECTION II

CEREBRAL VESSELS

The Role of Ultrasound in the Management of Cerebrovascular Disease

ANDREI V. ALEXANDROV, MD, RVT

Stroke is a major social and healthcare burden, with more than 700,000 people suffering from it annually in the United States. It is the leading cause of permanent disability, and its annual cost to patients, hospitals, and society is estimated at 51 billion U.S. dollars.[1] Cerebrovascular ultrasound has established applications in the detection of stroke risk factors and mechanisms, screening for therapeutic, surgical, and catheter-based interventions, and monitoring of arterial lesions responsible for stroke symptoms. Ultrasound provides a fast, portable, noninvasive, repeatable, and inexpensive technique for vascular diagnosis. Ultrasound in stroke care directly impacts on clinical decision-making in the following situations:[2]

- The early detection, quantification, and characterization of extracranial atherosclerosis and occlusive disease, especially at the carotid bifurcation
- The consequences of proximal arterial occlusive disease on the distal cerebral vasculature
- The detection of microemboli associated with cardiac and aortic pathology and carotid artery surgical manipulation (and perhaps gauging response to antiplatelet therapy)
- Selection of children with sickle cell disease for blood transfusion as an effective tool in primary stroke prevention
- The natural history and response to treatment of acute arterial occlusion that causes hyperacute stroke

- The time course and reversibility of cerebral vasospasm after subarachnoid hemorrhage

This chapter describes the use of cerebrovascular ultrasound tests in elective screening; i.e., outpatient diagnostic work-up, and at bedside for patients with acute neurologic problems.

DEFINITIONS OF TRANSIENT ISCHEMIC ATTACK AND STROKE

Transient ischemic attack (TIA) is a medical emergency, since well-documented measures help prevent stroke if they are implemented in a timely manner. The complete resolution of focal cerebral ischemic symptoms within 24 hours has been used to differentiate between the diagnosis of stroke and TIA. However, the majority of TIAs resolve within minutes, and advanced neuroimaging studies demonstrate that longer-lasting symptoms are likely, in fact, to be strokes.[3] TIAs have a more serious prognostic implication then previously appreciated. After a TIA occurs, about 10% of patients will have a stroke in the next 3 months, and almost half of these strokes will develop within the first 2 days after the initial symptoms.[4] Since TIA is a highly predictive risk factor for stroke, patients with TIA need to be evaluated in a timely and comprehensive manner when the diagnosis is suspected. Clinical history, knowledge of neurologic symptoms, and timely performance of brain imaging tests are essential in the work-up of these patients.

Data from the National Institutes of Neurological Disorders and Stroke (NINDS) rt-PA Stroke Study is helpful to draw an arbitrary time line between TIA and stroke. In this pivotal trial of thrombolytic therapy for ischemic stroke, half of patients with acute symptoms of cerebral ischemia received a placebo, and all of them had persisting neurologic deficits for at least 1 hour. At 24 hours after symptom onset, only 2.6% had recovered completely in the placebo group.[5] Therefore, from a clinical perspective, patients who have symptoms lasting for at least 1 hour have a 97% chance of having a stroke and should be evaluated emergently. The current time window for initiating the only approved therapy, systemic tissue plasminogen activator (TPA), is 3 hours after symptom onset. However, the majority of stroke patients arrive at a hospital outside this strict time window. Despite this, diagnostic testing of patients with symptoms lasting longer than 3 hours should be prioritized and accomplished in a timely manner, since effective measures to prevent stroke recurrence exist and depend on knowledge of the stroke pathogenic mechanism.[6]

Elective Cerebrovascular Ultrasound Testing

Screening for Carotid Artery Disease

Classic Neurologic Manifestations of Ischemic Stroke or TIA

Carotid arteries supply the middle cerebral and anterior cerebral arteries of the brain, and these territories are responsible for so-called anterior circulation symptoms such as unilateral weakness (arm more than leg), aphasia (difficulties with word finding or understanding), hemianopsia (partial loss of visual field), and amaurosis fugax (transient monocular blindness).

As illustrated in Chapter 6, the vertebral arteries unite to form the basilar artery, and together, these vessels supply the brainstem, cerebellum, midbrain, and visual cortex— vascular territories known as the posterior circulation. Symptoms attributable to the posterior circulation include unilateral weakness, dysarthria (slurred speech), dizziness, ataxia (disturbance of movement coordination), loss of consciousness, and cortical blindness.

Although general recognition of stroke symptoms is a relatively easy task, localization of the ischemic process may be challenging, even for neurologists, since both arterial distributions (anterior and posterior) may present with similar symptoms. Upon admission, a stroke patient undergoes computed tomography of the brain to differentiate bleeding (hemorrhagic stroke) from ischemia. Clinical localization of stroke symptoms is usually confirmed using magnetic resonance imaging of the brain, which shows better than CT the brain areas affected by ischemia.

Mechanisms of Ischemic Stroke or TIA

Stroke neurologists commonly use the so-called TOAST classification of stroke pathogenic mechanisms:[7]

- Large vessel athero-thrombotic stroke
- Cardio-embolic stroke
- Lacunar stroke
- Other (dissection, coagulopathy, paradoxical embolism, etc)
- Undetermined

Patients with large vessel athero-thrombotic stroke have imaging evidence of diameter reduction of the vessel by plaque or thrombus of more than 50%. These patients may suffer stroke due to hypoperfusion when severe proximal internal carotid artery (ICA) stenosis is coupled with poor collateralization. Alternatively, stroke may result from artery-to-artery embolization, commonly from a thrombogenic plaque surface, with variable degree of carotid stenosis. As many as 90% of ischemic strokes occur in the carotid artery territories. These patients represent the target group for screening the carotid arteries with ultrasound.

Patients with cardiogenic strokes suffer from embolism that originates in heart chambers. For example, patients with atrial fibrillation ("irregular-irregular" heart rhythm) are at high risk of forming a thrombus and embolizing brain vessels. This risk is reduced by anticoagulation with warfarin.[8] Carotid plaque and stenosis may also be found in these patients.

Patients suffering from so-called lacunar strokes develop occlusive lesions in the small perforating vessels of the brain that are currently below the resolution of ultrasound imaging systems. Nevertheless, strokes in the small vessel territory still require diagnostic work-up to exclude concomitant large vessel atherosclerosis as a potential contributing risk factor.

The first three types of stroke pathogenesis listed above account for approximately 30%, 35%, and 10% of all strokes, respectively, while other stroke types usually represent 10% of cases. In about 15% of stroke patients, clinical, radiologic, and other diagnostic studies reveal no identifiable risk factor, and the stroke mechanism in these patients remains undetermined.

Overall, the indications for first-ever carotid duplex ultrasound examination include:

1. Symptoms of stroke or TIA attributable to carotid artery distribution
2. Carotid bruit
3. Suspicion of carotid stenosis from other imaging tests such as magnetic resonance angiography
4. Preoperative screening for carotid stenosis
5. Assessment of a high cardiovascular risk patient

Carotid Endarterectomy Trials

Carotid endarterectomy (CEA) trials played a pivotal role in finding effective stroke prevention measures in patients with carotid atherosclerosis.[9-11] They established the levels of ICA stenosis in patients with a history of stroke or TIA when surgery is beneficial (i.e., >70%), when surgery is potentially better that antiplatelet therapy (50%–69%), and when medical therapy is better than surgical intervention (i.e., <50%) in the affected carotid artery distribution. Table 5–1 shows the increasing risk of stroke with increasing degree of extracra-.

Table 5–1. The Risk of Stroke and the Severity of Carotid Stenosis in Symptomatic Patients in the NASCET Trial

ICA Stenosis*	Medical Group[†]	Surgical Group[‡]	NNT[§]
70%–99%	26.1%	12.9%	8
50%–69%	22.2%	15.7%	15
<50%	18.7%	14.9%	26

*ICA stenosis is expressed as percent diameter reduction of the residual lumen on digital subtraction angiography measured by the North American (N) method.
[†]The "Medical Group" received antiplatelet therapy to prevent stroke.
[‡]The "Surgical Group" underwent CEA within 6 mo after TIA or minor stroke.
[§]NNT is the number of patients needed to treat to prevent one stroke.
CEA, carotid endarterectomy; ICA, internal carotid artery; TIA, transient ischemic attack.
From North American Symptomatic Carotid Endarterectomy Trial Collaborators: Beneficial effect of carotid endarterectomy in symptomatic patients with high-grade carotid stenosis. N Engl J Med 325:445–453, 1991, and Barnett HJ, Taylor DW, Eliasziw M, et al: Benefit of carotid endarterectomy in patients with symptomatic moderate or severe stenosis. North American Symptomatic Carotid Endarterectomy Trial Collaborators. N Engl J Med 339:1415–1425, 1998.

nial ICA stenosis and risk reduction with CEA. Risk of perioperative stroke and death is higher in patients with widespread leukoaraiosis, those with occlusion of the contralateral internal carotid artery, and those with intraluminal thrombus.[12] However, these patients still benefit from treatment. Patients with 50% to 69% stenosis experience lesser benefit, and some other groups may even be harmed by carotid endarterectomy, including women and patients with only transient monocular blindness.[12] Finally, a high-risk group for CEA is identified by the presence of severe coronary artery disease, chronic obstructive lung disease, or renal insufficiency, in whom CEA is associated with higher perioperative risk of stroke and death.[13]

In asymptomatic patients with ICA stenosis of more than 60%, CEA reduces absolute risk of first-ever stroke from 2% per year to 1% per year. This translates into the "number needed to treat," which is equal to 83 patients that need to undergo CEA to prevent one stroke in 2 years.[12] Furthermore, patient life expectancy should exceed 5 years to accumulate any significant benefit from this procedure. Performance of CEA in controlled clinical trials had a better safety profile than it did community practice. Increased perioperative risks may completely outweigh benefits of CEA in asymptomatic patients.[12,14] Nevertheless, selected patients with asymptomatic carotid stenosis may undergo CEA if they are found to have a "high-risk" plaque on B-mode ultrasound, frequent distal embolization, or impaired vasomotor reactivity on transcranial Doppler (TCD). These ancillary criteria were derived from smaller controlled cohort or observational studies that are discussed in the following subsections.

Although carotid endarterectomy is a durable procedure,[12] its use in a community setting may yield higher perioperative risks,[14] and the appropriate patient selection is of paramount importance. Initial diagnostic work-up with a combination of ultrasound and magnetic resonance angiography is a common clinical pathway that results in low carotid stenosis misclassification rates compared with catheter-based digital subtraction angiography.[15] However, in an attempt not to miss severe stenosis, digital subtraction angiography may still be used in selected patients, particularly when magnetic resonance angiography and ultrasound are discrepant.[16,17]

Carotid interventions to prevent stroke, such as angioplasty and stenting, are emerging as alternatives to CEA.[18] Carotid stenting can be offered to patients with high risk of peri-procedural complications of CEA (e.g., those with coronary, pulmonary, or renal diseases) or in a situation when carotid atheromas extend beyond the accessible surgical field. Otherwise, the safety and efficacy of stenting are now being compared in randomized clinical trials, and the indications for CEA and stenting will be redefined in the near future.

It is extremely important to carefully apply the results of the clinical trials in clinical practice to minimize risks associated with CEA. These steps include risk factor assessment[12] and application of the specific methods of measuring carotid stenosis in selecting patients for surgery.[19,20] Local criteria for grading carotid stenosis with ultrasound should be validated and set to predict an operable range of carotid stenosis, as defined by pivotal clinical trials.[9-11,21] These randomized trials used digital subtraction angiography as the definitive diagnostic test to measure the degree of carotid stenosis, expressed as the percent *linear diameter* reduction of the vessel as measured by strict and specific methods. To apply these methods, only one view of the tightest residual lumen (d) was selected and compared with the normal diameter (n). The stenosis is calculated using the formula:

$$\text{ICA Diameter Reduction} = (1 - d/n) \times 100\%,$$

where d and n are the diameter measurements made on a hard copy film in millimeters.

The **North American (N) method**, or the **"distal" degree of stenosis**, was used in the Asymptomatic Carotid Atherosclerosis Study (ACAS) and the North American Symptomatic Carotid Endarterectomy Trial (NASCET). In these trials, the denominator, n, refers to the distal ICA.[19] The measurement is made using a jeweler's eyepiece and calipers at the segment of the far-distal ICA with parallel walls, well beyond the carotid bulb and any post-stenotic dilation.

The **European (E) method**, or the **"local" degree of stenosis**, was employed in the European Carotid Surgery Trial (ECST) and requires drawing an imaginary outline of the ICA bulb to estimate the normal dimensions of the vessel at the site of the tightest narrowing.[10] Although there is no objective way to decide where exactly the normal vessel wall is supposed to be on the digital subtraction angiography image, the E method showed good reproducibility between experienced observers and provides stenosis values closer to anatomic stenosis than the N method. For instance, a 70% N stenosis is equal to an 84% E stenosis and a 90% area stenosis.[20,22,23] This is largely due to the fact that the ICA bulb diameter estimate is greater than the diameter of the distal ICA in the normal vessel and its segment beyond the stenosis.

These methods of measuring carotid stenosis represent indexes rather than precise measurements of the disease severity, since they are based on the diameter reduction estimates derived from a single angiographic projection. The N method is now the most widely used for measuring carotid stenosis, predicting the risk of stroke, selecting patients for carotid endarterectomy, and evaluating the accuracy parameters of ultrasound screening. The Society of Radiologists in Ultrasound has developed multispecialty consensus criteria concerning the proper method for predicting the operable range (N method) of carotid stenosis from carotid duplex examination (Table 5–2). The Consensus Panel determined a set of criteria most suitable for grading a focal stenosis in the proximal ICA.[24] It is recommended to use these criteria if a laboratory is new and seeking a set of most applicable criteria for prospective validation. If a laboratory has previously developed a set of their own criteria, validated them, and continues to successfully use them in clinical practice, then there is no need to change diagnostic criteria.[24]

After CEA, carotid ultrasound should be used for noninvasive follow-up. If a patient remains asymptomatic, yearly follow-up is generally sufficient. If a patient had bilateral disease prior to CEA, an earlier follow-up at 3 to 6 months can be used to assess the degree of carotid stenosis contralateral to CEA. If a patient becomes symptomatic any time after CEA, carotid ultrasound should be repeated to identify possible thrombosis (with early symptom recurrence) or restenosis.

High-Risk Carotid Plaque

Severe carotid stenosis is found in only 14% to 21% of patients with hemispheric cerebral symptoms, and its prevalence varies with ethnicity.[25] The majority of stroke patients have mild or moderate carotid plaques. Some of these plaques may also cause symptoms and may be more prone to progression, rupture, and thrombosis. Brightness-modulated (B-mode) ultrasound imaging can directly visualize and characterize plaque burden and potentially identify high-risk carotid plaques early, during the presymptomatic stage. In clinical studies,[26–30] the following types of asymptomatic carotid plaque predicted higher risk of subsequent cerebral ischemic events:

- Hypoechoic plaque
- Types 1 and 2 echolucent plaques,[31] particularly with echolucent area adjacent to the lumen
- Heterogeneous plaque

Table 5–2. The Society of Radiologists in Ultrasound Consensus Criteria for Grading Carotid Stenosis

Stenosis Range N Method	ICA PSV	ICA/CCA PSV Ratio	ICA EDV	Plaque
Normal	<125 cm/sec	<2.0	<40 cm/sec	None
<50%	<125 cm/sec	<2.0	<40 cm/sec	<50% diameter reduction
50%–69%	125–230 cm/sec	2.0–4.0	40–100 cm/sec	>50% diameter reduction
70–near occlusion	>230 cm/sec	>4.0	>100 cm/sec	>50% diameter reduction
Near occlusion	May be low or undetectable	Variable	Variable	Significant, detectable lumen
Occlusion	Undetectable	Not applicable	Not applicable	Significant, no detectable lumen

CCA, common carotid artery; EDV, end-diastolic velocity; ICA, internal carotid artery; N, North American; PSV, peak systolic velocity.

The role of B-mode imaging in screening for carotid plaques is to characterize plaque location, length, composition, and surface. In addition to carotid stenosis measurement, B-mode provides information about plaque extent in symptomatic patients that can be helpful in surgical considerations. Plaque typing can be used to identify high-risk asymptomatic patients with significant stenosis who are suitable for surgery.[29,30] Emboli detection with TCD also provides additional evidence for active emboligenic plaque surfaces, and these emboli-positive plaques are associated with higher risk of cerebral ischemic events.[32] Figure 5–1 shows a heterogeneous plaque with real-time evidence of artery-to-artery embolization in the middle cerebral artery, as well as multiple cortical embolic strokes.

Carotid duplex is often used as a sole screening test before carotid endarterectomy, particularly at ultrasound facilities with documented and sustained accuracy.[33–36] However, positive identification of surgical candidates is only one of several outcomes of cerebrovascular ultrasound testing. Patients who had an ischemic cerebral event may also have bilateral (Fig. 5–2), tandem carotid lesions, distal carotid and intracranial arterial lesions, as well as variable sufficiency of collateral supply and vasomotor reserve. This additional information allows stroke neurologists to identify stroke mechanisms and to select management options besides surgery for stroke prevention. At our laboratory at the University of Texas Stroke Treatment Team in Houston, we routinely perform carotid/vertebral duplex scanning together with TCD in practically all patients admitted with stroke or TIA to identify multiple potential stroke mechanisms.

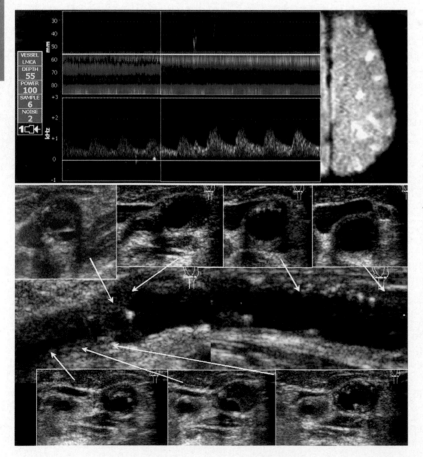

FIGURE 5–1. B-mode scans in the *lower panels* show longitudinal and transverse images of a heterogeneous plaque. *Arrows* show the locations of the transverse images. *Upper left and center panels* show transcranial power Doppler recordings of flow in the middle cerebral artery (MCA). Note the increase in velocity from the first to the second MCA segment, which is the result of a partially obstructing embolus from the internal carotid artery stenosis. The diffusion-weighted magnetic resonance image (*upper right panel*) shows multiple embolic strokes, also of carotid origin.

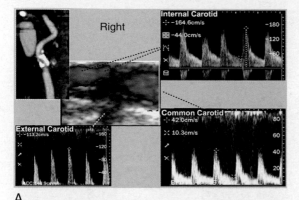

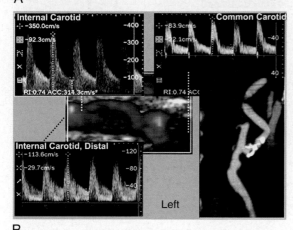

FIGURE 5–2. Bilateral carotid stenoses of 70% or more. The right internal carotid artery (ICA) (*A*) is more severely stenosed than the left ICA (*B*), which shows a compensatory velocity increase. Although peak systolic velocity in the right ICA is only 165 cm/sec compared with 350 cm/sec on the left, the ICA/common carotid artery (CCA) systolic velocity ratio is approximately 4.0 on both sides. This is due to greater reduction of the right CCA peak systolic velocity (PSV) 42 cm/sec compared with the left side, where CCA has a PSV of 84 cm/sec). Furthermore, lesion location in the right carotid system is more proximal and affects the right common carotid bifurcation, as shown by computed tomographic angiography (*image inserts*). Transcranial Doppler examination (not included here) showed that the left carotid system was providing collateral supply not only to the right carotid but also to the posterior circulation vessels, due to severe proximal basilar artery stenosis.

Other Roles of Extracranial Duplex Screening

Duplex technology can be used to determine if stroke patients have carotid lesions other than atherosclerosis. Examples include carotid thromboembolism, dissection, fibromuscular dysplasia, and radiation injury. These lesions have distinctively different appearances on B-mode ultrasound,

and their hemodynamic significance is determined using Doppler spectral data. When found, these lesions point to a specific stroke mechanism other that large vessel atherosclerosis,[37] and determination of such mechanisms can change treatment options for stroke patients.

Another role of extracranial duplex scanning is to determine the presence of verterbral arterial lesions in patients with neurologic symptoms that refer to the posterior cerebral circulation. Duplex ultrasound allows segmental assessment of the vertebral artery flow between transverse processes and visualization of the vertebral artery origins.[38,39] These segments should be thoroughly evaluated in patients with strokes or TIAs in the posterior circulation. The spectrum of vertebral pathology detectable by duplex scanning includes

- Vertebral artery stenosis (origin, V2, V3, and V4 segments)
- Vertebral artery occlusion or absence of flow due to congenital aplasia
- Hypoplastic vertebral artery
- Subclavian steal

If duplex ultrasound shows significant (>50%) vertebral stenosis or occlusion, along with evidence of plaque formation, this indicates that the mechanism of cerebral ischemic symptoms is likely large vessel atheromatous disease. Infrequently, duplex examination may show vertebral artery dissection,[40] and further testing is necessary to determine if it is an isolated vertebral dissection or an extension of aortic arch dissection. Further consideration should be given as to whether this dissection is spontaneous or trauma related.

Finally, the finding of subclavian steal (Fig. 5–3) is most often a harmless hemodynamic phenomenon that indicates the presence of atherosclerotic stenosis or occlusion in the subclavian artery. Occasionally, however, subclavian steal can produce symptoms related to transient hypoperfusion in the basilar artery.[41,42]

Screening for Intracranial Disease

The Warfarin Aspirin Intracranial Disease (WASID) trial[43,44] was terminated due to

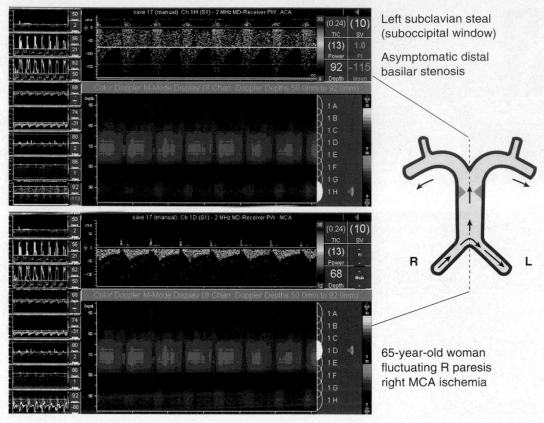

FIGURE 5–3. Transcranial Doppler spectral and motion mode findings in a 65-year-old woman with a fluctuating neurologic deficit due to ischemia in the right middle cerebral artery (MCA) distribution. M-mode transcranial Doppler shows alternating flow signal due to an asymptomatic right-to-left subclavian steal. More importantly, there is a focal velocity increase (2 : 1 compared with the terminal vertebral artery) and a bruit in the distal basilar artery, indicating stenosis of more than 50%.

excessive hemorrhagic complications and lack of efficacy for warfarin over aspirin to prevent recurrent stroke in patients with symptomatic intracranial stenoses of 50% or more. Nevertheless, intracranial vessel disease is recognized as an independent risk factor for stroke,[45–47] and attempts are continuing to develop therapies other than anticoagulation.[48–50]

Detection of intracranial stenoses using TCD is most reliable for the middle cerebral artery, terminal internal carotid artery, and basilar artery.[51–53] Various velocity thresholds have been introduced to predict significant intracranial stenosis. Since symptomatic middle cerebral artery (MCA) stenosis of 50% or more bears approximately 7% risk of recurrent stroke per year,[43] we have adjusted our criteria to optimize screening with TCD to predict the presence

of these lesions.[54] We use the cut-off of 100 cm/sec or more for the mean flow velocity (MFV) and the prestenotic-to-stenotic ratio 1 : >2 for defining diameter reduction of the MCA of 50% or more[54] (Fig. 5–4). Other groups developed their own velocity criteria for transcranial duplex imaging[55] and TCD.[56,57] When applying these published criteria, it is important to establish how the investigators measured percent stenosis angiographically and if angle correction was employed with duplex scanning.

Performance of TCD requires evaluation of vessels other than MCA, since in one study,[57] increasing the number of vessels with significant intracranial stenoses linearly increases the risk of subsequent stroke to the point that all symptomatic Chinese patients with six or more stenotic vessels suffered a stroke during follow-up.

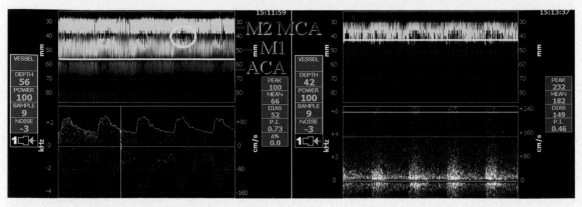

Proximal M1 MCA MFV 66 cm/sec   Distal M1/prox M2 MCA MFV 182 cm/sec

FIGURE 5–4. Power M-mode and spectral Doppler appearance of a distal M1/proximal M2 segment middle carotid artery (MCA) stenosis. *Left*, Spectral analysis at a depth of 56 mm shows proximal M1 MCA mean flow velocity (MFV) of 66 cm/sec and diversion of flow to the anterior cerebral artery (ACA; ACA MFV > MCA MFV). Note the appearance of a systolic bruit at a depth of 40 mm on M-mode display (*circle*). *Right*, Spectral Doppler measurement of the distal MCA shows a MFV of 182 cm/sec with stenotic to prestenotic ratio of 2.8 : 1 indicating MCA stenosis of more than 50%.

Transcranial Doppler can also be used as an inexpensive follow-up tool to demonstrate continuing artery-to-artery embolization, despite antiplatelet or anticoagulant therapy, as well as progression and regression of stenosis severity with combination therapies including angiotensin-converting enzyme (ACE) inhibitors and statins.[57,59–61] If TCD shows recurrent embolization and/or increasing degree of intracranial stenosis, with fluctuating neurologic deficit or recurrent events despite best medical therapy, these patients may be considered for experimental intracranial angioplasty stenting procedures.[49]

Shunt and Emboli Detection

Ultrasound can detect, quantify, and localize embolization in real time, and this subject has been particularly well studied in cerebral vessels with TCD[62–66] Detection of emboli with TCD is based on the definition of microembolic signals (MES) provided by the International Cerebral Hemodynamics Society consensus.[67] MES have the following characteristics on spectral Doppler analysis (Fig. 5–5):
1. Random occurrence during the cardiac cycle
2. Brief duration (usually <0.1 sec)

3. High intensity (>3 dB over background)
4. Primarily unidirectional signals (if fast Fourier transformation is used)
5. Audible component (chirp, pop)

The power motion–mode Doppler (power M-mode) adds extra dimensions to the process of emboli detection. It shows tracks of emboli in time and space and provides simultaneous real-time assessment of emboli passing through different vessels (Fig. 5–5), thereby increasing the yield of emboli detection with a single transducer.[68] Practically all MES detected by TCD are asymptomatic, since the size of the particles producing them is usually comparable to the diameter of brain capillaries or even smaller.[69] However, their cumulative count is related to the incidence of neurophycological deficits after cardiopulmonary bypass and stroke after carotid endarterectomy.[70–75] Furthermore, the significance of MES as a risk factor for ischemic stroke and as a parameter for platelet inhibition efficacy is emerging.[76]

Strict standards should be followed when an interpreter documents and reports microemboli on TCD.[77] The gold standard for MES identification still remains the on- or off-line interpretation of real-time, videotaped or digitally taped flow signals.[77–79] If spectral TCD is used, recordings should be obtained with minimal gain

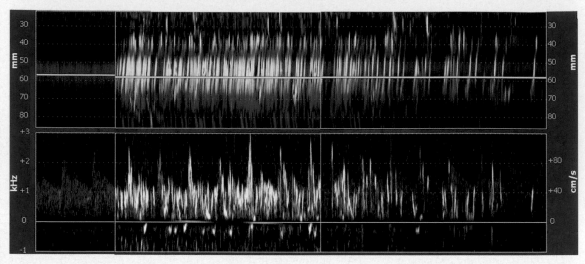

FIGURE 5–5. Positive "bubble" test for right-to-left shunt in a patients with large and functional patent foramen ovale confirmed by transesophageal echocardiography. The Valsalva maneuver induced a "curtain" of embolic signals in the middle cerebral artery. (Images courtesy of Dr. Zsolt Garami.)

at a fixed angle of insonation and with a small (<10 mm) sample volume. The probe should be maintained with a fixation device during monitoring for detection of spontaneous embolization for at least 0.5 to 1 hour. Prolonged monitoring times, two-channel simultaneous registration, and the use of power M-mode can improve the yield of emboli detection. Differentiation of embolic signals from artifacts is now possible using commercially available software.

Testing for right-to-left shunt is essential in patients when stroke or transient ischemic attack is thought to result from paradoxical embolization.[80,81] Although TCD cannot localize the shunt; i.e., patent foramen ovale or atrial septal defect, it provides information that complements transesophageal echocardiography. For instance, "bubble" testing with TCD can be done in a matter of minutes at bedside, with minimal or no discomfort to the patient. TCD can offer results of shunt detection with accuracy equal to echocardiography for detection of functional patent foramen ovale and may detect shunts even when transesophageal echocardiography is negative; i.e., in cases of pulmonary arteriovenous malformation or inability of the patient to perform Valsalva maneuver during echocardiography.[81,82]

To optimize TCD performance for right-to-left shunt, the following protocol should be followed:

1. Patient is in the supine position, and an 18-gauge needle is inserted into the cubital vein
2. A three-way stop-cock connector with two 10-ml syringes is connected to intravenous access
3. Nine-milliliter isontonic (preferably bacteriostatic) saline is forcefully mixed with 1 cc of air
4. Less than 1 ml of patient blood may be suctioned into syringe for better bubble formation with agitation
5. At least one MCA is monitored with TCD
6. The first bolus injection of agitated saline is made with the patient breathing normally
7. The second bolus injection of similarly prepared, and agitated saline is made with a 10 sec Valsalva maneuver initiated 5 sec after beginning the saline injection
8. If negative, TCD monitoring is extended up to 1 min to detect potentially late-arriving bubbles suggesting a pulmonary shunt

A four-level categorization is proposed by the International Consensus Criteria:[82]

1. No microembolic signals were detected (negative "bubble"-test)

2. An MES of 1 to 10 was detected (positive "bubble"-test)
3. An MES of 10 or more was detected with no curtain
4. A curtain is detected (test indicates the presence of a large and functional shunt) (Fig. 5–5)

The report should comment on whether a MES or bubbles were detected at rest or were provoked by the Valsalva maneuver. If few single bubbles were detected at rest and a curtain appeared with the Valsalva maneuver (Fig. 5–5), this also must be reflected in the report.

Clinical interest in shunt testing with TCD is increasing. Besides stroke patients with paradoxical embolism, functional patent formaen ovale may play a significant negative role in altitude decompression, in patients undergoing hip replacement, and in patients suffering from migraine with aura.[83–86] Noninvasive shunt detection, functional assessment, and percutaneous closure of the foramen open new possibilities in management of these patients.

Vasomotor Reactivity Testing

The main reason to evaluate vasomotor reactivity (VMR) of brain vessels is to identify patients at higher risk of stroke. VMR has been most extensively studied in the setting of carotid artery stenosis or occlusion. A variety of tests were introduced to evaluate intracranial hemodynamics using the phenomenon of VMR[87–92] including CO_2 reactivity with TCD, acetazolamide testing with TCD and cerebral blood flow scanning techniques, and the breath-holding index (BHI). The BHI is the simplest way of challenging VMR if the patient is compliant and capable of a 30-second breath hold.[92] This index is calculated using the mean flow velocities obtained by TCD before breath-holding (baseline) and at the end of 4 sec of breathing after 30 sec of breath-holding:

$$BHI = \frac{MFV_{baseline} - MFV_{end}}{MFV_{baseline}} \times \frac{100}{\text{seconds of breath-holding}}$$

The patient should be able to hold his or her breath voluntarily for at least 24 sec and preferably for 30 sec. The following steps can help the patient complete this task. First, explain in detail what needs to be accomplished, and demonstrate yourself that no major chest excursions should be made at the beginning and end of breath-holding. Major chest volume changes associated with forced breathing change intrathoracic pressure and may affect velocity and flow pulsatility. Second, announce the duration of breath holding to the patient at 10-sec intervals after breath-holding has started. This helps the patient to be more confident that he or she can complete the task. Use envelope or average mean velocities beginning 4 sec after the patient resumed breathing (i.e., the optimized signals from the entire display if the sweep speed was set at 4–5 sec).

Breath-holding index values of less than 0.69 are predictive of risk of stroke in patients with asymptomatic, severe ICA stenoses and symptomatic occlusions.[93,94] If a patient has a reduction in asymptomatic proximal ICA stenosis diameter of 70% or more and a BHI less than 0.69, his or her risk of subsequent stroke is at least three times greater than that of a similar patient with normal vasomotor reactivity. This information, together with other findings such as blunting of the MCA waveform,[95] plaque morphology[26–30] and emboli, (32) can identify asymptomatic patients at particularly high risk of stroke who are therefore more suitable for surgery.

Breath-holding with TCD does not require any gas monitoring equipment or intravenous injections. Although the subjectivity of patient effort and the unknowns of blood gas concentration potentially limit reliability, the BHI has been prospectively validated to predict clinical outcomes in stenoocclusive ICA disease, and BHI represents a simple screening test that can be used in the outpatient clinic to identify patients with impaired vasomotor reactivity. Further clinical trials will determine the need for bypass surgery based on vasomotor reserve findings, particularly in patients with chronic ICA occlusions.[96]

Bedside Testing

Subarachnoid Hemorrhage

The most common cause of subarachnoid hemorrhage (SAH) is spontaneous rupture of cerebral aneurysms.[97–99] Vasospasm is a common complication of SAH that may lead to delayed ischemic neurologic deficits.[100–103] The term *vasospasm* refers to a delayed, sustained contraction of the cerebral arteries, which can be induced by blood products that remain in contact with the cerebral vessel wall following subarachnoid hemorrhage.[100,101] SAH can also occur after head injury and following neurosurgical operations for other lesions. Post-traumatic vasospasm is now increasingly recognized as a clinical entity with potentially significant consequences.[103–106] Martin and colleagues[107] suggested that patients with significant post-traumatic subarachnoid hemorrhage be examined frequently with TCD for the presence of vasospasm as well as hypoperfusion or hyperperfusion states after brain injury.

Vasospasm will occur in most patients following nontraumatic SAH and will cause some degree of vessel narrowing.[100,101,103] The clinical severity of SAH, as measured with the Hunt-Hess Grades[108] or the Glasgow Coma Scale,[109,110] is generally predictive of vasospasm development and progression to delayed neurological deficits, as are other parameters, including the clot burden and hydrocephalus on computed tomography[111] and velocity changes on TCD.[112] However, the majority of patients with SAH do not develop vessel narrowing to the point of reducing blood flow to ischemic levels. Most patients develop mild or moderate vasospasm that spontaneously resolves without significant neurological consequences. Severe vasospasm causes greater vessel narrowing, with reduction of blood flow to an ischemic threshold and the development of delayed ischemic neurological deficits.[113]

One of the first clinical applications of TCD was the detection of cerebral vasospasm after SAH.[114,115] Although TCD velocity does not allow measurement of cerebral blood flow,[116] TCD can be used to

1. Detect the onset of asymptomatic vasospasm
2. Follow spasm progression and facilitate hypertension-hemodilution-hypervolemia therapy
3. Identify patients with severe vasospasm and select patients for angioplasty/papaverine
4. Monitor the effect of therapies and interventions
5. Detect spasm resolution[117–121]

Baseline TCD measurements should be obtained in patients with SAH on admission and after invasive angiography or surgical clipping of the aneurysm. TCD should be repeated frequently (daily or every other day) throughout the hospital stay. Lindegaard and coworkers[117] showed that a vasospastic MCA usually demonstrates velocities greater than 120 cm/sec, with the velocity being inversely related to arterial diameter. They also showed that velocities greater than 200 cm/sec are predictive of residual MCA lumen diameter of 1 mm or less. (Normal MCA diameter is approximately 3 mm.)

The changes in TCD velocity have been correlated with vessel narrowing measured angiographically, and the best correlations are in the MCA.[117,118] Sloan and colleagues[122,123] evaluated the sensitivity and specificity of TCD for vasospasm in the MCA and the vertebrobasilar system. By recording velocity in the MCA and extracranial ICA with the same 2-MHz transducer, a Lindegaard ratio[124,125] (mean MCA velocity/mean ICA velocity) can be calculated, which may help to determine spasm severity and the relative benefit of hyperemia or hypertension-hemodilution-hypervolemia therapy.

Typical proximal vasospasm after SAH affects the MCA and the terminal ICA (Fig. 5–6), followed in frequency by bilateral A1 anterior cerebral artery spasm and spasm of the basilar artery stem. Newell and associates[126] showed that vasospasm can be limited to distal vascular distributions in a relatively small percentage of cases and can therefore be missed by TCD. Although TCD is insensitive for detecting far distal vasospasm (i.e., M3 MCA subdivision), distal spasm affecting proximal

M2 segments of the MCA can be detected. Far distal spasm can often be anticipated by the distribution of blood in more distal locations on the initial computed tomographic scan following subarachnoid hemorrhage.

Although asymptomatic patient selection with TCD for early angioplasty to prevent the onset of delayed ischemic neurologic deficits remains controversial, balloon angioplasty, with or without papaverine, is the most common endovascular therapy employed in the treatment of cerebral vasospasm.[127,128] Two studies performed in 2000[129,130] also showed that TCD and other variables can be used to monitor hypertension-hemodilution-hypervolemia therapy and predict outcomes after subarachnoid hemorrhage.

Cerebral Circulatory Arrest

Brain edema or mass effect can lead to increasing intracranial pressure that compresses small and large intracranial arteries, eventually culminating in cerebral circulatory arrest. Absence of brain perfusion correlates with an oscillating (reverberating) flow pattern, systolic spike, or absent flow signals in basal cerebral arteries.[131-143] The term *oscillating* flow signal means that blood pushed intracranially during systoli is pushed out of the brain during diastoli (Fig. 5–7). This state of cerebral circulatory arrest leads to brain death that is established as a clinical diagnosis.[144] TCD is a reliable tool for confirming brain death through the demonstration of cerebral circulatory arrest, with accuracy parameters close to 100% at experienced centers.[131-143]

Based on previous published reports[131-143] and our own clinical experience, we have developed the following algorithm if cerebral circulatory arrest is suspected:

1. Document arterial blood pressure at the time of TCD examination.
2. Positive (toward the brain) MCA or basilar artery end-diastolic flow means no cerebral circulatory arrest.
3. Absent end-diastolic flow means uncertain cerebral circulatory arrest (too early or too late).
4. Reversed minimal end-diastolic flow means possible cerebral circulatory arrest (continue monitoring).
5. Reverberating flow means probable cerebral circulatory arrest. (Confirm in both MCAs at 50–60 mm and basilar artery at 80–90 mm, then monitor arrest for 30 min.)

Transcranial Doppler cannot be used exclusively to diagnose brain death, since this is a clinical diagnosis.[144] As a confirmatory tool, TCD can be used to demonstrate cerebral circulatory arrest in adults and children, except in infants younger than 6 months.[131-143] TCD can be used to monitor progressive flow changes toward cerebral circulatory arrest. Once a reverberating signal is found, it should be monitored for at least 30 min in both MCAs and the basilar artery to avoid false-positive findings. Also, avoid insonation of arterial bifurcations; i.e., MCA/anterior cerebral artery, since bidirectional, reverberating signals may overlap, creating an illusion of positive end-diastolic flow.

Transcranial Doppler can also be used to determine the appropriate time for other confirmatory tests (i.e., to minimize the need for nuclear flow studies with residual cerebral blood flow, often required by organ harvesting transplant protocols) and to discuss the consequent issues with the patient's family.

Acute Ischemic Stroke

Intravenous TPA is currently the only Food and Drug Administration–approved therapy for ischemic stroke, but TPA must be administered within 3 hr from symptom onset.[5] Non-contrast computed tomography is the first-line imaging test for differentiation of hemorrhagic and ischemic events. Based on clinical and computed tomography examinations, TPA can be given without confirmation of the presence of an arterial occlusion.[5] However, this treatment strategy, without confirmation of arterial occlusion, has been criticized.[145] More centers are now attempting vascular imaging to determine the presence, or persistence, of occlusion or reocclusion that has been linked to

Transcranial Doppler

UT

S T A T

Stroke Treatment Team

S T A T Neurosonology Service
phone (713) 500 **** pager (713) 648 ****

Patient Information: 45 y.o. woman   SAH   R Pcomm aneurysm   H-H Grade II   Day 0: 03/25/03

	Day	2	3	4	5	6	7	8	9	10	11	12	13	14	15
	Time	15:00	11:15	10:20	09:30	08:00	08:00	08:00	09:00	10:15	11:00	11:30	:	:	:
Right	dMCA	62/0.8	91/0.8	125/0.8	163/0.7	172/0.6	165/0.6	178/0.5	108/0.9	100/0.9	101/0.9	99/0.9	d/c		
	pMCA	65/0.9	100/0.9	136/0.7	177/0.8	200/0.7	212/0.6	259/0.5	112/0.8	107/0.9	105/0.9	108/0.9			
	ACA	58/0.8	78/0.9	91/0.8	102/0.8	130/0.8	152/0.7	163/0.6	92/0.8	83/0.8	85/0.7	87/0.8			
	PCA	34/1.1	38/1.1	47/1.0	45/1.0	52/1.0	55/0.9	63/0.8	60/0.9	63/0.9	57/1.0	50/0.9			
	VA	30/1.2	33/1.2	41/1.1	40/1.1	42/1.1	47/1.2	40/0.9	51/1.1	43/1.0	47/1.0	43/1.2			
	ICA/ratio	30/2	35/2.6	38/3.6	47/3.8	45/4.4	37/5.7	33/7.8	50/2.2	51/2.1	45/2.3	50/2.2			
Left	dMCA	55/1.0	67/0.9	77/0.9	75/0.9	89/0.8	97/0.8	93/0.9	74/0.8	79/0.8	81/0.8	79/0.9			
	pMCA	68/0.7	73/0.8	81/0.9	88/0.9	110/0.8	115/0.7	112/0.8	86/0.9	84/1.0	90/0.8	85/1.0			
	ACA	67/0.8	82/0.8	83/0.7	113/0.7	142/0.6	148/0.6	135/0.6	100/0.8	82/0.8	89/0.7	91/0.8			
	PCA	41/1.0	42/1.0	38/0.9	48/1.0	45/1.0	47/1.0	45/1.0	43/1.1	47/1.0	39/1.0	40/0.9			
	VA	35/0.9	37/0.8	39/1.0	45/0.9	43/1.0	38/1.0	43/0.8	44/1.0	47/1.1	42/0.9	45/0.9			
	ICA/ratio	35/1.9	36/2.6	38/2	43/2	47/2.3	45/2.6	46/2.4	49/1.8	45/1.9	47/1.9	43/2			
	dBA	48/0.9	45/1.0	49/1.0	51/1.1	48/1.0	56/0.8	68/0.8	60/1.0	55/1.0	53/1.0	51/0.9			
	pBA	51/0.8	50/0.9	54/1.1	49/1.0	54/1.1	64/0.9	75/0.9	63/1.1	60/1.1	59/1.1	63/1.0			
	MABP	93	91	93	110	112	123	129	94	91	92	90			
	ICP	8	6	8	10	9	8	8	6	d/c					
	CVP	5	4	5	11	12	12	12	9	7	6	d/c			
	Wedge	9	7	9	15	16	16	16	13	12	10	d/c			
	Card. output	3.7	3.2	3.6	4.8	4.9	5.1	5.2	4.5	4.2	4.0	d/c			
	Hematocrit	39	38	37	33	32	32	31	32	33	33	34			
	Cardiac index	2.3	2.0	2.3	3.0	3.1	3.2	3.3	2.8	2.6	2.5	d/c			
	HHH (y/no)	no	no	no	yes	yes	yes	yes	no	no	no	no			

FIGURE 5–6. Typical course of the terminal internal carotid artery (ICA)/middle carotid artery (MCA) vasospasm on daily transcranial Doppler monitoring in a 45-year-old woman with a right posterior communicating artery aneurysm clipped on day 2 after headache onset. Data are shown as mean flow velocity/pulsatility index (MFV/PI). The *bold numbers* indicate MFVs and Lindegaard ratios that are diagnostic of spasm in the right terminal ICA/MCA. The *bold italic values* offer indirect evidence of vasospasm due to compensatory velocity increase or mild spasm development on the contralateral side. The *bold values* show early increase of velocities predictive of spasm development.

Daily interpretation: Day 2: Baseline normal values; no vasospasm. Day 3: Slight increase of mean flow velocities on the side of aneurysm; no significant vasospasm.

Day 4: Mild vasospasm; elevated velocities and Lindegaard ratio right MCA and anterior carotid artery (ACA) (suggests terminal ICA /MCA vasospasm location). Days 5 and 6: Low to moderate right terminal ICA/MCA vasospasm with unilateral and contralateral velocity increase. The latter may be from compensatory flow or mild left ACA/MCA vasospasm.

Days 7 and 8: Moderate (day 7) and severe (day 8) right terminal ICA/MCA vasospasm.

Day 9: No significant vasospasm after balloon angioplasty; hyperemic velocity/ratio values. Days 10–12: No vasospasm; low resistance flows after discontinuation of ventricular drainage. (Case presentation developed with Dr. Anne Wojner.)

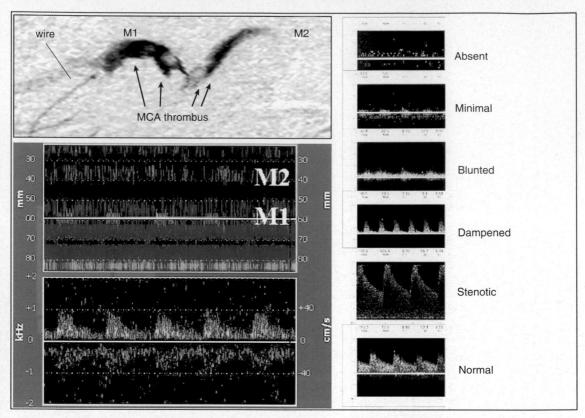

FIGURE 5-7. Acute thromboembolism of the middle cerebral artery (MCA; *upper left image* obtained during invasive angiography). *Lower left image,* Residual flow signals at acute MCA occlusion location by power M-mode Doppler. *Right images,* The Thrombolysis in Brain Ischemia (TIBI) flow grading system.

poor prognosis and may necessitate further (experimental) intra-arterial interventions.[146,147] Various tests can be used for this purpose, including invasive digital subtraction angiography, magnetic resonance angiography, computed tomographic angiography, and ultrasound.[148,149] Ultrasound has an advantage of being a quick and inexpensive method for patency assessment and monitoring that can be used at the bedside. The key to the application of transcranial ultrasound in the often restless acute stroke patient is a "fast-track" insonation protocol.[150] An experienced sonographer can use this method, guided by a physician's clinical assessment, to determine the presence and location of intracranial occlusion within minutes. Bedside assessment should begin with TCD, since acute arterial obstruction that is responsible for cerebral ischemia is almost always intracranial. Once completed, the TCD examination can be supplemented with a

rapid carotid/vertebral duplex assessment to determine the presence of an extracranial stenosis of 50% or more, an extracranial thrombus, or a thrombus, which is often the cause of artery-to-artery embolism or hypoperfusion. As compared with emergency catheter angiography, the accuracy of combined intracranial and extracranial ultrasound examination, performed by expert sonographers in the emergency department, can be 100% for detection of lesions amenable to intervention.[151]

Transcranial Doppler Criteria for Acute Arterial Occlusion

Previously published criteria for intracranial occlusions focused on the absence of flow signals at a presumed thrombus location or velocity asymmetry between homologous segments, mostly the MCAs.[152–154] Indeed, complete arterial occlusion should produce no detectable flow signals, as well as dampening of velocity in the proximal vessels. This is the case with chromic extracranial occlusions found in the ICA with duplex ultrasound. However with acute intracranial occlusion, some residual flow to or around the thrombus may exist due to its irregular shape, relatively soft thrombus composition, and elevated systolic pressures that cause additional distension of muscular arterial walls. An acute occlusion, therefore, may produce a variety of waveforms representing this residual flow.[155]

The Thrombolysis in Myocardial Infarction (TIMI) flow grading system was developed to assess the residual flow in coronary vessels with invasive angiography.[156] The amount of residual flow predicts the success of both coronary and intracranial thrombolysis,[156,157] since TPA binds to fibrin sites at the thrombus surface in proportion to its plasma concentration and the residual flow (Fig. 5–7). Increasing amounts of residual flow bring more TPA to the thrombus. We have developed the Thrombolysis in Brain Ischemia (TIBI) flow grading system to evaluate residual flow noninvasively and to monitor thrombus dissolution in real time.[155] The TIBI system expands previous definitions of acute arterial occlusion by focusing the examiner's attention on relatively weak signals with abnormal flow waveforms that can be found along arterial stems filled with thrombi (Fig. 5–7). TIBI flow grades correlate with stroke severity and mortality, as well as the likelihood of recanalization and clinical improvement.[155] Recently, an angiographic classification specific to intracranial vessels was proposed, called the Thrombolysis In Cerebral Infarction (TICI) system.[158]

Acute intracranial arterial occlusion is a dynamic process, since thrombus can propagate, break up, or rebuild within seconds or minutes, thereby changing the degree of arterial obstruction and affecting the correlation between ultrasound and angiography. When the term *acute occlusion* is applied to the interpretation of ultrasound findings, it means that there is a hemodynamically significant obstruction to flow and that if urgent angiography is performed, it will likely show an arterial lesion amendable to intervention. This lesion may be a complete occlusion (TIMI grades 0–1) or a partial occlusion corresponding to TIMI grade 2. The presence of a large vessel occlusion on TCD has to be confirmed by other findings, such as flow diversion to a branching vessel or a collateral channel.

Furthermore, ultrasound may suggest that more than one occlusion is present in the same patient; i.e., tandem lesions in the ICA and MCA. Tandem lesions are suspected when an abnormal TIBI flow grade is found in the MCA with signs of collateralization of flow via major channels (such as the anterior or posterior communicating artery, reversed ophthalmic artery flow) or when duplex ultrasound indicates the presence of an additional extracranial arterial lesion.[159]

Bedside ultrasound examination in acute cerebral ischemia can help to
1. Identify thrombus presence
2. Determine thrombus location(s)
3. Assess collateral supply
4. Find the worst residual flow signal
5. Monitor recanalization and reocclusion

Transcranial Doppler Monitoring and Ultrasound-Enhanced Thrombolysis

Transcranial Doppler monitoring of normothermic patients with acute ischemic stroke is safe:[160] In our prospective studies, 2 hr of TCD monitoring using Food and Drug Administration–approved devices set at full power at given insonation depth and tight transducer fixation resulted in hemorrhage rates lower than can be expected from the pivotal NINDS-rt-PA Stroke Study. Using TCD or transcranial duplex imaging, the evolution of MCA occlusion can be followed in real time and the recanalization process can be measured.[161–165] Early recanalization leads to clinical recovery from stroke, and ultrasound can identify early responders to thrombolytic therapy[164–166] as well as patients with persisting arterial occlusion or reocclusion[146,147] (Figure 5–8). Furthermore, ultrasound aimed at the re-

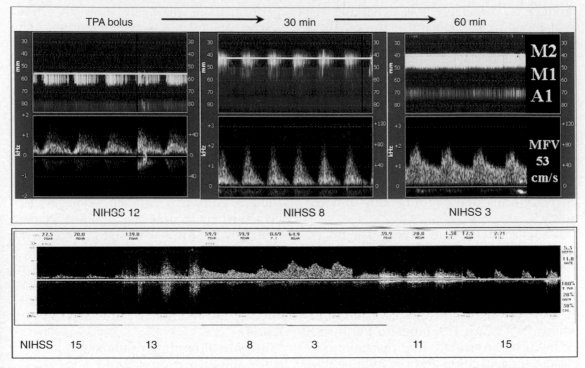

Figure 5–8. Examples of complete recanalization (*upper row*) and reocclusion (*bottom row*) during tissue plasminogen activator (TPA) infusion in acute ischemic stroke patients. Time-corresponding neurologic changes are described using the National Institutes of Health Stroke Scale (NIHSS). MFV, mean flow velocity.

sidual flow/thrombus interface can be used to further enhance the therapeutic activity of TPA.

In vitro and in vivo experiments showed that continuous thrombus exposure to ultrasound in the KHz-to-low-MHz frequency range enhances TPA activity.[167–171] Several mechanisms of ultrasound-enhanced thrombolysis were identified, including

1. Reversible disaggregation of uncross-linked fibrin fibers[167]
2. Microcavity formation in the shallow layer of thrombus[168]
3. Increased enzymatic transport of TPA[169,170]
4. Increased plasma flow through fibrin clots[171]

These effects of ultrasound improve penetration of TPA through the thrombus, thereby increasing the overall amount of TPA effectively delivered to the binding sites along the thrombus.

In a human cadaver skull model,[172] ultrasound shortened time to recanalization as follows: TPA alone, 29 min; TPA with 1-MHz commercial TCD, 17 min; and TPA with 185-KHz pulsed ultrasound, 14 min (p < 0.01). Significant flow improvement was demonstrated within 10 min of insonation with 185-KHz ultrasound, inducing faster reperfusion compared with 1-MHz ultrasound. Although KHz frequencies better facilitate TPA-induced lysis, as compared with MHz frequencies, probably due to better skull penetration,[172] the concern remains that longer wavelength of KHz ultrasound makes the effect more mechanically driven, causing thrombus and surrounding tissues to vibrate and stretch. The clinical phase II trial of low- and mid-KHz frequencies to enhance systemic TPA therapy, called THRUMBI,[173] was halted because of an unacceptably high rate of symptomatic hemorrhage (Daffersthoffer M, personal communication). On the contrary, MHz frequencies have shorter wavelength and shorter path, and therefore, pressure waves can be focused on the thrombus/residual flow interface, leaving brain structures unaffected.

Based on our pilot clinical studies,[160,166] we designed the CLOTBUST trial (Combined *Lysis* of *Thrombus* in *Brain* ischemia using transcranial *Ultrasound* and *Systemic TPA*). In this multicenter, phase II randomized clinical trial, we sought to determine the rates of complete recanalization and early dramatic recovery, as well as the rate of symptomatic intracerebral hemorrhage in patients receiving thrombolysis as well as externally applied TCD, as compared with systemic thrombolysis without continuous ultrasound monitoring. TPA infusion combined with 2 hours of TCD monitoring results in 19% more patients experiencing complete recanalization or dramatic clinical recovery from stroke. This trial confirms positive biological activity of 2 MHz diagnostic ultrasound aiding systemic thrombolytic therapy.[174]

References

1. Centers for Disease Control: Public health and aging: Hospitalizations for stroke among adults aged ≥ 65 years: United States, 2000. Morbid Mortal Wkly Rep 52:586–589, 2003.
2. Grotta JC: Ultrasound: What's in the waveforms? In Alexandrov AV (ed): Cerebrovascular Ultrasound in Stroke Prevention and Treatment. New York, Blackwell Publishing-Futura, 2003, pp ii–iii.
3. Albers GW, Caplan LR, Easton JD, et al: Transient ischemic attack—proposal for a new definition. N Engl J Med 347:1713–1716, 2002.
4. Johnston SC, Gress DR, Browner WS, Sidney S: Short-term prognosis after emergency department diagnosis of TIA. JAMA 284:2901–2906, 2000.
5. The National Institutes of Neurological Disorders and Stroke rt-PA Stroke Study Group: Tissue plasminogen activator for acute ischemic stroke. N Engl J Med 333:1581–1587, 1995.
6. Adams HP Jr, Adams RJ, Brott T, et al: Guidelines for the early management of patients with ischemic stroke: A scientific statement from the Stroke Council of the American Stroke Association. Stroke 34:1056–1083, 2003.
7. Adams HP Jr, Bendixen BH, Leira E, et al: Antithrombotic treatment of ischemic stroke among patients with occlusion or severe stenosis of the internal carotid artery: A report of the Trial of Org 10172 in Acute Stroke Treatment (TOAST). Neurology 53:122–125, 1999.
8. Hart RG: Antithrombotic therapies for stroke prevention in atrial fibrillation. Adv Neurol 92:249–256, 2003.
9. North American Symptomatic Carotid Endarterectomy Trial Collaborators: Beneficial effect of carotid endarterectomy in symptomatic patients with high-grade carotid stenosis. N Engl J Med 325:445–453, 1991.
10. European Carotid Surgery Trialists' Collaborative Group: Randomised trial of endarterectomy for recently symptomatic carotid stenosis: Final results of the MRC European Carotid Surgery Trial (ECST). Lancet 351:1379–1387, 1998.
11. Executive Committee of the Asymptomatic Carotid Atherosclerosis Study: Endarterectomy for asymptomatic carotid artery stenosis. JAMA 273:1421–1428, 1995.
12. Barnett HJ, Meldrum HE, Eliasziw M for the North American Symptomatic Carotid Endarterectomy Trial (NASCET) collaborators: The appropriate use of carotid endarterectomy. CMAJ 166:1169–1179, 2002.
13. Ouriel K, Hertzer NR, Beven EG, et al: Preprocedural risk stratification: Identifying an appropriate population for carotid stenting. J Vasc Surg 33:728–732, 2001.
14. Chaturvedi S, Aggarwal R, Murugappan A: Results of carotid endarterectomy with prospective neurologist follow-up. Neurology 55:769–772, 2000.
15. Johnston DC, Goldstein LB: Clinical carotid endareterectomy decision-making: Noninvasive vascular imaging versus angiography. Neurology 56:1009–1015, 2001.
16. Norris JW, Rothwell PM: Nonivasive carotid imaging to select patients for endarterectomy: Is it really safer than conventional angiography? Neurology 56:990–991, 2001.
17. Qureshi AI, Suri MF, Ali Z, et al: Role of conventional angiography in evaluation of patients with carotid artery stenosis demonstrated by Doppler ultrasound in general practice. Stroke 32:2287–2291, 2001.
18. Gomez CR: Carotid angioplasty and stenting: New horizons. Curr Atheroscler Rep 2:151–159, 2000.
19. Fox AJ: How to measure carotid stenosis? Radiology 186:316–318, 1993.
20. Alexandrov AV, Bladin CF, Maggisano R, Norris JW: Measuring carotid stenosis: Time for a reappraisal. Stroke 24:1292–1296, 1993.
21. Barnett HJ, Taylor DW, Eliasziw M, et al: Benefit of carotid endarterectomy in patients with symptomatic moderate or severe stenosis. North American Symptomatic Carotid Endarterectomy Trial Collaborators. N Engl J Med 339:1415–1425, 1998.
22. Alexandrov AV, Bladin CF, Murphy J, et al: Clinical applicability of methods to measure

carotid stenosis. J Stroke Cerebrovasc Dis 4:258–261, 1994.

23. Rothwell PM, Gibson RJ, Slattery J, et al: Equivalence of measurements of carotid stenosis. A comparison of three methods on 1001 angiograms. European Carotid Surgery Trialists' Collaborative Group. Stroke 25:2435–2439, 1994.

24. Grant E, Benson C, Moneta G, et al: Carotid artery stenosis: Gray-scale and Doppler US diagnosis—Society of Radiologists in Ultrasound Consensus Conference. Radiology 229:340–346, 2003.

25. Mast H, Thompson JL, Lin IF, et al: Cigarette smoking as a determinant of high-grade carotid artery stenosis in Hispanic, black, and white patients with stroke or transient ischemic attack. Stroke 29:908–912, 1998.

26. Bluth EI: Evaluation and characterization of carotid plaque. Semin Ultrasound CT MR 18:57–65, 1997.

27. Polak JF, Shemanski L, O'Leary DH, et al: Hypoechoic plaque at US of the carotid artery: An independent risk factor for incident stroke in adults aged 65 years or older. Cardiovascular Health Study. Radiology 208:649–654, 1998.

28. Mathiesen EB, Bonaa KH, Joakimsen O: Echolucent plaques are associated with high risk of ischemic cerebrovascular events in carotid stenosis: The tromso study. Circulation 103:2171–2175, 2001.

29. Aburahma AF, Thiele SP, Wulu JT Jr: Prospective controlled study of the natural history of asymptomatic 60% to 69% carotid stenosis according to ultrasonic plaque morphology. J Vasc Surg 36:437–442, 2002.

30. Nicolaides AN: High risk carotid plaque. Ultrasound Med Biol 29:S38, 2003.

31. Geroulakos G, Ramaswami G, Nicolaides A, et al: Characterization of symptomatic and asymptomatic carotid plaques using high-resolution real-time ultrasonography. Br J Surg 80:1274–1277, 1993.

32. Molloy J, Markus HS: Asymptomatic embolization predicts stroke and TIA risk in patients with carotid artery stenosis. Stroke 30:1440–1443, 1999.

33. Moneta GL, Edwards JM, Chitwood RW, et al: Correlation of North American Symptomatic Carotid Endarterectomy Trial (NASCET) angiographic definition of 70% to 99% internal carotid artery stenosis with duplex scanning. J Vasc Surg 17:152–157, 1993.

34. Moneta GL, Edwards JM, Papanicolaou G, et al: Screening for asymptomatic internal carotid artery stenosis: Duplex criteria for discriminating 60% to 99% stenosis. J Vasc Surg 21:989–994, 1995.

35. Ranger WR, Glover JL, Bendick PJ: Carotid endarterectomy based on preoperative duplex ultrasound. Am Surg 61:548–554, 1995.

36. Logason K, Karacagil S, Hardemark HG, et al: Carotid artery endarterectomy solely based on duplex scan findings. Vasc Endovascular Surg 36:9–15, 2002.

37. Adams HP, Bendixen BH, Kappelle LJ, et al: Classification of subtype of acute ischemic stroke. Definitions for use in a multicenter clinical trial. TOAST. Trial of Org 10172 in Aucte Stroke Treatment. Stroke 24:35–41, 1993.

38. Bartels E, Fuchs HH, Flugel KA: Duplex ultrasonography of vertebral arteries: Examination, technique, normal values, and clinical applications. Angiology 43:169–180, 1992.

39. Bartels E: Color-Coded Duplex Ultrasonography of the Cerebral Vessels. Stuttgart, Schattauer, 1999.

40. Bartels E, Flugel KA: Evaluation of extracranial vertebral artery dissection with duplex color-flow imaging. Stroke 27:290–295, 1996.

41. Toole JF: Cerebrovascular Disorders, 4th ed. New York, Raven Press, pp 199–123.

42. Bornstein NM, Norris JW: Subclavian steal: A harmless haemodynamic phenomenon? Lancet 2:303–305, 1986.

43. Chimowitz MI, Kokkinos J, Strong J, et al: The Warfarin-Aspirin Symptomatic Intracranial Disease Study. *Neurology* 45:1488–1493, 1995.

44. Samuels OB, Joseph GJ, Lynn MJ, et al: A standardized method for measuring intracranial arterial stenosis. AJNR Am J Neuroradiol 21:643–646, 2000.

45. Sacco RL, Kargman DE, Gu Q, Zamanillo MC: Race-ethnicity and determinants of intracranial atherosclerotic cerebral infarction. The Northern Manhattan Stroke Study. Stroke 26:14–20, 1995.

46. Wityk RJ, Lehman D, Klag M, et al: Race and sex differences in the distribution of cerebral atherosclerosis. Stroke 27:1974–1980, 1996.

47. Wong KS, Huang YN, Gao S, et al: Intracranial stenosis in Chinese patients with acute stroke. Neurology 50:812–813, 1998.

48. Chimowitz MI: Antithrombotic therapy for atherosclerotic intracranial arterial stenosis. Adv Neurol 92:271–274, 2003.

49. Gomez CR, Orr SC: Angioplasty and stenting for primary treatment of intracranial arterial stenoses. Arch Neurol 58:1687–1690, 2001.

50. Chimowitz MI: Angioplasty or stenting is not appropriate as first-line treatment of intracranial stenosis. Arch Neurol 58:1690–1692, 2001.

51. Lindegaard KF, Bakke SJ, Aaslid R, Nornes H: Doppler diagnosis of intracranial artery occlu-

sive disorders. J Neurol Neurosurg Psychiatry 49:510–518, 1986.

52. de Bray JM, Joseph PA, Jeanvoine H, et al: Transcranial Doppler evaluation of middle cerebral artery stenosis. J Ultrasound Med 7:611–616, 1988.

53. Ley-Pozo J, Ringelstein EB: Noninvasive detection of occlusive disease of the carotid siphon and middle cerebral artery. Ann Neurol 28:640–647, 1990.

54. Felberg RA, Christou I, Demchuk AM, et al: Screening for intracranial stenosis with transcranial Doppler: The accuracy of mean flow velocity thresholds. J Neuroimaging 12:9–14, 2002.

55. Baumgartner RW, Mattle HP, Schroth G: Assessment of >/=50% and <50% intracranial stenoses by transcranial color-coded duplex sonography. Stroke 30:87–92, 1999.

56. Rother J, Schwartz A, Rautenberg W, Hennerici M: Middle cerebral artery stenoses: Assessment by magnetic resonance angiography and transcranial Doppler ultrasound. Cerebrovasc Dis 4:273–279, 1994.

57. Wong KS, Li H, Lam WW, et al: Progression of middle cerebral artery occlusive disease and its relationship with further vascular events after stroke. Stroke 33:532–536, 2002.

58. Schwarze JJ, Babikian V, DeWitt LD, et al: Longitudinal monitoring of intracranial arterial stenoses with transcranial Doppler ultrasonography. J Neuroimaging 4:182–187, 1994.

59. Segura T, Serena J, Castellanos M, et al: Embolism in acute middle cerebral artery stenosis. Neurology 56:497–501, 2001.

60. Arenillas JF, Molina CA, Montaner J, et al: Progression and clinical recurrence of symptomatic middle cerebral artery stenosis: A long-term follow-up transcranial Doppler ultrasound study. Stroke 32:2898–2904, 2001.

61. Gao S, Wong KS: Characteristics of microembolic signals detected near their origins in middle cerebral artery stenoses. J Neuroimaging 13:124–132, 2003.

62. Babikian VL, Feldmann E, Wechsler LR, et al: Transcranial Doppler ultrasonography: Year 2000 update. J Neuroimaging 10:101–115, 2000.

63. Spencer MP, Campbell SD, Sealey JL, et al: Experiments on decompression bubbles in the circulation using ultrasonic and electromagnetic flowmeters. J Occup Med 11:238–244, 1969.

64. Padayachee TS, Gosling RG, Bishop CC, et al: Transcranial measurement of blood velocities in the basal cerebral arteries using pulsed Doppler ultrasound: A method of assessing the Circle of Willis. Ultrasound Med Biol 12:5–14, 1986.

65. Deverall PB, Padayachee TS, Parsons S, et al: Ultrasound detection of micro-emboli in the middle cerebral artery during cardiopulmonary bypass surgery. Eur J Cardiothorac Surg 2:256–260, 1988.

66. Spencer MP, Thomas GI, Nicholls SC, Sauvage LR: Detection of middle cerebral artery emboli during carotid endarterectomy using transcranial Doppler ultrasonography. Stroke 21: 415–423, 1990.

67. The International Cerebral Hemodynamics Society Consensus Statement: Stroke 26:1123, 1995.

68. Moehring MA, Spencer MP: Power M-mode transcranial Doppler ultrasound and simultaneous single gate spectrogram. Ultrasound Med Biol 28:49–57, 2002.

69. Brucher R, Russel D: Background and principles. In Tegeler CH, Babikian VL, Gomez CR (eds): Neurosonology. St Louis, Mosby, 1996, pp 231–234.

70. Clark RE, Brillman J, Davis DA, et al: Microemboli during coronary artery bypass grafting. Genesis and effect on outcome. J Thorac Cardiovasc Surg 109:249–257, 1995.

71. Diegeler A, Hirsch R, Schneider F, et al: Neuromonitoring and neurocognitive outcome in off-pump versus conventional coronary bypass operation. Ann Thorac Surg 69:1162–1166, 2000.

72. Spencer MP: Transcranial Doppler monitoring and causes of stroke from carotid endarterectomy. Stroke 28:685–691, 1997.

73. Jansen C, Moll FL, Vermeulen FE, et al: Continuous transcranial Doppler ultrasonography and electroencephalography during carotid endarterectomy: A multimodal monitoring system to detect intraoperative ischemia. Ann Vasc Surg 7:95–101, 1993.

74. Ackerstaff RG, Jansen C, Moll FL, et al: The significance of microemboli detection by means of transcranial Doppler ultrasonography monitoring in carotid endarterectomy. J Vasc Surg 21:963–969, 1995.

75. Ackerstaff RG, Moons KG, van de Vlasakker CJ, et al: Association of intraoperative transcranial doppler monitoring variables with stroke from carotid endarterectomy. Stroke 31:1817–1823, 2000.

76. Kaposzta Z, Clifton A, Molloy J, et al: S-nitrosoglutathione reduces asymptomatic embolization after carotid angioplasty. Circulation 106:3057–3062, 2002.

77. Ringelstein EB, Droste DW, Babikian VL, et al: Consensus on microembolus detection by TCD. International Consensus Group on Microembolus Detection. Stroke 29:725–729, 1998.

78. Cullinane M, Reid G, Dittrich R, et al: Evaluation of new online automated embolic signal

detection algorithm, including comparison with panel of international experts. Stroke 31:1335–1341, 2000.

79. Markus HS: Transcranial Doppler ultrasound. Br Med Bull 56:378–388, 2000.

80. Lechat P, Mas JL, Lascault G, et al: Prevalence of patent foramen ovale in patients with stroke. N Engl J Med 318:1148–1152, 1988.

81. Zanette EM, Mancini G, De Castro S, et al: Patent foramen ovale and transcranial Doppler: Comparison of different procedures. Stroke 27:2251–2255, 1996.

82. Jauss M, Zanette E: Detection of right-to-left shunt with ultrasound contrast agent and transcranial Doppler sonography. Cerebrovasc Dis 10:490–496, 2000.

83. Foster PP, Boriek AM, Butler BD, et al: Patent foramen ovale and paradoxical systemic embolism: A bibliographic review. Aviat Space Environ Med 74:B1–B64, 2003.

84. Colonna DM, Kilgus D, Brown W, et al: Acute brain fat embolization occurring after total hip arthroplasty in the absence of a patent foramen ovale. Anesthesiology 96:1027–1029, 2002.

85. Anzola GP, Magoni M, Guindani M, et al: Potential source of cerebral embolism in migraine with aura: A transcranial Doppler study. Neurology 52:1622–1625, 1999.

86. Wilmshurst PT, Nightingale S, Walsh KP, Morrison WL: Effect on migraine of closure of cardiac right-to-left shunts to prevent recurrence of decompression illness or stroke or for haemodynamic reasons. Lancet 356:1648–1651, 2000.

87. Bishop CCR, Powell S, Insall M, et al: Effect of internal carotid artery occlusion on middle cerebral artery blood flow at rest and in response to hypercapnia. Lancet 29:710–712, 1986.

88. Ringelstein EB, Sievers C, Ecker S, et al: Non-invasive assessment of CO_2-induced cerebral vasomotor response in normal individuals and patients with internal carotid artery occlusions. Stroke 19:962–969, 1988.

89. Sorteberg W, Lindegaard KF, Rootwelt K, et al: Effect of acetazolamide on cerebral blood flow velocity and regional cerebral blood flow in normal subjects. Acta Neurochir 97:139–145, 1989.

90. Kleiser B, Widder B: Course of carotid artery occlusions with impaired cerebrovascular reactivity. Stroke 23:171–174, 1992.

91. Webster MW, Makaroun MS, Steed DL, et al: Compromised cerebral blood flow reactivity is a predictor of stroke in patients with symptomatic carotid artery occlusive disease. J Vasc Surg 21:338–344, 1995.

92. Markus HS, Harrison MJ: Estimation of cerebrovascular reactivity using transcranial Doppler, including the use of breath-holding as the vasodilatory stimulus. Stroke 23:668–673, 1992.

93. Silvestrini M, Vernieri F, Pasqualetti P, et al: Impaired cerebral vasoreactivity and risk of stroke in patients with asymptomatic carotid artery stenosis. JAMA 283:2122–2127, 2000.

94. Vernieri F, Pasqualetti P, Matheis M, et al: Effect of collateral flow and cerebral vasomotor reactivity on the outcome of carotid artery occlusion. Stroke 32:1552–1558, 2001.

95. Hartmann A, Mast H, Thompson JL, et al: Transcranial Doppler waveform blunting in severe extracranial carotid artery stenosis. Cerebrovasc Dis 10:33–38, 2000.

96. Adams HP, Powers WJ, Grubb RL, et al: Preview of a new trial of extracranial-to-intracranial arterial anastomosis: The carotid occlusion surgery group. Neurosurg Clin N Am 12:613–624, 2001.

97. Oldenkott P, Stolz C: Subarachnoid hemorrhage. The diagnostic guiding symptom: The blood containing liquor. Cause, clinical aspects, treatment problems and prognosis (in German). Med Welt 23:1326–1331, 1969.

98. Niizuma H, Kwak R, Otabe K, Suzuki J: Angiography study of cerebral vasospasm following the rupture of intracranial aneurysms: Part II. Relation between the site of aneurysm and the occurrence of the vasospasm. Surg Neurol 11:263–267, 1979.

99. Reynolds AF, Shaw CM: Bleeding patterns from ruptured intracranial aneurysms: An autopsy series of 205 patients. Surg Neurol 15:232–235, 1981.

100. Weir B, Grace M, Hansen J, Rothberg C: Time course of vasospasm in man. J Neurosurg 48:173–178, 1978.

101. Sloan MA: Cerebral vasoconstriction: physiology, pathophysiology, and occurrence in selected cerebrovascular disorders. In Caplan LR (ed): Brain Ischemia: Basic Concepts and their Clinical Relevance. London, Springer-Verlag: 1994, pp 151–172.

102. Fleischer AS, Raggio JF, Tindall GT: Aminophylline and isoproterenol in the treatment of cerebral vasospasm. Surg Neuro l8:117–121, 1977.

103. Kistler JP, Crowell RM, Davis KR, et al: The relation of cerebral vasospasm to the extent and location of subarachnoid blood visualized by CT scan: A prospective study. Neurology 33:424–436, 1983.

104. Lee JH, Martin NA, Alsina G, et al: Hemodynamically significant cerebral vasospasm and outcome after head injury: A prospective study. J Neurosurg 87:221–233, 1997.

105. Zubkov AY, Pilkington AS, Bernanke DH, et al: Posttraumatic cerebral vasospasm: Clinical

and morphological presentations. J Neuro-trauma 16:763–770, 1999.

106. Zubkov AY, Lewis AI, Raila FA, et al: Risk factors for the development of post-traumatic cerebral vasospasm. Surg Neuro l53:126–130, 2000.

107. Martin NA, Patwardhan RV, Alexander MJ, et al: Characterization of cerebral hemody-namic phases following severe head trauma: Hypoperfusion, hyperemia, and vasospasm. J Neurosurg 87:9–19, 1997.

108. Hunt WE, Hess RM: Surgical risk as related to time of intervention in the repair of intra-cranial aneurysms. J Neurosurg 28:14–20, 1968.

109. Teasdale G, Jennett B: Assessment of coma and impaired consciousness—a practical guide. Lancet 2:81–84, 1974.

110. Teasdale GM, Murray L: Revisiting the Glasgow Coma Scale and Coma Score. Inten-sive Care Med 26:153–154, 2000.

111. Black PM: Hydrocephalus and vasospasm after subarachnoid hemorrhage from ruptured intracranial aneurysms. Neurosurgery 18: 12–16, 1986.

112. Seiler RW, Grolimund P, Aaslid R, et al: Cere-bral vasospasm evaluated by transcranial ultrasound correlated with clinical grade and CT-visualized subarachnoid hemorrhage. J Neurosurg 64:594–600, 1986.

113. Yamakami I, Isobe K, Yamaura A, et al: Vasospasm and regional cerebral blood flow (rCBF) in patients with ruptured intracranial aneurysm: Serial rCBF studies with the xenon-133 inhalation method. Neurosurgery 13: 394–401, 1983.

114. Aaslid R, Markwalder TM, Nornes H: Non-invasive transcranial Doppler ultrasound recording of flow velocity in basal cerebral arteries. J Neurosurg 57:769–774, 1982.

115. Lindegaard KF, Nornes H, Bakke SJ, et al: Cere-bral vasospasm after subarachnoid haemor-rhage investigated by means of transcranial Doppler ultrasound. Acta Neurochir (Wien) 42(suppl):P81–P84, 1988.

116. Clyde BL, Resnick DK, Yonas H, et al: The rela-tionship of blood velocity as measured by transcranial doppler ultrasonography to cere-bral blood flow as determined by stable xenon computed tomographic studies after aneurys-mal subarachnoid hemorrhage. Neurosurgery 38:896–904, 1996.

117. Lindegaard KF, Nornes H, Bakke SJ, et al: Cere-bral vasospasm after subarachnoid haemor-rhage investigated by means of transcranial Doppler ultrasound. Acta Neurochir Suppl (Wien) 42:81–84, 1988.

118. Sloan MA: Transcranial Doppler monitoring of vasospasm after subarachnoid hemorrhage. In Tegeler CH, Babikian VL, Gomez CR (eds): Neurosonology. St Louis, Mosby, pp 156–171, 1996.

119. Giller CA, Purdy P, Giller A, et al: Elevated transcranial Doppler ultrasound velocities fol-lowing therapeutic arterial dilation. Stroke 26:123–127, 1995.

120. Lewis DH, Eskridge JM, Newell DW, et al: Brain SPECT and the effect of cerebral angioplasty in delayed ischemia due to vasospasm. J Nucl Med 33:1789–1796, 1992.

121. Rajendran JG, Lewis DH, Newell DW, Winn HR: Brain SPECT used to evaluate vasospasm after subarachnoid hemorrhage: Correlation with angiography and transcranial Doppler. Clin Nucl Med 26:125–130, 2001.

122. Sloan MA, Haley EC, Kassell NF, et al: Sensi-tivity and specificity of transcranial Doppler ultrasonography in the diagnosis of vaso-spasm following subarachnoid hemorrhage. Neurology 39:1514–1518, 1989.

123. Sloan MA, Burch CM, Wozniak MA, et al: Transcranial Doppler detection of verte-brobasilar vasospasm following subarachnoid hemorrhage. Stroke 25:2187–2197, 1994.

124. Lindegaard KF, Nornes H, Bakke SJ, et al: Cerebral vasospasm diagnosis by means of angiography and blood velocity measure-ments. Acta Neurochir (Wien) 100:12–24, 1989.

125. Lindegaard KF: The role of transcranial Doppler in the management of patients with subarachnoid haemorrhage: A review. Acta Neurochir (suppl)72:59–71, 1999.

126. Newell DW, Grady MS, Eskridge JM, Winn HR: Distribution of angiographic vasospasm after subarachnoid hemorrhage: implications for diagnosis by transcranial Doppler ultra-sonography. Neurosurgery 27:574–577, 1990.

127. Kaku Y, Yonekawa Y, Tsukahara T, Kazekawa K: Superselective intra-arterial infusion of papaverine for the treatment of cerebral vasospasm aftcr subarachnoid hemorrhage. J Neurosurg 77:842–847, 1992.

128. Kassell NF, Helm G, Simmons N, et al: Treatment of cerebral vasospasm with intra-arterial papaverine. J Neurosurg 77:848–852, 1992.

129. Quereshi AI, Suarez JI, Bhardwaj A, et al: Early predictors of outcome in patients receiving hypervolemic and hypertensive therapy for symptomatic vasospasm after subarachnoid hemorrhage. Crit Care Med 28:824–829, 2000.

130. Quereshi AI, Sung GY, Razumovsky AY, et al: Early identification of patients at risk for symptomatic vasospasm after aneurismal sub-rachnoid hemorrhage. Crit Care Med 28: 984–990, 2000.

131. Grolimund P, Seiler RW, Mattle H: Possibilities and limits of transcranial Doppler sonography (in German). Ultraschall Med 8:87–94, 1987.

132. Klingelhofer J, Conrad B, Benecke R, Sander D: Intracranial flow patterns at increasing intracranial pressure. Klin Wochenschr 65:542–545, 1987.

133. Kirkham FJ, Levin SD, Padayachee TS, et al: Transcranial pulsed Doppler ultrasound findings in brain stem death. J Neurol Neurosurg Psychiatry 50:1504–1513, 1987.

134. Ropper AH, Kehne SM, Wechsler L: Transcranial Doppler in brain death. Neurology 37:1733–1735, 1987.

135. Hassler W, Steinmetz H, Gawlowski J: Transcranial Doppler ultrasonography in raised intracranial pressure and in intracranial circulatory arrest. J Neurosurg 68:745–751, 1988.

136. Bode H, Sauer M, Pringsheim W: Diagnosis of brain death by transcranial Doppler sonography. Arch Dis Child 63:1474–1478, 1988.

137. Newell DW, Grady MS, Sirotta P, Winn HR: Evaluation of brain death using transcranial Doppler. Neurosurgery 24:509–513, 1989.

138. Petty GW, Mohr JP, Pedley TA, et al: The role of transcranial Doppler in confirming brain death: Sensitivity, specificity, and suggestions for performance and interpretation. Neurology 40:300–303, 1990.

139. van der Naalt J, Baker AJ: Influence of the intra-aortic balloon pump on the transcranial Doppler flow pattern in a brain-dead patient. Stroke 27:140–142, 1996.

140. Hennerici M, Neuerburg-Heusler D: Vascular Diagnosis With Ultrasound: Clinical References with Case Studies. Stuttgart, Thieme, 1998, p 120.

141. Ducrocq X, Hassler W, Moritake K, et al: Consensus opinion on diagnosis of cerebral circulatory arrest using Doppler-sonography: Task Force Group on cerebral death of the Neurosonology Research Group of the World Federation of Neurology. J Neurol Sci 159:145–150, 1998.

142. Ducrocq X, Braun M, Debouverie M, et al: Brain death and transcranial Doppler: Experience in 130 cases of brain dead patients. J Neurol Sci 160:41–46, 1998.

143. Hadani M, Bruk B, Ram Z, et al: Application of transcranial doppler ultrasonography for the diagnosis of brain death. Intensive Care Med 25:822–828, 1999.

144. Wijdicks EF: The diagnosis of brain death. N Engl J Med 344:1215–1221, 2001.

145. Caplan LR, Mohr JP, Kistler JP, Koroshetz W: Should thrombolytic therapy be the first-line treatment for acute ischemic stroke? Thrombolysis—not a panacea for ischemic stroke. N Engl J Med 337:1309–1310, 1997.

146. Alexandrov AV, Grotta JC: Arterial re-occlusion in stroke patients treated with intravenous tissue plasminogen activator. Neurology 59:862–867, 2002.

147. Lewandowski CA, Frankel M, Tomsick TA, et al: Combined intravenous and intra-arterial r-TPA versus intra-arterial therapy of acute ischemic stroke: Emergency Management of Stroke (EMS) Bridging Trial. Stroke 30:2598–2605, 1999.

148. Warach S: Stroke neuroimaging. Stroke 34:345–347, 2003.

149. Xavier AR, Qureshi AI, Kirmani JF, et al: Neuroimaging of stroke: A review. South Med J 96:367–379, 2003.

150. Alexandrov AV, Demchuk A, Wein T, Grotta JC: The yield of transcranial Doppler in acute cerebral ischemia. Stroke 30:1605–1609, 1999.

151. Chernyshev O, Garami Z, Calleja S, et al: Yield and accuracy of emergent combined carotid/transcranial ultrasound examination in acute cerebral ischemia [abstract]. Stroke 35:28a, 2004.

152. Zanette EM, Fieschi C, Bozzao L, et al: Comparison of cerebral angiography and transcranial Doppler sonography in acute stroke. Stroke 20:899–903, 1989.

153. Razumovsky AY, Gillard JH, Bryan RN, et al: TCD, MRA, and MRI in acute cerebral ischemia. Acta Neurol Scand 99:65–76, 1999.

154. Kaps M, Damian MS, Teschendorf U, Dorndorf W: Transcranial Doppler ultrasound findings in the middle cerebral artery occlusion. Stroke 21:532–537, 1990.

155. Demchuk AM, Burgin WS, Christou I, et al: Thrombolysis in Brain Ischemia (TIBI) TCD flow grades predict clinical severity, early recovery and mortality in intravenous TPA treated patients. Stroke 32:89–93, 2001.

156. The TIMI Study Group: The Thrombolysis in Myocardial Infarction (TIMI) Trial: Phase I findings. N Engl J Med 312:932–936, 1985.

157. Labiche LA, Malkoff M, Alexandrov AV: Residual flow signals predict complete recanalization in stroke patients treated with TPA. J Neuroimaging 13:28–33, 2003.

158. Higashida RT, Furlan AJ: Trial Design and Reporting Standards for Intra-Arterial Cerebral Thrombolysis for Acute Ischemic Stroke. Stroke 34:1923–1924, 2003.

159. Alexandrov AV (ed): Cerebrovascular Ultrasound in Stroke Prevention and Treatment. New York, Blackwell Publishing/Futura, 2003.

160. Alexandrov AV: Ultrasound-enhanced thrombolysis for stroke: Clinical significance. Eur J Ultrasound 16:131–140, 2002.

161. Kaps M, Link A: Transcranial sonographic monitoring during thrombolytic therapy. Am J Neuroradiol 19:758–760, 1998.

162. Burgin WS, Malkoff M, Felberg RA, et al: Transcranial Doppler ultrasound criteria for recanalization after thrombolysis for middle cerebral artery stroke. Stroke 31:1128–1132, 2000.

163. Molina CA, Montaner J, Abilleira S, et al: Time course of tissue plasminogen activator-

induced recanalization in acute cardioembolic stroke: A case-control study. Stroke 32:2821–2827, 2001.

164. Alexandrov AV, Burgin WS, Demchuk AM, et al: Speed of intracranial clot lysis with intravenous TPA therapy: Sonographic classification and short term improvement. Circulation 103:2897–2902, 2001.

165. Eggers J, Koch B, Meyer K, et al: Effect of ultrasound on thrombolysis of middle cerebral artery occlusion. Ann Neurol 53:797–800, 2003.

166. Alexandrov AV, Demchuk AM, Felberg RA, et al: High rate of complete recanalization and dramatic clinical recovery during TPA infusion when continuously monitored by 2 MHz transcranial Doppler monitoring. Stroke 31:610–614, 2000.

167. Braaten JV, Goss RA, Francis CW: Ultrasound reversibly disaggregates fibrin fibers. Thromb Haemost 78:1063–1068, 1997.

168. Kondo I, Mizushige K, Ueda T, et al: Histological observations and the process of ultrasound contrast agent enhancement of tissue plasminogen activator thrombolysis with ultrasound exposure. Jpn Circ J63:478–484, 1999.

169. Francis CW, Onundarson PT, Carstensen EL, et al: Enhancement of fibrinolysis in vitro by ultrasound. J Clin Invest 90:2063–2068, 1992.

170. Francis CW, Blinc A, Lee S, Cox C: Ultrasound accelerates transport of recombinant tissue plasminogen activator into clots. Ultrasound Med Biol 21:419–424, 1995.

171. Siddiqi F, Blinc A, Braaten J, Francis CW: Ultrasound increases flow through fibrin gels. Thomb Haemost 21:419–424, 1995.

172. Behrens S, Spengos K, Daffertshoffer M, et al: Transcranial ultrasound-improved thrombolysis: Diagnostic versus therapeutic ultrasound. Ultrasound Med Biol 27:1683–1689, 2001.

173. Daffertshoffer M, Hennerici M: Ultrasound in the treatment of ischaemic stroke. Lancet Neurology 2:283–290, 2003.

174. Alexandrov AV: CLOTBUST: Results of a Multi-center Randomized Trial of Ultrasound Enhanced Thrombolysis for Acute Ischemic Stroke. Presentation at the 29th International Stroke Conference, San Diego, CA, February 5–7, 2004.

Chapter 6

Normal Cerebrovascular Anatomy and Collateral Pathways

EDWARD B. DIETHRICH, MD

The vascular system of the human brain differs significantly, both anatomically and physiologically, from other organs in the body. Although it accounts for only 2% of the body weight, the brain receives 15% of the cardiac output and consumes 20% of the body's oxygen supply in the basal state.[1] Cerebral arteries are little influenced by sympathetic nerves, unlike other arteries, but they are markedly affected by chemical changes in the blood.

Obstructive disease afflicting the cerebrovascular system can produce a wide array of sometimes ambiguous symptoms. Clinicians must attempt to identify the exact areas involved in the disease process; however, this is often made difficult by individual variability in the cerebral vasculature. Indeed, the extent of clinical symptoms is entirely dependent on the ability of the collateral circulation to maintain adequate cerebral perfusion. Therefore, understanding the normal and collateral anatomy and the mechanisms of cerebral blood flow is essential to the diagnosis of obstructive disease in the cerebrovascular system.

This chapter addresses the anatomic and physiologic principles that influence the investigation of the vascular supply to the brain. It is important to stress the significance of appreciating the hemodynamics of the brain. Individuals vary considerably in their ability to compensate for alterations in cerebral blood flow, and the physician must be aware of the potential mechanisms for cerebrovascular collateralization to carry out a judicious evaluation protocol.

As new treatment modalities become available for both extracranial and intra-cranial pathologies, a basic appreciation of normal anatomy, congenital variations, and collateral vascular pathways is extremely important. Angioplasty and stenting are now being used frequently to treat intracranial atherosclerotic disease, aneurysms, and stroke, and these techniques require extremely specialized knowledge of the vascular anatomy.

VASCULAR ANATOMY

The brain is supplied directly by four vessels: the two internal carotid arteries and the vertebral arteries. Any discussion of the cerebrovascular system must begin at the origins of these vessels, because obstructive disease, stenoses, ulcerative plaques, aneurysms, or anomalies anywhere in these arteries may produce a stroke or symptoms of vascular insufficiency.

The blood supply for the central nervous system[1-3] derives from the three great vessels arising from the aortic arch in the superior mediastinum—the brachiocephalic, the left common carotid, and the left subclavian arteries (Fig. 6–1). The brachiocephalic artery travels upward, slightly posterior from the arch to the right of the neck for its 4- to 5-cm length, dividing into the right common carotid artery and the right subclavian artery at the upper border of the right sternoclavicular junction. The left common carotid artery ascends from the arch and passes beneath the left sternoclavicular joint. Neither common carotid has collateral branches, but each divides into the internal and external carotid arteries at

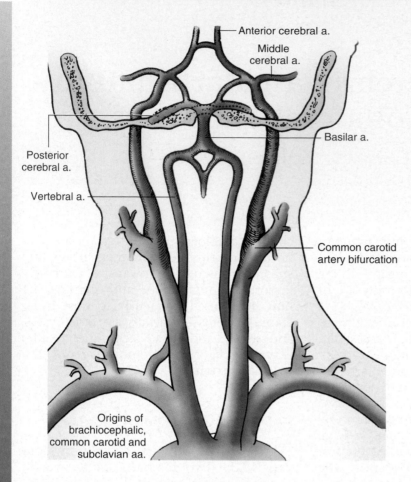

Anterior cerebral a.

Middle
cerebral a.

Basilar a.

Posterior
cerebral a.

Vertebral a.

Common carotid
artery bifurcation

Origins of
brachiocephalic,
common carotid and
subclavian aa.

FIGURE 6–1. Extracranial cerebro-vascular anatomy showing major arterial pathways to the brain.

the level of the upper border of the thyroid cartilage.

The internal carotids supply most of the anterior circulation to the cerebrum (Fig. 6–2). In their cervical portion, the internal carotid arteries may be relatively straight or may curve tortuously as they travel to the base of the skull. There are no branches of the internal carotid arteries in the neck. As they proceed intracranially, the internal carotid arteries give rise to the caroticotympanic branches in the petrous bone, the meningohypophyseal branches in the cavernous sinus region, and the ophthalmic arteries immediately distal to the cavernous sinus. Eight millimeters beyond the clinoid process, within the dura mater, the internal carotid arteries give rise to the posterior communicating arteries, which join with the posterior cerebral arteries. Further cephalad, the internal carotid arteries divide into the middle and anterior cerebral arter-

ies and give rise posteriorly to the anterior choroidal arteries.

The external carotid arteries normally supply no blood to the brain. However, several of their branches can become important collateral pathways if occlusion occurs in the internal carotid or vertebral arteries. The branches of the external carotid artery are the ascending pharyngeal, the superior thyroid, the lingual, the external maxillary, the occipital, the facial, the posterior auricular, the internal maxillary, the transverse facial, and the superficial temporal arteries. The external carotid branches most vital to collateral circulation are those in communication with the ophthalmic artery and those that interconnect between the muscular branches of the occipital and vertebral arteries (Fig. 6–3).

The posterior circulation to the brain is supplied in large part by the vertebral arteries arising from the subclavian arteries. The

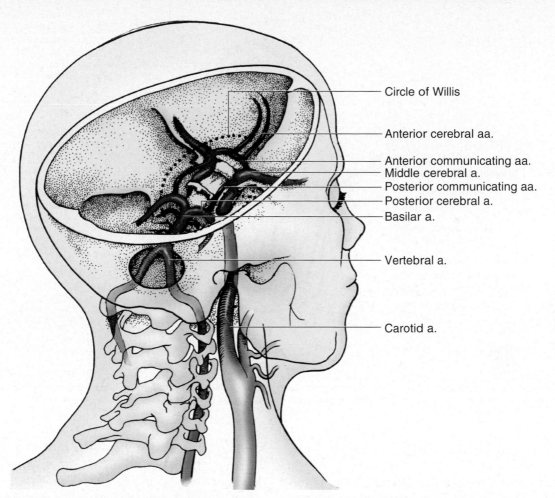

Circle of Willis

Anterior cerebral aa.

Anterior communicating aa.
Middle cerebral a.
Posterior communicating aa.
Posterior cerebral a.
Basilar a.

Vertebral a.

Carotid a.

FIGURE 6–2. Intracranial cerebrovascular anatomy showing anastomotic connections of the circle of Willis. Note that the principal blood supply to intracranial structures is through the carotid arteries.

vertebrals lie within the foramina transversarium of the upper cervical vertebrae and wind anteriorly into the subarachnoid space at the side of the medulla oblongata at the level of the atlanto-occipital interspace. They proceed cephalad and anteriorly until they reach the pontomedullary level, where they join to form the basilar artery. Four branches arise from the basilar artery as it courses upward before dividing into the posterior cerebral arteries. Branches of the basilar artery supply the entire pons and the superior and anterior aspects of the cerebellum. Branches of the vertebral arteries supply the medulla and the interior surface of the cerebellum.

The cerebral branches of the internal carotids and vertebral arteries are joined at the base of the brain by an arterial circle known as the circle of Willis. This anastomosis is the most important element in intracranial collateral circulation and is also a common site of aneurysmal formation. It is a hexagonal arrangement of arteries composed of the anterior, middle, and posterior cerebral arteries, which are joined together by the anterior and posterior communicating arteries (see Fig. 6–2). Under normal circumstances, there is little mixing of blood through the communicating arteries. However, in instances of arterial occlusion in carotid or vertebrobasilar vessels, this circle opens to function as a vital collateral pathway (see later).

Component arteries of the circle of Willis can vary greatly in size, and there are at least

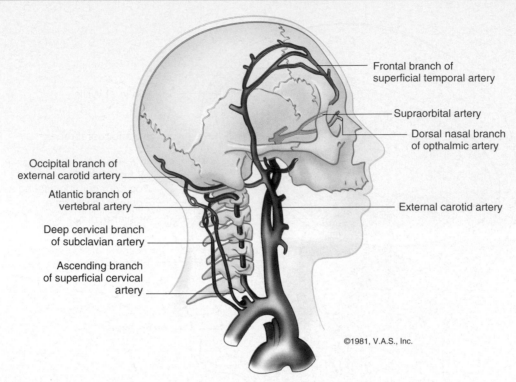

FIGURE 6–3. Extracranial cerebrovascular anatomy. Note the anastomotic connections between the external and internal carotid arteries and among the occipital, cervical, and vertebral arteries.

nine congenital variations in the structure of the circle (Fig. 6–4). The most common anomalies involve the absence or hypoplasia of one or both communicating arteries. An anomalous origin of the posterior cerebral artery from one or both internal carotid arteries has also been commonly encountered. Anomalies in the anterior portion of the circle are less commonly found, although among these, absence or hypoplasia of the proximal segment of the anterior cerebral artery between the internal carotid and anterior communicating arteries is more usual. Among the variations, the most significant in terms of decreasing collateral potential are those in which the anterior or posterior communicating arteries are absent or impervious. These conditions may isolate the anterior and posterior circulations or the left and right hemispheric carotid territories.

Normal arch formation is shown in Figure 6–5A. Anomalous formations can occur in the extracranial circulation, most commonly involving the origins of the carotid and vertebral arteries. Most frequent is a sharing or close association between of the origin of the brachiocephalic artery with the left common carotid artery (Fig. 6–5B). Less often, the left common carotid artery may arise from the brachiocephalic artery (Fig. 6–5C). Also seen is the anomalous origin of the left vertebral artery on the aortic arch between the left common carotid and subclavian arteries (Fig. 6–5D). Rarely, the right subclavian artery may have an aberrant origin on the aortic arch. Other abnormalities may occur in the cervical region, such as agenesis of the internal carotid arteries, but these are rare. Abnormalities in the vertebral arteries are usually limited to variations in size between the left and right, a common occurrence.

CEREBRAL HEMODYNAMICS

Before discussing the potential collateral pathways in the cerebrovascular system, it is best to explain the dynamics of cerebral blood flow[1,4] to help gain an appreciation of the importance of collateralization.

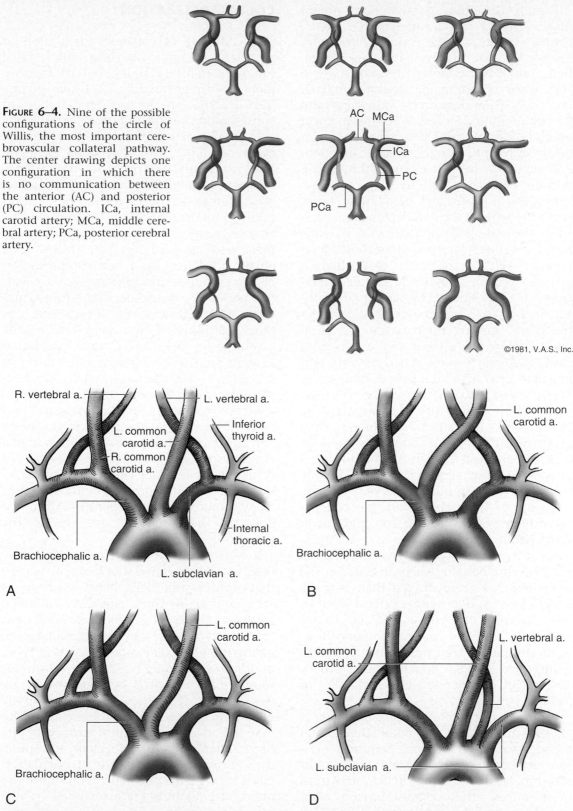

FIGURE 6–4. Nine of the possible configurations of the circle of Willis, the most important cerebrovascular collateral pathway. The center drawing depicts one configuration in which there is no communication between the anterior (AC) and posterior (PC) circulation. ICa, internal carotid artery; MCa, middle cerebral artery; PCa, posterior cerebral artery.

©1981, V.A.S., Inc.

FIGURE 6–5. *A,* Normal arch configuration. *B,* Sharing or close association of the origin of the brachiocephalic artery with the left common carotid artery. *C,* Left common carotid artery arising from the brachiocephalic artery. *D,* Anomalous origin of the left vertebral artery on the aortic arch between the left common carotid and subclavian arteries.

Despite the brain's large apportionment of the body's blood supply (15% of the cardiac output), there is little circulatory reserve because of the brain's high metabolic rate. Furthermore, the brain has no significant oxygen or glucose stores, making it entirely dependent on the vascular system for maintenance.[1,2] This is why even short episodes of interrupted cerebral flow can bring on symptoms of cerebral dysfunction, and cellular death can occur within 3 to 8 minutes of vascular failure.

Extrinsically, cerebral blood flow varies with the effective arterial perfusion pressure. Adequate perfusion relies on systemic blood pressure, cardiac output, and blood volume. Within the range of fluctuation possible for these extrinsic factors, blood flow can be modulated by a group of intrinsic factors that control cerebral vascular resistance. Among these factors are intracranial pressure, arterial oxygen tension, carbon dioxide tension, blood viscosity, and vascular tone. Although the cerebral vessels are supplied with nerves, there has been little evidence that they play other than a minor role in controlling blood flow. Oxygen and carbon dioxide concentrations play the greatest roles in modulating cerebrovascular resistance, with carbon dioxide being the more significant factor.

Variations in cerebral blood gas concentrations serve to provide constant blood flow within a wide range of systemic pressures and also provide local control to areas with varying demands.[1] For instance, if the brain requires more oxygen than is being supplied, it produces more carbon dioxide. This increase in carbon dioxide causes vasodilatation and increases blood flow until enough oxygen has been supplied to reduce the carbon dioxide concentration. This effect can happen either globally or locally.

Compensatory cerebral vasodilatation is also the mechanism that maintains cerebral blood flow when cerebral perfusion pressure drops as a person assumes an upright position. However, if the circulation is compromised by atherosclerotic disease, compensation may be insufficient, leading to symptoms of regional or diffuse hypoxia or anoxia.

COLLATERALIZATION

The vital role of collateral circulation in vascular occlusion has been appreciated for more than a century, but its involvement in cerebrovascular occlusive disease has become an increasingly important consideration as treatment of extracranial and intracranial pathologies has become more common. The advent of angiography[4-6] certainly improved our understanding of treatment options and, more recently, other diagnostic techniques such as duplex ultrasound, four-vessel selective arch intracranial angiography, and magnetic resonance angiography (MRA) have all provided us with a better appreciation of the existence and importance of collateral pathways. Clinicians evaluating symptoms of cerebrovascular insufficiency or other pathologies must be aware of the extent of (or lack of) collateral circulation as they prepare for modern interventional procedures. For example, when contemplating carotid stenting with embolic protection, one must consider the condition of the contralateral internal carotid artery and its contribution to the intracranial circulation (Fig. 6–6). In the presence of contralateral internal carotid artery occlusion, the cerebral protection device most likely should be one that permits continued flow on the ipsilateral side during the procedure.

It was once believed that arteries in the brain were end arteries, but it is now known that capillary and precapillary anastomoses are common. To appreciate these collateral pathways better, it should be noted that there are two types of arterial branches supplying the brain. The more important types in terms of neuronal function and nutrient supply for the central nervous system are the penetrating arteries. However, it is the diffuse circumferential or superficial arteries that spread over the entire surface of the cervical hemispheres, brain stem, and spinal cord through which collateral circulation takes place. The circle of Willis and the major arterial trunks are included in this superficial system.

The routes for intracranial collateral circulation can be divided into three

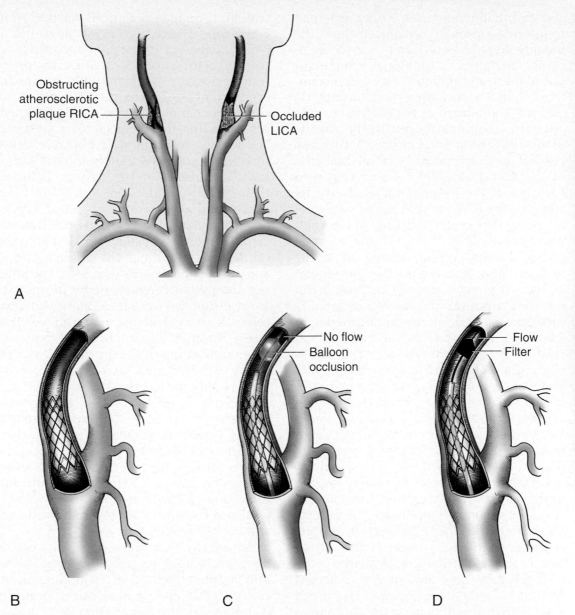

FIGURE 6–6. *A,* Obstructing atherosclerotic plaque in the right internal carotid artery and an occluded left internal carotid artery. *B,* Proposed treatment is internal carotid artery stenting with embolic protection. *C,* Balloon occlusive device eliminates flow. *D,* Filter device permits flow while trapping emboli and is probably a better choice in this case.

categories: large interarterial connections, intracranial-extracranial anastomoses, and small interarterial communications. The major pathway is the circle of Willis, providing communication between the two carotid arteries or between the basilar artery and the right or left carotid artery. As described earlier, the anatomic variations possible within this arterial circle are normally of little importance unless occlusion in one of the cervical vessels occurs, demanding collateral blood flow.

Second only to the circle of Willis in importance are the complex intracranial-extracranial or prewillisian anastomoses. Perhaps the best-known prewillisian anastomosis is that between the external and internal carotid arteries, through the orbital and ophthalmic arteries. Other external-to-internal carotid collaterals include the meningohypophyseal and caroticotympanic branches. Additional important prewillisian anastomoses may be encountered clinically, including the following: (1) the occipital branch of the external carotid artery in communication with the atlantic branch of the vertebral artery; (2) the deep cervical and ascending cervical branches of the subclavian artery connecting with branches of the lower vertebral artery, the atlantic branch of the upper vertebral artery, and the occipital branch of the internal carotid artery; and (3) the external carotid arteries communicating across the midline. Also included in the prewillisian group is the rete mirabile or "wonderful net" of transdural anastomoses across the subdural space from the dural arteries to arteries on the surface of the brain.

Of lesser importance are the leptomeningeal collaterals forming the meningeal border zone network. These connect the terminal cortical branches of the main cerebral arteries across the border zones along each vascular territory. Although these are not major collateral pathways, they may be sufficiently developed to interfere with the diagnosis of cerebrovascular insufficiency. Indeed, arterial occlusions may not become symptomatic because of adequate perfusion by the leptomeningeal anastomoses in the portion of the thrombosed artery's distribution. Similarly, excellent collateral flow around a thrombosed cortical vessel may induce rapid clearing of a neurologic deficit, leading the clinician to believe an extracranial occlusive process is involved.

It should be noted that there are no effective anastomotic pathways between neighboring cerebral artery branches, deep penetrating arteries, or the superficial and deep branches of the cerebral arteries.

The opening of collateral pathways is dependent largely on the age of the individual and the time sequence of occlusion. In older individuals, collateral pathways are more likely to be hypoplastic or involved in the atherosclerotic process. Even collateral vessels of sufficient luminal size are often not able to adapt rapidly

enough to sudden occlusions, such as from embolism. Hence, collateral flow has a better chance of developing adequately in persons with slowly evolving atherosclerotic occlusions. When multiple atherosclerotic lesions are present, the adequacy of the collateral channels may be greatly lessened. Also affecting the adequacy of a collateral bed are the availability of multiple rather than single collateral sources and the pathologic conditions of the vessels, reducing their capacity for dilation.

Extracranially, there are numerous cervicocranial collaterals. Occlusion of an internal carotid produces collateral circulation to the carotid siphon through the external carotid and ophthalmic arteries (Fig. 6–7). The anterior and middle cerebral arteries in this case are also supplied from the opposite anterior cerebral artery and the posterior cerebral artery through the anterior and posterior communicating arteries. In the case of vertebral occlusion near its origin (Fig. 6–8), flow is shunted to the thyrocervical and costocervical axes, with compensatory enlargement of the opposite vertebral artery. Collateral circulation arising from occlusion of large branches of the aortic arch is through the intercostal and internal mammary arteries to the subclavian, and then through the branches of the thyrocervical and costocervical axes to the vertebral and carotid arteries (Fig. 6–9).

Historically, a number of procedures have been used to judge collateral flow. The simplest method of estimating intracranial collateral potential was a 5-minute common carotid compression test. Today, though, with the advent of angiography and magnetic resonance angiography techniques, such procedures are rarely used. Indeed, the ability to actually visualize collateral flow in pathologic conditions and create a "road map" for interventional correction has changed diagnosis and treatment considerably.

CONCLUSIONS

The vascular system of the human brain can be afflicted by obstructive disease, which produces a variety of often nebulous

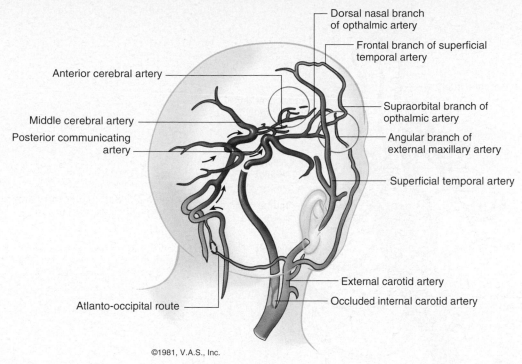

FIGURE 6–7. Major external carotid and vertebral collateral pathways associated with internal carotid occlusion.

symptoms. In attempting to evaluate these symptoms and define the areas of disease involvement, the clinician must have a thorough knowledge of the vascular anatomy and an appreciation of the individual variability that may be encountered.

The physician must also be cognizant of cerebral hemodynamics and the availability of collateral flow to interpret test results, characterize symptoms, and arrive at an accurate diagnosis. Modern treatments using endoluminal technologies have

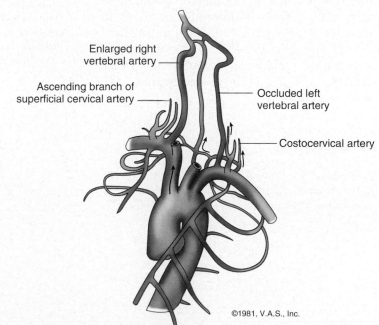

FIGURE 6–8. Major collateral pathways in vertebral occlusion.

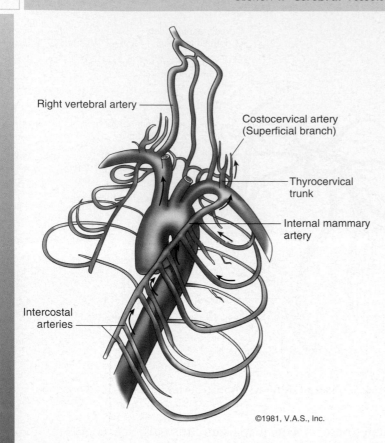

Right vertebral artery

Costocervical artery
(Superficial branch)

Thyrocervical
trunk

Internal mammary
artery

Intercostal
arteries

©1981, V.A.S., Inc.

Figure 6–9. Major collateral pathways in proximal subclavian occlusion.

accentuated the need for a better understanding of vascular anatomy and its variations and collateral pathways.

This chapter has presented an in-depth review of normal cerebrovascular anatomy and commonly encountered anomalies, with a discussion of hemodynamics as it applies to the potential for collateralization. Commonly encountered extracranial and intracranial collateral circulation has been defined, and its clinical significance has been emphasized.

References

1. Stephens RB, Stilwell DL: Arteries and Veins of the Human Brain. Springfield, IL, Charles C Thomas, 1969.
2. McVay CB: Anson and McVay Surgical Anatomy, 6th ed. Philadelphia, WB Saunders, 1984.
3. Clemente CD (ed): Gray's Anatomy of the Human Body, 30th American ed. Philadelphia, Lea & Febiger, 1985.
4. Meyer JS (ed): Modern Concepts of Cerebrovascular Disease. New York, Spectrum Books, 1975.
5. Fields WS, Breutman ME, Weibel J: Collateral Circulation to the Brain. Baltimore, Williams & Wilkins, 1965.
6. Strandness DE Jr: Collateral Circulation in Clinical Surgery. Philadelphia, WB Saunders, 1969.

Chapter 7

Normal Findings and Technical Aspects of Carotid Sonography

WILLIAM J. ZWIEBEL, MD

NORMAL CAROTID WALL STRUCTURE

The walls of all arteries consist of three distinct layers. The innermost layer is the *intima*, or epithelial lining of the artery. The middle layer is the *media*, or muscular layer, which gives the artery its stiffness, elasticity, and strength. The outer layer is the *adventitia*, which is composed of loose connective tissue. As illustrated in Figure 7–1, all three layers are represented in ultrasound images.[1–3] The intima and adventitia produce parallel echogenic lines, with an intervening echo void that represents the media. Please note that the intimal reflection is only a reflection! The thickness of this reflection exceeds the actual thickness of the intima. Histologic studies have shown that the thickness of the media and adventitia are more accurately depicted on ultrasound images.[1]

The intimal reflection should be straight, thin, and parallel to the adventitial layer. Significant undulation and thickening of the intima indicate plaque deposition (see Chapter 8) or, rarely, fibromuscular hyperplasia. After endarterectomy, the intimal reflection is missing at the surgical site, because the intima is removed with the plaque. The neointima that covers the endarterectomy site is not visible sonographically.

Seeing the intimal reflection on longitudinal images ensures that the image plane passes through the long axis (diameter) of the vessel. Similarly, in transverse sections, visualization of the intima indicates that the image plane is perpendicular to the vessel axis. A false impression of arterial wall thickening may occur with off-axis longitudinal images, as illustrated in Figure 7–2.

The carotid bulb is the widened portion of the distal common and proximal internal carotid arteries. Thus, the carotid bulb does not merely lie in the internal carotid, as is sometimes thought, but spans the junction of both vessels. The degree to which the carotid arteries widen at the carotid bulb varies from one individual to another. Usually the widening is slight, but some normal individuals have capacious carotid bulbs that may harbor large plaques in the absence of significant carotid stenosis.

NORMAL FLOW CHARACTERISTICS

In normal arteries that are relatively straight, blood flow is *laminar*, meaning that blood cells move in parallel lines. As shown in Figure 7–3, the laminar flow pattern can sometimes be seen on color flow images, with slower velocities near the vessel wall and faster velocities near the lumen center producing different colors. It is important to recognize that flow is not always laminar in normal vessels. As noted in Chapter 3, the laminar pattern may be disturbed by vessel tortuosity, kinks, or branching. These normal flow disturbances are shown by mixtures of colors on color flow images and by Doppler spectral broadening. The most noteworthy normal flow disturbance occurs at the carotid bifurcation (Fig. 7–4), where a vortex is established in the bulbous portions of the common carotid artery (CCA) and

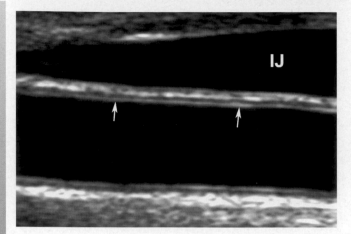

FIGURE 7–1. Normal arterial anatomy. This longitudinal image of the common carotid artery demonstrate a sharp line (specular reflection) that emanates from the intimal surface (*arrows*). The black line peripheral to this reflection represents the media of the artery. The outermost white line is the adventitia of the artery. Note that no wall structure is visible in the adjacent internal jugular vein (IJ), because vein walls have a very thin muscular layer and are much thinner, overall, than arterial walls.

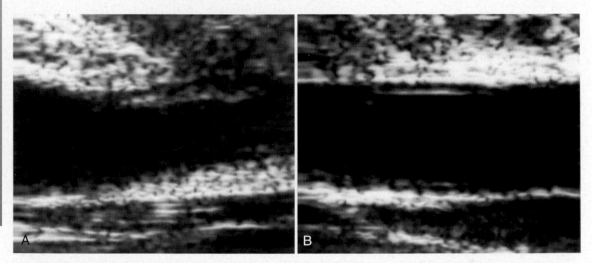

FIGURE 7–2. False positive plaque diagnosis due to off-axis image plane. *A*, It appears that plaque is present, resulting in stenosis, in this off-diameter section of the common carotid artery. *B*, The same artery is shown to be normal by moving the transducer very slightly so that the plane of the section passes through the long axis (diameter) of the vessel. Note the clearly seen intimal reflections.

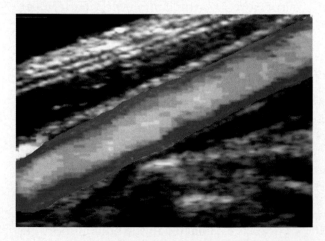

FIGURE 7–3. Laminar flow pattern. Darker red shades are seen at the periphery of this common carotid artery, because flow is slower near the wall. Lighter colors are present throughout the rest of the vessel, in which flow is faster.

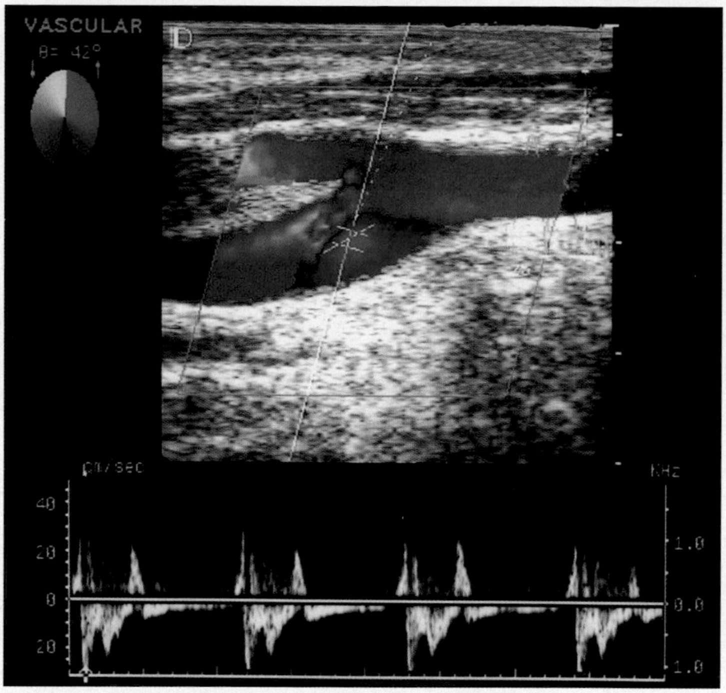

FIGURE 7–4. Long-axis view of the carotid bifurcation. The blue area in the bulbous portion of the internal carotid artery represents the normal flow reversal zone. The Doppler spectrum seen at the base of the image shows a disturbed, to-and-fro pattern caused by simultaneous forward and reverse flow in this area.

internal carotid artery (ICA).[4-7] The size of the vortex appears to be related to anatomic factors, including the diameter of the artery lumen and the degree of angulation between the ICA and the external carotid artery (ECA).

The normal pulsatility features of the CCA, ICA, and ECA, as depicted with spectral Doppler, are of considerable diagnostic importance and require close attention. Normal pulsatility features are used to distinguish between the ICA and ECA; furthermore, altered carotid pulsatility is an important clue about the presence of carotid occlusive disease. In some cases, pulsatility changes are the *only* indication of significant carotid abnormality. Please review the normal carotid pulsatility features illustrated in Figure 7–5. This material is not repeated elsewhere in the text.

The normal range of velocities in the CCA, ICA, and ECA has not been studied extensively,[8-11] and velocities may vary with physiologic differences among individuals. Peak systolic velocity in the CCA is not well documented, but clinical experience indicates that velocities exceeding 100 cm/sec are uncommon. It is noteworthy that the CCA peak systolic velocity increases as one

proceeds proximally from the carotid bifurcation (toward the aortic arch).[12] Peak systolic velocity increases about 9 cm/sec for each centimeter of distance. This observation is of considerable importance, as the measured systolic velocity ratio (ICA stenosis/CCA; see Chapter 9) may vary from one examination to another if the CCA measurement is made at various distances from the carotid bifurcation. The general recommendation is to measure the CCA velocity at a standardized distance below the "crotch" of the carotid bifurcation. We use 4 cm, because this is the length of the ultrasound transducer that we use for carotid artery examination. The ultrasound transducer, therefore, becomes a handy measuring stick. The CCA velocity is measured one transducer length from the crotch of the bifurcation.

Peak systolic velocity in the ICA is reported to range from 54 to 88 cm/sec in normal adults (mean population values). It should be noted that these values apply to the postbulbar region of the ICA. Values observed within the bulbous portion of the ICA are lower, and, as noted in Chapter 3, the spectral waveforms in the bulb may have a peculiar to-and-fro appearance. Peak

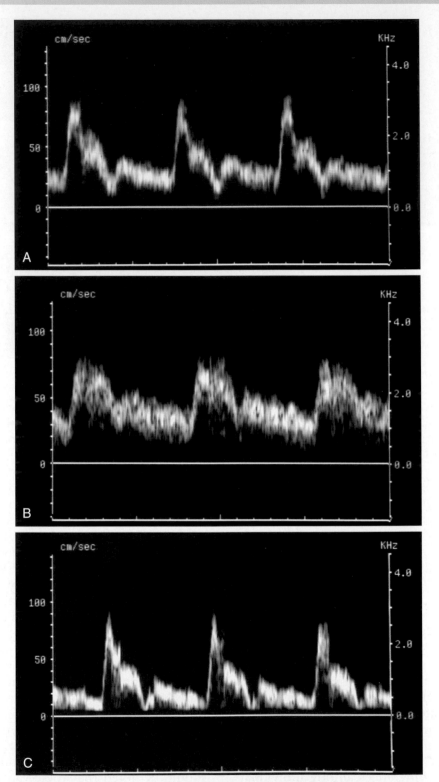

FIGURE 7–5. Normal carotid artery Doppler waveforms. *A,* Waveforms in the common carotid artery have moderately broad systolic peaks and a moderate amount of flow throughout diastole. *B,* The internal carotid artery waveforms have broad systolic peaks and a large amount of flow throughout diastole. *C,* External carotid artery waveforms have sharp systolic peaks and relatively little flow in diastole.

Table 7–1. Features That Identify the External and Internal Carotid Arteries

Features	Carotid Arteries	
	External	*Internal*
Size	Usually smaller	Usually larger
Branches	Yes	No
Orientation	Proceeds anteriorly, toward the face	Proceeds posteriorly, toward the mastoid process
Doppler characteristics	High-resistance flow pattern	Low-resistance flow pattern
Temporal artery tap	Waveform deflections	No deflections

systolic ICA velocities as high as 120 cm/sec have been reported in some normal individuals, but these values are exceptional, and an ICA velocity exceeding 100 cm/sec should be viewed as potentially abnormal.

Peak systolic velocity in the ECA is reported as 77 cm/sec (mean) in normal individuals, and the maximum velocity does not normally exceed 115 cm/sec. Considerable patient-to-patient variability occurs in ECA flow velocity in normal individuals because pulsatility varies considerably from one person to another. (Some individuals have a sharply spiked systolic peak, while others have a more blunted peak.) Moreover, ECA velocity may be elevated substantially if the ECA is serving as a collateral that circumvents an ipsilateral or contralateral ICA stenosis. Therefore, high ICA velocities may occasionally be encountered in the absence of ECA stenosis.

VESSEL IDENTITY

The correct identification of the ECA and ICA is of utmost importance, because significant diagnostic error may occur if these vessels are misidentified. All of the findings listed in Table 7–1 are useful for distinguishing between the ICA and ECA, but among these, the Doppler findings are of greatest importance. The ICA has a low-resistance flow pattern, whereas the ECA has a high-resistance pattern. If the identity of the carotid bifurcation branches is uncertain, move the Doppler sample volume back and forth between the branches. The Doppler signals from the two vessels should look and sound *different* if one of the vessels is the ICA and the other is the ECA. If the Doppler signals look and *sound* the same in both vessels, then the vessels identified are probably two ECA branches, and the ICA is probably occluded. Most importantly, tapping on the superficial temporal artery, in front of the ear, causes notches in the ECA Doppler spectrum (Fig. 7–6). Tapping does not affect the ICA spectrum, since the superficial temporal artery is not a tributary of the ICA. When all efforts fail and bifurcation branch identity remains uncertain, do not guess! Indicate to the interpreting sonologist that you are not sure whether you have actually identified the ECA and ICA and that you may instead have imaged

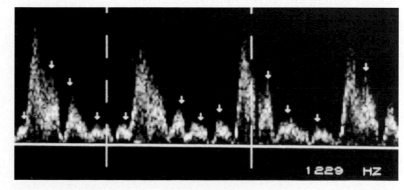

FIGURE 7–6. Temporal artery tapping identifies the external carotid artery. The taps of the examiner's finger generate sharp deflections (*arrows*) on the external carotid artery waveform.

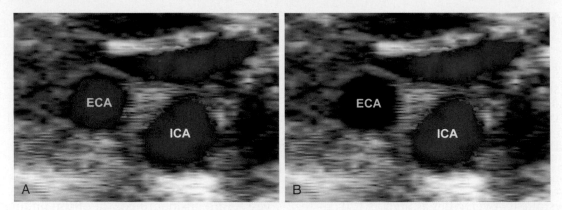

FIGURE 7–7. Color Doppler visualization of pulsatility patterns. *A*, In systole, flow is evident (red color) in both the internal (ICA) and external (ECA) carotid arteries. *B*, In diastole, flow is absent in the external carotid artery (ECA) but persists in the internal carotid artery (ICA). When seen in real time, the color in the ECA "blinks" on and off, whereas color undulates in brightness in the ICA.

two branches or the ECA. In such a case, occlusion of the ICA is implied. It is better to say that you are uncertain than to make a major diagnostic error, such as overlooking ICA occlusion.

Differences in ECA and ICA pulsatility are also manifested in the color flow image (Fig. 7–7). Flow continues throughout the entire cardiac cycle in the CCA and ICA. As a result, color is always present in these vessels, although the brightness *undulates* from diastole to systole. In the ECA, flow is markedly diminished or absent in diastole; consequently, color *flickers* off and on in this vessel.

EXAMINATION PROTOCOL

An examination protocol should be established within each vascular laboratory to ensure that carotid sonography is performed consistently, comprehensively, and accurately. The ultrasound protocols described here are used in our vascular laboratory. These techniques may be modified to match the needs of specific patients or vascular laboratories. In all cases, however, the protocol should meet or exceed the standards established by the *American Institute of Ultrasound in Medicine,** the *Intersocietal Commission for the Accreditation*

of Vascular Laboratories,[†] or the *American College of Radiology*.[‡] The standards of these organizations are substantially the same.

INSTRUMENTATION

The carotid duplex examination should be performed only with appropriate instrumentation. The current standard of practice in the United States includes the following equipment: (1) high-frequency transducers with short focal distances designed for near-field work; (2) color flow imaging; (3) pulsed, directional Doppler, with velocity measurement capabilities; and (4) frequency spectrum analysis. A large number of instruments are available that provide these features.

PATIENT POSITION

We examine the carotid arteries with the patient in the supine position and with the examiner seated at the patient's head. Some sonographers choose to sit next to the patient rather than at the patient's head. In some institutions, the patient is examined in a reclining chair equipped with a headrest, such as a dental chair. In any case, exposure of the neck should be maximized by having the patient drop the ipsilateral

*American Institute of Ultrasound in Medicine, 14750 Sweitzer Lane, Suite 100, Laurel, MD 20707; http://www.aium.org.

[†]Intersocietal Commission for Accreditation of Vascular Laboratories, 8840 Stanford Boulevard, Suite 4900, Columbia, MD 21045; http://www.icavl.org.
[‡]American College of Radiology, 1891 Preston White Drive, Reston, VA 20191; http://www.acr.org.

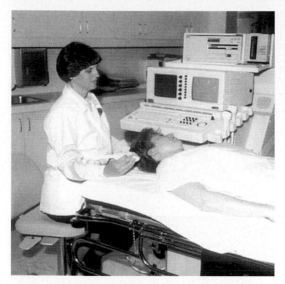

FIGURE 7–8. Patient and technologist positions for carotid ultrasound examination.

shoulder as far as possible. (Tell the patient, "Reach down for your hip.") Neck exposure is also optimized by tilting and rotating the head away from the side being examined (Fig. 7–8). Do not hesitate to vary the position of the head and neck during the examination to facilitate visualization of the vessels. Be creative!

TRANSDUCER POSITION

Several transducer positions are used to examine the carotid arteries in long-axis (longitudinal) planes, as illustrated in Figure 7–9. Generally, the posterolateral and far-posterolateral positions are most useful for showing the carotid bifurcation and the ICA, but, in some cases, an anterior or lateral approach works best. Short-axis (transverse) views of the carotid arteries are obtained from an anterior, lateral, or posterolateral approach, depending on which best shows the vessels.

The *far*-posterolateral approach often provides the best images of the distal reaches of the ICA. To use this view effectively, it is necessary to turn the patient's head far to the contralateral side and to place the transducer posterior to the sternomastoid muscle (see Fig. 7–9D). Neophyte sonographers generally have difficulty imaging the ICA, because they fail to approach the vessel from a sufficiently posterior location.

CAROTID ARTERY VERSUS JUGULAR VEIN

The CCA lies immediately adjacent to the jugular vein, but the two vessels are easily differentiated. First, flow in the carotid artery is toward the head and pulsatile. In contrast, flow in the jugular vein is toward the feet and has typical venous flow features (low velocity, undulating flow pattern, "windstorm" sound). Also, the caliber of the carotid artery is fairly uniform, whereas the caliber of the jugular vein varies markedly from moment to moment, in response to respiration. Finally, the carotid arteries are thick walled, and a distinct intimal reflection is visible. The jugular vein wall is thin (invisible), and the vein collapses with slight pressure from the transducer.

IMAGE ORIENTATION

Consistent with internationally accepted conventions, we orient longitudinal images with the patient's head to the left. Likewise, transverse images generally are oriented as if viewed from the patient's feet, with the patient's right side on the left side of the image. Admittedly, we are not terribly particular about transverse image orientation, but we label the vessels accurately.

RECORDING

In the past, we routinely recorded the entire carotid ultrasound examination on videotape, but we no longer do this, as color hard-copy imaging has improved, and reviewing taped studies is cumbersome. Many ultrasound instruments can record short video clips, often in conjunction with digital picture archiving systems. These clips are very helpful for illustrating dynamic features of the carotid examination. In western nations, digital picture archiving systems are now in common use for ultrasound recording, but transparent film or color (paper) prints also remain in widespread use. In either case, it is important to conduct the examination in a consistent pattern. We start with the right carotid bifurcation and then go to the left.

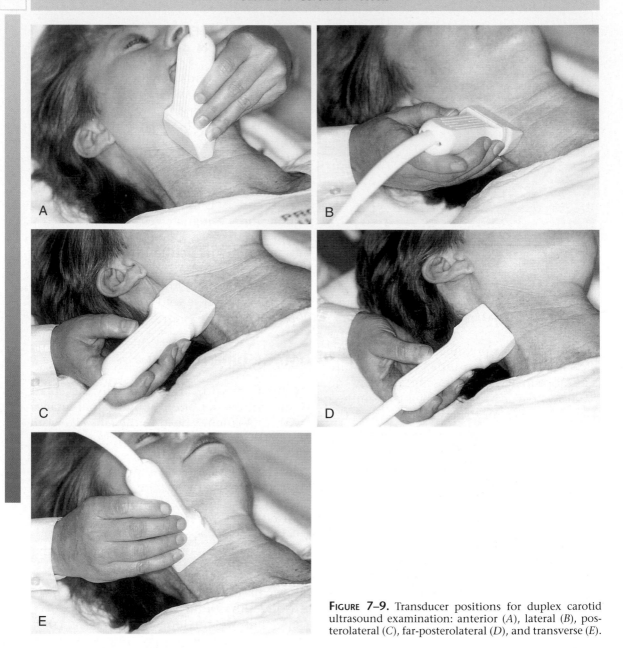

FIGURE 7–9. Transducer positions for duplex carotid ultrasound examination: anterior (*A*), lateral (*B*), posterolateral (*C*), far-posterolateral (*D*), and transverse (*E*).

All segments of the examination are recorded in sequence, beginning with the CCA and proceeding into the ICA and then the ECA. With this patterned approach, hard-copy images are recorded in an orderly, predictable way, which greatly simplifies interpretation of the studies. The patterned recording approach, furthermore, reduces the potential for diagnostic error, because the interpreter is less apt to mistake one Doppler waveform or vessel for another.

In addition to hard-copy images, we routinely use a report form (Fig. 7–10), on which the sonographer writes important information, including the patient history, blood flow velocity data (derived from spectrum analysis), and notations concerning plaque location and severity. This form is filed permanently in the vascular laboratory. A dictated report is included in the hospital chart and is transmitted to the referring clinician.

Department of Veterans Affairs

Vascular Laboratory
VA Medical Center
Salt Lake City, Utah

Carotid Artery Duplex Ultrasound

PATIENT IDENTIFICATION

Date: ____________ Technologist: ______ Tape # ______ Requested By: ________________

History: ____

Slurred Speech	❑	Amaurosis Fugax	R / L
Vertigo	❑	Blurred Vision	R / L
Drop Attack	❑	Hemiplegia	R / L
Memory Impairment/Confusion	❑	Weakness-Numbness Arm/Leg	R / L
		Previous Carotid Surgery	R / L

Prior Duplex or Angio Resuts______________________________

Right Carotid

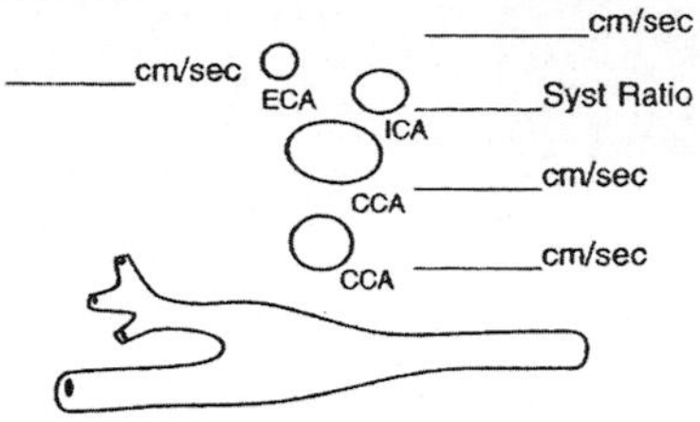

Left Carotid

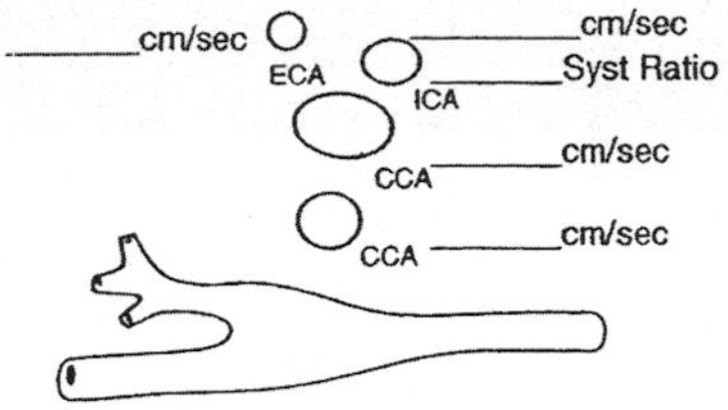

Right Vertebral

Diameter ______ mm ______ cm/sec Ante/Retro

Left Vertebral

Diameter ______ mm ______ cm/sec Ante/Retro

Technologist Comments: ______________________________

Right	**Preliminary**	**Final**	**Left**	**Preliminary**	**Final**
CCA	________	________	CCA	________	________
ICA	________	________	ICA	________	________
ECA	________	________	ECA	________	________
Progression	Y / N	Y / N	Progression	Y / N	Y / N

4-Part – White: Radiology - Pink: Preliminary Copy - Yellow: Medical Records - Goldenrod: MD

VA Form 10-44/C (114/660)
August 1994

FIGURE 7–10. Report form for carotid ultrasound examination. CCA, common carotid artery; ECA, external carotid artery; ICA, internal carotid artery.

THE EXAMINATION SEQUENCE

According to our department protocol, carotid examinations follow these steps:

Step 1. *Get oriented!* Choose the transducer position that best displays the carotid vessels in a longitudinal view. Generally, the posterolateral approach, as shown in Figure 7–9*D*, is most advantageous.

Step 2. *Record a velocity spectrum* from the CCA (Fig. 7–11). A recording site that is free of disease is preferred, and the following points should be noted: (1) The

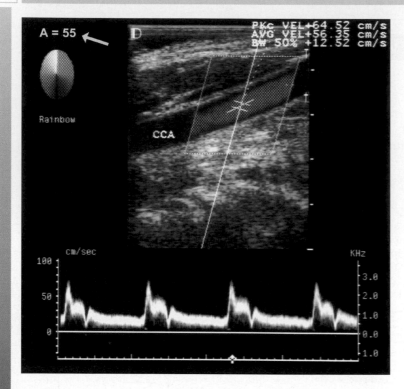

FIGURE 7–11. Accurate common carotid artery (CCA) velocity measurement. The CCA is clearly visualized; the Doppler sample volume is central in the artery and below the bulbous portion. The Doppler angle (*arrow*, left upper corner) is 60 degrees or less, and the Doppler signal (waveform) is strong and clear. AVG VEL, average velocity; BW, bandwidth; PKc VEL, peak systolic velocity.

measurement point should be 4 cm below the crotch of the carotid bifurcation (for reasons described previously); (2) care should be taken that the sample volume is squarely within the center of the vessel; and (3) the Doppler angle must be sufficient (60–70 degrees is best) to accurately measure the peak systolic velocity (see Chapter 3). These conditions are extremely important, as improper sampling of the CCA may artifactually raise or lower the peak systolic velocity, in turn skewing the systolic velocity ratio used to estimate ICA narrowing (see Chapters 3 and 9). The result could be inaccurate diagnosis of clinically significant carotid narrowing.

Step 3. Survey the carotid bifurcation with color flow imaging. Begin at the clavicle with longitudinal images, proceed to the carotid bifurcation, and, from there, continue into the ECA and ICA. Then repeat the process with transverse images. The purpose of this survey is to confirm the patency of the arteries, to identify and localize plaque and associated flow abnormalities, and to define the junction of the ECA and ICA (so that plaque location can be determined correctly).

Step 4. Confirm the identity of the ICA and ECA by their Doppler spectral signatures (see Fig. 7–5), by anatomic features summarized in Table 7–1, and by tapping on the superficial temporal artery (Fig 7–6). The proper identification of the branch vessels is essential, as ECA stenoses usually are not subject to treatment, while significant ICA stenoses usually are treated.

Step 5. With the survey completed and the identity of the ICA and ECA confirmed, *scrutinize significant areas of plaque formation*, documenting with hard copy the thickness of plaque, the degree of lumen reduction, and other plaque features (as discussed in subsequent chapters). Images transverse to the vessel axis are essential for assessment of plaque thickness and luminal narrowing, and gray-scale images often show plaque features better than color flow images.

A view that simultaneously shows both the ECA and the ICA, as seen in Figure 7–4,

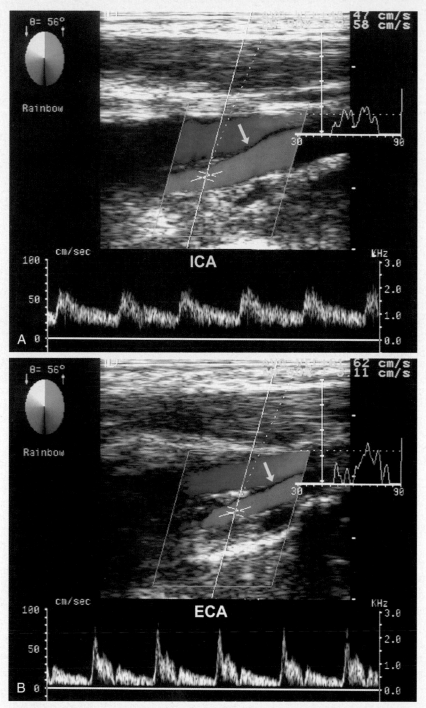

FIGURE 7–12. Identifying the internal and external carotid arteries. By shifting back and forth between the internal (*A*) and external (*B*) carotid arteries (ICA and ECA, respectively), the sonographer has determined that the junction of the vessels is at the approximate location of the *arrows*. The pulsatility of the ICA is clearly different from that of the ECA.

is very useful for localizing plaque. Unfortunately, this view cannot frequently be achieved (due to an unfavorable orientation of the carotid bifurcation). As an alternative, plaque location may be determined by shifting the image back and forth between the bifurcation branches and noting the point at which they come together (Fig. 7–12). This operation can be documented with a video clip.

Step 6. When a stenosis is present, *record angle-corrected velocity spectra in the stenosis* (as discussed in Chapter 3) also obtain color flow images that illustrate the location and length of the stenosis, as well as the flow disturbances present in the stenotic and poststenotic regions. If possible, obtain cross-sectional images showing the degree of luminal narrowing. Video clips of the color flow and spectral components can provide dynamic information of value to the interpreting sonologist.

Step 7. *Evaluate vertebral artery flow*, as discussed in Chapter 11. Record an image of the inter-transverse portion of each vertebral artery and representative Doppler spectral waveform, including measurement of the peak systolic velocity.

Step 8. *Assess subclavian artery flow*, to detect stenosis or occlusion of these vessels. Each subclavian artery is imaged from a long-axis perspective, from either a supraclavicular approach or a transpectoral approach (see Chapter 16). This can be done at the beginning or the end of the ipsilateral carotid examination. A representative Doppler spectral waveform is recorded in each vessel. These waveforms should show a high-resistance flow pattern and be slightly pulsatile. A low-resistance or damped pattern, and lack of pulsatility, suggests stenosis or occlusion proximal to the point of Doppler examination. In some cases, a subclavian stenosis may be visualized directly. In such instances, color Doppler images of the stenosis should be recorded, and Doppler spectral measurement should be obtained in and distal to the stenosis, in the same manner as for carotid stenosis.

References

1. Wolverson MK, Bashiti HM, Peterson GJ: Ultrasonic tissue characterization of atheromatous plaques using a high resolution real time scanner. Ultrasound Med Biol 6:669–709, 1983.
2. Pignoli P, Tremoli E, Poli A, et al: Intimal plus medial thickness of the arterial wall: A direct measurement with ultrasound imaging. Circulation 6:1399–1406, 1986.
3. Poli A, Tremoli E, Colombo A, et al: Ultrasonographic measurement of the common carotid arterial wall thickness in hypercholesterolemic patients. Atherosclerosis 70:253–261, 1988.
4. Zwiebel WJ: Duplex examination of the carotid arteries. Semin Ultrasound CT MR 11:97–135, 1990.
5. Zierler RE, Phillips DJ, Beach KW, et al: Noninvasive assessment of normal carotid bifurcation hemodynamics with color flow ultrasound imaging. Ultrasound Med Biol 13:471–476, 1987.
6. Merritt CRB: Doppler blood flow imaging: Integrating flow with tissue data. Diagn Imaging 11:146–155, 1986.
7. Middleton WD, Foley WD, Lawson TL: Flow reversal in the normal carotid bifurcation: Color Doppler flow imaging analysis. Radiology 167:207–210, 1988.
8. Blackshear WM, Phillips JD, Chikos PM, et al: Carotid artery velocity patterns in normal and stenotic vessels. Stroke 11:67–71, 1980.
9. Zbornikova V, Lassvik C: Duplex scanning in presumably normal persons of different ages. Ultrasound Med Biol 12:371–378, 1986.
10. Ku DN: A review of carotid scanning. Echocardiography 5:53–69, 1988.
11. Paivansalo MJ, Sinituoto TMJ, Tikkakoski TA, et al: Duplex ultrasound of the external carotid artery. Acta Radiology 37:41–43, 1996.
12. Meyer JI, Khalil RM, Obuchowski NA, Baus LK: Common carotid artery: Variability of Doppler US velocity measurements. Radiology 204:339–341, 1997.

Chapter 8

Ultrasound Assessment of Carotid Plaque

WILLIAM J. ZWIEBEL, MD

Diagnostic ultrasound is capable of conveniently evaluating the composition of atherosclerotic plaque in a clinical setting, in the course of routine carotid examinations. Magnetic resonance imaging is also capable of assessing plaque composition, but at present, only in a research setting where special high-resolution equipment is available. In spite of the availability of ultrasound instruments capable of plaque assessment, few ultrasound practitioners evaluate carotid plaque on a regular basis, and the concept of plaque assessment has been received with mixed levels of enthusiasm in the research community—praised by some and condemned as worthless by others. The root of this controversy is concern about the accuracy of ultrasound plaque assessment and uncertainty about the clinical implications of carotid plaque findings. For many years now, the potential value of ultrasound plaque assessment has been stated in the medical literature, but the clinical realization of this potential has been elusive. Nevertheless, ultrasound instrumentation has improved substantially in the last decade, and it may well be that the promised benefit of carotid plaque evaluation is close to realization. It is worthwhile, therefore, to review this matter in some detail.

DETECTION

Atherosclerotic plaque is initially revealed sonographically by an increase in the combined thickness of the intima and media layers, and subsequently by echogenic material that encroaches on the arterial lumen.[1-9] Homa and colleagues[8] found that the normal intima-media thickness in the common carotid artery, as measured in areas void of plaque, increases linearly with age from a mean of 0.48 at age 40 yr to 1.02 at age 100 yr follows the formula $(0.009 \times age) + 0.116$. In addition to age-related change, the intima-media thickness also increases in response to early plaque formation, and this measurement is used, therefore, as a marker for cardiovascular risk in a variety of clinical settings.[3,5-7,9-13] For the most part, the intima-media measurement has been used for research, but it can be used in a clinical setting as a marker for cardiovascular risk. In literature reports, the intima-media thickness has been measured variously in the tubular and bulbous portions of the common carotid and in the proximal internal carotid artery. Typically, longitudinal images are used that clearly depict the intimal reflection and the media, as shown in Figure 8–1A. The cut points for intima-media thickness between normal and abnormal populations have varied among reported studies, and therefore it is difficult to establish a single cut point that defines abnormality. Additionally, the age-related variance described previously must be considered. It is a reasonable assumption, however, that an intima-media thickness of 0.9 or more is abnormal and is likely to be associated with sonographically visible plaque. Please note that older studies tended to include areas of visible plaque in the measurements of intima-media thickness, which is no longer recommended. The intima-media thickness

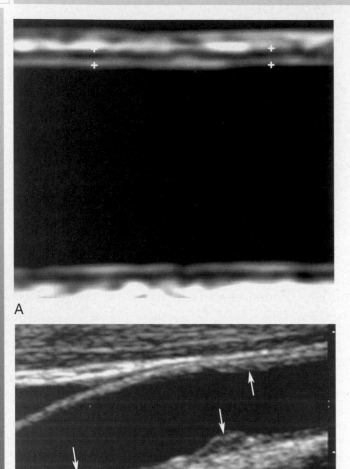

A

B

Figure 8–1. Intima-media thickness and small plaques. *A,* Measurement points (*cursors*) for determining the intima-medial thickness are shown on this highly magnified common carotid artery image. Two measurement locations are shown that clearly display the boundaries of the intima and media. *B,* Small plaques (*arrows*) are seen on this long axis image spanning the distal common- and proximal internal carotid arteries.

measurement should not include grossly visible plaque.

Thickening of the intima-media complex implies occult plaque formation, but plaque may, of course, be seen directly with ultrasound when it achieves sufficient size to protrude into the carotid artery lumen (Fig. 8–1B). Small carotid artery plaques are very commonly present in individuals older than 50 yr,[6–8,11,13] and the prevalence of plaque increases with age to a high of 80+% for men between the ages of 80 and 100 yr. (The prevalence is somewhat lower for women.) Because of its prevalence, the significance of small carotid plaques is uncertain. Large and potentially dangerous plaque occurs uncommonly, with a reported incidence in large population-based studies of 2% or less for men and women 50 yr and older.[6]

The interobserver variation for plaque detection ranges from fair to good among reported studies.[10–13,14] The causes of such variation include the technologists' skill level, ultrasound image quality, failure to examine the same vascular segment, and lack of a uniform definition of findings indicating the presence of plaque. With improvements in instrumentation and methods, interobserver variation may be expected to improve with time, but technical diligence and quality assurance methods are required to ensure accurate plaque detection.

EXTENT, SEVERITY, AND FOLLOW-UP

Having detected carotid plaque, we are faced with the need to describe it in a way that accurately represents its extent and severity. For evaluating plaque progression over time in a clinical or research setting, precise ultrasound images are needed to show the longitudinal and circumferential extent of plaque, as well as its thickness.[4–6,8,15–18] To this end, three dimensional ultrasound imaging holds considerable promise.[15,16,19] For day-to-day clinical assessment of the carotid arteries, as conducted in most community hospitals, such detail is unnecessary, and in such circumstances, a general description of plaque extent and severity is adequate. In my reports of carotid ultrasound studies, I separately describe plaque extent and severity. By *extent,* I mean the length of the vessel (cephalocaudad) affected by plaque. I report plaque extent descriptively (e.g., "Plaque extends from the distal common carotid artery into the proximal internal carotid artery."). By *severity,* I mean the thickness of plaque. This is more difficult to define sonographically, because plaque varies in thickness from one location to another, so I define the maximum plaque thickness at whatever location(s) it occurs. The best means for assessing carotid plaque thickness is from *transverse* (short-axis) images, which most accurately show the maximum thickness of the plaque and the resultant degree of luminal narrowing. *Plaque severity can be grossly overestimated or underestimated from longitudinal images,* as illustrated in Figures 8–2 and 8–3. When reporting plaque severity, I usually use generic terms, such as *minimal, moderate,* and *severe.* For situations in which greater precision is desirable, I report the plaque thickness in millimeters, and I note whether the plaque is eccentric or circumferential (i.e., extending around the circumference of the lumen). In our vascular laboratory, we generally do not follow up patients on the basis of plaque measurements per se. Instead, we recommend a follow-up interval based on Doppler assessment of stenosis severity. In essence, measuring plaque or stenosis amounts to the same thing, however, for the degree of stenosis indirectly indicates the severity of plaque formation.

PLAQUE PATHOGENESIS

Current theory holds that atherosclerosis is a response to injury that is mediated (or directed) by the endothelial cells that line the arteries.[14,20–23] Three processes occur in the course of plaque formation. First, lipids from the blood accumulate in the subendothelium. Second, the lipid material is ingested by macrophages, forming foam cells, so named because of their foamy microscopic appearance. Finally, smooth muscle cells migrate from the muscular layer to the subendothelial layer and become transformed into fibroblasts. These form a collagenous (fibrous) matrix within the plaque and also form a fibrous cap on the lumenal side of the plaque, below the intimal layer. Up to this point, the plaque structure is stable.

There is increasing evidence that inflammation plays an important pathogenic role in the evolution of plaque.[20] Beginning at the foam cell stage, an inflammatory process is apparent. Ongoing inflammation causes the breakdown of foam cells and other components of plaque and the accumulation of inflammatory debris. The inflammatory process disrupts the structure of the plaque, weakens the fibrous cap, and extends to the intima. Evidence has also been uncovered in recent years suggesting that bacterial infection may play a role in plaque formation.[24–26] The role of infection and the relationship of infection to the inflammatory response is presently debated.

These are exciting times in the field of atherosclerosis research. The investigation of inflammation and bacterial infection are two of many exciting developments

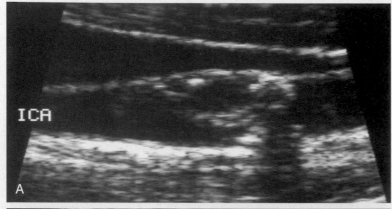

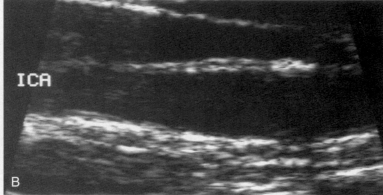

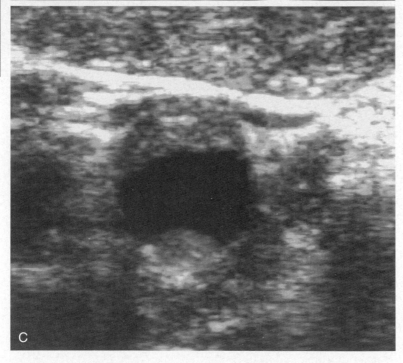

FIGURE 8–2. Incorrect plaque assessment from longitudinal images. *A,* The internal carotid artery (ICA) appears to be largely filled with plaque on this longitudinal image. *B,* Another longitudinal image from a different perspective shows very little plaque. *C,* A transverse views at the same location accurately display the thickness and circumferential extent of plaque.

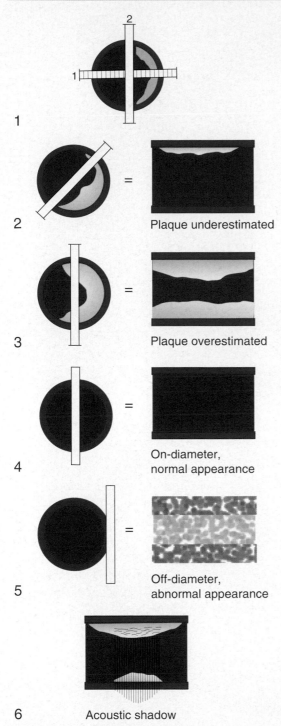

1

2 Plaque underestimated

3 Plaque overestimated

4 On-diameter,
normal appearance

5 Off-diameter,
abnormal appearance

6 Acoustic shadow

FIGURE 8–3. Causes for misinterpretation of carotid plaque severity. *1*, Plaque is not seen in the horizontal image plane but is accurately represented in the vertical image plane. *2*, This image plane underestimates plaque thickness. *3*, Plaque thickness and luminal narrowing are overestimated. *4*, A scan through the vessel axis (diameter) generates a normal appearance, but an off-axis scan (*5*) simulates pathology. *6*, Pathology is obscured by an acoustic shadow.

in research on plaque formation. Perhaps we are finally getting closer to an understanding of plaque pathogenesis, and perhaps this will lead to better methods of prevention and treatment of atherosclerosis.

As suggested previously, there are two broad catagories of atherosclerotic plaque, *uncomplicated* and *complicated* (Fig. 8–4). Uncomplicated, or stable, plaque is uniform in composition, for the most part, and is covered by a subintimal fibrous cap. The architecture of complicated plaque is not uniform. Instead the plaque is disturbed by inflammation-induced degenerative processes, resulting in plaque necrosis, hemorrhage into the plaque substance, calcification, thinning or disruption of the fibrous cap, disruption of the endothelial layer, and plaque ulceration.

Among the degenerative changes cited previously, the most important are disruption of the fibrous cap and the endothelium, which may directly cause embolization, through the shedding of plaque contents into the bloodstream. Embolization also is caused by the adherence of platelets or thrombus to denuded plaque surface. This material is subsequently shed into the bloodstream and thence to the brain, where it may occlude cerebral arteries and cause ischemia or infarction.

Central to current thinking about plaque evolution is the concept that stable, uncomplicated plaque tends to be transformed into complicated plaque through chronic inflammation and an injury process that includes plaque necrosis and hemorrhage.[20,23,27-30] It appears, furthermore, that repeated cycles of injury and repair occur in many plaques. Hence, large plaques tend to be complicated histologically, whereas small plaques tend to be uncomplicated. As a correlate, large plaques are prone to cause embolization, and small plaques are less likely to do so. Large plaques cause stenosis, while small plaques do not. Therefore, the presence of high-grade carotid stenosis indicates the presence of large plaques that are apt to be complicated and prone to embolization. This fact has been verified histolgically and sonographically, with direct observations of plaque

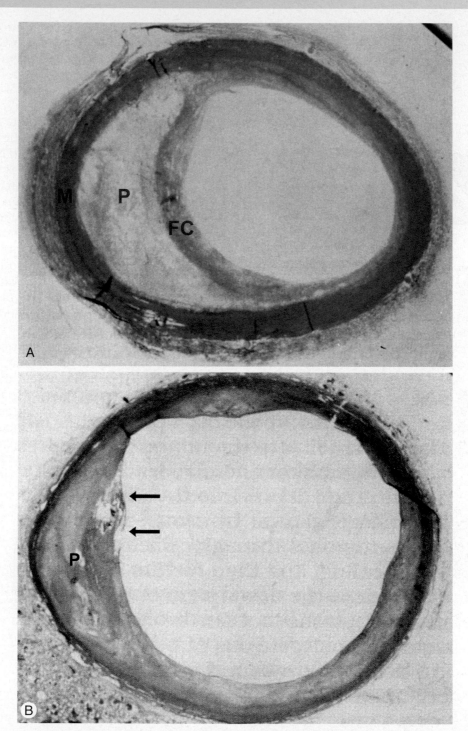

FIGURE 8–4. Plaque histology. *A,* Microscopic section of an uncomplicated plaque. The fibrous cap (FC) is intact, and the plaque contents (P) are homogeneous. *B,* Microscopic section of a complicated plaque. The fibrous cap is ruptured and an area of cavitation is present (*arrows*). The plaque contents (P) are heterogeneous. (From O'Leary D, Glagov S, Zarins C, Giddens D: Carotid artery disease. In Rifkin MD, Charboneau JW, Laing FC [eds]: Ultrasound 1991: Special Course Syllabus, 77th Scientific Assembly and Annual Meeting. Oak Park, IL, RSNA Publications, 1991, pp 189–200. Reproduced with the kind permission of Daniel O'Leary, MD.)

complications, including fibrous cap disruption and ulceration, in the presence of high-grade carotid stenosis.[16,19,31,32]

It is important to note here that although most vascular laboratories judge plaque severity indirectly, based on the severity of stenosis, some patients may have large carotid plaques that nevertheless generate relatively little stenosis. This occurs when the bulbous portions of the distal common and proximal internal carotid arteries are unusually large. The capacious carotid bulb can harbor a large volume of potentially complicated and clinically dangerous plaque in the absence of significantly elevated flow velocity. It is important, therefore, to get a sense of the carotid plaque volume in the course of sonographic examination, as well as the severity of stenosis. In my opinion, the presence of a large volume of plaque should be reported to the referring clinician, even if high-grade stenosis is absent.

PLAQUE CHARACTERIZATION

As noted previously, the primary role of carotid sonography is the detection and assessment of carotid stenosis. Nevertheless, much has been made of the ability of ultrasound to characterize plaque composition, and therefore, ultrasound practitioners should be familiar with plaque characterization concepts, which may have importance in a clinical setting.[27–30,32–60] In general terms, plaque can be characterized as *low, medium,* or *high* in echogenicity and as *homogeneous* or *heterogeneous* in texture. The histologic correlates of these characteristics are as follows.

Low Echogenicity

Fibrofatty plaque (Fig. 8–5A), which contains a large amount of lipid material, is low in echogenicity. This type of plaque is less echogenic than the nearby sternomastoid muscle, and in some cases fibrofatty plaque is so echo poor that it is difficult to see with ultrasound. Visualization difficulties, however, are ameliorated with color flow or B-flow imaging, because a flow void is visible even if the plaque is not well seen. Plaque that is low in echogenicity is less cellular than more echogenic plaque and is associated with elevated serum levels of low-density lipoprotein, plaque ulceration, and increased risk of cerebral ischemic symptoms.*

Moderate Echogenicity

As the collagen and cellular content of plaque increases relative to the fat content, ultrasound echogenicity also increases. Hence, fibrous plaque, in which collagen is a prominent component, is moderately echogenic (Fig. 8–5B). Fibrous plaque is easy to see with ultrasound. Its echogenicity equals or exceeds that of the sternomastoid muscle, but it is less echogenic than the arterial adventitia. Moderately echogenic plaque is less associated with cerebral ischemic symptoms than plaque that is diffusely low in echogenicity or that which is heterogeneous, as discussed later.

Strong Echogenicity

Dystrophic calcification occurs in plaque, and such calcification generates strong reflections, accompanied by distal acoustic shadows (Fig. 8–5C). These reflections equal or exceed the brightness of any other object in the image. High-resolution sonography is extremely sensitive to the presence of calcification, and areas on the order of 1 mm in diameter may be detected. Plaque calcification may be focal or diffuse, and large calcification may generate acoustic shadows that obscure the arterial lumen, interfering with ultrasound diagnosis. Although it is assumed that calcification is a consequence of plaque complications previously described, an association between plaque calcification and symptomatology has not been established, apparently because the calcified areas represent healed or dormant processes of no immediate threat to the fibrous cap or endothelium.

*See references 27–29, 32, 33, 37–40, 43, 44, 48, 49, 51, 52, 54–56,60

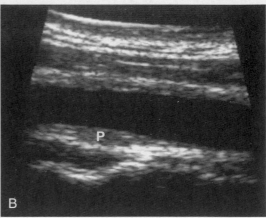

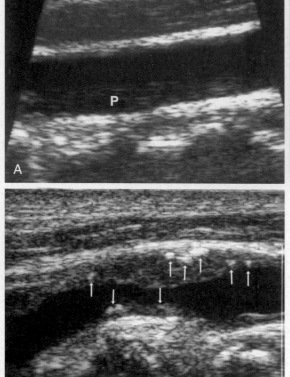

FIGURE 8–5. Ultrasound plaque characterization. *A,* Low-echogenicity, high lipid content plaque (P). *B,* Moderately echogenic fibrous plaque (P). *C,* Strongly echogenic calcifications (*arrows*) are present throughout this plaque.

Homogeneous Versus Heterogeneous

It has long been noted that, from an ultrasound perspective, some plaque is homogeneous, and some plaque is heterogeneous. Calcification is one cause of heterogeneity, but as noted previously, no correlation has been reported between calcification and neurologic symptoms. Two other types of heterogeneity have been discussed widely in the literature, namely, focal and scattered areas of *low* echogenicity (Fig. 8–6). Clinical interest has centered on reports that hemispheric neurologic symptoms, including transient ischemia and stroke, are more common in patients with heterogeneous plaque than in those with homogeneous, medium-echogenicity (fibrous) plaque. In theory, focal or diffuse plaque heterogeneity is related to complicated plaque histology and potentially with degeneration of the fibrous

cap and endothelium. Thus, heterogeniety is linked with increased potential for embolization, as discussed previously. Plaque heterogeneity, therefore, is postulated as a precursor of hemispheric neurologic symptoms.*

The principal method for assessing plaque echogenicity/homogeneity is visual, which is convenient and requires no special equipment beyond a high-resolution ultrasound instrument. A widely used method for visual assessment is that proposed by Gray-Weale and colleagues[43] and by Geroulakos and coworkers[44] that employs five easily defined plaque categories. The risk level associated with each plaque catagory is shown in Table 8–1. Although this is a straightforward method of plaque assessment, questions have been raised about

*See references 28, 29, 32, 33, 37–40, 43, 44, 48–52, 56, 60

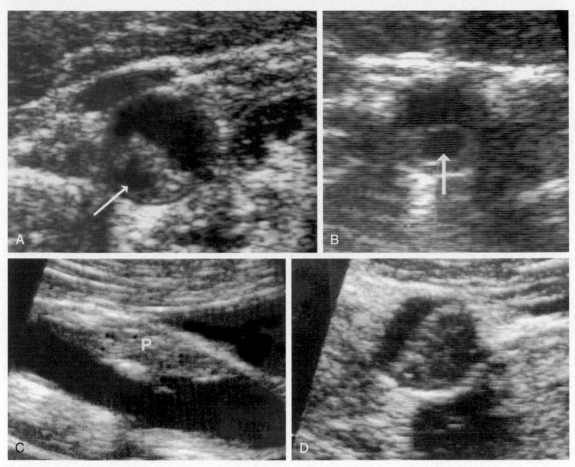

FIGURE 8–6. Heterogeneous plaque. *A* and *B,* Large focal hypoechoic areas are present (*arrows*). *C* and *D,* The plaque (P) is diffusely heterogeneous, with multiple areas of low echogenicity. A focal crypt with an overhanging edge is present in *C,* consistent with ulceration.

Table 8–1. Carotid Plaque Types

Type	Characteristics	Risk of Symptoms
1	Uniformly echolucent	High
2	Predominantly echolucent (>50% of plaque structure)	High
3	Predominantly echogenic (>50% of plaque structure)	Lower
4	Uniformly echogenic	Lowest
5	Unclassified due to calcification or poor visualization (partially visualized plaque may be classified on the basis of the region that is seen)	Unknown

interobserver variation in plaque category assignment. There are several sources for such variability, including intrinsic instrument differences, variance in instrument settings, and sonologist experience. Nevertheless, it has been shown that excellent results may be obtained with visual plaque assessment with proper attention to imaging details.[61]

Concerns about interobserver variability led to the development of less subjective methods of plaque assessment, first reported by El Atrozy and associates[62] and subsequently refined by others.[45,48–50,53,61] These methods measure the sonographic or optical density of plaque, which in turn is expressed either as a median gray-scale/density level (called the gray-scale median) for the entire plaque or as the difference between the highest and lowest values within a plaque. These methods provide an objective, measurable value that describes plaque echogenicity, eliminating the subjectivity of visual plaque assessment, and there is evidence that interobserver variability is good to excellent with these techniques, especially when ultrasound instrument adjustment is standardized. Reports of excellent correlation of gray-scale median and symptomatology also have been published. The difficulty with this method is the need for off-line computer equipment to analyze plaque gray-scale or optical density levels. Such assessment is time consuming, and the necessary equipment is currently available only in a research setting. It is likely; however, that a measurement package designed to evaluate plaque echogenicity could be incorporated into ultrasound instruments or picture archiving system, facilitating clinical application.

Points of Controversy

The concept of plaque characterization with ultrasound was first discussed in the late 1970s yet has remained controversial to this day. In large measure, this controversy is based on the inconsistent results obtained when ultrasound findings are compared with plaque histology, as derived from endarterectomy specimens.[27–30,33–41,43,50,51,53,56,63,64] General correlation between plaque echogenicity and composition is well accepted; namely, that low-echogenicity plaque is fatty and moderately echogenic plaque is more fibrous. For specific plaque features, such as necrosis, hemorrhage, and lipid deposits, however, correlation is shaky. Generally, the reported sonographic-histologic correlation is fair to good but rarely excellent. More importantly, some studies, including recent publications, find poor correlation or no correlation at all between sonographic and histologic findings.[42,46,47,63]

The association of symptomatology, assessed retrospectively or prospectively, with ultrasound plaque features generally has been more reliable than the association between histology and ultrasound findings. High-risk plaque types, as defined in Table 8–1, have been associated with increased risk of symptoms and conversely are seen at endarterectomy, more commonly in patients with symptoms than in those without. Nevertheless, even this aspect of ultrasound plaque evaluation has come into question, with several studies, including some performed with up-to-date equipment, showing no association between ultrasound patterns and the incidence of hemispheric symptoms.[23,29,47,64]

The reasons for discrepant results published with respect to ultrasound plaque characterization are obscure. Nevertheless, I believe it is important to proceed with research in this field. The capabilities of ultrasound instruments improve continuously, and ultimately, I believe, ultrasound plaque findings will have a place in clinical patient management. For the present, however, I am reluctant to recommend that any therapeutic action be taken solely on the basis of plaque composition features.

PLAQUE SURFACE FEATURES

It is well established that embolic occlusion of intracranial arteries is the primary cause of stroke, as opposed to the immediate hemodynamic effects of carotid stenosis or occlusion.[64–66] It has further been established that denuded or ulcerated carotid plaque surfaces are common sources of cerebral emboli that cause stroke or other neurologic events. Therefore, ultrasound assessment of plaque surface features is of considerable diagnostic interest.[1,15,16,19,27,28,64,67–70] Unfortunately, the performance of sonography for plaque surface assessment has been somewhat disappointing. A few series of meaningful size have shown that ultrasound is effective for detecting ulcers.[15,16,19,27] Other histologically verified studies[28,67,68,71] have shown either no correlation, or poor ultrasound results, for ulcer detection (33%–67% sensitivity and 31%–84% specificity). The problem, it

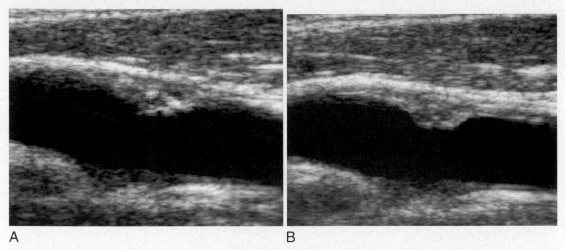

A   B

FIGURE 8–7. Spurious plaque ulceration. *A,* The plaque on the wall nearest to the transducer appears to have an irregular surface. *B,* With slight adjustment of the image plane, the plaque is visualized better and instead has a smooth surface. Which version correctly represents the plaque surface?

appears, is the inability of ultrasound to differentiate between small ulcer craters and other plaque deformities, as illustrated in Figures 8–7 and 8–8. Even the angiographic depiction of plaque ulceration is unreliable, as indicated by the deletion of this parameter from the North American Symptomatic Carotid Endarterectomy Trial.[1]

In my opinion, disappointing literature reports concerning ulcer detection result from emphasis on detecting *all ulcers*. Truly, it would be useful if we could detect all ulcers, but technical limitations described previously prevent this. I believe, however, that sonography can successfully identify *large ulcers* that are depicted as sharply defined excavations, as shown in Figure 8–9. Before I call something an ulcer, however, I must be convinced of the following: (1) the cavity is truly within a plaque; (2) the cavity is sharply marginated (perhaps with overhanging edges, as in Figs. 8–6C and 8–9); and (3) there is blood flow within the cavity, confirmed either with color- or B-flow imaging (Fig. 8–10). The first two features help to exclude a pseudoulcer caused by adjacent plaques, and the third feature excludes a focal hypoechoic region (e.g., plaque hemorrhage) that could mimic an ulcer on casual observation. I do not feel that one can accurately diagnose smaller

ulcers with standard clinical ultrasound equipment, but perhaps we will be able to do so in the future with three-dimensional imaging and reconstructed surface displays of the vessel lumen.[16]

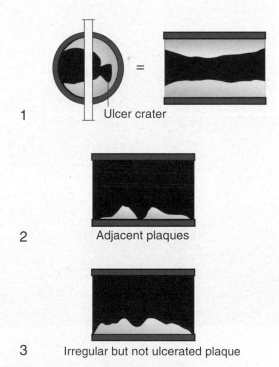

1   Ulcer crater

2   Adjacent plaques

3   Irregular but not ulcerated plaque

FIGURE 8–8. Sources of error in ulcer diagnosis: *1,* The image plane (*vertical bar*) does not include the ulcer. *2,* Adjacent plaques simulate ulceration. *3,* The plaque surface is irregular but not ulcerated.

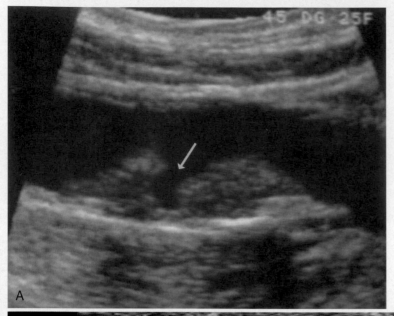

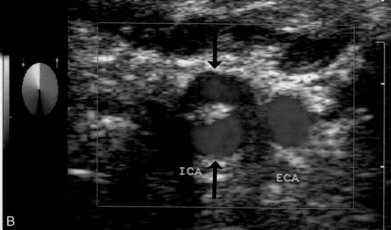

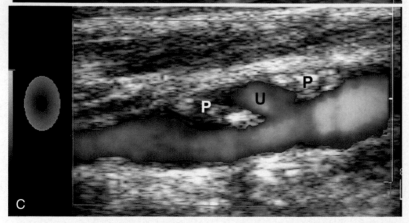

FIGURE 8–9. Large plaque ulcers. *A,* A discrete crypt (*arrow*) is clearly present within this plaque. *B,* A large ulcer creates a "pseudodissection" on this transverse image of an internal carotid artery (*arrows*). The blue area is the ulcer crater and the red area is the arterial lumen. ECA, external carotid artery; ICA, internal carotid artery. *C,* Power Doppler in the same patient confirms the presence of a large ulcer (U). P, plaque.

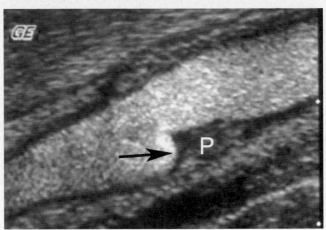

FIGURE 8–10. B-flow plaque image. This carotid plaque is nicely outlined using B-flow. The plaque has a concave border (*arrow*), and the adjacent edge is acutely angulated, but I could not say whether this is an ulcer or not. (Courtesy of the General Electric Co., Milwaukee WI.)

References

1. Streiffler JY, Benavente AJ, Fox AJ: The accuracy of angiographic detection of carotid plaque ulceration: Results from the NASCET study [abstract]. Stroke 22:149, 1991.
2. Pignoli P, Tremoli E, Poli A, et al: Intimal plus medial thickness of the arterial wall: A direct measurement with ultrasound imaging. Circulation 6:1399–1406, 1986.
3. Poli A, Tremoli E, Colombo A, et al: Ultrasonographic measurement of the common carotid arterial wall thickness in hypercholesterolemic patients. Atherosclerosis 70:253–261, 1988.
4. Riley WA, Barnes RW, Applegate WB, et al: Reproducibility of noninvasive ultrasonic measurement of carotid atherosclerosis. The Asymptomatic Carotid Artery Plaque Study. Stroke 23:1062–1068, 1992.
5. Bond MG, Wilmoth SK, Enevold GL, et al: Detection and monitoring of asymptomatic atherosclerosis in clinical trials. Am J Med 86:33–36, 1989.
6. Ebrahim S, Papacosta O, Whincup P, et al: Carotid plaque, intima media thickness, cardiovascular risk factors, and prevalent cardiovascular disease in men and women: The British Regional Heart Study. Stroke. 30: 841–850, 1999.
7. Sun Y, Cheng-Huai L, Chien-Jung L, et al: Carotid atherosclerosis, intima media thickness and risk factors—an analysis of 1781 asymptomatic subjects in Taiwan. Atherosclerosis 164:89–94, 2002.
8. Homa S, Nobuyoshi H, Ishida H, et al: Carotid plaque and intima-media thickness assessed by B-mode sonography in subjects ranging from young adults to centenarians. Stroke 32:830–835, 2001.
9. Sakaguchi M, Kitagawa K, Nagai Y, et al: Equivalence of plaque score and intima-media thickness of carotid ultrasonography for predicting severe coronary artery lesion. Ultrasound Med Biol 29:367–371, 2003.
10. Li R, Cai J, Tegeler C, et al: Reproducibility of extracranial carotid atherosclerotic lesions assessed by B-mode ultrasound: The atherosclerosis risk in communities study. Ultrasound Med Biol 22:791–799, 1996.
11. Salonen R, Seppanen K, Rauremaa R, Salonen JT: Prevalence of carotid atherosclerosis and serum cholesterol levels in eastern Finland. Arteriosclerosis 8:788–792, 1988.
12. Sutton-Tyrrell K, Wolfson SK, Thompson T, Kelsoey SF: Measurement variability in Duplex scan assessment of carotid atherosclerosis. Stroke 23:215–220, 1992.
13. Prati P, Vanuzzo D, Casaroli M, et al: Prevalence and determinants of carotid atherosclerosis in a general population. Stroke 23:1705–1711, 1992.
14. Gibbons GH, Dzau VJ: The emerging concept of vascular remodeling. N Engl J Med 330: 1431–1438, 1994.
15. Wijeyaratne SM, Jarvis S, Stead LA, et al: A new method for characterizing carotid plaque: multiple cross-sectional view echomorphology. J Vasc Surg. 37:778–784, 2003.
16. Schminke U, Motsch L, Hilker L, Kessler C: Three-dimensional ultrasound observation of carotid artery plaque ulceration. Stroke 31: 1651–1655, 2000.
17. Kozakova M, Morizzo C, Andreucetti F, et al: Quantification of extracranial carotid artery stenosis by ultrafast three-dimensional ultrasound. J Am Soc Echocardiography 14: 1203–1211, 2001.
18. Yao J, van Sambeek MR, Dall'Agata A, et al: Three-dimensional ultrasound study of carotid arteries before and after endarterectomy; analysis of stenotic lesions and surgical impact on the vessel. Stroke 29:2026–2031, 1998.
19. Palombo C, Kozakova M, Morizzo C, et al: Ultrafast three-dimensional ultrasound:

Application to carotid artery imaging. Stroke 29:1631–1637, 1998.

20. Libby P: The fire within. Scientific American 286:46–55, 2002.

21. Ross R, Glomset JA: The pathogenesis of atherosclerosis (Part 1). N Engl J Med 295:369–377, 1976.

22. Ross R, Glomset JA: The pathogenesis of atherosclerosis (Part 2). N Engl J Med 295:420–425, 1976.

23. O'Leary D, Glagov S, Zarins C, Giddens D: Carotid artery disease. In Rifkin MD, Charboneau JW, Laing FC (eds): Ultrasound 1991: Special Course Syllabus, 77th Scientific Assembly and Annual Meeting. Oak Park, IL, RSNA Publications, 1991, pp 189–200.

24. Neureiter D, Heuschmann P, Stintzing S, et al: Detection of *Chlamydia pneumoniae* but not of *Helicobacter pylori* in symptomatic atherosclerotic carotids associated with enhanced serum antibodies, inflammation and apoptosis rate. Atherosclerosis 168:153–162, 2003.

25. Ezzahiri R, Stassen FR, Kurvers HA, et al: *Chlamydia pneumoniae* infection induces an unstable atherosclerotic plaque phenotype in LDL-receptor, ApoE double knockout mice. Eur J Vasc Endovasc Surg 26:88–95, 2003.

26. Sessa R, Di Pietro M, Schiavoni G, et al: *Chlamydia pneumoniae* DNA in patients with symptomatic carotid atherosclerotic disease. J Vasc Surg 37:1027–1031, 2003.

27. O'Donnell TR Jr, Erodoes L, Mackey WC, et al: Correlation of B-mode ultrasound imaging and arteriography with pathologic findings at carotid endarterectomy. Arch Surg 120:443–449, 1985.

28. Lusby RJ, Ferrel LD, Ehrenfeld WK, et al: Carotid plaque hemorrhage. Arch Surg 117:1479–1487, 1981.

29. Reilly LM: Importance of carotid plaque morphology. In Bernstein EF (ed): Vascular Diagnosis, 4th ed. St. Louis, Mosby–Year Book, 1993, pp 333–340.

30. Bassiouny HS, Sakaguchi Y, Mikucki SA, et al: Juxtalumenal location of plaque necrosis and neoformation in symptomatic carotid stenosis. J Vasc Surg 26:585–594, 1977.

31. AbuRahma AF, Wulu JT Jr, Crotty B: Carotid plaque ultrasonic heterogeneity and severity of stenosis. Stroke 33:1772–1775, 2002.

32. Pedro LM, Fernandes e Fernandes J, Pedro MM: Ultrasonographic risk score of carotid plaques. Eur J Vasc Endovasc Surg 24:492–498, 2002.

33. Bluth EI: Evaluation and characterization of carotid plaque. Semin Ultrasound CT MR 18:57–65, 1997.

34. Weinberger J, Marks SJ, Gaul JJ, et al: Atherosclerotic plaque at the carotid artery bifurcation: Correlation of ultrasonographic imaging with morphology. J Ultrasound Med 6:363–366, 1987.

35. Edwards JH, Kricheff II, Gorstein F, et al: Atherosclerotic subintimal hematoma of the carotid artery. Radiology 133:123–129, 1987.

36. Seeger JM, Klingman N: The relationship between carotid plaque composition and neurologic symptoms. J Surg Res 43:78–85, 1987.

37. Imparato AM, Riles TS, Gorstein F: The carotid bifurcation plaque: Pathologic findings associated with cerebral ischemia. Stroke 3:238–245, 1979.

38. Reilly M, Lusby RF, Highes L, et al: Carotid plaque histology using real time ultrasonography: Clinical and therapeutic implications. Arch Surg 120:1010–1012, 1985.

39. Bluth EI, Kay D, Merritt CRB, et al: Sonographic characterization of carotid plaque: Detection of hemorrhage. Am J Neuroradial 7:311–314, 1986.

40. Imparato AM, Riles TS, Mintzer K, et al: The importance of hemorrhage in the relationship between gross morphologic characteristics and cerebral symptoms in 376 carotid artery plaques. Ann Surg 197:195–198, 1983.

41. Widder B, Paulat K, Hackspacher J, et al: Morphological characterization of carotid artery stenosis by ultrasound duplex scanning. Ultrasound Med Biol 16:349–354, 1990.

42. Ratiff DA, Gallagher PJ, Hames TK, et al: Characterization of carotid artery disease: Comparison of duplex scanning with histology. Ultrasound Med Biol 11:835–840, 1985.

43. Gray-Weale AC, Graham JC, Burnett JR, et al: Carotid artery atheroma: Comparison of preoperative B-mode ultrasound appearance with carotid endarterectomy specimen pathology. J Cardiovasc Surg 29:676–681, 1988.

44. Geroulakos G, Ramaswami G, Nicolaides A, et al: Characterization of symptomatic and asymptomatic carotid plaques using high-resolution real-time ultrasonography. Br J Surg 80:1274–1277, 1993.

45. el-Barghouty N, Nicolaides A, Bahal V, et al: The identification of the high risk carotid plaque. Eur J Vasc Endovasc Surg 11:470–478, 1996.

46. Droste DW, Karl M, Bohle RM, Kaps M: Comparison of ultrasonic and histopathological features of carotid artery stenosis. Neurol Res 19:380–384, 1997.

47. Hatsukami TS, Ferguson MS, Beach KW, et al: Carotid plaque morphology and clinical events. Stroke 28:95–100, 1977.

48. Biasi GM, Sampaolo A, Mingazzini P, et al: Computer analysis of ultrasonic plaque echolucency in identifying high risk carotid bifurcation lesions. Eur J Vasc Endovasc Surg 17:476–479, 1999.

49. Tegos TJ, Sabetai MM, Nicolaides AN, et al: Comparability of the ultrasonic tissue charac-

teristics of carotid plaques. J Ultrasound Med 19:399–407, 2000.

50. Aly S, Bishop CC: An objective characterization of atherosclerotic lesion: An alternative method to identify unstable plaque. Stroke 31: 1921–1924, 2000.

51. Schulte-Altedorneburg G, Droste DW, Haas N, et al: Preoperative B-mode ultrasound plaque appearance compared with carotid endarterectomy specimen histology. Acta Neurol Scand 101:188–194, 2000.

52. Mathiesen EB, Bonaa KH, Joakimsen O: Low levels of high-density lipoprotein cholesterol are associated with echolucent carotid artery plaques: The tromso study. Stroke 32:1960–1965, 2001.

53. Ciulla MM, Paliotti R, Ferrero S, et al: Assessment of carotid plaque composition in hypertensive patients by ultrasonic tissue characterization: A validation study. J Hypertens 20:1589–1596, 2002.

54. Gronholdt ML, Nordestgaard BG, Bentzon J, et al. Macrophages are associated with lipid-rich carotid artery plaques, echolucency on B-mode imaging, and elevated plasma lipid levels. J Vasc Surg 35:137–145, 2002.

55. Gronholdt ML, Nordestgaard BG, Schroeder TV, et al: Ultrasonic echolucent carotid plaques predict future strokes. Circulation 104:68–73, 2001.

56. Goncalves I, Moses J, Pedro LM, et al: Echolucency of carotid plaques correlates with plaque cellularity. Eur J Vasc Endovasc Surg 26:32–38, 2003.

57. Denzel C, Fellner F, Wutke R, et al: Ultrasonographic analysis of arteriosclerotic plaques in the internal carotid artery. Eur J Ultrasound 16:161–167, 2003.

58. Bicknell CD, Cheshire NJ: The relationship between carotid atherosclerotic plaque morphology and the embolic risk during endovascular therapy. Eur J Vasc Endovasc Surg 26:17–21, 2003.

59. Cave EM, Pugh ND, Wilson RJ, et al: Carotid artery duplex scanning: Does plaque echogenicity correlate with patient symptoms? Eur J Vasc Endovasc Surg 10:77–81, 1995.

60. Polak JF, Shemanski L, O'Leary DH, et al: Hypoechoic plaque at US of the carotid artery: an independent risk factor for incident stroke in adults aged 65 years or older. Cardiovascular Health Study. Radiology 208:649–654, 1998. [Erratum in Radiology 209:288–289, 1998.]

61. Mayor I, Momjian S, Lalive P, Sztajzel R: Carotid plaque: comparison between visual and greyscale median analysis. Ultrasound Med Biol 29:961–966, 2003.

62. El Atrozy T, Nicolaides A, Tegos, et al: The effect of B-mode standardization on the echogenicity of symptomatic and asymptomatic carotid bifurcation plaque. Int Angiol 17:179–186, 1998.

63. Wolverson MK, Bashiti HM, Peterson GJ: Ultrasonic tissue characterization of atheromatous plaques using a high resolution real time scanner. Ultrasound Med Biol 6:669–709, 1983.

64. Carr S, Farb A, Pearce WH, et al: Atherosclerosis plaque rupture in symptomatic carotid artery stenosis. J Vasc Surg 12:755–766, 1996.

65. Brown PB, Zwiebel WJ, Call CK: Degree of cervical carotid artery stenosis and hemispheric stroke: Duplex sonographic US findings. Radiology 170:541–543, 1989.

66. Carroll BA: Duplex sonography in patients with hemispheric stroke symptoms. J Ultrasound Med 8:535–539, 1989.

67. Bluth EI, McVay LV, Merritt CRB, Sullivan MA: The identification of ulcerative plaque with high resolution duplex sonographic carotid scanning. J Ultrasound Med 7:73–76, 1988.

68. O'Leary DH, Holen J, Ricotta JJ, et al: Carotid bifurcation disease: Prediction of ulceration with B-mode ultrasound. Radiology 162: 523–525, 1987.

69. Hallam MJ, Reid JM, Cooperberg PL: Color flow Doppler and conventional duplex scanning of the carotid bifurcation: Prospective, double-blinded, correlative study. Am J Radiol 153: 1101–1105, 1989.

70. Steinke W, Kloetzsch C, Hehherici M: Carotid artery disease assessed by color Doppler flow imaging: Correlation with standard Doppler sonography and angiography. Am J Radiol 154:1061–1068, 1990.

71. Sitzer M, Wolfram M, Jorg R, et al: Color flow Doppler-assisted duplex imaging fails to detect ulceration in high-grade internal carotid artery stenosis. J Vasc Surg 24:461–465, 1996.

Chapter 9

Ultrasound Assessment of Carotid Stenosis

ERICA L. MITCHELL, MD, AND GREGORY L. MONETA, MD

This chapter provides an overview of the traditional and evolving criteria used for grading carotid artery stenosis, as well as the clinical relevance of sonography in the management of symptomatic and asymptomatic carotid disease. Also included are discussions of carotid restenosis after endarterectomy and the diagnostic difficulties imposed by internal carotid coils and kinks and bilateral high-grade carotid stenosis.

TECHNICAL NOTES

The technical aspects of carotid sonography are presented in detail in Chapter 7. Nevertheless, a few technical points are included here to present our perspective on the carotid ultrasound examination.

We begin the carotid artery duplex examination by recording the indication for the examination. The patient's carotid and subclavian arteries are then auscultated for bruits, and the carotid and radial pulses are palpated bilaterally. Brachial systolic and diastolic blood pressures are measured in each arm. The carotid duplex ultrasound examination includes the carotid and vertebral arteries bilaterally, as stipulated by vascular laboratory accrediting organizations. It is important to perform bilateral carotid examinations, because the flow characteristics in one carotid artery may be influenced significantly by the status of the contralateral carotid artery. A very-high-grade stenosis or occlusion of one common or internal carotid artery can result in increased compensatory flow in the opposite vessel.[1] This leads to velocity readings in the patent artery that are higher than expected and

may suggest a greater degree of stenosis than is actually present.

The ultrasound examination should include both longitudinal and transverse scans of the vessels. Vessel diameter measurements, visual assessment of stenosis severity, and plaque assessments should be done in the transverse plane. Doppler waveforms should be generated from the longitudinal plane. Gray-scale images alert the examiner to the presence of plaque in the arterial wall, while changes in the hue of the color flow pattern suggest the presence of stenosis.

Detailed characterization of carotid plaques for routine clinical duplex scanning is controversial (see Chapter 8). Advances in duplex scanning technology have allowed better elucidation and characterization of carotid plaque; however, there are currently no definite therapeutic recommendations that can be made from ultrasound plaque characteristics.

Interpretative criteria for carotid stenosis are based primarily on the Doppler-derived velocity waveforms. Errors in Doppler position and errors in angle correction will therefore lead to serious errors in diagnosis. The Doppler waveform should be obtained with an angle of insonation not exceeding 60 degrees and preferably as close to 60 degrees as possible. Measurements obtained with an angle of insonation greater than 60 degrees are likely to be inaccurate, even with the appropriate angle adjustment. In our department, we routinely obtain spectral Doppler waveforms from the common carotid artery (CCA) low in the neck; from the CCA just proximal to the carotid bifurcation; from the proximal, mid-, and distal (cervical) internal carotid artery (ICA); and from the origin of the external carotid artery (ECA). Additional waveforms are obtained from any areas of suspected stenosis, as suggested by gray-scale or color flow images. When evaluating the CCA, a spectral waveform should always be generated from the most proximal, straight segment of the vessel that is accessible to the scan head. For calculating the systolic velocity ratio (discussed later), the common carotid peak systolic velocity (PSV) should be measured at a standardized distance from the point at which the ICA and ECA divide, as discussed in Chapter 7. We also measure spectral Doppler waveforms across the transverse axis of the carotid bulb to document flow patterns indicating normality. Unidirectional flow is found along the flow divider of the bifurcation in normal carotid arteries. There is transient reversal of flow at peak systole near the center stream and at the outer wall opposite the flow divider, and the velocities along the outer wall may drop to zero at the end of diastole. These normal flow patterns are used in conjunction with the absence of visible plaque to indicate a normal carotid bulb.

Velocity measurements are recorded routinely from the proximal, mid-, and distal cervical portions of the ICA. The flow pattern should be that of a typical low-resistance vessel. Normal flow disturbances of the carotid bulb may extend into the mid-ICA and can be reflected in waveforms obtained at that level. The distal ICA includes the segment at least 3 cm above the bifurcation. Atherosclerosis usually develops within the first 2 cm of the bifurcation and rarely is isolated in the distal portion of the vessel. There are, however, a few circumstances, such as fibromuscular hyperplasia, where velocity increases are localized to the distal ICA, without the presence of proximal ICA plaque.

DETECTING AND ASSESSING STENOSIS

Doppler diagnosis of carotid stenosis focuses on three areas, the prestenotic region, the stenosis itself, and the post-stenotic region. Although the most important Doppler findings are observed within a carotid stenosis, diagnostically significant findings also are present in the pre- and poststenotic regions, as discussed in the following sections.

CCA Waveform Findings

The character of the normal CCA Doppler velocity waveform is that of a low-resistance vessel, as 80% of the CCA flow is into the ICA. The CCA end-diastolic velocity (EDV) should be above zero in normal individuals and should be similar to the EDV of the contralateral common carotid taken at approximately the same level in the neck.

In the great majority of cases, carotid stenosis or occlusion occurs in the proximal ICA. As a result, the CCA exhibits Doppler waveform findings typical of the prestenotic region. In the presence of very-high-grade ICA stenosis or ICA occlusion, outflow is primarily through the higher-resistance external carotid circulation. Under such circumstances the CCA waveform takes on the high-flow-resistance characteristics of an ECA (Fig. 9–1), with flow to zero, or nearly zero, in end-diastole. In addition, the PSV and the overall flow velocity may be substantially lower than normal due to reduced carotid artery flow. By merely observing these changes in the CCA, one can reliably predict the presence of high-grade stenosis or occlusion of the ICA. For this and other reasons mentioned later, it is good practice to begin the interpretation of carotid ultrasound studies by comparing side to side the Doppler waveforms in the CCAs.

The CCA contralateral to an ICA stenosis or occlusion may demonstrate increased flow velocity overall, with particular elevation of the EDV. These changes represent a compensatory increase in blood flow volume in the nonobstructed ICA in response to reduced cerebral perfusion. As this compensatory hemodynamic change can be substantial, stenosis-related flow velocities may be artificially elevated on the side with compensatory high-volume flow. This problem is addressed later in this chapter.

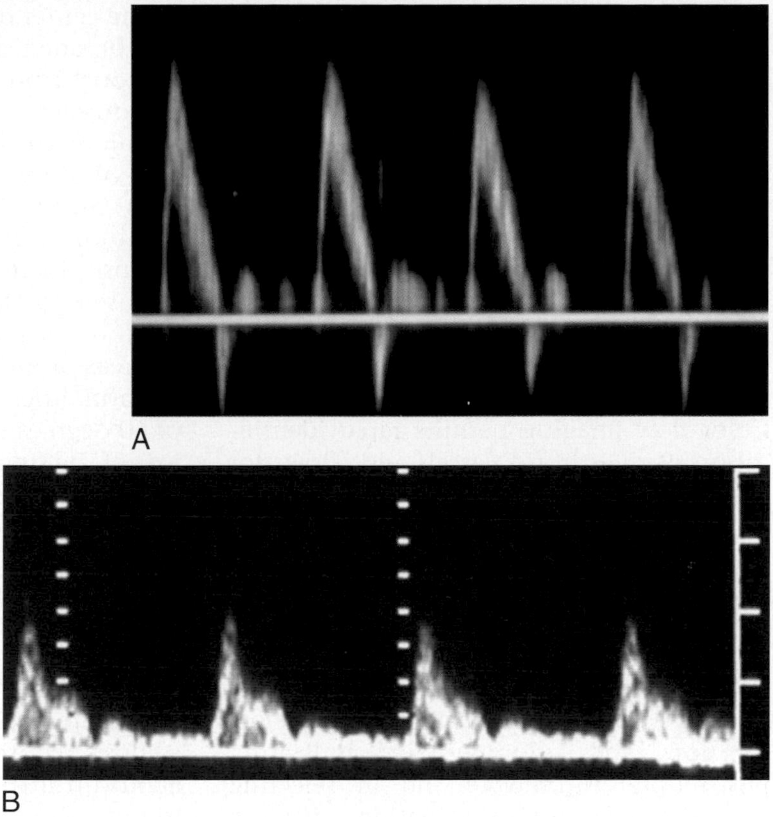

FIGURE 9–1. High-resistance flow proximal to severe occlusive disease. *A*, This common carotid Doppler waveform has a high-resistance, triphasic configuration due to internal carotid artery (ICA) occlusion. *B*, High resistance is manifested in this ICA waveform due to distal ICA occlusive disease at the base of the skull.

In the presence of a significant stenosis at the origin of the CCA or the right brachiocephalic artery, the ipsilateral CCA waveform may be dampened, with low velocity overall and a slower rise to peak systole when compared with the contralateral common carotid waveform (Fig. 9–2). The cervical CCA, in such cases, represents the poststenotic region, rather than the prestenotic region, as occurs in ICA stenosis. It is very important to note the CCA waveform findings caused by proximal stenosis, as they often are the only indicator of clinically significant carotid occlusive disease that may be treatable. The CCA flow changes seen with proximal stenoses are also important diagnostically because the overall reduction in flow velocity may artificially lower velocities in an ipsilateral ICA stenosis, leading to underestimation of stenosis severity. In some cases of proximal CCA or innominate artery stenosis, the ipsilateral common carotid waveform may exhibit poststenotic turbulence low in the neck, representing disturbed flow distal to the stenosis. An illustration with such findings is included in Chapter 16.

When low-velocity, damped Doppler waveforms are seen in the CCA, one should initially ascertain if the finding is unilateral

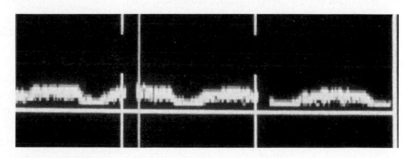

FIGURE 9–2. Markedly damped Doppler waveforms due to proximal common carotid artery occlusive disease.

or bilateral. If it is unilateral, it is likely that the cause is a CCA origin or bracheocephalic artery stenosis, as discussed previously. If the finding is bilateral, however, the etiology is cardiac, either in the form of critical aortic stenosis or severely diminished myocardial function accompanied by a low ejection fraction.

Doppler Findings in the Stenosis

Color flow imaging permits rapid identification of the carotid vessels and allows for easier recognition of flow abnormalities that suggest the presence of stenosis. Color flow imaging also more accurately identifies ICA occlusion than does gray-scale imaging alone and is essential for distinguishing ICA occlusion from very-high-grade stenosis, as discussed in the following chapter. The presence of color shifts, indicating high velocity flow, and color mosaics, indicating poststenotic turbulence, aid in selecting potential areas for examination with the pulsed Doppler.

Although color flow and gray-scale imaging are important for identifying stenosis and for accurate placement of the Doppler sample volume, hemodynamic quantification of the severity of carotid stenosis is still primarily achieved by analysis of Doppler spectral waveforms. The specific measurements used for this purpose are the PSV and EDV and the systolic velocity ratio, as illustrated in Figure 9–3. As a stenosis develops, the PSV first becomes elevated; therefore, PSV is a principal measure of stenosis severity. EDV lags behind, relatively speaking, as stenosis severity progresses but rises rapidly as the stenosis becomes severe (diameter reduction of $\geq 60\%$). Thus, EDV is a good marker for high-grade stenosis. The systolic velocity ratio is a very important measure of stenosis severity, as it compensates for abnormally high and low flow states that skew the PSV and EDV upward or downward, as discussed later.

To accurately measure flow velocity, the sample volume must be properly placed within the area of greatest stenosis. Originally, this meant placing the sample volume in the center of the vessel to minimize spectral broadening. Color flow, however, has demonstrated that the orientation of the stenotic jet within a stenosis is frequently not along the longitudinal axis of the vessel. This finding has resulted in controversy with regard to the proper technique of obtaining velocity waveforms at sites of stenosis. In areas of mild to moderate stenosis, use of a Doppler angle of 60 degrees to the long axis of the vessel is recommended. In areas of more severe stenosis and/or wall abnormalities, however, the Doppler angle of 60 degrees should be defined by the long axis of the stenotic flow jet, as demonstrated by color flow (Fig. 9–3A). The sample volume size should be kept as small as possible, usually 1.5 mm, to detect discrete changes in flow velocity. This is important, as the highest velocities may be localized to a small area in the flow stream that emanates from the stenosis. In practice, the sonographer, having identified the stenosis, gently moves the sample volume about until the point of highest velocity is found.

Although color flow sonography is not the primary means for measuring the severity of carotid stenosis, the flow image represents an important safeguard for preventing diagnostic error. In all cases, the Doppler and color flow findings should be cross-checked for concordance. If there is disagreement between the impression obtained with the color and Doppler examinations (e.g., color Doppler suggests high-grade stenosis but velocities are only moderately elevated), the findings of both should be reviewed to resolve the discrepancy. Frequently, the cause of such discrepancies is abnormally high or low flow volume, as discussed previously in the section on CCA waveform findings.

Doppler Findings Distal to the Stenosis

Damping of Doppler velocity waveforms may be seen in the region distal to carotid stenosis when the lesion is severe and flow reducing (Fig. 9–3C). This finding was discussed and illustrated previously with

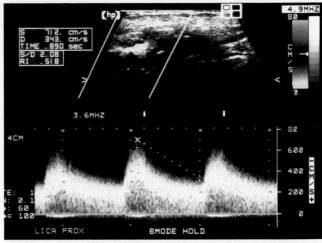

A

FIGURE 9–3. Internal carotid artery (ICA) stenosis exceeding 70% diameter reduction. *A,* Color Doppler indicates considerable narrowing of the ICA. Extremely high systolic and diastolic velocities are present in the stenosis (peak systole, 721 cm/sec; end diastole, 343 cm/sec). *B,* Severely disturbed flow is evident in the poststenotic region, indicated by poor definition of the spectral border and simultaneous forward and reverse flow in systole. *C,* ICA Doppler waveforms distal to the stenosis are damped, with delayed acceleration to peak systolic velocity and disproportionate diastolic flow.

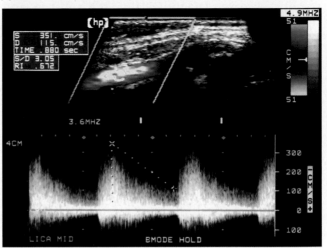

B

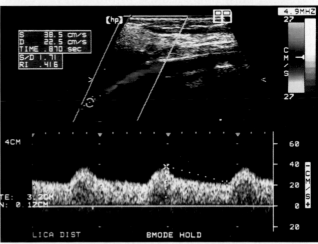

C

respect to carotid origin stenosis. Severely damped Doppler signals may be seen distal to near-occlusive stenoses of the internal carotid, as illustrated in the chapter that follows.

The most common abnormality seen distal to carotid stenosis is spectral broadening caused by disturbed blood flow or frank turbulence. Poststenotic flow disturbance is at best a qualitative measure of arterial stenosis; nevertheless, its detection is of importance. Fill-in of the Doppler spectral waveform generally indicates the presence of carotid stenosis with diameter reduction of at least 50%, but this level of disturbed flow occasionally can be seen with non-stenotic disease. Diagnostically, the most significant poststenotic flow disturbance produces simultaneous forward and reverse spectral Doppler signal, accompanied by poor definition of the upper spectral border, as illustrated in Chapter 3. This form of disturbed flow implies the presence of severe carotid stenosis and should not be disregarded. In patients with markedly calcified carotid plaque, severely disturbed flow distal to the plaque may be the only substantial evidence of the presence of clinically significant stenosis.

The use of a large sample volume that incorporates flow from many points within the vessel in the generation of the spectral waveform may give the false impression of disturbed flow, potentially leading to the misdiagnosis of moderate disease in an otherwise normal vessel. This becomes particularly important when spectral broadening is a parameter in distinguishing normal arteries from those with mild or moderate degrees of atherosclerotic plaque. When spectral broadening is used to assess the degree of carotid artery stenosis, careful attention must also be paid to the gain settings. If the gain is set too high, spectral broadening will occur as an artifact.

GRADING CAROTID STENOSIS

Many factors contribute to the clinical importance of a carotid plaque. These include plaque composition,[2-5] hemorrhage,[6] ulceration,[7] the state of the fibrous cap overlying the plaque, and the severity of lumen reduction. Of these factors, however, only the severity of stenosis has been unequivocally demonstrated to predict stroke. It is the ability of duplex scanning to accurately categorize carotid artery stenosis that has made duplex ultrasound the primary modality for evaluating carotid artery disease.

Duplex criteria for quantifying carotid artery stenosis have been developed primarily through comparisons of duplex-derived spectral waveforms and contrast arteriograms. Fine differences in the degree of stenosis, as measured by angiography, cannot be delineated with duplex scanning, and duplex-derived categories of stenosis are therefore relatively broad. Sensitivities and specificities for spectral analysis of duplex-derived waveforms for detecting an ICA stenosis of 50% to 99% or greater are between 90% and 95%.[8,9] At this time, detection of specific threshold levels of ICA stenosis appears to be most important clinically.

There are numerous spectral criteria for classifying stenosis in the ICA. Some focus on categories of stenosis, while others focus on threshold levels of stenosis. One of the most widely accepted classification schemes for categories of ICA stenosis was developed at the University of Washington under the direction of Dr. Eugene Strandness. These criteria have been useful in the study of the natural history of carotid atherosclerosis and in clinical practice (Table 9–1). In the University of Washington system, velocity waveform analysis and spectral criteria are used to classify ICA angiographic stenosis as normal, 1% to 15%, 16% to 49%, 50% to 79%, and 80% to 99% stenosis and occlusion.[10] Prospective validation of these criteria has demonstrated an overall agreement of 82% with contrast angiography. The ability to recognize normal arteries (specificity) is 84%, and the sensitivity of the criteria to detect carotid disease is 99%.[11,12]

Carotid Endarterectomy Trials

All diagnostic tests, including carotid artery duplex scanning, must undergo continued

Table 9–1. University of Washington Duplex Criteria for Internal Carotid Artery Stenosis

Diameter Reduction (%)	Velocity	Spectral Characteristics
0	PSV < 125 cm/sec	No spectral broadening
1–15	PSV < 125 cm/sec	Spectral broadening in systolic deceleration
16–49	PSV > 125 cm/sec	Spectral broadening through out systole
50–79	PSV > 125 cm/sec	Extensive spectral broadening
80–99	PSV > 125 cm/sec and EDV > 140 cm/sec	Extensive spectral broadening
Occluded	No ICA flow detected	Min diastolic flow or reversed flow in ipsilateral CCA

CCA, common carotid artery; EDV, end-diastolic velocity; ICA, internal carotid artery; PSV, peak systolic velocity.

reevaluation to remain relevant to current clinical practice. Prospective randomized trials of the efficacy of carotid endarterectomy (CEA; e.g., the North American Symptomatic Carotid Endarterectomy Trial [NASCET][13] and the Asymptomatic Carotid Atherosclerosis Study [ACAS][14]) have had a profound impact on validating the indications for CEA in patients with carotid bifurcation atherosclerosis. Not surprisingly, the results of these trials have also changed the way many interpret and report carotid duplex examinations.

In NASCET, symptomatic patients with ICA stenosis of 70% to 90% diameter reduction treated with a combination of medical management and CEA had an ipsilateral fatal and nonfatal stroke rate of 7.0% at 18 months, compared with an ipsilateral fatal and nonfatal stroke rate of 24% at 18 months when treated with medical management alone. The difference was highly significant ($P < 0.001$). This represents an absolute reduction in risk of 17% in favor of surgical management and a relative risk reduction of 71%, favoring a combination of medical and surgical management over medical management alone, by the end of 18 months. Patients with symptomatic stenosis of the ICA of 50% to 69% diameter reduction were also studied in this trial. The stroke and death rate at 5 yr was 15.7% for patients treated with a combination of medical management and CEA versus 22% for patients treated with medical management alone. There was no benefit of CEA in

patients with symptoms and ICA stenosis of less than 50% diameter reduction. Overall, with regard to symptomatic ICA stenosis, CEA for ICA stenosis of 70% to 99% has the highest therapeutic index, while the therapeutic index for CEA in patients with ICA stenosis of 50% to 69% is relatively modest.

The ACAS established surgical benefit for prophylactic CEA in good-risk patients with ICA asymptomatic stenosis of 60% to 99%.[15] In this study, there was a 5.9% absolute and a 53% relative risk reduction in patients treated with CEA and medical management versus patients treated with medical management alone. After a mean follow-up of 2.7 yr, the aggregate risk over 5 yr for ipsilateral stroke and death was 11% for patients treated only medically and 5.1% for patients treated with CEA and medical management. Thus, 19 patients would need to undergo CEA to prevent one stroke over a 5-yr interval. Therefore, the benefit of operation in asymptomatic patients is not large, and the therapeutic index for CEA is quite narrow in patients with even high-grade asymptomatic ICA stenosis.

In both the NASCET and ACAS studies, ICA stenosis was calculated from arteriograms by comparing the diameter of the minimal residual lumen to the diameter of the presumably disease-free distal cervical ICA,[16,17] as illustrated in Figure 9–4. The University of Washington duplex criteria, which preexisted the endarterectomy trials, were also obtained by comparing duplex

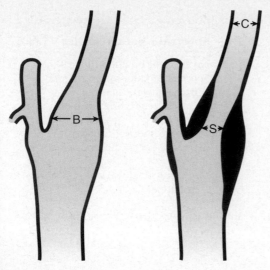

FIGURE 9–4. North American Symptomatic Carotid Endarterectomy Trial (NASCET) and Asymptomatic Carotid Atherosclerosis Study (ACAS) stenosis measurement method. The least diameter of the stenosis (S) is compared with the postbulbar ICA diameter (C). Percent stenosis is S/C × 100. The University of Washington criteria were obtained by comparing the diameter of the residual stenotic lumen (S) with the diameter of the ICA bulb (B) estimated as if free of disease.

waveforms with contrast carotid angiograms. However, in developing the University of Washington criteria, carotid artery stenosis was estimated by comparing the diameter of the residual lumen at its narrowest point with an estimate of the diameter of the ICA bulb if it were free of atherosclerosis. Because the bulb has a greater diameter than the distal ICA, the two methods of measurement do not give the same calculated percentage of angiographic stenosis for the same lesion. Calculations of angiographic stenosis using the distal ICA as the reference vessel result in lower calculated stenosis percentages than calculations using the bulb as the reference site. This effect is particularly striking for more modest lesions.

In a review of 1001 internal carotid angiograms, 34% of the ICAs were classified as stenosis of 70% to 99% using the ICA bulb as the reference vessel. In contrast, when the distal cervical ICA was used as the reference site, only 16% of the ICAs were classified as 70% to 99% stenosis. More than

99% of distal ICA-based calculations of stenosis were less than bulb-based calculations.[17] Thus, the duplex stenosis criteria developed at the University of Washington using the bulb as the reference vessel are not directly applicable to the results of NASCET or ACAS. In addition, many duplex criteria, including the University of Washington criteria, do not specifically address the 60% and 70% threshold levels used in ACAS and NASCET.

NASCET/ACAS–Based ICA Stenosis Criteria

Since the randomized CEA trials were completed, new duplex criteria for noninvasively determining ICA stenosis have been developed that are directly relevant to NASCET and ACAS.[18,19] These new criteria should not replace the University of Washington criteria that very accurately quantify atherosclerosis in the carotid bulb. Rather, they are most useful in aiding selection of patients for CEA, because they are directly applicable to the threshold levels of carotid stenosis addressed in the NASCET and ACAS trials.

The initial studies addressing this issue were performed at the Oregon Health & Science University. Duplex results in more than 300 internal carotid arteries were compared with angiograms, with angiographic stenosis calculated according to the NASCET and ACAS method. Using receiver-operator characteristics (ROC) curves and analysis of many duplex variables, it was determined that a systolic velocity ratio (the ratio of the maximal ICA [PSV] to maximal CCA PSV low in the neck) of 4.0 or more provided the highest accuracy in identifying a NASCET stenosis of 70% to 99%.[18] These data were later confirmed in a prospective study utilizing duplex scans and angiographic studies from our institution and from the University of Washington. In this study, duplex scans and angiograms were compared from 158 ICAs. Forty-two percent of the ICAs had an angiographic stenosis of 70% to 99% calculated according to the NASCET method. A systolic velocity ratio of 4.0 or higher was able to predict ICA stenosis of 70% to 99% with 91% sensitivity, 90% specificity, and an overall accuracy of 90%.[20]

Duplex velocity criteria were also developed at Oregon Health & Science University for asymptomatic patients, defining the ICA stenosis threshold of 60% or greater utilized by ACAS.[19] ICA angiograms and duplex examinations were again compared. ROC curves for many different duplex variables were derived, and the combination of a PSV of 260 cm/sec or greater and an EDV of 70 cm/sec or greater provided the highest accuracy for identifying an angiographic ICA stenosis of 60% to 99% (84% sensitivity, 94% specificity, positive predictive value of 92%, overall accuracy of 90%). Similar results were obtained with a systolic velocity ratio of 3.2 or greater. Because a duplex scan suggesting ICA stenosis of 60% to 99% in an asymptomatic patient may lead to an angiogram or operation and noting the modest therapeutic benefit of CEA in asymptomatic patients, it was reasoned that under many clinical circumstances, criteria for asymptomatic patients should have an even higher positive predictive value than for symptomatic patients. A 95% positive predictive value for ICA angiographic stenosis of 60% to 99% could be achieved in the same database with a combination of an ICA PSV of 290 cm/sec or greater and an EDV of 80 cm/sec or greater. To provide maximal current clinical relevance to referring physicians, our vascular laboratory now reports the results of carotid artery duplex scanning using both the University of Washington criteria and these more recently derived threshold criteria for asymptomatic ICA stenosis of 60% to 99% or more and symptomatic ICA stenosis of 70% to 99% or more.

Different duplex devices are known to vary in their estimation of standardized velocities tested in a phantom model. Careful analysis of data from several centers by Fillinger and colleagues[21] suggests that differences in patient composition at each center and slight variations in measured velocities from duplex devices of different manufacturers account for this finding.

Clearly, no specific duplex criteria for a threshold level of angiographic carotid stenosis can be both 100% sensitive and specific. Proper interpretation of carotid artery duplex examinations requires recognition that criteria for predicting a specific level of angiographic ICA stenosis may vary with the duplex scanner utilized and that any given velocity criteria will be associated with some false negatives and some false positives.

Consensus Committee ICA Stenosis Criteria

Recognizing that duplex criteria from different centers differ for the threshold levels of angiographic stenosis determined by ACAS and NASCET, a panel of authorities from a variety of medical specialties assembled to review the carotid ultrasound literature. This group, which convened in 2002, focused on previously untreated atherosclerotic stenosis of the proximal ICA. The panel developed a consensus regarding the key components of the carotid ultrasound examination and reasonable criteria for stratification of ICA stenosis.[22]

The consensus committee recommended that all carotid examinations be performed with gray-scale imaging, color Doppler, and spectral Doppler. The examination should be performed by a credentialed vascular technologist in accordance with the standards of one of the accrediting bodies. Doppler waveforms should be measured with an insonation angle as close to 60 degrees as possible but not exceeding 60 degrees, and the sample volumes should be placed within the area of maximal stenosis. The panelists also noted that reporting of the degree of ICA stenosis varies from laboratory to laboratory, among different readers within the same laboratory, and even with the same individual.[23-27] The consensus panelists recommended that laboratories establish protocols for stratifying the degree of ICA stenosis based on Doppler measurements and that, once established, these criteria should apply to all readers within the laboratory. With the understanding that ultrasound is most accurate when lesions are classified as lying above or below a single level, such as 60% stenosis or 70% stenosis, the panelists recommended the consistent use of relatively broad diagnostic strata to estimate the degree of ICA stenosis with ultrasound.[28] They also recognized that Doppler is relatively inaccurate for subcategorizing stenoses of less than 50% and recommended that these stenoses be reported under a single category as stenosis of less than 50%. It was suggested that subcategories for minor degrees of stenosis not be used.

Based on extensive discussions and review of numerous studies (Table 9–2A and B),[18,19,23,28–45] the consensus panel recommended stratifying the degree of ICA stenosis, based on Doppler and imaging results, into the following strata: normal (no hemodynamic or gray-scale evidence of atherosclerosis); stenosis of less than 50%; stenosis of 50% to 69%; stenosis of 70% or more but less than near occlusion; near occlusion; and occlusion. The diagnosis of near occlusion and occlusion should be based on Doppler measurements of velocity as well as gray-scale and color Doppler findings. The stenosis thresholds of 50% and 70% were chosen because they were felt to be thresholds used by many surgeons for operative intervention.

The panel noted that many Doppler parameters are used for the evaluation of ICA stenosis, including ICA PSV, ICA EDV, the ICA/CCA PSV ratio, and the ICA/CCA EDV ratio. The panel recommended that the ICA PSV and the presence of plaque on gray-scale and/or color Doppler imaging should be the primary parameters used to diagnose and grade ICA stenosis.

ICA PSV is easy to obtain and seems reasonably reproducible. However, data suggest that the reproducibility of PSV, even among experienced vascular technologists, is sufficiently poor that PSVs should not be used as a continuous variable in clinical carotid duplex scanning.[44] The degree of stenosis estimated by ICA PSV and the degree of narrowing of the ICA lumen seen on gray-scale and color Doppler should correlate. Furthermore, additional parameters such as

ICA/CCA PSV ratio and ICA EDV should be employed as internal checks and are especially useful when ICA PSV may not be representative of the extent of disease. Such situations include the presence of tandem lesions, contralateral high-grade stenosis, discrepancy between visual assessment of the plaque and ICA PSV, elevated CCA velocities, hyperdynamic cardiac states, or low cardiac output.

The consensus panel recommended the following criteria stratifying ICA stenosis. These criteria have not been subjected to retrospective or prospective evaluation and do not represent the results of any one laboratory or study (Table 9–3).

- The ICA is considered **normal** when the ICA PSV is less than 125 cm/sec and there is no visible plaque or intimal thickening. Normal arteries should also have an ICA/CCA ratio of less than 2.0 and ICA EDV of less than 40 cm/sec.

- **ICA stenosis of less than 50%** is present when the ICA PSV is less than 125 cm/sec and there is visible plaque or intimal thickening. Such arteries should also have an ICA/CCA PSV ratio of less than 2.0 and an ICA EDV of less than 40 cm/sec.

- **ICA stenosis of 50% to 69%** is present when the ICA PSV is 125 to 230 cm/sec and there is visible plaque. Such arteries should also have an ICA/CCA PSV ratio of 2.0 to 4.0 and an ICA EDV of 40 to 100 cm/sec.

- **ICA stenosis of 70% or more** but less than near occlusion is present when the ICA PSV is more than 230 cm/sec and there is visible plaque with lumen narrowing on gray-scale and color Doppler imaging. (The higher the PSV, the greater the likelihood [positive predictive value] of severe disease.) Such stenoses should also have an ICA/CCA ratio of more than 4 and an ICA EDV of more than 100 cm/sec.

- In cases of **near occlusion** of the ICA, the velocity parameters may not apply. "Preocclusive" lesions may be associated with high, low, or undetectable velocity measurements. The diagnosis of near occlusion is therefore established primarily by demonstration of a markedly

Table 9–2A. Review of Literature for Diagnosing Internal Carotid Artery Stenosis with Doppler Thresholds

Author	Ref	Year	N	Threshold % Stenosis*	PSV	EDV	Ratio†	Performance % Sens	% Spec	% PPV	% NPV	% Acc
Huston J et al	29	2000	915	50	130		1.6	92	90	90	91	91
Huston J et al	29	2000	915	70	230	70	3.2	86	90	83	92	89
Soulez G et al	40	1999		60			2.9	94	80	72	96	
AbuRahma AF et al	31	1998		50	140			92	95	97	89	93
AbuRahma AF et al	31	1998		60	150	65		82	97	96	86	90
AbuRahma AF et al	31	1998		70	150	90		85	95	91	92	92
Carpenter JP et al	32	1996	110	70	210			94	77	68	96	83
Carpenter JP et al	32	1996	110	70		70		92	60	73	86	77
Carpenter JP et al	32	1996	110				3.3	100	65	65	100	79
Hood DB et al	33	1996	457	70	130	100		78	97	88	94	93
Carpenter JP et al	34	1995		60	230			98	87	88	98	92
Carpenter JP et al	34	1995		60		40		97	52	86	86	86
Carpenter JP et al	34	1995		60			2.0	97	73	78	96	76
Carpenter JP et al	34	1995		60	230	40	2.0	100	100	100	100	100
Browman MW et al	35	1995	75	70	175			91	60			
Moneta GL et al	19	1995	176	60	260	70	3.2–3.5	84	94	92	88	90
Neale ML et al	36	1994	60	70	270	110		96	91			93
Moneta GL et al	18	1993		70	325	130		83	90	80	92	88

*Degree of stenosis set as cutoff for diagnosis.
†Ratio of internal carotid artery peak systolic velocity to common carotid artery peak systolic velocity.
Acc, accuracy; EDV, internal carotid artery end-diastolic velocity; N, number of patients; NPV, negative predictive value; PPV, positive predictive value; PSV, internal carotid artery peak systolic velocity; Ref, reference; sens, sensitivity; spec, specificity.

narrowed lumen with color Doppler. In some near occlusive lesions, color Doppler can distinguish between near occlusion and occlusion by demonstrating a thin wisp of color traversing the lesion.

• **Occlusion** of the ICA is present when there is no detectable patent lumen on gray-scale imaging and no flow with spectral, color, or power Doppler. Near occlusive lesions may be misdiagnosed as occlusions when only gray-scale

Table 9–2B. Review of Literature for Diagnosing Internal Carotid Artery Stenosis with Doppler-Studies Not Providing Sensitivities, Specificities, and Predictive Values

Author	Ref	Year	N	Threshold Chosen % Stenosis*	PSV	EDV	Ratio[†]	Performance Assessment and Results
Umemura A & Yamada K	37	2000	60	Variable thresholds				Evaluated B-flow without Doppler
Perkins JM et al	38	2000						
Grant EG et al	28	2000						Doppler performs poorly for estimating degree of stenosis, better for differentiating above and below a single degree of stenosis
Beebe HG et al	39	1999						Color and gray-scale perform well alone; Doppler helps for mid-range lesions
Grant EG et al	30	1999	303	60	200		3	Asymptomatic patients; outcome better than sensitivity/specificity/accuracy
Grant EG et al	30	1999		70	175		2.5	Symptomatic patients; outcome better than sensitivity/specificity/accuracy
Ranke C et al	23	1999		70				Ratio of ICA PSV at stenosis to ICA PSV distal to stenosis; sensitivity 94%, specificity 98%
Soulez G et al	40	1999		70				Ratio of ICA PSV at stenosis to ICA PSV distal to stenosis; sensitivity 94%; specificity 81%; PPV 62%; NPV 98%
Derdeyn CP & Powers WJ	41	1996		60	230			Simulator
Griewig B et al	42	1996						Power Doppler better than color Doppler (not quantified)
Srinivasan J et al	43	1995	164					Doppler poor for differentiating degree of stenosis for values <50%
Hunink MG et al	44	1993	60					PSV best parameter for predicting stenosis >70%
Bluth EI et al	45	1988						EDV best, but did not use NASCET criteria for angiography

*Degree of stenosis set as cutoff for diagnosis.
[†]Ratio of internal carotid artery peak systolic velocity to common carotid artery peak systolic velocity.
EDV, internal carotid artery end-diastolic velocity; ICA, internal carotid artery; N, number of patients; NASCET, North America Symptomatic Carotid Endarterectomy Trial; NPV, negative predictive value; PPV, positive predictive value; PSV, internal carotid artery peak systolic velocity; Ref, reference; sens, sensitivity; spec, specificity.

Table 9–3. Consensus Panel Table of Ultrasound and Doppler Criteria for Diagnosis of Internal Carotid Artery Stenosis

Primary Parameters			Additional Parameters	
Degree of Stenosis	ICA PSV	Plaque Estimate*	ICA/CCA PSV Ratio	ICA EDV
Normal	<125 cm/sec	None	<2.0	<40 cm/sec
<50%	<125 cm/sec	<50% diameter reduction	<2.0	<40 cm/sec
50%–69%	125–230 cm/sec	≥50% diameter reduction	2.0–4.0	40–100 cm/sec
≥70 but less than near occlusion	≥230 cm/sec	≥50% diameter reduction	>4.0	>100 cm/sec
Near occlusion	High, low, or undetectable	Visible	Variable	Variable
Total occlusion	Undetectable	Visible, no detectable lumen	Not applicable	Not applicable

*Plaque estimate with the gray-scale ultrasound and the color Doppler imaging.
CCA, common carotid artery; EDV, end-diastolic velocity; ICA, internal carotid artery; PSV, peak systolic velocity.

ultrasound and spectral Doppler are used.

OTHER TOPICS RELEVANT TO CAROTID ARTERY DUPLEX SCANNING

Surveillance of Asymptomatic Disease

A retrospective analysis of more than 300 patients performed at our institution determined that symptomatic patients with less than 60% diameter ICA stenosis and an ICA PSV of more than 175 cm/sec on initial duplex examination had a significantly higher rate of progression to ICA stenosis of 60% to 99% than asymptomatic patients with ICA PSVs of less than 175 cm/sec.[46] Based on this finding, a prospective evaluation of 407 patients was performed, representing 640 patent, nonoperated ICA stenoses less than 60%.[47] Symptomatic progression of ICA stenosis was infrequent in this group. Only three patients, at a mean of 21 mo, developed hemispheric symptoms (transient ischemic attack in all) and had ipsilateral atherosclerosis progression. In addition, one ICA progressed to occlusion at 54 mo, with a resulting transient

ischemic attack. No patient had neurologic symptoms *without* ipsilateral progression of ICA stenosis.

Asymptomatic progression to ICA stenosis of 60% to 99% was detected in 10% of patients and 7% of ICAs at a mean of 18 months, and such progression correlated with the patients' initial duplex examination. The mean PSV, mean EDV, and mean ICA/CCA PSV ratio were all higher initially in those whose plaque/stenoses subsequently progressed, versus those in whom atherosclerosis remained stable. Asymptomatic progression to ICA stenosis of 60% to 99% occurred in 4% of ICAs with initial PSVs of less than 175 cm/sec, while 26% of ICAs with initial PSVs of more than 175 cm/sec progressed to stenosis of 60% to 99% (P < 0.0001, Table 9–4). The mean time of progression to ICA stenosis of more than 60% to 99% was 21 ± 10 months with initial PSVs of less than 175 cm/sec, as compared with 14 ± 9 months in those with initial PSVs of more than 175 cm/sec. By life table analysis, freedom from progression to ICA stenosis of 60% to 99% was significantly higher for those patients with an initial ICA PSV of less than 175 cm/sec, versus those with an initial ICA PSV of more than 175 cm/sec.

Thus, asymptomatic patients (who have not had a previous ipsilateral endarterec-

Table 9–4. Comparison of Initial Duplex Parameters in ICAs Progressing and Not Progressing From ICA Stenosis of <60% to ICA Stenosis of 60%–99%

Initial Duplex Value	Nonprogressing Arteries (N = 587)	Progressing Arteries (N = 46)	P Value
Mean PSV	110 ± 47	166 + 55	<0.0001
Mean EDV	36 ± 15	55 + 22	<0.0001
Mean ICA/CCA PSV ratio	1.40 ± 0.68	2.21 + 1.00	<0.0001

CCA, common carotid artery; EDV, end-diastolic velocity; ICA, internal carotid artery; PSV, peak systolic velocity.

tomy) with ICA stenosis of less than 60% and duplex scan–determined ICA PSV of less than 175 cm/sec can be safely followed with serial scans at examination intervals of 1 yr. Patients with ICA stenosis of less than 60% and PSVs of 175 cm/sec or higher on initial duplex examination are significantly more likely to progress asymptomatically to ICA stenosis of 60% to 99%. Progression in this subgroup is sufficiently frequent to warrant follow-up duplex studies at 6-mo intervals.

Recurrent Carotid Stenosis

As with primary stenosis and occlusion, ultrasound can be used to demonstrate or rule out recurrent carotid stenosis after CEA, patch grafting, bypass surgery, and carotid stenting. Three patterns of ICA stenosis following CEA have been recognized. Lesions present within 1 mo of CEA are likely residual lesions and represent a technically imperfect operation. Early recurrences following a technically adequate operation occur within the first 2 yr after CEA, usually within the first 12 mo and result from myointimal hyperplasia. Late recurrences occur 2 yr or more following endarterectomy and are due to recurrent atherosclerosis.

Over the past three decades, there have been more than 160 publications on recurrent carotid artery stenosis following CEA. These publications encompass more than 62,000 carotid endarterectomies. The incidence of carotid restenosis in these series averaged 6% (range: 0%–50%). The mean incidence of asymptomatic carotid resteno-

sis detected noninvasively is 9%, more than four times the 2% incidence of symptomatic recurrent stenosis. In recent years, the performance of routine patch angioplasty by many surgeons has lowered the rate of carotid restenosis. Restenosis develops in a mean of 12% of arteries closed primarily versus 5% of those closed with a patch. Overall, it appears that approximately 20% of carotid restenoses are due to residual stenosis at the time of surgery. Stenoses that occur within the first 2 yr represent about 50% of carotid restenoses. The remaining 30% of restenoses occur more than 2 yr after operation. Fewer than 25% of carotid restenoses ever become symptomatic, and only about 7% ever cause stroke. One study of 380 patients followed up to 16 yr or more found that the overall incidence of recurrent carotid stenosis equaling or exceeding 50% was 10.8%. Incidences at 1, 3, 5, and 10 yr were 5.8%, 9.9%, 13.9%, and 23.4%, respectively.[48] Only 2.1% developed severe (>80%) recurrent stenosis.

Several studies have examined the optimal timing and frequency of duplex sonography after surgery, to detect both recurrent carotid stenosis and contralateral atherosclerotic disease progression. The value of early duplex scanning after CEA in patients with a normal intraoperative completion study is limited, as shown by a retrospective study of 380 CEAs with intraoperative completion angiography, duplex scans, or both.[49,50] Follow-up ICA duplex scans were normal in 95.8% of patients after CEA. There were no severe recurrent ICA stenoses. Overall, only 0.5% of the patients with operated ICAs developed even moderate restenosis within the first 6 mo. This study demonstrated that duplex surveillance in the first 6 mo postoperatively is unproductive when intraoperative completion studies are normal.

Recent studies have found that after CEA, contralateral progression of atherosclerosis is a much more important problem than ipsilateral ICA restenoses. In a study of 221 patients who underwent CEA, progression of contralateral disease, rather than restenosis, was the most common finding that resulted in the need for reintervention during a mean follow-up period of 27.4 mo.[50] Only 2.7% of the patients with operated ICAs had asymptomatic recurrent stenosis of more than 50% diameter by duplex scanning, and only 1 of 221 patients had recurrent stenosis of more than 75%, requiring reoperation. The yield for post-CEA surveillance in the operated artery was less than 1%, while progression of contralateral disease occurred in 12% of patients, leading to seven CEAs for high-grade stenosis. Importantly, disease progression to stenosis of more than 75% was five times as frequent in patients with ICA stenosis of more than 50% initially. All patients but one who eventually required contralateral endarterectomy for disease progression had ICA stenosis of more than 50% when first seen. The authors concluded that duplex scanning at *1- to 2-yr intervals* after CEA is adequate when an uncomplicated CEA is achieved, based on surgical completion studies, and minimal contralateral disease (<50% stenosis) is present.

These data show that following CEA, the likelihood of finding significant carotid restenosis requiring repair is quite low. If reoperation is indicated only for symptomatic recurrent lesions and selected high-grade asymptomatic restenoses, the frequency of subsequent follow-up examinations can be dictated primarily by the status of the contralateral, nonoperated carotid artery or by the development of neurologic symptoms. Generally, patients with CEA who have normal intraoperative completion studies and stenosis of less than 50% in the contralateral artery can be safely followed with carotid duplex scanning at 1-yr intervals. Patients with less than technically perfect results of CEA or stenosis of

more than 50% in the contralateral unoperated ICA should undergo follow-up duplex scanning at 6 mo.

Bilateral High-Grade Stenosis

Doppler-derived flow velocities from the ICA opposite an ICA occlusion or high-grade stenosis may suggest a higher degree of narrowing, due to collateralization, than is observed angiographically. Several investigators have found that contralateral occlusion leads to overestimation of ICA stenosis with standard Doppler criteria.[51-53] Until recently, no studies have addressed the effectiveness of CEA performed on the basis of ACAS-based Doppler criteria for ICA stenosis contralateral to high-grade ICA stenosis or occlusion. This information is important in planning CEA when duplex scanning is used as the sole means of preoperative stenosis assessment.

A study conducted in our laboratory over an 8-yr period determined the effects of unilateral CEA on the duplex scan findings in the contralateral ICA in patients with bilateral carotid stenosis.[54] Four hundred and sixty patients underwent CEA for ICA stenosis of 60% to 99%, and 107 of these had an asymptomatic contralateral ICA stenosis of 50% to 99% by standard Doppler criteria (PSV > 125 cm/sec). Among these asymptomatic stenoses, 38 met Doppler criteria for ICA stenosis of 60% to 99% preoperatively. Following surgery, there was a mean decrease of 48 cm/sec (10.1%) in PSV and 36 cm/sec (19.3%) in the EDV in the unoperated, asymptomatic stenoses. In 8 of 38 patients (21.1%), the unoperated ICA lesions of 60% to 99% were reclassified as less than 60% on postoperative duplex scanning. Six of 69 patients with asymptomatic ICA stenosis who did not meet criteria for narrowing of 60% to 99% prior to contralateral CEA met these criteria on their first postoperative examination. All of these patients were close to the Doppler threshold on preoperative testing. It follows that when duplex scanning is used as the sole imaging modality before CEA, patients with severe bilateral carotid stenosis must have an additional duplex examination after the initial CEA to reassess stenosis severity and the need for surgery of the unoperated ICA.

Our findings with respect to bilateral ICA stenosis were similar to those of Busuttil and coworkers,[51] who found that duplex scanning, in comparison to angiography, overestimated the degree of stenosis in 27% of ICAs contralateral to a high-grade stenosis. These investigators observed an average decrease in peak systolic frequency of 1175 Hz (approximately 36 cm/sec) and end-diastolic frequency of 475 Hz (approximately 15 cm/sec) after contralateral CEA. Overall, 51% of patients had a one-category decrease in the Doppler-estimated severity of ICA stenosis following contralateral CEA. Fujitani and associates[1] further noted that duplex scan overestimation of stenosis is more common in less-severe categories of stenosis than in higher-severity categories.

ICA Coils and Kinks

Tortuosity of the ICA is a common finding in elderly patients and may be difficult to distinguish from carotid artery aneurysm on physical examination. Occasionally, ICA tortuosity is associated with fibromuscular dysplasia.[55] In essence, tortuosity comes in two forms: coiling of the ICA and kinking, and both may occur together. While very unusual, marked ICA kinking, with an inside angle of less than 90 degrees, may result in neurologic symptoms if there is either flow reduction imposed by the kink or concomitant plaque formation at the site of the kink that results in distal embolization.[56] A history of neurologic symptoms associated with head motion, or the presence of an abnormal pulsation in the neck, should lead the clinician to suspect the presence of a kink, and these observations are indication for further workup.

Internal carotid artery kinks and coils may cause problems with respect to duplex examination (Fig. 9–5). The course of the tortuous ICA can usually be traced with color flow imaging, and real-time B-mode ultrasound can readily image concurrent atheromatous plaque in the tortuous segment. In addition, color flow can help distinguish a tortuous vessel from a carotid artery aneurysm in a patient with a pulsating neck mass. It is difficult, nonetheless, to interpret Doppler frequency shifts and spectral analysis findings in tortuous carotid

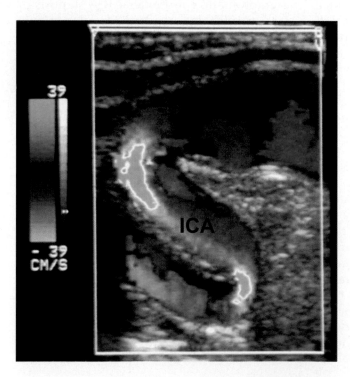

Figure 9–5. Color Doppler image of a tortuous internal carotid artery (ICA). By better identifying the course of a tortuous ICA with color flow, the Doppler angle can be more accurately determined, resulting in more reliable velocity measurements.

arteries because of distorted flow patterns and angulations. Flow in the tortuous artery inevitably is quite disturbed, and marked turbulence may occur in kinked ICAs, yet the clinical importance of such disturbances is unknown. Color flow allows for reasonably accurate determination of the Doppler angle and placement of the sample volume, leading to more reliable velocity measurements when stenosis is suspected, but in some cases it is not clear that the ascribed Doppler angle is sufficiently accurate for diagnosis. Unfortunately, we cannot provide solutions to the diagnostic dilemmas imposed by ICA kinks and coils. A potential solution to these problems may lie with high-resolution, contrast-enhanced magnetic resonance or computed tomographic angiography. These methods now offer image resolution of 1 mm or less and the capacity to reconstruct the image in any plane of section. These capabilities are likely to provide the most accurate assessment of tortuosity-related ICA stenosis currently available.

CCA and ECA Stenosis

The velocity criteria used for classifying disease in the internal carotid artery have not been tested for application to the ECA or the CCA. However, as with the ICA, relative degrees of stenosis may be determined by the presence of plaque with B-mode imaging, aberration in color flow on duplex examination, spectral broadening, and increase in PSV. Although not specifically tested, stenosis of more than 50% can be inferred by the presence of a focally increased velocity followed by poststenotic turbulence. Normally, the CCA has attributes of the ICA and ECA. The CCA will take on the quality of the "normal" vessel (ICA or ECA) when the other is occluded. If there is a proximal CCA (or right innominate artery) high-grade stenosis or occlusion, the ipsilateral CCA Doppler flow quality will be dampened with low PSVs, as compared with the contralateral side. Poststenotic turbulence also may be seen. There are no widely employed validated criteria to give a diameter reduction for stenosis in the CCA. Stenosis of greater than 50% is inferred by PSV of more than 125 cm/sec associated with poststenotic turbulence. As noted previously, a focal high-grade stenosis or multiple lesions within the CCA can result in diminished PSVs and EDVs in the ICA, with resulting underestimation of degree of stenosis within the ICA.

CONCLUSION

Duplex scanning remains the most accurate and clinically useful method to noninvasively evaluate the extracranial carotid artery. The addition of color flow to gray-scale imaging and pulse Doppler examination facilitates performance of the examination and, in some cases, improves accuracy. Performance and interpretation of duplex studies must, however, change with increased knowledge of carotid artery disease and its therapy. Only through continual reassessment and careful investigation will duplex scanning remain the pre-eminent noninvasive method for assessing the carotid artery.

References

1. Fujitani RM, Mills JL, Wang LM, Taylor SM: The effect of unilateral internal carotid arterial occlusion upon contralateral duplex study: Criteria for accurate interpretation. J Vasc Surg 16:459–467; discussion, 467–468, 1992.
2. Goes E, Janssens W, Maillet B, et al: Tissue characterization of atheromatous plaques: Correlation between ultrasound image and histological findings. J Clin Ultrasound 18:611–617, 1990.
3. Gray-Weale AC, Graham JC, Burnett JR, et al: Carotid artery atheroma: Comparison of preoperative B-mode ultrasound appearance with carotid endarterectomy specimen. J Cardiovasc Surg 29:115–123, 1988.
4. Block RW, Lusby RJ: Carotid plaque morphology and interpretation of echolucent lesion. In Diagnostic Vascular Imaging. London, Arnold, 1992, pp 225–236.
5. El-Barghouty N, Geroulakos G, Nicolaides A, et al: Computer assisted carotid plaque characterization. Eur J Vasc Endovasc Surg 9:389–393, 1995.
6. Lennihan L, Krupsky WJ, Mohr JP, et al: Lack of association between carotid plaque hematoma

and ischemic cerebral symptoms. Stroke 18:879–881, 1987.

7. Comerota AJ, Katz ML, White JV, et al: The preoperative diagnosis of the ulcerated carotid atheroma. J Vasc Surg 11:505–510, 1990.

8. Colhoun E, Macerlean D: Carotid artery imaging using duplex scanning and bi-directional arteriography: A comparison. Clin Radiol 35:101–106, 1984.

9. Eikelboom BC, Ackerstaff RG, Ludwig JW, et al: Digital video subtraction angiography and duplex scanning in assessment of carotid artery disease: Comparison with conventional angiography. Surgery 94:821–825, 1983.

10. Strandness DE Jr: Duplex scanning in vascular disorders. New York, Raven Press, 1990, pp 92–120.

11. Roederer GO, Langlois YE, Jager KA, et al: A simple spectral parameter for accurate classification of severe carotid artery disease. Bruit 3:174–178, 1989.

12. Roederer GO, Langlois YE, Chan AT, et al: Ultrasonic duplex scanning of the external carotid arteries: Improved accuracy using new features from the carotid artery. J Cardiovasc Ultrasonography 1:373–380, 1982.

13. North American Symptomatic Carotid Endarterectomy Trial Collaborators: NASCET: Beneficial effect of carotid endarterectomy in patients with high-grade carotid stenosis. N Engl J Med 325:445–453, 1991.

14. Executive Committee for Asymptomatic Carotid Atherosclerosis Study: Endarterectomy for asymptomatic carotid artery stenosis. JAMA 273:1421–1428, 1995.

15. Asymptomatic Carotid Atherosclerosis Study Group: ACAS: Study design for randomized prospective trial of carotid endarterectomy for asymptomatic atherosclerosis. Stroke 20:844–849, 1989.

16. North American Symptomatic Carotid Endarterectomy Trial (NASCET) Steering Committee: North American symptomatic carotid endarterectomy trial: Methods, patient characteristics, and progress. Stroke 1991:711–720, 1991.

17. Rothwell PM, Gibson RJ, Slattery J, et al: Equivalence of measurements of carotid stenosis: A comparison of three methods on 1001 angiograms. Stroke 25:2435–2439, 1994.

18. Moneta GL, Edwards JM, Chitwood RW, et al: Correlation of North American Symptomatic Carotid Endarterectomy Trial (NASCET): Angiographic definition of 70% to 99% internal carotid artery stenosis with duplex scanning. J Vasc Surg 17:152–157; discussion 157–159, 1993.

19. Moneta GL, Edwards JM, Papanicolaou G, et al: Screening for asymptomatic internal carotid artery stenosis: Duplex criteria for discriminating 60% to 99% stenosis. J Vasc Surg 21:989–994, 1995.

20. Edwards JM, Moneta GL, Papanicolaou G, et al: Prospective validation of a new duplex ultrasound criteria for 70%–99% internal carotid stenosis. JEMU 16:3–7, 1995.

21. Fillinger MF, Baker RJ Jr, Zwolak RM, et al: Carotid duplex criteria for a 60% or greater angiographic stenosis: Variation according to equipment. J Vasc Surg 24:856–864, 1996.

22. Grant EG, Benson CB, Moneta GL, et al: Carotid Artery Stenosis: Gray-scale and Doppler US diagnosis—Society of Radiologists in Ultrasound Consensus Conference (online). Radiology, September 18, 2003.

23. Ranke C, Creutzig A, Becker H, Trappe HJ: Standardization of carotid ultrasound: A hemodynamic method to normalize for interindividual and interequipment variability. Stroke 30:402–406, 1999.

24. Alexandrov AV, Brodie DS, McLean A, et al: Correlation of peak systolic velocity and angiographic measurement of carotid stenosis revisited. Stroke 28:339–342, 1997.

25. Fillinger MF, Baker RJ Jr, Zwolak RM, et al: Carotid duplex criteria for 60% or greater angiographic stenosis: Variation according to equipment. J Vasc Surg 24:856–864, 1996.

26. Howard G, Baker WH, Chambless LE, et al: An approach for the use of Doppler ultrasound as a screening tool for hemodynamically significant stenosis (despite heterogeneity of Doppler performance). A multicenter experience. Asymptomatic Carotid Atherosclerosis Study Investigators. Stroke 27:1951–1957, 1996.

27. Kuntz KM, Polak JF, Whittermore AD, et al: Duplex ultrasound criteria for the identification of carotid stenosis should be laboratory specific. Stroke 28:597–602, 1997.

28. Grant EG, Duerinckx AJ, El Saden SM, et al: Ability to use duplex US to quantify internal carotid stenoses: Fact or fiction? Radiology 214:247–252, 2000.

29. Huston J 3rd, James E, Brown RD Jr, et al: Redefined duplex ultrasonographic criteria for the diagnosis of carotid artery stenosis. Mayo Clin Proc 75:1133–1140, 2000.

30. Grant EG, Duerinckx AJ, El Saden S, et al: Doppler sonographic parameters for the detection of carotid stenosis. Am J Roentgenol 172:1123–1129, 1999.

31. AbuRahma AF, Robinson PA, Stickler DL, et al: Proposed new duplex classification for threshold stenoses used in various symptomatic and asymptomatic carotid endarterectomy trials. Ann Vasc Surg 12:349–358, 1998.

32. Carpenter JP, Lexa FJ, Davis JT: Determination of duplex Doppler ultrasound criteria appropriate to the North American Symptomatic

Carotid Endarterectomy Trial. Stroke 27:695–699, 1996.

33. Hood DB, Mattos MA, Mansour A, et al: Prospective evaluation of new duplex criteria to identify 70% internal carotid artery stenosis. J Vasc Surg 23:254–261, 1996.

34. Carpenter JP, Lexa FJ, Davis JT: Determination of 60% or greater carotid artery stenosis by duplex Doppler ultrasonography. J Vasc Surg 22:697–703, 1995.

35. Browman MW, Cooperberg PL, Harrison PB, et al: Duplex ultrasonography criteria for internal carotid stenosis of more than 70% diameter: Angiographic correlation and receiver operating characteristic curve analysis. Can Assoc Radiol J 46:291–295, 1995.

36. Neale ML, Chambers JL, Kelly AT, et al: Reappraisal of duplex criteria to assess significant carotid stenosis with special reference to reports from the North American Symptomatic Carotid Endarterectomy Trial and the European Carotid Surgery Trial. J Vasc Surg 20:642–649, 1994.

37. Umemura A, Yamada K: B-mode flow imaging of the carotid artery. Stroke 32:2055–2057, 2000.

38. Perkins JM, Galland RB, Simmons MJ, Magee TR: Carotid duplex imaging: Variation and validation. Br J Surg 87:320–322, 2000.

39. Beebe HG, Salles-Cunha SX, Scissons RP, et al: Carotid arterial ultrasound scan imaging: A direct approach to stenosis measurement. J Vasc Surg 29:838–844, 1999.

40. Soulez G, Therasse E, Robillard P, et al: The value of internal carotid systolic velocity ratio for assessing carotid artery stenosis with Doppler sonography. Am J Roentgenol 172:207–212, 1999.

41. Derdeyn CP, Powers WJ: Cost-effectiveness of screening for asymptomatic carotid artery disease. Stroke 27:1944–1950, 1996.

42. Griewig B, Morganstern C, Driesner F, et al: Cerebrovascular disease assessed by color flow and power Doppler ultrasonography. Comparison with digital subtraction angiography in internal carotid artery stenosis. Stroke 27:95–100, 1996.

43. Srinivasan J, Mayberg MR, Weiss DG, Eskridge J: Duplex accuracy compared with angiography in the Veterans Affairs Cooperative Studies Trial for Symptomatic Carotid Stenosis. Neurosurgery 36:648–653, 1995.

44. Hunink MG, Polak JF, Barlan MM, O'Leary DH: Detection and quantification of carotid artery stenosis: Efficacy of various Doppler velocity parameters. Am J Roentgenol 160:619–625, 1993.

45. Bluth EI, Stavros AT, Marich KW, et al: Carotid duplex sonography: A multicenter recommendation for standardized imaging and Doppler criteria. Radiographics 6:487–506, 1988.

46. Nehler MR, Moneta GL, Lee RW, et al: Improving selection of patients with less than 60% asymptomatic internal carotid stenosis for follow-up carotid artery duplex scanning. J Vasc Surg 24:580–585, 1996.

47. Lovelace TD, Moneta GL, Abou-Zamzam AM Jr, et al: Optimizing duplex follow-up in patients with an asymptomatic internal carotid artery stenosis of less than 60%. J Vasc Surg 33:56–61, 2001.

48. Mattos MA, van Bemmelen PS, Barkmeier ID, et al: Routine surveillance after carotid endarterectomy: Does it affect clinical management? J Vasc Surg 17:819–830, 1993.

49. Roth SM, Back MR, Bandyk DF, et al: A rational algorithm for duplex scan surveillence after carotid endarterectomy. J Vasc Surg 31:838–839, 1999.

50. Pross C, Shortsleeve CM, Baker JD, et al: Carotid endarterectomy with normal findings from a completion study: Is there need for early duplex scan? J Vasc Surg 33:963–967, 2001.

51. Busuttil SJ, Franklin DP, Youkey JR, et al: Carotid duplex overestimation of stenosis due to severe contralateral disease. Am J Surg 172:144–148, 1996.

52. Hayes AC, Johnson KW, Baker WH, et al: The effect of contralateral disease on carotid Doppler frequency. Surgery 103:19–23, 1988.

53. van Everdingen KJ, Kapelle LJ: Overestimation of a stenosis in the internal carotid artery by duplex sonography caused by an increase in flow volume. J Vasc Surg 27:479–485, 1998.

54. Abou-Zamzam AM Jr, Moneta GL, Edwards JM, Yeager RA, Taylor LM Jr, Porter JM: Is a single preoperative duplex scan sufficient for planning bilateral carotid endarterectomy? J Vasc Surg 31:282–288, 2000.

55. Effeney DJ, Ehrenfeld WK, Stoney RJ, et al: Fibromuscular dysplasia of the internal carotid artery. World J Surg 3:179, 1979.

56. Sarkari NB, Bickerstaff ER: Neurological manifestations associated with internal carotid loops and kinks in children. J Neurol Neurosurg Psychiatry 33:194, 1973.

Chapter 10

Carotid Occlusion, Unusual Carotid Pathology, and Tricky Carotid Cases

WILLIAM J. ZWIEBEL, MD, AND JOHN S. PELLERITO, MD

CAROTID OCCLUSION

Arterial occlusion is diagnosed with ultrasound through the following observations: (1) absence of arterial pulsations; (2) echogenic material filling the arterial lumen; (3) absence of flow (color flow or spectral Doppler); and (4) small vessel size (chronic occlusion).[1-7] The typical findings of internal carotid occlusion are shown in Fig. 10–1.

At first glance, the diagnosis of occlusion appears to be an easy matter, but false-positive diagnoses may occur when the artery is obscured by acoustic shadowing, when image quality is poor, when Doppler signals are weak, and especially when the vessel is nearly occluded and only a "trickle" of flow is present. The latter problem is of considerable clinical importance, for an occluded vessel is irremediable, whereas a nearly occluded vessel may be treated with endarterectomy if the stenosis is localized and the distal vessel is of good caliber. A nearly occluded internal carotid artery (ICA) often produces the angiographic "string sign" (Fig. 10–2A). It is important to realize that the apparent small caliber of the arterial lumen represented by the "string" of contrast is an artifact. The string sign results from puddling of the slow-moving contrast agent in the dependent (posterior) portion of the arterial lumen with the patient supine. The lumen, in fact, is widely patent, and the stenosis is localized at the ICA origin.

Differentiation between highly stenosed and occluded carotid arteries was a major problem for ultrasound in the pre–color flow days, but now, through the use of color and power Doppler sonography, stenosis and occlusion can be accurately differentiated (see Fig. 10–2B, C). The use of power Doppler imaging is particularly advocated because of its sensitivity to low flow rates, and studies using color or power Doppler[6,7] report close to 100% sensitivity and specificity in the diagnosis of near occlusion of the ICA. To attain this level of accuracy, however, several technical details must be followed. First, adjust the instrument to detect minimum flow velocity. The pulse repetition frequency should be as low as possible, and the low-frequency filter should be minimized so that low-frequency signals are not excluded. Second, obtain the best possible view of the occluded vessel and scrutinize the lumen for any hint of

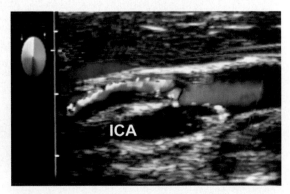

FIGURE 10–1. Internal carotid artery (ICA) occlusion. No flow is present in the ICA, and the vessel is filled with minimally echogenic material. These are typical features of carotid occlusion. The external carotid artery (upper vessel) is stenotic.

blood flow. Remember that the view chosen should optimize the Doppler angle of the color flow image. I generally prefer power Doppler, but color Doppler may work better in some cases, especially when movement artifacts are a problem. Third, interrogate the visualized segments of the carotid artery with spectral Doppler imaging. The signals obtained may be very weak, so high Doppler gain settings often are needed. Remember, pulsed Doppler is more sensitive than color Doppler for the detection of slow- or low-velocity flow. Do not mistake the highly damped arterial flow signals for venous flow. (Check the flow direction.)

Finally, look at the occluded vessel from several transducer approaches, including the transverse plane, before concluding that flow is absent.

Atherosclerosis is by far the most common cause of carotid artery occlusion, but fibromuscular dysplasia and arterial dissection (discussion follows) are additional causes. Most occlusions in the carotid system occur in the ICA, but occlusion also may occur in the common (CCA) or external (ECA) carotid artery. The incidence of CCA occlusion occurs approximately one tenth as often as ICA occlusion,[5] but this incidence is sufficiently large for

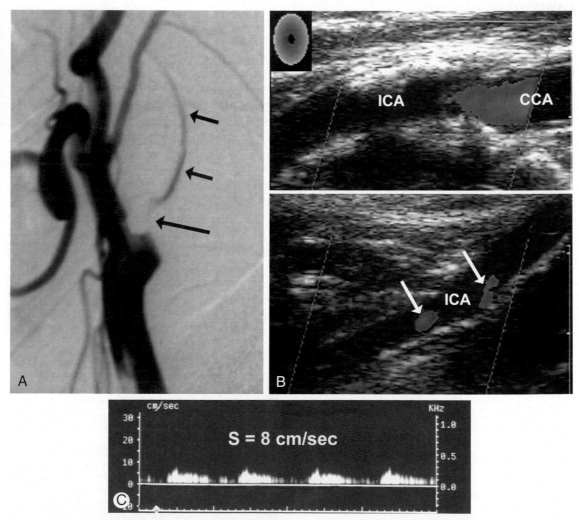

FIGURE 10–2. Near occlusion of the internal carotid artery (ICA). *A,* Only a trickle of flow is present in the ICA, producing the arteriographic "string sign" (*short arrows*). The area of narrowing is actually confined to the ICA origin (*long arrow*), and the rest of the vessel is widely patent. The string results from puddling of the contrast agent against the posterior wall of the vessel with the patient supine. *B,* At first glance (*top*) it appears that the ICA is occluded, but with diligent scanning, flow is identified by focal areas of color (*bottom*). *C,* Doppler shows markedly damped flow signals and low peak systolic velocity (S) in the areas of color. CCA, common carotid artery.

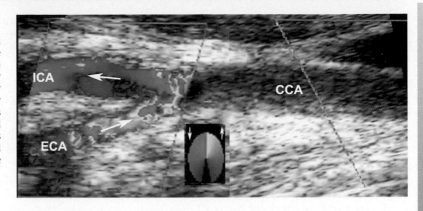

FIGURE 10–3. Common carotid artery occlusion. A composite image (note the two *color boxes*) shows absence of blood flow in the common carotid artery (CCA), which contains mildly echogenic material. Flow is reversed in the external carotid artery (ECA), which supplies blood to the internal carotid artery (ICA). (*Arrows* indicate flow direction.)

the occasional diagnosis of CCA occlusion in a typical community-based vascular practice. CCA occlusion is frequently accompanied by stroke or other neurologic events but may also be encountered in the absence of neurologic symptoms.[5] The ICA may remain patent in spite of CCA occlusion (Fig. 10–3), because collateral supply to the ICA develops through the ECA branches. Flow reverses in the collateral ECA branches and remains cephalad in the ICA.

CAROTID ARTERY DISSECTION

Arterial dissection refers to the entry of blood into the wall of the artery, separating the layers of the wall and creating a false lumen through which blood flows.[8–14] For blood to enter the wall and cause dissection, there must be a rent in the intima, which may be caused by violent trauma, iatrogenic trauma, or an underlying weakness of the muscular layer that allows the intima to tear. The location at which the wall layers separate varies. In some cases, only the intima is dissected from the wall, while in other cases, portions of the media or the media and adventitia may delaminate. Thus, the thickness of the membrane separating the true and false lumens varies. Dissection at the adventitial layer may permit pseudoaneurysm formation adjacent to the artery.

Arterial dissection produces a false lumen that may be blind-ended or may reconnect with the true lumen at a site distal to the point of dissection. A blind-ended false

lumen will thrombose (occlude) and bulge into the true lumen, causing stenosis or occlusion. Blood continues to flow in the false lumen if its distal end reconnects with the true lumen. Consequent to either form of dissection, embolization or reduced flow may cause thrombosis of intracranial vessels and brain damage. Less commonly, false aneurysm formation occurs when dissection extends to the serosal layer of the carotid artery.

Carotid artery dissection usually originates in the aortic arch and extends only to the carotid bifurcation, but dissection can extend into the ICA. Three to seven percent of aortic arch dissections are complicated by stroke or transient cerebral ischemia.[12–14] Common carotid extension most commonly occurs with ascending arch dissection (Stanford's type A), which usually is age related but also may be caused by elastic tissue degeneration, as seen with Marfan's or Ehlers-Danlos syndromes. Stanford's type B dissection, occurring distal to the aortic arch, usually does not affect the carotid arteries. Considering that neurologic symptoms are uncommon when carotid dissection extends from the aortic arch, such dissection may occasionally be an incidental finding at carotid sonography.

Carotid dissection may also originate within the ICA, usually beginning at the skull base and extending downward to the carotid bifurcation.[8,10] This dissection may occur either spontaneously or following trauma. Some "spontaneous" dissections may not really be spontaneous and may actually result from nonviolent trauma, such as unusually strenuous exercise or rapid neck motion. In some cases, the precipitating trauma may be unrecognized by the patient. Arterial pathology may also lead to atraumatic ICA dissection, including fibromuscular hyperplasia, Marfan syndrome, cystic medial necrosis, and Ehlers-Danlos syndrome. Unlike CCA dissection, the false lumen of ICA dissection is almost always occluded by thrombus.

Seventy percent of spontaneous ICA dissections or those following minimal trauma occur in patients 35 to 50 years of age, with an equal incidence in men and women. Systemic hypertension is present in one of three cases and is considered a predisposing factor. Presentation includes headache, neck and facial pain, hemispheric ischemic symptoms, and cranial nerve palsy. Seventy percent of ICA dissections resolve with mild or no neurologic deficit, but 25% of patients suffer disabling neurologic consequences and 5% of cases are fatal.[8,10] Spontaneous restoration of ICA flow occurs in many cases of high-grade stenosis or occlusion through retraction of the thrombus in the false lumen, relieving compression of the true lumen. Typically, the only therapies employed for carotid dissection are antithrombotic and antihypertensive medications.

Carotid dissection resulting from violent trauma most commonly originates with direct injury to the ICA, either from stretching of the artery across cervical spine structures or from direct arterial compression by cervical spine elements or the mandible.[11,13] Trauma causes a rent in the intima and an injury that weakens the underlying wall structure, permitting delamination. Serious neurologic consequences are more common with traumatic carotid dissection than with atraumatic dissection.[10]

The ultrasound findings associated with carotid dissection[9,10,12] may be dramatic when the intima is separated from the rest of the wall and flutters in the flow stream with each cardiac cycle (Fig. 10–4). Severe flow disturbances are caused by the fluttering intima. However, if the tissue between the true and false lumens is thick, the intervening membrane is stiffer and dissection is indicated simply by duplication of the carotid lumen (Fig. 10–5).

The classic sonographic presentation of ICA dissection is a smooth, tapering stenosis (Fig. 10–6) occurring in a patient who is younger than the typical patient with atherosclerotic stenosis (i.e., ≤50 years of age). Regardless of age, however, consider dissection in any patient with a smooth, tapering ICA stenosis *without visible atherosclerotic plaque*. In other cases of ICA dissection, the sonographic findings may be subtle and easily overlooked. The ICA lumen may be *normal* in the area just above the bifurcation if dissection beginning at the skull base does not extend down to the point of sonographic visualization. In such instances, the only detectable abnormality is increased flow resistance seen in the Doppler waveforms and possibly reduced flow velocity overall due to distal ICA obstruction. In some cases, a thin intimal flap may not be appreciated during color Doppler examination due to color blooming artifact. That is, the color will write over the thin flap, and only the color flow disturbance is seen. The flap is better seen when the examiner turns off the color display and examines the vessel with grayscale imaging. Another presentation is ICA *occlusion* with no apparent cause. Again, the absence of atherosclerotic plaque or youthful presentation should suggest the diagnosis of dissection.

When carotid dissection is recognized, the sonographer should try to perform as much of the following as possible. First, the extent of dissection should be ascertained, which in turn may indicate whether dissection originated in the aortic arch or the ICA. Second, the presence, direction, and characteristics of flow in the true and false lumen should be documented. Third, the patency of the ECA and ICA should be determined, and Doppler waveforms should be scrutinized in both vessels to assess the status of the ICA circulation and the presence of ECA collateralization. Finally, if dissection causes stenosis, the degree of narrowing should be evaluated both visually (color flow) and with Doppler velocity

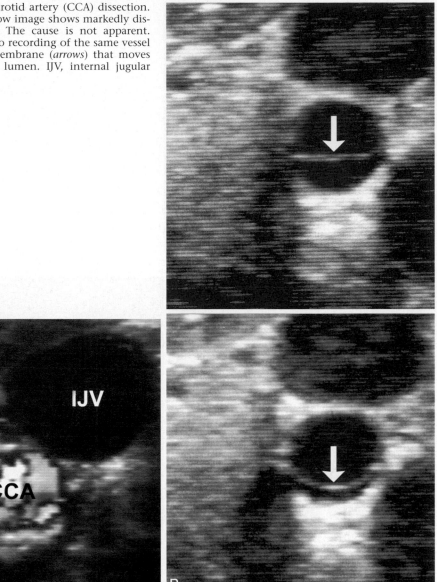

FIGURE 10–4. Common carotid artery (CCA) dissection. *A*, This short-axis, color flow image shows markedly disturbed flow in the CCA. The cause is not apparent. *B*, Two frames from a video recording of the same vessel show a thin dissection membrane (*arrows*) that moves freely within the arterial lumen. IJV, internal jugular vein.

measurements. Further evaluation with angiography, magnetic resonance angiography, or computed tomographic angiography usually is necessary to appreciate the full extent of dissection.

CAROTID PSEUDOANEURYSM

A pseudoaneurysm, or false aneurysm, is in fact a soft-tissue hematoma into which blood circulates from a hole in the arterial wall. A true aneurysm is one in which the artery walls are intact but stretched. Carotid pseudoaneurysms[15–22] most often result from violent trauma (usually penetrating), but also occur iatrogenically in the course of attempted percutaneous jugular vein catheterization or during therapeutic/diagnostic arteriography. Additional causes are carotid dissection or pathologies that weaken the arterial wall, such as vasculitis, fibrous dysplasia, Marfan syndrome, and Ehlers-Danlos syndrome.

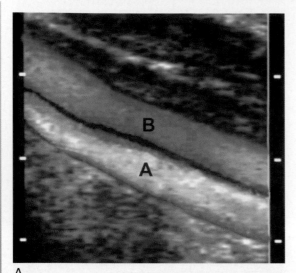

A

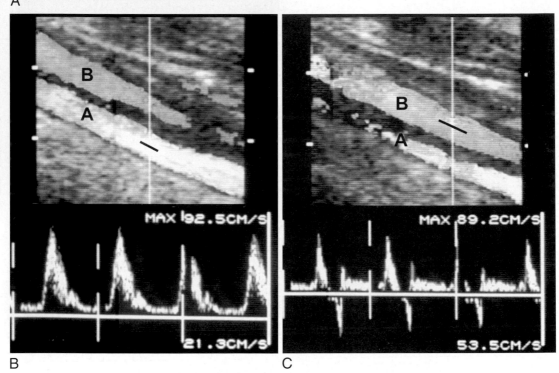

B   C

FIGURE 10–5. Common carotid artery dissection. *A*, This long-axis, color flow view shows division of the common carotid artery into two lumens (marked *A* and *B*). In this case, the dissection membrane was thick and moved very little with each arterial pulse. *B*, Doppler waveforms in lumen A have continuous forward flow throughout the cardiac cycle, suggesting that this is the true lumen. *C*, To-and-fro flow is present in lumen B.

Iatrogenic and post-traumatic pseudoaneuryms are usually accompanied by considerable ecchymosis or other trauma-associated findings. Pseudoaneurysms caused by nonpenetrating trauma, arterial diseases, or catheterization may present only with a palpable, and possibly pulsatile, mass, neck pain, or cranial nerve palsy. Neurologic symptoms of any kind, including cerebral ischemia/stroke, are reported in 40% of cases, and these may be accompanied by imaging evidence of cerebral infarction. Perhaps the most dramatic consequence of carotid pseudoaneurysm is rupture (blow out) and life-threatening soft tissue hemorrhage, but this occurs only rarely. Until recently, therapy for carotid pseudoaneurysm has been surgery, but clinically stable lesions may now be treated nonsurgically with covered wall stents.

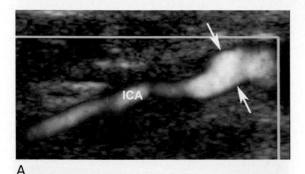

A

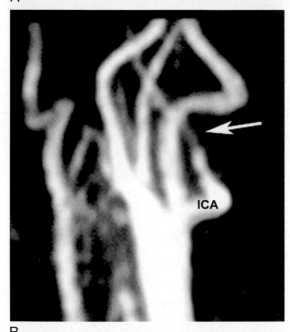

B

FIGURE 10–6. Spontaneous internal carotid artery (ICA) dissection. *A*, The ICA abruptly tapers from its normal size (*arrows*) at its origin. It is smoothly narrowed throughout its length (power Doppler image). *B*, Magnetic resonance angiography in the same patient shows diffuse narrowing of the ICA (*arrow*) beyond its origin, consistent with dissection.

Sonographically, carotid pseudoaneurysms are spherical masslike lesions into which blood is seen to circulate from the carotid artery (Fig. 10–7). The size of the lesion is variable, as is the relative proportion of thrombus and circulating blood within the aneurysm. Some pseudoaneurysms may be largely thrombosed, with only a small amount of blood flow. Others may show large areas of swirling blood flow with little thrombus. In all cases, however, a to-and-fro flow pattern should be seen in the neck of the pseudoaneurysm

on spectral Doppler examination. The distance of the pseudoaneurysm from the carotid artery also is variable, and the length of the "neck" connecting the two varies from one case to another. The diameter of the neck also varies. It is likely that pseudoaneurysms with short, fat necks and large arterial openings are more dangerous clinically than those with long, skinny necks, but no data have been collected to support this assumption.

In assessing a pseudoaneurysm sonographically (carotid or elsewhere), the following information should be gathered: (1) the size and location of the lesion; (2) the presence of to-and-fro flow in the pseudoaneurysm neck, confirming that the lesion is indeed a pseudoaneurysm; (3) the length and diameter of the neck; and (4) the proportion of thrombus and flowing blood. The latter two findings are potentially important, as they may influence the choice of therapy. A small pseudoaneurysm with little flow and a long, thin neck may safely occlude spontaneously and require no therapy. Follow-up Doppler sonography is used to follow pseudoaneurysm to assess for thrombosis or interval growth.

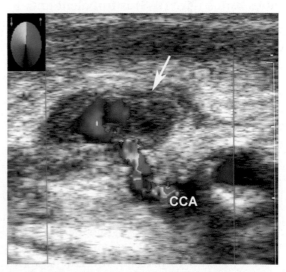

FIGURE 10–7. Carotid pseudoaneurysm. (Neck swelling and ecchymosis following attempted internal jugular vein catheterization.) Color flow examination shows a pseudoaneurysm (*arrow*) connected with the common carotid artery (CCA) by a thin neck.

CAROTID ARTERIOVENOUS FISTULA

A fistula is an opening that connects two epithelialized structures. In the case of an arteriovenous fistula (AVF),[15-22] communication occurs between an artery and a vein. An AVF almost always results from trauma, either violent or iatrogenic. The most likely site of occurrence is between the femoral artery and vein, because this is a common location for vascular catheterization, but AVFs can occur elsewhere, including the carotid artery. In carotid cases, the cause may be blunt trauma, penetrating trauma, or attempted jugular vein catheterization. The actual pathology in AVF cases may be a combination of AVF and pseudoaneurysm. Because the carotid artery and the internal jugular vein lay side-by-side, they are subject to AVF formation, but a fistula may occur with other neck veins as well. Clinical carotid AVF presentations include visible neck trauma; ecchymosis; a palpable hematoma; a palpable or audible thrill; and a dilated, hyperdynamic draining vein. High-output cardiac failure may occur with large fistulas. Treatment is surgical or angiographic. In the latter case, a covered wall stent is installed in the artery at the fistula site.

The ultrasound hallmark of an arteriovenous fistula (Fig. 10–8) is turbulent and, in some cases, pulsatile venous flow. The turbulence often is powerful and dramatic, and on color flow imaging, it may generate a "visible color bruit" adjacent to the vein, caused by vibration of surrounding soft tissues. In the absence of dramatic venous turbulence, the diagnosis of arteriovenous fistula should be questioned. With large AVFs, high-volume venous flow is apparent, as indicated by high-Doppler-velocity measurements. In some cases, the actual arteriovenous communication may be visible sonographically, but visualization of the fistula is not always possible because the opening may be small, or turbulent effects may obscure the fistula. Nevertheless, the correct diagnosis can be made from the venous Doppler findings described previously. Ancillary findings that may accompany an AVF include soft tissue fluid

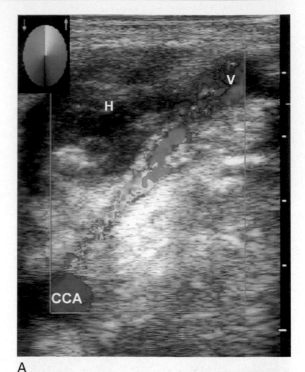

A

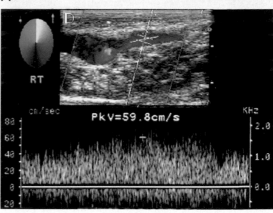

B

FIGURE 10–8. Carotid arteriovenous fistula. (Extensive ecchymosis and neck swelling following attempted internal jugular vein catheterization.) *A*, This transverse color flow image shows a lengthy tract connecting the common carotid artery (CCA) with a superficial vein (V). A soft tissue hematoma (H) also is visible. *B*, Doppler interrogation of the draining vein shows turbulent, high-velocity flow (almost 60 cm/sec).

(ecchymosis), a hematoma, or a pseudoaneurysm.

FIBROMUSCULAR DYSPLASIA

Fibromuscular dysplasia (FMD)[23-25] is a disorder of unknown etiology that affects medium-sized arteries. Women are affected by the disease three times more commonly than men, and the disorder usually presents in adults 25 to 50 years old. Although familial association is reported in 11% of cases, FMD is not a genetic disorder in strict terms. The renal arteries are the most common site for FMD, with the internal carotid artery a distant second. Other medium-sized arteries are occasionally involved. The most common presenting clinical symptom in FMD patients is systemic hypertension, caused by renal artery stenosis. With carotid involvement, transient cerebral ischemia is the usual presentation, although stroke can also occur. About 30% of FMD patients have aneurysms of the intracranial cerebral arteries; hence, an additional presentation may be cerebral hemorrhage.

FMD is a dysplastic disorder, not degenerative or inflammatory. The pathologic process is overgrowth of smooth muscle cells and fibrous tissue within the arterial wall. In the most common form, seen in 85% of cases, the media is primarily involved, and in the remaining cases, either the adventitia or the intima is the primary site. The medial form has a characteristic "string-of-beads" angiographic appearance (Fig. 10–9C) caused by alternating areas of medial fibroplasia and focal aneurysmal dilatation. Sonographically, this classical FMD form produces a series of ridges in the arterial wall (usually the ICA), as shown in Fig. 10–9A. This may be best seen with power Doppler imaging. However, there are two other imaging presentations of FMD: a long, tubular ICA stenosis or asymmetrical ICA out-pouching. In all cases, however the ICA is selectively involved, and the affected area tends to be relatively high in the ICA.

When FMD exhibits the classic string-of-beads appearance, differentiation from other carotid pathology generally is not difficult. The "long stenosis" presentation is a different story, however. This form is not specific and may be mistaken for atherosclerosis or dissection. The latter is particularly problematic, as ICA dissection is said to complicate about 20% of FMD cases. Differentiation from atherosclerosis generally is on the basis of age, as FMD usually presents at a younger age than does atherosclerosis. Many cases of FMD will require correlation with arteriography, magnetic resonance angiography, or computed tomographic angiography for confirmation or definitive diagnosis.

CAROTID BODY TUMOR

The normal carotid body is a tiny ovoid structure 1 to 1.5 mm in size located in the adventitia of the carotid bifurcation. The function of the carotid body is not well understood, but it is a component of the autonomic nervous system that participates in the control of arterial pH, blood gas levels, and blood pressure.[11]

Carotid body tumors[11,26,27] are paragangliomas of relatively low malignant potential that arise in the carotid body. The most common presentation is a palpable neck mass with headache. Neck pain is the second most common presentation. These are rare tumors, and because of their rarity, up to 25% are initially thought to be enlarged lymph nodes before surgical biopsy (which can lead to substantial hemorrhage of these highly vascular tumors). Although the malignant potential of carotid body tumors is small, resection is standard therapy to prevent local adverse effects, such as laryngeal nerve palsy and invasion of the carotid arteries. Local recurrence occurs in 6% of cases and distant metastasis in 2% of cases.

On sonographic examination, carotid body tumors are highly vascular masses nestled within the "crotch" of the carotid bifurcation, as seen in Figure 10–10. In some cases, the tumor may encase or surround the ECA or ICA, causing stenosis or potentially complicating surgical excision. It is useful, therefore, to assess the relationship of the tumor to the bifurcation vessels. Ultrasound may also be used to follow the growth of small tumors if surgery is not anticipated (e.g., in an elderly person with limited life expectancy or a poor surgical candidate). Most carotid body tumors are surgically resected to prevent invasion of the carotid arteries or the nearby recurrent laryngeal nerve. Untreated, they may cause carotid

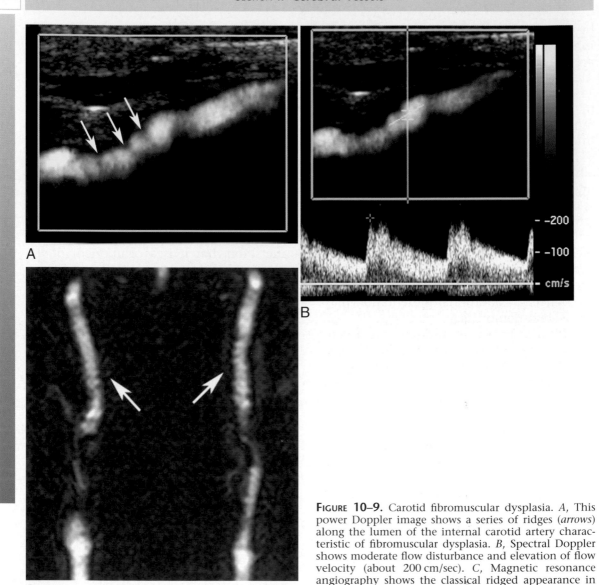

FIGURE **10–9.** Carotid fibromuscular dysplasia. *A,* This power Doppler image shows a series of ridges (*arrows*) along the lumen of the internal carotid artery characteristic of fibromuscular dysplasia. *B,* Spectral Doppler shows moderate flow disturbance and elevation of flow velocity (about 200 cm/sec). *C,* Magnetic resonance angiography shows the classical ridged appearance in both internal carotid arteries (*arrows*).

stenosis or occlusion or may result in carotid rupture. Arteriography is usually performed preoperatively, and the tumor may be embolized angiographically to reduce vascularity in anticipation of surgery.

TRICKY CAROTID CASES

The editors of this text have, over the years, encountered cases that have surprised us or others. Our goal here is to present examples of these tricky cases so that, hopefully, the readers of this text will not succumb to

the features of these cases that make them difficult.

Case 1

Introduction

This 68-year-old man presented with a right cervical bruit. He had undergone left carotid endarterectomy 8 years previously. His *left* common carotid artery is occluded, as shown in Figure 10–3. The findings on the right side are shown in Figure 10–11. Please

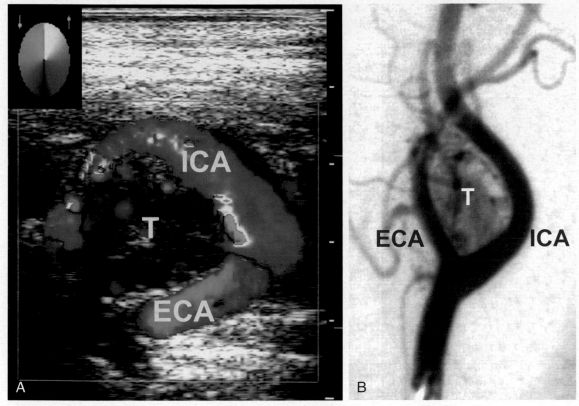

FIGURE 10–10. Carotid body tumor. *A,* This longitudinal color flow image shows a homogeneous, hypoechoic tumor (T), which splays the internal (ICA) and external (ECA) carotid artery branches. Blood flow (*color areas*) was easily detected in the tumor. *B,* Carotid arteriography in the lateral projection shows the highly vascular nature of the mass.

review this information and determine the severity of the right ICA stenosis.

Analysis

At first glance, the peak systolic velocity (257 cm/sec) and the end-diastolic velocity (115 cm/sec) suggest a high-grade stenosis whose diameter has been reduced by 70% or more, but notice that the color flow image is not consistent with that level of narrowing. If you calculate the systolic velocity ratio (ICA/CCA), you get 2.1, which is well below the 4.0 level usually seen with narrowing of 70% or more. The reason for the spuriously high velocities is the contralateral CCA occlusion. Notice the peak systolic velocity of 121 cm/sec in the right CCA. This is well above the normal level,

which rarely reaches 100 cm/sec. This phenomenon is called *compensatory flow* through the normal or less severely involved carotid artery. The carotid artery opposite the high-grade stenosis or occlusion demonstrates increased peak systolic velocities, which appear out of proportion to the degree of narrowing identified on gray-scale and color Doppler examination. The systolic velocity ratio (ICA/CCA) performs better, therefore, than the ICA peak systolic velocity alone in grading stenosis severity. In this case, the right carotid vessels are serving as collaterals that make up for diminished left carotid blood flow. The higher volume of blood flow skews all velocities upward in the right carotid system, including the ICA stenosis velocity. One important clue to the diagnosis of compensatory flow is elevation of peak systolic

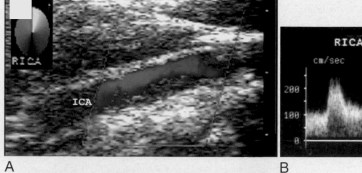

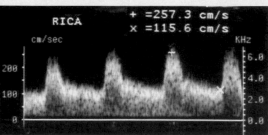

A

B

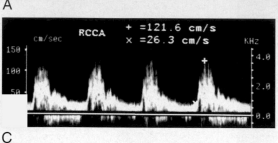

C

FIGURE 10–11. Case 1. *A*, Right internal carotid artery (RICA) color flow image. *B*, RICA Doppler spectrum. *C*, Right common carotid artery (RCCA) Doppler spectrum.

velocities throughout the entire contralateral CCA and ICA.

Diagnosis

Approximately 50% ICA stenosis with exaggerated flow velocity due to collateralization.

Points to Remember

1. High-flow states, regardless of cause, increase peak systolic velocity, possibly causing overestimation of stenosis severity.
2. Always look at the "big picture," not just an isolated velocity measurement. Think about what is happening in the entire carotid/vertebral system and remember that altered flow physiology in one area may affect Doppler findings in other areas.
3. Always consider the systolic velocity ratio when you diagnose stenosis severity.
4. Always compare the spectral Doppler, gray-scale, and color flow findings. If they do not correspond, ask yourself, "Does this make sense, or am I making a mistake?"

Case 2

Introduction

This 78-year-old man presented with a left cervical bruit. Gray-scale and color flow images (not included here) showed only minimal bifurcation plaque bilaterally. Please review the Doppler findings, shown in Figure 10–12, and make a diagnosis.

Analysis

Note that all of the Doppler waveforms on the left side are damped and of lower velocity than on the right. This pulsus parvus and tardus appearance always indicates that you are downstream from a stenosis. Because the findings are unilateral, they indicate that the stenosis is on the left only. The narrowing must be in the proximal, nonvisualized segment of the CCA, because we noted that only minimal plaque was seen in the visualized portions.

Diagnosis

High-grade, proximal left common carotid artery stenosis.

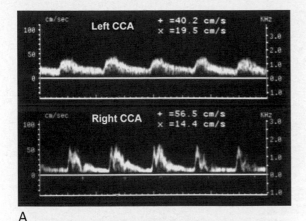

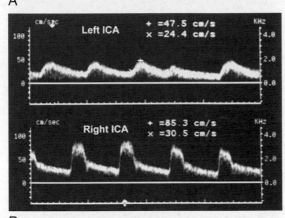

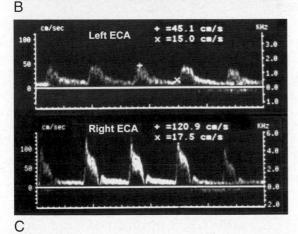

FIGURE 10–12. Case 2. *A*, Left and right common carotid artery (CCA) Doppler spectrum. *B*, Left and right internal carotid artery (ICA) Doppler spectrum. *C*, Left and right external carotid artery (ECA) Doppler spectrum.

Points to Remember

Important arterial pathology may exist that is outside the range of direct carotid visualization (either proximal or distal). Such pathology is revealed only by Doppler findings.

1. Always compare the waveform shape and Doppler velocity measurements from both carotid arteries side to side. Differences may not be as obvious as in this case, but even subtle differences should be treated as suspicious.
2. Stenoses occur commonly at the aortic origin of the brachiocephalic arteries. The most frequent sites are the left common carotid and the left subclavian arteries.

Case 3

Introduction

This 73-year-old woman suffered a right hemispheric stroke but had a good recovery. Take a look at the Doppler signals derived from the right carotid bifurcation branches (Fig. 10–13*A* and *B*). Decide which is the ICA and which is the ECA *before* you look at the angiogram in the same figure (part *C*).

Analysis

The right ICA is occluded, but this fact was missed by the inexperienced sonographer and sonologist involved with this case. It is easy, in retrospect, to understand why this misdiagnosis occurred. The two Doppler waveforms shown in Figure 10–13 are virtually identical because they both are from ECA branches. Unfortunately, the similarity of the waveforms was not appreciated. In addition, the sonographer did not tap on the superficial temporal artery. If she had, the fact that both vessels were, in fact, ECA branches may have been apparent.

The pulsatility of the Doppler waveforms is another observation that might have prevented this error. Both waveforms are *more* pulsatile than normally seen in the ICA, yet they are *less* pulsatile than the usual ECA waveforms. The diminished pulsatility results from collateralization to the low-resistance cerebral circulation.

Finally, an anatomic factor contributing to the error was the large size of the primary

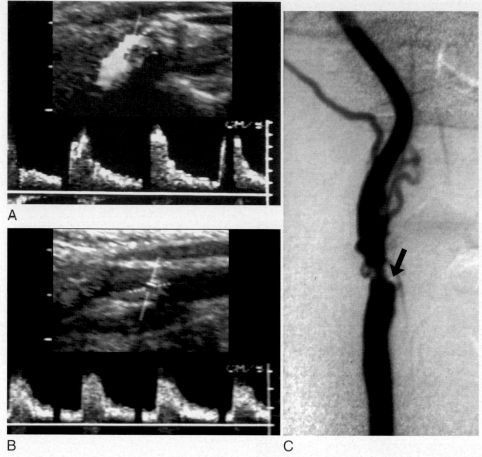

FIGURE 10–13. Case 3. *A* and *B*, Right carotid bifurcation branches. *C*, Right carotid arteriogram. *Arrow* indicates the stump of the occluded ICA.

ECA collateral, which made the sonographer believe that this vessel was the ICA.

Diagnosis

Internal carotid artery occlusion with ECA collateralization.

Points to Remember

1. The Doppler signals in the ICA and ECA should always sound different, and the waveforms should always look different.
2. The sonographer should tap on the superficial temporal artery in front of the ear to identify the ECA, and the resulting Doppler spectrum should be recorded as part of each carotid ultrasound examination.
3. If you cannot decide if one bifurcation vessel is the ECA and the other is the ICA, *do not guess*! It is better to say that you are unsure than to make a diagnostic error. When in doubt, our sonographers label the carotid branches A and B, rather than ECA and ICA, and we, the physicians, take it from there. Basically, we have two options: bring the patient back and look for ourselves, or refer the patient for another imaging study such as magnetic resonance or computed tomographic arteriography.
4. Misidentification of the ICA and ECA can be very important in cases of stenosis. Patient management may be inappropriate if an ECA stenosis is attributed to the

ICA or vice versa. (In the case presented here, the misdiagnosis did not affect clinical management, as the ICA was occluded.)

Case 4

Introduction

A screening carotid ultrasound was ordered on this 55-year-old man prior to cardiac surgery. With gray-scale and color flow imaging, only a few small plaques were seen in the cervical portions of the carotid arteries. Please review the Doppler waveform findings shown in Figure 10–14 and make a diagnosis.

Analysis

The Doppler waveforms are uniformly damped, and flow velocity is low in all areas, indicating a "global" physiologic disorder. The two principal considerations are aortic valve disease and poor myocardial function. In this case, the patient was awaiting aortic valve replacement for severe aortic stenosis. Had the problem been severe aortic insufficiency, a to-and-fro flow pattern might be seen in the Doppler waveforms.

Diagnosis

Aortic valve stenosis causing global damping of carotid Doppler waveforms.

Points to Remember

1. Global low velocity and damping is usually caused by aortic valve disease or poor myocardial function.
2. Cardiac function can profoundly affect carotid Doppler findings. If this patient had a carotid stenosis, velocities in the stenosis would have been substantially lower than in an individual without heart disease. As in the case of compensatory flow (Case 1), the ICA/CCA

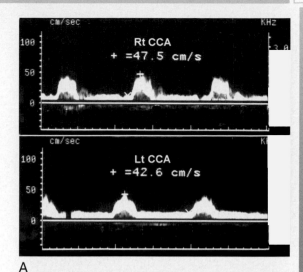

A

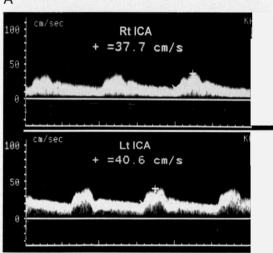

B

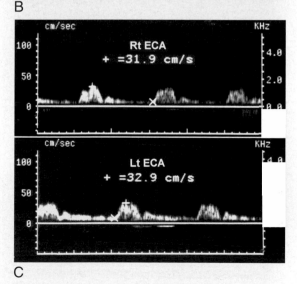

C

FIGURE 10–14. Case 4. *A*, Right and left common carotid artery (CCA) Doppler spectrum. *B*, Right and left internal carotid artery (ICA) Doppler spectrum. *C*, Right and left external carotid artery (ECA) Doppler spectrum.

systolic velocity ratios approximate the level of disease better than ICA peak velocity used independently.

3. Always consider the "global" view of cardiovascular physiology when interpreting carotid ultrasound studies.

Case 5

Introduction

This 77-year-old man presented with right hemispheric transient cerebral ischemia. Look at the findings presented in Figure 10–15 and grade the right ICA stenosis.

Assessment

By merely looking at the right common carotid Doppler waveform, you can diagnose high-grade stenosis or occlusion of the right ICA, because the waveform provides evidence of very high flow resistance indicated by absence of flow late in diastole. In addition, peak systolic velocity (21.5 cm/sec) is very low, because the obstruction has reduced the volume of blood flowing through the right CCA.

The confusing thing about this case is the relatively low peak systolic velocity of 178 cm/sec in the ICA stenosis, as well as the absence of end-diastolic velocity elevation. The peak systolic velocity would ordinarily be consistent with a 50% to 69% stenosis, but this degree of narrowing does not correlate with the high-resistance CCA Doppler waveforms or the color flow image, which clearly suggests a high degree of ICA narrowing.

So, what is going on here? Why is the peak velocity measurement so out of line with the other findings? There are two reasons for the discrepancy. First, the color flow image shows that this is an unusually

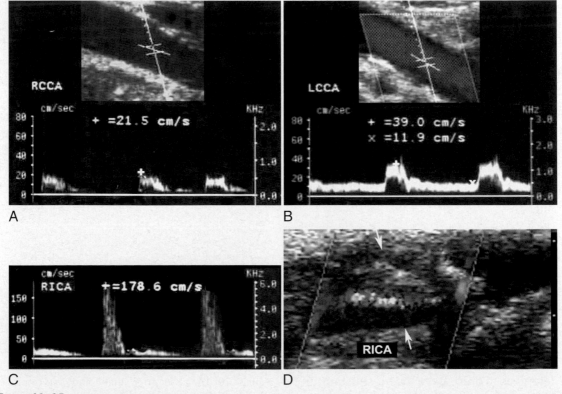

FIGURE 10–15. Case 5. *A*, Right common carotid artery (RCCA) Doppler spectrum. *B*, Comparison left CCA (LCCA) Doppler spectrum. *C*, Right internal carotid artery (RICA) Doppler spectrum. *D*, Long-axis color flow view of the RICA. (*Arrows* indicate the arterial wall, which is not clearly seen.)

long stenosis. The flow resistance imposed by a stenosis is directly proportional to its length. In long stenoses, the resistance is so great that the flow velocity may be substantially lower than that seen in a short stenosis. The second reason for the low velocity is evident in the left CCA Doppler findings. Peak CCA systolic velocity is only 39 cm/sec, which is much lower than the usual 60 or 70 cm/sec. This man has reduced cardiac function, due to ischemic myocardial damage, which causes reduced flow velocity in all parts of his cerebral vessels, including the right ICA stenosis.

Did you calculate the ICA/CCA systolic ratio? If you did, you would have found a very high ratio of 8.5, clearly consistent with high-grade stenosis.

Diagnosis

Severe (>70%) ICA stenosis with unusually low stenotic zone velocity.

Points to Remember

1. Low-flow states (e.g., cardiac dysfunction or proximal arterial obstruction) generally reduce stenosis velocity. The systolic velocity ratio generally compensates for this.
2. Peak systolic and end-diastolic velocity are lower than anticipated in long stenoses (>2 cm).
3. As stated previously, always consider the "big picture" of cardiovascular physiology to avoid overestimating or underestimating stenosis severity.
4. Always compare the gray-scale, color flow, and Doppler findings. If they do not match, investigate the possibility of diagnostic error.

Case 6

Introduction

This is a follow-up examination in a 52-year-old man who had undergone innominate artery stenting 8 mo previously. Please review the Doppler findings in Figure 10–16. What is the cause of the strange carotid waveforms on the right side? What other vessels would you look at to confirm your diagnosis?

Assessment

The right CCA and ICA Doppler waveforms are biphasic, indicating that to-and-fro blood flow is present in these vessels. ECA flow is cephalad but with an odd waveform pattern. What could cause biphasic carotid artery signals? There are two possibilities. If both the right and left carotid signals were biphasic, aortic insufficiency would be the cause. With unilateral, right-sided biphasic signals, the cause is innominate artery stenosis. During systole, blood flows forward into the carotid system, while in diastole, it flows backward into the right subclavian artery and arm. In this case, the innominate stenosis is severe enough to cause flow reverses in the CCA and ICA. With less severe stenosis, CCA and ICA flow remains cephalad, but the Doppler waveforms are oddly shaped, similar to the ECA waveforms seen in this case. This odd waveform shape has been called the "crouching bunny." The head and ears are on the right and the body on the left. You don't see a crouching bunny? Look at the waveforms on the right side of the spectrum.

If the innominate artery were occluded, flow would be persistently reversed in the carotid arteries, or perhaps the CCA would be occluded by thrombus. If the stenosis were at the CCA origin, damped flow signals would be seen, similar to Case 2.

The other vessels to look at in this case are the right vertebral and the subclavian arteries. The vertebral artery would have biphasic, or reversed, Doppler waveforms, and the subclavian artery would have monophasic, damped waveforms. These are the standard findings of vertebral-to-subclavian steal, which are illustrated in the next chapter. In addition, you could angle the ultrasound image down beneath the clavicle in an attempt to directly visualize high flow velocity and turbulence in the stenotic innominate artery. (We tried but could not see far enough.)

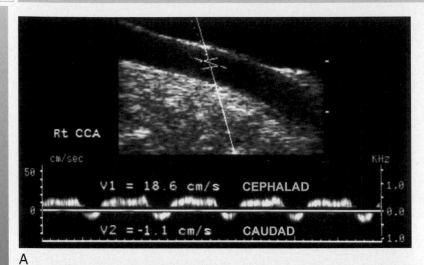

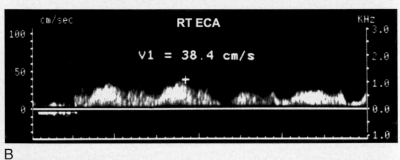

A

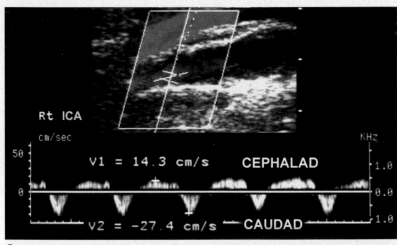

B

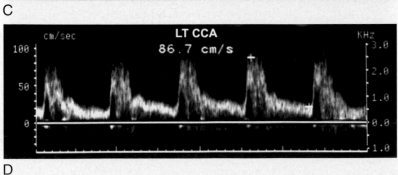

C

D

FIGURE 10–16. Case 6. *A–C*, Right common carotid artery (CCA), external carotid artery (ECA), and internal carotid artery (ICA) Doppler spectrum, respectively. *D* and *E*, Left CCA and ICA Doppler spectrum, respectively.

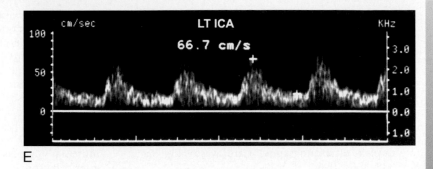

FIGURE 10–16—cont'd.

E

Diagnosis

Right carotid steal caused by innominate artery stenosis.

Points to Remember

1. Biphasic or "crouching bunny" carotid waveforms result from innominate stenosis.
2. Innominate occlusion causes flow reversal in the right carotid arteries or secondary CCA occlusion.
3. Carotid steal occurs only on the right side, where the carotid and subclavian arteries have a common origin from the innominate artery. The left CCA arises directly from the aortic arch.
4. If you see odd waveforms in the right carotid system or in the vertebral arteries, look for associated subclavian artery Doppler abnormalities and measure the blood pressure in both arms. (A 20-mm Hg side-to-side difference indicates subclavian or innominate obstruction.)

References

1. Middleton WD, Foley WD, Lawson TL: Color flow Doppler imaging of carotid artery abnormalities. Am J Roentgenol 150:419–425, 1988.
2. Erickson SJ, Middleton WD, Mewissen MW, et al: Color Doppler evaluation of arterial stenoses and occlusions involving the neck and thoracic inlet. Radiographics 9:389–406, 1989.
3. Hallam MJ, Reid JM, Cooperberg PL: Color flow Doppler and conventional duplex scanning of the carotid bifurcation: Prospective, double-blinded correlative study. Am J Roentgenol 152:1101–1105, 1989.
4. Steinke W, Kloetzsch C, Hennerici M: Carotid artery disease assessed by color Doppler flow imaging: Correlation with standard Doppler sonography and angiography. Am J Roentgenol 154:1061–1068, 1998.
5. Chang YJ, Lin SK, Ryu SJ, Wai YY: Common carotid artery occlusion: Evaluation with duplex sonography. Am J Neuroradiol 16:1099–1105, 1995.
6. Lee DH, Gao FQ, Rankin RN, et al: Duplex and color Doppler flow sonography of occlusion and near occlusion of the carotid artery. Am J Neuroradiol 17:1267–1274, 1996.
7. Mattos MA, Hodgson KJ, Ramsey DE, et al: Identifying total carotid occlusion with colour flow duplex scanning. Eur J Vasc Surg 6:204–210, 1992.
8. Petro GR, Witwer GA, Cacayorin ED, et al: Spontaneous dissection of the cervical internal carotid artery: Correlation of arteriography, CT, and pathology. Am J Neuroradiol 148:393–398, 1987.
9. Hennerei M, Steinke W, Rautenberg W: High-resistance Doppler flow pattern in extracranial carotid dissection. Arch Neurol 46:670–672, 1989.
10. Provenzale JM: Dissection of the internal carotid and vertebral arteries: Imaging features. Am J Roentgenol 165:1099–1104, 1995.
11. Cottrell ED, Smith LL: Management of uncommon lesions affecting the extracranial vessels. In Rutherford RB (ed): Vascular Surgery, vol II. Philadelphia, WB Saunders, 1995, pp 1622–1636.
12. Zieliński T, Wołkanin-Bartnik J, Janaszek-Sitkowska H, et al: Persistent dissection of carotid artery in patients operated on for type A acute aortic dissection—carotid ultrasound follow-up. Int J Cardiol 70:133–139, 1999.
13. Sturzenegger M, Mattle HP, Rivoir A, Baumgartner RW: Ultrasound findings in carotid artery dissection: Analysis of 43 patients. Neurology 45:691–698, 1995.

14. Walker PJ, Sarris GE, Miller DC: Peripheral vascular manifestations of acute aortic dissection. In Rutherford RB (ed): Vascular Surgery, vol II. Philadelphia, WB Saunders, 1995, pp 1087–1102.

15. El-Sabrout R, Cooley DA: Extracranial carotid artery aneurysms: Texas Heart Institute experience. J Vasc Surg 31:702–712, 2000.

16. Kuzniec S, Kauffman P, Molnar LJ, et al: Diagnosis of limbs and neck arterial trauma using duplex ultrasonography. Cardiovasc Surg 6:358–366, 1998.

17. Munera F, Soto JA, Palacio DM, et al: Penetrating neck injuries: Helical CT angiography for initial evaluation. Radiology 216:356–362, 2000.

18. Takeuchi Y, Numata T, Suzuki H, et al: Differential diagnosis of pulsatile neck masses by Doppler color flow imaging. Ann Otol Rhinol Laryngol 104:633–638, 1995.

19. Needleman L, Nack TL: Vascular and nonvascular masses. J Vasc Technol 18:299–306, 1994.

20. Goldberg BB: Iatrogenic femoral arteriovenous fistula: Diagnosis with cold Doppler imaging. Radiology 170:749–752, 1989.

21. Biffl WL, Ray CE Jr, Moore EE, et al: Treatment-related outcomes from blunt cerebrovascular injuries: Importance of routine follow-up arteriography. Ann Surg 235:699–706, 2002.

22. Redekop G, Marotta T, Weill A: Treatment of traumatic aneurysmal and arteriovenous fistulas of the skull base by using endovascular stents. J Neurosurg 95:412–419, 2001.

23. Moore WS: Vascular surgery: A comprehensive review, 6th ed. Philadelphia, WB Saunders, 142–143, 295, 306–307, 1999.

24. Van Damme H, Sakalihasan N, Limet R: Fibromuscular dysplasia of the internal carotid artery: Personal experience with 13 cases and literature review. Acta Chir Belg 99:163–168, 1999.

25 Stewart MT, Moritz MW, Smith RB 3rd: The natural history of carotid dysplasia. J Vasc Surg 3:305–310, 1986.

26. Rao AB, Koeller KK, Adair CF: Paragangliomas of the head and neck: Radiologic-pathologic correlation. RadioGraphics 19:1605–1632, 1999.

27. Muhm M, Polterauer P, Gstottner W, Temmel A, et al: Diagnostic and therapeutic approaches to carotid body tumors: Review of 24 patients. Arch Surg 132:279–284, 1997.

Chapter 11

Ultrasound Assessment of the Vertebral Arteries

PHILLIP J. BENDICK, PHD

The relationship between carotid athero-sclerotic disease and lateralizing symptoms of cerebrovascular ischemia, such as transient ischemic attacks, amaurosis fugax, and stroke, is well established, and carotid endarterectomy has been shown to be effective in the management of selected groups of these patients.[1–3] However, no consistently successful diagnostic and management techniques are available for those patients who present with a more confusing clinical picture of nonlocalizing symptoms of transient cerebral ischemia, such as blurred vision, ataxia, vertigo, syncope, or generalized extremity weakness. It can be difficult to determine whether the symptoms arise from carotid artery thromboembolic disease, generalized ischemia resulting from carotid or vertebrobasilar artery occlusive disease (or both), or some factor not directly related to the cerebral vasculature, such as cardiac disease.[4–6] Symptomatology of posterior circulation ischemia is typically multiple and varied, and the potential contribution of vertebrobasilar insufficiency may be difficult to evaluate. Although surgical reconstruction of the vertebral arteries is a successful and relatively safe procedure,[7,8] the selection of appropriate patients for such reconstruction can be confounded by the previously mentioned diagnostic uncertainties, as well as by the fact that symptoms of posterior circulation ischemia frequently improve following carotid artery endarterectomy or reconstruction.[9,10]

Angiography, performed on the basis of the patient's clinical history data, histori-cally has been the definitive diagnostic procedure to identify significant vertebrobasilar obstructive lesions.[11,12] The use of duplex ultrasound as a primary diagnostic technique for the diagnosis of vertebrobasilar insufficiency has been limited. Routine evaluation of the vertebral arteries is an accreditation requirement for the Extracranial Cerebrovascular System by the Intersocietal Commission for the Accreditation of Vascular Laboratories,* as well as other accrediting organizations, but this assessment typically is limited to the presence or absence of flow and flow direction. Standard textbooks have limited reference to the vertebral arteries, despite the fact that the vertebrobasilar system is responsible for 20% to 30% of intracranial blood flow. For example, in Strandness's textbook on vascular disorders, only two paragraphs of the entire chapter on extracranial arterial disease deal with the vertebral arteries, and then only to discuss qualitative waveform evaluation.[13]

Duplex ultrasound has been shown to be an effective noninvasive technique for the evaluation of the extracranial segments of the vertebral arteries.[14–18] Adequate imaging and quantitative spectral Doppler velocity data can be obtained from some portion of the mid-segment of the extracranial vertebral arteries in more than 98% of patients and vessels.[16,19,20] It is possible to collect imaging and spectral Doppler velocity data from the origin of the right

*8840 Stanford Boulevard, Suite 4900, Columbia, MD 21045; www.icavl.org.

vertebral artery in more than 80% of patients and from the origin of the left vertebral artery in approximately two thirds of patients. The sections below describe appropriate duplex ultrasound evaluation techniques, the qualitative and quantitative data that can be obtained, and the interpretation and possible clinical significance of these results.

EXAMINATION TECHNIQUES

Because most hemodynamically significant lesions of the vertebral arteries occur at their origin (Region V1, defined as the segment from the origin of the vertebral artery to its entrance into the foramen of the transverse process, which occurs at the level of the sixth cervical vertebra in approximately 90% of cases), it would seem that this would be the logical site to begin the duplex ultrasound examination. Anatomically, however, this approach can be technically difficult (if not technically impossible) in as many as one third of patients, as the origin of the vertebral artery may lie deep to the skin surface and visualization may be obstructed by the clavicle, which interferes with the necessary probe position. Additionally, as the first major branch off the subclavian artery, the vertebral artery origin may be markedly tortuous, making proper angle correction for velocity measurements very difficult. Finally, the origin and proximal segment of the vertebral artery may be confused with other large branches arising from the proximal subclavian artery, such as the thyrocervical trunk.

A more reliable approach to assessment of the vertebral arteries is to initially evaluate the vessel near its mid-segment, or Region V2 (the segment of the vertebral artery that courses cranially through the foramina to the transverse process of the axis). This segment of vessel is typically quite straight, with minimal tortuosity; does not have any significant taper or diameter changes; has no immediately adjacent blood vessels, except the vertebral vein; and has no significant branching segments that would make flow velocity measurements unreliable. In addition, Region V2 of the vertebral arteries is only rarely involved with atherosclerotic obstructive disease. Further distally, the vertebral artery may be interrogated using a suboccipital approach and transcranial Doppler techniques, but Region V3 (the segment that extends from the artery's exit at the axis to its entrance into the spinal canal) and Region V4 (extending from the point of perforation of the dura to the origin of the basilar artery) are generally inaccessible to duplex ultrasound during an extracranial cerebrovascular examination.

Imaging of Region V2 is most easily accomplished by first obtaining a good longitudinal view of the mid–common carotid artery at the approximate level of the third through fifth cervical vertebrae. Once this image has been obtained, a slight lateral rocking motion of the probe will bring the vertebral artery into view. The vertebral artery is readily identified by the prominent anatomic landmarks of the transverse processes of the cervical spine, which appear as bright echogenic lines in the image, beyond which deeper-lying tissues are obscured by acoustical shadowing (Fig. 11–1). Between these anechoic, rectangular-shaped regions of acoustic shadowing lie an anechoic band representing the vertebral artery, as seen with gray-scale sonography. Color flow Doppler imaging helps to identify the vertebral artery by the pulsatile pattern of color flow within the anechoic band. The color flow image also distinguishes the vertebral artery from the adjacent vertebral vein, but typically the gray-scale image, with its anatomic landmarks, is sufficient for identifying the vertebral artery. Once an image of the artery has been obtained, the spectral Doppler sample volume can be placed in mid-vessel (Fig. 11–2) to obtain qualitative and quantitative data for the evaluation of local hemodynamics. If these data appear abnormal, the vertebral artery can be followed back toward its origin as far as possible (Fig. 11–3), using combined gray-scale and color Doppler imaging, to assess flow hemodynamics in the proximal segment of the artery.

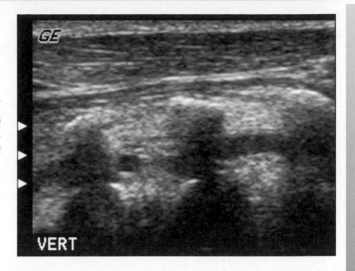

FIGURE 11–1. Normal vertebral artery. Longitudinal gray-scale image of a normal vertebral artery segment at the approximate level of C3–C5 (Region V2) showing the acoustic shadowing from the adjacent bony transverse processes of the spine.

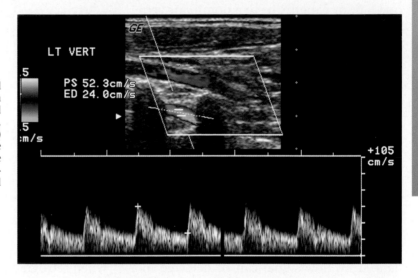

FIGURE 11–2. Normal spectral Doppler velocity waveform from the mid-segment of a vertebral artery. Peak systole is well defined, with a peak systolic velocity (PS) of 52 cm/sec. Sustained antegrade flow is present throughout the cardiac cycle, similar to the normal flow patterns in the internal carotid artery.

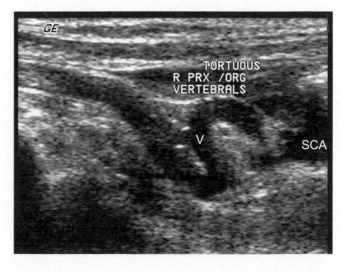

FIGURE 11–3. Longitudinal gray-scale image of the origin of a normal vertebral artery. Note the tortuosity of the proximal segment (Region V1) of the artery.

VERTEBRAL ARTERY HEMODYNAMICS: QUALITATIVE ASSESSMENT

Normal Findings

Qualitatively, the spectral Doppler velocity waveform in the vertebral artery should appear as a scaled-down version of flow in the internal carotid artery, since both directly supply the low-resistance intracranial vascular system. The waveform should have a well-defined systolic peak with sustained flow throughout diastole, as seen in Figure 11–2. There is wide variability in the absolute peak systolic velocity in normal patients, with a range of 20 cm/sec to 60 cm/sec.[15] From one third to one half of patients have a dominant vertebral artery, which demonstrates larger size and higher flows than the contralateral side. In such cases, the nondominant, anatomically small vertebral artery may demonstrate flow characteristics of increased vascular resistance, with diminished flow velocities at peak systole and throughout diastole.

Absence of Flow

Abnormalities in vertebral artery flow hemodynamics can be detected readily from the spectral Doppler velocity waveform and data. If no flow signal can be detected in a vertebral artery that is adequately imaged, that is diagnostic of a vertebral artery occlusion, as with any other blood vessel. While the occlusion is typically at the origin of the artery, there may be only a segmental occlusion, and this should be verified whenever possible by more proximal evaluation of the vertebral artery, as close to the origin as can be accomplished.

Flow Reversal

A more common finding in the vertebral artery is reversed flow, or subclavian steal, illustrated in Figure 11–4. This is a simple diagnosis to make with duplex ultrasound

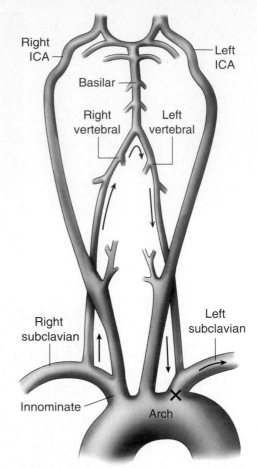

FIGURE 11–4. Illustration of the route of flow in the left vertebral steal. *X* indicates the point of subclavian artery obstruction. ICA, internal carotid artery.

when retrograde vertebral artery flow is seen throughout the cardiac cycle (Fig. 11–5), although one must be careful not to confuse the pulsatile flow signal in the vertebral vein with reversed vertebral artery flow. In 90% of cases, reversed vertebral flow (due to subclavian steal) occurs on the left side. When vertebral flow reversal is seen on the right side, it is important to determine whether the source of the steal is the subclavian artery, which affects only vertebral artery flow, or the innominate artery, which has a significant effect on both the right common carotid and vertebral arteries. As a secondary diagnostic finding in patients with subclavian steal, it should also be possible to document abnormal flow velocity waveforms in the distal segment of the affected

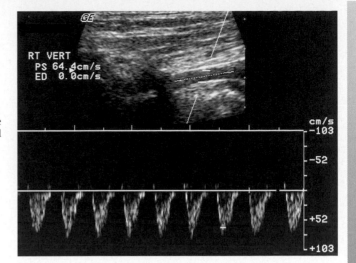

FIGURE 11–5. Reversed vertebral flow. The spectral Doppler velocity signal shows reversed flow secondary to subclavian steal.

subclavian artery (Fig. 11–6). Typically, patients with subclavian steal have a systolic pressure difference greater than 15 to 20 mm Hg between the normal and affected arms. An additional secondary finding may be increased vertebral artery size and flow contralateral to the subclavian steal. Due to the great degree of variability in normal vertebral artery size and flow velocity cited previously, however, these findings are not diagnostic as isolated observations.

Frequently, in cases of subclavian steal, there may be a subclavian artery obstruction at its origin that is significant but not so severe as to cause a complete reversal of flow in the ipsilateral vertebral artery. The changing balance of hemodynamic forces during the cardiac cycle causes systolic flow deceleration in the vertebral artery, which if severe enough, is manifest as bidirectional flows (Fig. 11–7). During peak systole, a significant pressure drop occurs across the subclavian artery stenosis in association with a high-velocity flow jet. At the same time, normal systolic pressure is present in the contralateral vertebral artery and basilar artery. As a result, there is a net pressure gradient, from distal to proximal, across the vertebral artery on the side of the subclavian stenosis, which causes deceleration during systole or even transient reversal of flows. During the diastolic phase of the cardiac cycle, flow velocities across the subclavian artery lesion are diminished and no significant pressure drop occurs across the stenosis; thus, during diastole, the net pressure gradient within the affected vertebral artery is essentially normal and produces antegrade flows with diminished absolute flow velocities.

When the balance of hemodynamic forces produces a bidirectional flow pattern, the overall effect is a net volume blood flow in the vertebral artery that is very small, on the order of only a few milliliters per minute. This net flow may be either antegrade or retrograde, and angiographically, the low flow rate may result in nonvisualization of the vertebral artery, mimicking occlusion.[21]

Elevated Velocity

There are a number of hemodynamic conditions that might lead to abnormally strong or highly accelerated flow patterns in the vertebral arteries. The most common was mentioned previously; namely, the presence of a dominant vertebral artery, most often seen on the left side. Significantly increased vertebral artery flows also may be seen when one or both vertebral arteries are the compensatory mechanism for occlusive disease elsewhere in the cerebrovascular system (Fig. 11–8). This may be a consequence of occlusion or near occlusion of an internal carotid artery or the

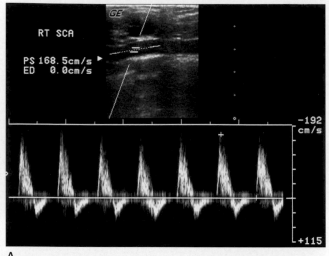

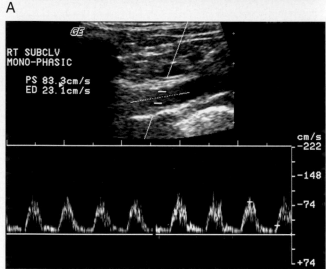

A

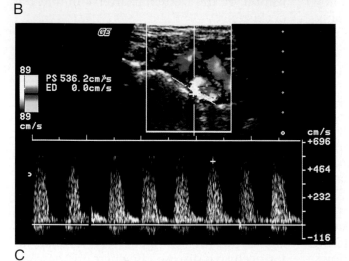

B

FIGURE 11–6. Subclavian steal Doppler findings. *A*, Spectral Doppler velocity signal from a normal subclavian artery shows the characteristic high-resistance multiphasic waveform. *B*, Spectral Doppler velocity signal from the distal subclavian artery of the patient with subclavian steal (shown in Fig. 11–5). The waveform is monophasic, significantly diminished, and damped, characteristic of severe proximal obstruction at the origin of the subclavian artery. *C*, Spectral Doppler velocity signal from the origin of the subclavian artery showing a characteristic stenotic, turbulent flow signal with markedly elevated peak systolic velocity (PS, 536 cm/sec).

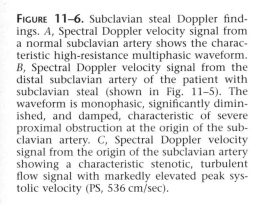

C

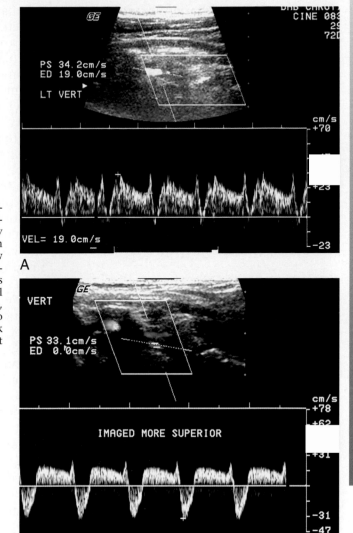

FIGURE 11–7. Vertebral waveform abnormalities ipsilateral to subclavian steal. *A,* This spectral Doppler vertebral signal shows early systolic deceleration. The point of minimum flow, where the spectral trace hits the zero-flow baseline, occurs at peak systole, when the pressure drop across the subclavian artery stenosis is maximum. *B,* Spectral Doppler vertebral signal shows bidirectional flow. In this case, the subclavian stenosis is severe enough to cause transient reversal of flow during peak systole, with resumption of diminished but antegrade flows during diastole.

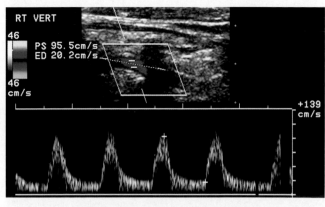

FIGURE 11–8. Contralateral compensatory flow. Elevated right vertebral artery flow (peak systole, PS, 95.5 cm/sec) is evident in a patient with a left subclavian steal. Compensatory flow accounts for the reversed flows in the contralateral vertebral artery.

contralateral vertebral artery, or may represent compensatory flow from a subclavian steal in the contralateral vertebral artery. An anatomically small vertebral artery may have elevated peak systolic velocities because of the small lumen, but, typically, diastolic velocities will be diminished as well, because of the elevated vascular resistance of a small-caliber vessel (Fig. 11–9). Rarely, high-velocity turbulent flow patterns may be detected in the mid-segment of a vertebral artery because of extrinsic compression from the bony spine (often associated with changes in head or neck position) or, even more rarely, because of a mid-vertebral atherosclerotic stenosis.

VERTEBRAL ARTERY HEMODYNAMICS: QUANTITATIVE ASSESSMENT

In addition to the qualitative evaluation of vertebral artery flow hemodynamics, it is possible to quantitate volume flows in the vertebrobasilar arterial system. This may provide clinically helpful information in some cases, as the majority of posterior circulation symptoms are thought to represent ischemia, unlike the thromboembolic nature of most carotid artery territory symptoms. Technically, the ability to calculate vertebral artery volume flows is present on most duplex ultrasound instruments. It requires a combination of spectral Doppler velocity data, from which a time-averaged velocity for a complete cardiac cycle can be

calculated, and a measurement of the vessel lumen diameter, from which cross-sectional area can be calculated (Fig. 11–10). These two measurements can be combined to give volume flow in milliliters per minute. Measurement accuracy approaches +/– 10% in a vessel segment such as the mid-vertebral artery, which is relatively straight and non-tapering and is without significant branches at the measurement site.[16] Our own experience[16] has shown that it is technically possible to measure volume flow in more than 99% of vertebral arteries (1491 of 1500 consecutive patients). As with peak systolic velocities, patients with normal physiology show a wide variation in volume flows, ranging from less than 75 mL/min to more than 150 mL/min. When both vertebral arteries are considered together, however, the normal total (right plus left) vertebral artery flow is approximately 200 mL/min or greater. Patients with nonlocalizing cerebrovascular symptoms suggestive of posterior circulation ischemia are much more likely to have overall diminished (<200 mL/min) vertebrobasilar system flow than asymptomatic patients or those with lateralizing, hemispheric symptoms. This is particularly true if there is only minimal or no obstructive disease in the carotid artery systems, thus identifying a group of symptomatic patients with potentially true posterior circulation ischemia secondary to poor vertebrobasilar system hemodynamics.

The clinical importance of diminished vertebrobasilar flow depends on the underlying cause of poor flow and whether it can

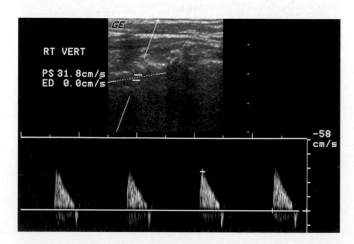

FIGURE 11–9. Diminished flow (peak systole, PS, 31.8 cm/sec) in an anatomically small vertebral artery (lumen diameter approximately 2 mm). The spectral Doppler velocity waveform also exhibits characteristics of a high-resistance flow signal, with an absence of any diastolic flow, caused by the increased vascular resistance of the small vessel lumen.

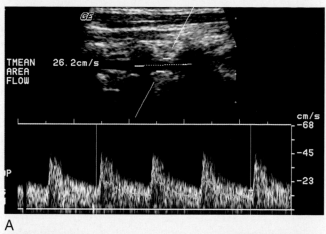

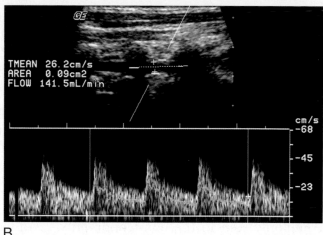

FIGURE 11–10. Vertebral volume flow measurement. *A*, Spectral Doppler velocity signal from a normal vertebral artery showing machine-calculated, time-averaged mean velocity (TMEAN 26 cm/sec) over three consecutive cardiac cycles. The time-averaged velocity is used for the determination of volume flows in the vessel. *B*, Cursors have been placed on the image shown in part *A*, identifying the lumen diameter at the site of the time-averaged velocity measurement, allowing calculation of volume flow (mean velocity times vessel cross-sectional area), in this case, 141 mL/min (FLOW).

be remedied. The vertebral arteries may be hypoplastic bilaterally and unable to support more flow; there may be poor cardiac output; or there may be an intracranial occlusion of the distal vertebral or basilar artery. Qualitative assessment of the spectral Doppler velocity flow waveform can be used to diagnose distal vertebral or basilar occlusion, because the absolute velocities in both systole and diastole are likely to be severely diminished because of elevated distal vascular resistance, even though the waveform shape may appear to be relatively normal. If an intracranial lesion is suspected as the underlying cause of diminished vertebral flow waveforms, this can be effectively evaluated by angiography, as newer technologies have made angioplasty and stenting of the basilar artery possible.

Severe, proximal vertebral artery obstructive disease may also be responsible for diminished vertebrobasilar system flow and cerebrovascular symptoms. In such cases, the spectral Doppler velocity waveform exhibits a "tardus-parvus" waveform, characteristic of damping (Fig. 11–11) (that is, a waveform with delayed onset of a rounded, poorly defined systolic peak, poor antegrade flows during diastole, and significantly diminished velocities throughout the cardiac cycle).

If damped Doppler waveforms are seen in a vertebral artery, a careful duplex ultrasound examination of the proximal segment and origin of the affected vertebral artery should be conducted to identify the site and severity of any obstructive lesion that may be present. Visible narrowing on color flow examination, accompanied by high-velocity color aliasing and the mosaic pattern characteristic of poststenotic disturbed flow (Fig. 11–12), are findings indicating vertebral artery stenosis. The

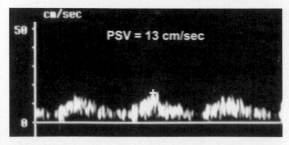

FIGURE 11–11. Diminished flow in midvertebral artery secondary to a proximal stenosis. The velocity waveform shows the classic "tardus-parvus" shape, with a rounded, poorly defined systolic peak and diminished velocities throughout the cardiac cycle. (Peak systolic velocity [PSV] is only 13 cm/sec.)

confirming evidence is high-velocity flow documented with spectral Doppler measurements. No velocity criteria are available to define the severity of vertebral artery stenoses; however, peak systolic velocity should be far above (typically at least a threefold increase) the normal range, the upper limit of which is 60 cm/sec. Ultrasound diagnosis of stenosis at the vertebral artery origin is complicated by the frequent occurrence of considerable tortuosity in the proximal 1 to 2 cm of the vertebral artery. Because of tortuosity, disturbed flow is commonly seen in the nonstenotic proxi-

mal vertebral artery, and kinking of the vessel may occur, generating elevated flow velocities. Tortuosity also may render angle-corrected Doppler velocity measurements unreliable. Considering these problems, ultrasound assessment of origin stenoses of the vertebral arteries must be considered qualitative. If damped signals are present distal to the stenosis, then one can be reasonably confident that the lesion is hemodynamically significant. Otherwise, the findings must often be regarded as suggestive of hemodynamic significance, and confirmation must be sought with angiography. Correct diagnosis is important, as modern surgical and interventional techniques have made it possible to directly address most proximal vertebral artery stenoses with good success.

DUPLEX ULTRASOUND VERSUS MAGNETIC RESONANCE ANGIOGRAPHY

While duplex ultrasound has replaced conventional angiography in most cases for the diagnosis of carotid artery atherosclerotic disease and management decisions regard-

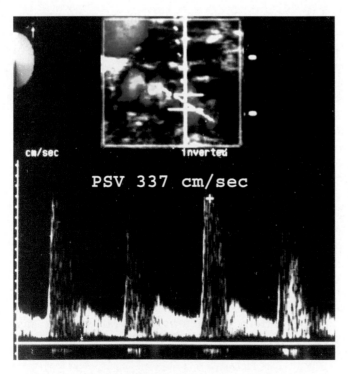

FIGURE 11–12. Vertebral origin stenosis. Turbulence is visible at the origin of the vertebral artery on the color flow image. Spectral Doppler shows markedly elevated peak systolic velocity (PSV; 337 cm/sec) and further evidence of flow turbulence.

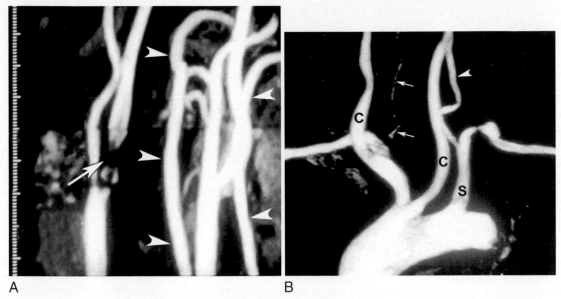

A   B

FIGURE 11–13. Magnetic resonance angiography (MRA) of the vertebral arteries. *A*, MRA clearly shows the vertebral arteries (*arrowheads*) despite signal dropout in the right carotid artery bifurcation region (*arrow*) due to flow turbulence. *B*, MRA of the aortic arch shows both proximal common carotid arteries (C) and the proximal left vertebral artery (*arrowhead*). The right vertebral artery (*arrows*) is hypoplastic with severely diminished flow and, consequently, is not well seen. Note the stenosis of the left subclavian artery (S) and poststenotic dilatation. As this stenosis lies beyond the vertebral origin, it would not affect vertebral artery flow.

ing carotid endarterectomy, the duplex ultrasound findings are often corroborated by magnetic resonance angiography (MRA). The same can be said for evaluation of the vertebral arteries as MRA techniques and contrast agents continue to evolve (Fig. 11–13). Vertebral artery stenosis and extrinsic vertebral arterial compression by the bony structures in Regions V2 and V3 are readily detected with MRA.[22] Particularly with the use of contrast-enhanced MRA and three-dimensional MRA image reconstruction, the visualization of the vertebral arteries improves significantly over standard two-dimensional time-of-flight MRA.[23,24] Additionally, phase contrast MRA measures actual vertebral artery flows and directly assesses vertebrobasilar arterial hemodynamics.[25] From a cost-effective perspective, duplex ultrasound remains the initial best choice for vertebral artery evaluation, but if there are equivocal ultrasound findings, contrast-enhanced three-dimensional MRA appears to be the best choice to acquire the needed diagnostic information. In particular, when duplex ultrasound findings suggest vertebral artery obstructive disease at a site not accessible to direct imaging, such as an inaccessible vertebral artery origin or a high-resistance flow waveform characteristic of more distal (Regions V3 or V4) disease, MRA is able to visualize the region of interest with minimal invasiveness. Rare findings such as vertebral artery dissection, which occurs most frequently in Region V4, or subsequent vertebral artery aneurysm formation are occasionally suggested by abnormal duplex ultrasound findings, but definitive diagnosis is best made by MRA.[26,27] The limitations of MRA for the vertebral arteries are much the same as those for the carotid arterial system. Not all patients are candidates for magnetic resonance procedures because of metallic implants or an inability to cooperate fully for the examination. The percentage of such patients increases with increasing age; unfortunately, so does the incidence of cerebrovascular disease involving the vertebrobasilar system. Signal dropout in regions of severe flow turbulence, such as that distal to a stenosis or in a region of very slow flow, as might be seen in a hypoplastic vessel, also limit the diagnostic capability of MRA in some cases (see Fig. 11–13*B*).

CONCLUSIONS

Duplex ultrasound provides a very reliable noninvasive technique for the evaluation of the vertebral arteries. Arterial flow hemodynamics can be evaluated qualitatively by assessing the presence or absence of flow, flow direction, and the characteristics of the spectral Doppler flow waveform itself for relative systolic/diastolic flows and systolic flow deceleration. In addition, quantitative volume flow measurements can be made in the vertebral arteries for those patients with symptoms of possible or suspected posterior circulation ischemia. Overall evaluation of vertebral artery hemodynamics provides useful clinical information in (1) assessing the hemodynamic status of the entire extracranial cerebrovascular system, (2) assessing the pathways and adequacy of compensatory collateral flows in patients with significant obstructive disease, (3) potentially identifying a subgroup of patients whose clinical presentation may be related strictly to the posterior circulation, and 4) identifying flow abnormalities in the vertebrobasilar system secondary to lesions that can be addressed and corrected surgically or with other interventional techniques, similar to what is presently done for carotid territory lesions.

References

1. North American Symptomatic Carotid Endarterectomy Trial Collaborators: Beneficial effect of carotid endarterectomy in symptomatic patients with high-grade carotid stenosis. N Engl J Med 325:445–453, 1991.
2. Executive Committee for the Asymptomatic Carotid Atherosclerosis Study: Endarterectomy for asymptomatic carotid artery stenosis. JAMA 273:1421–1428, 1995.
3. North American Symptomatic Carotid Endarterectomy Trial Collaborators: Benefit of carotid endarterectomy in patients with symptomatic moderate or severe stenosis. N Engl J Med 339:1415–1425, 1998.
4. Fisher CM, Gore I, Okabe N, White PD: Atherosclerosis of the carotid and vertebral arteries—extracranial and intracranial. J Neuropathol Exp Neurol 24:455–476, 1965.
5. Castaigne P, Lhermitte F, Gautier JC: Arterial occlusions in the vertebrobasilar system. Brain 96:133–154, 1973.
6. Ford JJ, Baker WH, Ehrenhaft JL: Carotid endarterectomy for nonhemispheric transient ischemic attacks. Arch Surg 110:1314–1317, 1975.
7. Berguer R, Feldman AJ: Surgical reconstruction of the vertebral artery. Surgery 93:670–675, 1983.
8. Reul GJ Jr, Cooley DA, Olson SK, et al: Long-term results of direct vertebral artery operations. Surgery 96:854–862, 1984.
9. Malone JM, Moore WS, Hamilton R: Combined carotid vertebral vascular disease. Arch Surg 115:783–785, 1980.
10. Bogousslavsky J, Regli F: Vertebrobasilar transient ischemic attacks in internal carotid artery occlusion or tight stenosis. Arch Neurol 42:64–68, 1985.
11. Pritz MB, Chandler WF, Kindt GW: Vertebral artery disease: Radiologic evaluation, medical management, and microsurgical treatment. Neurosurgery 9:524–530, 1981.
12. Imparato AM, Riles TS, Kim GE: Cervical vertebral angioplasty for brain stem ischemia. Surgery 90:842–852, 1981.
13. Strandness DE Jr: Extracranial artery disease. In Strandness DE Jr (ed): Duplex Scanning in Vascular Disorders, 2nd ed. New York: Raven Press, 1993, pp 113–157.
14. Ackerstaff RGA, Hoeneveld H, Slowikowski JM, et al: Ultrasonic duplex scanning in atherosclerotic disease of the innominate, subclavian and vertebral arteries: A comparative study with angiography. Ultrasound Med Biol 10:409–418, 1984.
15. Bendick PJ, Jackson VP: Evaluation of the vertebral arteries with duplex sonography. J Vasc Surg 3:523–530, 1986.
16. Bendick PJ, Glover JL: Vertebrobasilar insufficiency: Evaluation by quantitative duplex flow measurements. J Vasc Surg 5:594–600, 1987.
17. Bendick PJ, Glover JL: Hemodynamic evaluation of vertebral arteries by duplex ultrasound. Surg Clin North Am 70:235–244, 1990.
18. Welch HJ, Murphy MC, Raftery KB, Jewell ER: Carotid duplex with contralateral disease: The influence of vertebral artery blood flow. Ann Vasc Surg 14:82–88, 2000.
19. Ackerstaff RGA, Grosweld WJHM, Eikelboom BC: Ultrasonic duplex scanning of the prevertebral segment of the vertebral artery in patients with cerebral atherosclerosis. Eur J Vasc Surg 2:387–393, 1988.
20. Kuhl V, Tettenborn B, Eicke BM, et al: Color-coded duplex ultrasonography of the origin of

the vertebral artery: Normal values of flow velocities. J Neuroimaging 10:17–21, 2000.

21. Bendick PJ: Duplex examination. In Berguer R, Caplan LR (eds): Vertebrobasilar Arterial Disease. St. Louis: Quality Medical Publishers, 1992, pp 93–103.

22. Clifton AG: MR angiography. Br Med Bull 56:367–377, 2000.

23. Phan T, Huston J 3rd, Bernstein MA, et al: Contrast-enhanced magnetic resonance angiography of the cervical vessels: experience with 422 patients. Stroke 32:2282–2286, 2001.

24. Ersoy H, Watts R, Sanelli P, et al: Atherosclerotic disease distribution in carotid and vertebrobasilar arteries: Clinical experience in 100 patients undergoing fluoro-triggered 3D Gd-MRA. J Magn Res Imaging 17:5435–558, 2003.

25. Guppy KH, Charbel FT, Corsten LA, et al: Hemodynamic evaluation of basilar and vertebral artery angioplasty. Neurosurgery 51:327–333, 2002.

26. Shin JH, Suh DC, Choi CG, Leei HK: Vertebral artery dissection: spectrum of imaging findings with emphasis on angiography and correlation with clinical presentation. Radiographics 20:1687–1696, 2000.

27. Zuccoli G, Guidetti D, Nicoli F, et al: Carotid and vertebral artery dissection: Magnetic resonance findings in 15 cases. Radiol Med (Torino) 104:466–471, 2002.

Chapter 12

Ultrasound Assessment of the Intracranial Arteries

DARIUS G. NABAVI, MD, SHIRLEY M. OTIS, MD,
AND E. BERND RINGELSTEIN, MD

INTRODUCTION

In 1965, Miyazaki and Kato[1] first reported the use of continuous-wave Doppler ultrasound for the assessment of extracranial cerebral vessels. Despite its rapid development in other fields, this technique was not applied to the intracranial vessels until 1982. At that time, Aaslid and colleagues[2] developed a transcranial Doppler (TCD) device with a pulsed wave sound emission of 2 MHz that could successfully penetrate the skull and accurately measure blood flow velocities in the basal arteries of the circle of Willis. With the introduction of TCD, it became possible to record intracranial blood flow velocity directly, and TCD became an important noninvasive method for assessing cerebral hemodynamics and for evaluating intracranial cerebrovascular disease. The continuous development and refinement of ultrasonography during the past 2 decades has now established a large array of TCD techniques for clinical application. In 1990, the clinical use of transcranial color-coded duplex sonography (TCCS) was another important step forward. This technique combines B-mode imaging with frequency-based color coding and Doppler sonography.[3] By means of TCCS, direct on-line visualization of the basal cerebral arteries and their flow directions became possible, allowing for angle-corrected measurements of blood flow velocities at defined depths. Subsequently, power-based[4] and three-dimensional TCCS[5] were added, and ultrasound contrast agents were intro-

duced,[6] further enhancing the diagnostic capability of this technique.[7] (Also see Chapter 4.) Ultrasound contrast agents have likewise provided the opportunity to detect right-to-left cardiac shunts[8] and to perform perfusion studies of the brain parenchyma based on indicator dilution principles.[9] The detection of microembolic signals (MESs) by means of TCD constitutes another developmental landmark, allowing one to noninvasively detect and quantify microemboli circulating through the cerebral arteries.[10] One of the most exciting developments of transcranial ultrasonography represents the phenomenon of ultrasound-assisted thrombolysis (sonothrombolysis).[11] The latter may open a new era of *therapeutic* ultrasound. This chapter provides an overview of the main technical and clinical aspects of intracranial ultrasonography and briefly introduces the latest technical developments.

EXAMINATION TECHNIQUES

General Prerequisites

Two prerequisites should be fulfilled before performing a TCD examination: (1) the status of the extracranial arteries has to be known completely, and (2) the patient needs to rest comfortably to avoid major fluctuations of P_{CO_2} and movement artifacts. In addition, two main anatomic considerations must be dealt with by the examiner: (1) the accessibility of the ultrasonic "windows" within the skull that can be penetrated with the ultrasonic beam are often limited or not easily identified; and (2) the arteries at the base of the skull vary greatly in respect to size, course, development, and site of access.[12-15] The transmission of ultrasound through the cranium is a significant problem that has been extensively studied.[16-17] It depends on the skull structure, which consists of three layers, each of which influences ultrasound transmission in different ways. Grolimund[17] has performed a number of in vitro experiments showing that a wide range of energy loss occurs in different skull samples, and that the energy loss varies greatly from one location to another and among individuals. In no case was the power measured behind the skull greater than 35% of the transmitted power. It was further shown that the skull has the effect of an acoustic lens, and that refraction of the beam depends more on the variation of bone thickness than on the angle of insonation.

TCD and TCCS Devices

For transcranial ultrasound applications, the primary design consideration is an excellent signal-to-noise ratio. This is one of the reasons that available transcranial instruments have a lower bandwidth, and, therefore, a larger and less-defined sample volume than most other pulsed Doppler devices. Commercial TCD systems mostly use a 2-MHz, pulsed, range-gated Doppler device with good directional resolution. TCCS is performed with 1.8- to 3.6-MHz phased array sector transducer. Further instrumental requirements are (1) transmitting powers between 10 and 100 mW/cm/sec, (2) adjustable Doppler gate depth, (3) pulse repetition frequency up to 20 kHz, (4) focusing of the ultrasonic beam at a distance of 40 to 60 mm, and (5) on-line display of the time-averaged velocity and peak systolic velocity derived from spectral analysis of the ultrasonic signals. Many commercially available TCD machines are equipped with special headbands or helmets to enable continuous monitoring.

Ultrasonic Windows

Four main ultrasound approaches have been described to insonate the intracranial arteries: the transtemporal, transorbital, suboccipital (i.e., transforaminal), and submandibular approaches,[18] as illustrated in Figure 12–1. An extensive nomenclature has been developed for describing the segments of the intracranial cerebral arteries, and this terminology is used in this chapter. If you are unfamiliar with cerebral artery nomenclature, please refer to Figure 12–2.

Transtemporal Approach

The probe is placed on the temporal aspect of the head, cephalad to the zygomatic arch and immediately anterior and slightly superior to the tragus of the ear conch (Fig. 12–3, position *1*). This is usually the most promising examination site. A more-posterior window immediately cephalad and slightly dorsal to the first one (Fig. 12–3, position *2*) may be more appropriate in a minority of cases, especially for insonation of the P2 segment of the posterior cerebral arteries (PCAs). In some patients, a more frontally

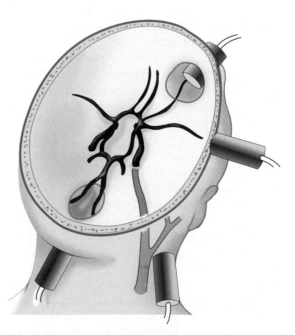

FIGURE 12–1. Relationship of ultrasonic probes to the available ultrasound windows and to the basal cerebral arteries.

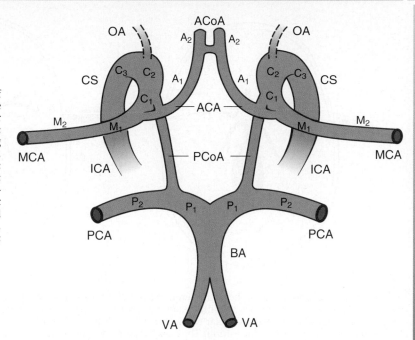

FIGURE 12–2. Nomenclature of the basal cerebral arteries of the circle of Willis. ACA, anterior cerebral artery (segments A_1, A_2); ACoA, anterior communicating artery; BA, basilar artery; CS, carotid siphon (segments C_1–C_3); ICA, internal carotid artery; MCA, middle cerebral artery (segments M_1, M_2); OA, ophthalmic artery; PCA, posterior cerebral artery (segments P_1, P_2); PCoA, posterior communicating artery; VA, vertebral artery.

located temporal ultrasonic window may be present (Fig. 12–3, position 3). By using these transtemporal approaches, the beam can be angulated anteriorly or posteriorly relative to the corresponding probe positions on the opposite side of the head. The *anterior* orientation of the beam allows for the insonation of the M_1 and M_2 segments of the middle cerebral arteries (MCAs), the C_1 segment of the carotid siphon (CS), the A_1 segment of the anterior cerebral artery (ACA), and often the anterior communicating artery (Fig. 12–4A). The *posteriorly* angulated beam insonates the P_1 and P_2 segments of the PCA, the top of the basilar artery (BA), and the posterior communicating arteries (Fig. 12–4B).

Transorbital Approach

Components of the anterior cerebral circulation may be evaluated by placing the transducer against the closed eyelid.[13] To avoid damage to the lenses of the eyes, the power of the ultrasound transmission has to be reduced. The ophthalmic artery can usually be insonated at depths of 45 to 50 mm, whereas the C_3 segment (anterior knee of the CS) is normally met at insonation depths of 60 to 65 mm (Fig. 12–5A). At slightly greater insonation depths of 70 to 75 mm, the C_2 segment shows flow away from the probe (downward deflection), and the C_4 segment shows flow toward the probe (upward deflection). These flow directions apply only when the beam is nearly sagittal (slight medial obliquity) and enters the skull through the supraorbital or infraorbital fissures. Typical insonation depths and velocities are shown in Figure 12–5B.

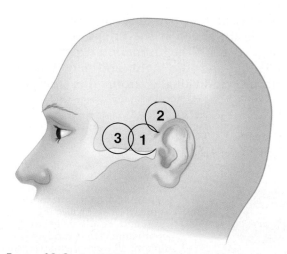

FIGURE 12–3. Available temporal ultrasonic windows and probe placement. *1*, Preauricular position; *2*, posterior window; *3*, anterior window. The probe should first be placed in the preauricular region to identify the middle cerebral artery. Very subtle meander-like movements of the probe should be performed in each position. If position *1* is not successful, position *2* should be tried next, before position *3* is chosen.

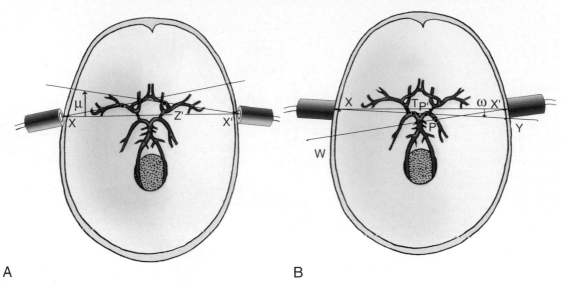

A   B

FIGURE 12–4. Position of the probe in the temporal region to insonate the anterior and posterior parts of the circle of Willis. *A,* Line *X–X'* indicates a frontal plane that runs through the regular placement of the probe on either side and, simultaneously, perpendicular to the sagittal midline of the skull. *Z'* indicates the site of the intracranial ICA (internal carotid artery) bifurcation. The *X'–Z'* distance is 63 ± 5 mm. The angle μ is the angle with which the probe is aimed more anteriorly toward the MCA (middle cerebral artery) and ACA (anterior cerebral artery) segments. This angle was found to be 6 ± 1.1 degrees. *B,* The angle ω indicates the angle with which the beam is directed more posteriorly to insonate the top (*T*) of the BA (basilar artery) and the P_1 segments (*P'*) on both sides. This angle was found to be 4.6 ± 1.2 degrees. The BA bifurcation could be insonated at depths of 78 ± 5 mm, corresponding to the distance *X–T* or *X'–T,* respectively. *Y* indicates the fictional point at which the pathway of the beam then transits the contralateral skull—that is, approximately 2 to 3 cm behind the external acoustic meatus. The P_2 segments (*P*) can also be insonated if the beam is directed even more posteriorly and slightly caudally (*line X'–P*). *W* lies approximately 5 cm behind the contralateral external acoustic meatus.

The transorbital approach is much less established and validated than the transtemporal or suboccipital approach.

Suboccipital Approach

The suboccipital (or transforaminal) approach is essential for screening the verte-

bral artery (VA) and the BA throughout their entire lengths. The probe is placed exactly between the posterior margin of the foramen magnum and the palpable spinous process of the first cervical vertebra, with the beam aimed at the bridge of the nose (Fig. 12–6*A*).[2] The insonation depth is set at 65 mm, and the right and left VAs are tracked individually from this (deepest)

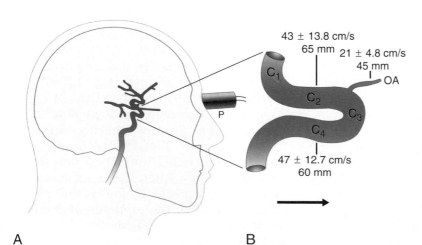

A   B

FIGURE 12–5. Insonation of the ophthalmic artery and carotid siphon by the transorbital approach. *A,* Probe (P) location and relationship to the ophthalmic artery and carotid siphon. *B,* Representative insonation depths and normal flow values within various segments of the carotid siphon (C_1–C_4) and ophthalmic artery (OA).

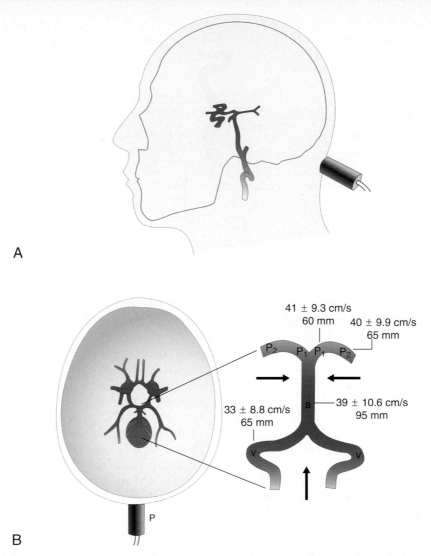

A

B

41 ± 9.3 cm/s
60 mm   40 ± 9.9 cm/s
                65 mm

P₂   P₁ P₁ P₂

33 ± 8.8 cm/s   B — 39 ± 10.6 cm/s
65 mm   95 mm

V   V

P

FIGURE 12–6. *A*, Transcranial Doppler examination of the vertebral system by the suboccipital approach. *B*, Representative insonation and normal flow values within the distal vertebral arteries (V) and the basilar trunk (B). The P_1 and P_2 velocities are measured transtemporally. P, probe.

point toward the foramen magnum, using progressively smaller insonation depths (from 50 down to 35 mm). As the depth decreases, the sound beam is angled more and more sharply toward the side of the head. The extradural part of the VA, on the posterior arch of the atlas, can also be screened. Flow is toward the transducer in this segment. The BA can be tracked cephalad from the point at which the VAs unite. The superior end of the BA is reached at a depth of approximately 95 to 125 mm. Flow in the VAs is normally directed away from the probe. Typical insonation depths and flow velocities are shown in Figure 12–6B.

Submandibular Approach

The submandibular approach completes the examination in that the retromandibular and more distal extradural parts (C5–C6 segments) of the internal carotid artery (ICA) can be evaluated. This particular examination is a useful complement to extracranial studies, because it facilitates the detection of ICA dissection and chronic ICA occlusion with abundant collateralization through the external carotid artery. With the transducer positioned as shown in Figure 12–7A, the beam is directed slightly medially and posteriorly. The ICA can regularly be tracked to

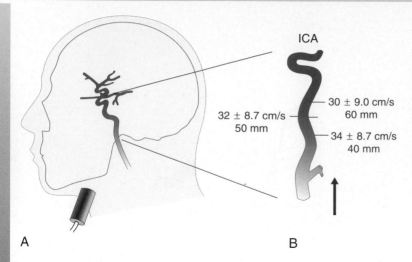

FIGURE **12–7.** *A,* Transcranial Doppler examination of the petrous portion of the internal carotid artery (ICA) by the submandibular approach. The ICA can be traced from depths of 25 to 80 mm, corresponding to the C5 segment of the ICA. *B,* Representative insonation depths and normal flow values within the distal intracranial ICA.

a depth of 80 to 85 mm, at which point it bends medioanteriorly to form the CS. Typical insonation depths and flow velocities are shown in Figure 12–7*B.*

Diagnostic Approach

Basic TCD Examination

In general, it is most convenient to start with transtemporal insonation, to identify the MCA on either side at an insonation depth of 50 to 55 mm, and then to track the ipsilateral arterial network, step by step, in various directions. Proof of traceability of the MCA is necessary for its unequivocal identification. This is also true for other arteries at the base of the brain. *Traceability*

refers to the fact that the MCA (and usually other arteries) can be tracked in incremental steps from a more shallow insonation depth (35 mm) to deeper sites (55 mm) without changes in the character of the flow profile and flow direction. When tracking the MCA medially (65–70 mm), an abrupt change in flow direction (away from, rather than toward the probe) indicates insonation of the A1 segment of the ACA. Flow signals *toward* the probe at this depth usually emanate from the CS at its junction with the MCA. Typical depths and flow velocities are shown in Figure 12–8.

By angling the beam more posteriorly from a transtemporal approach, the P1 segment of the PCA can be picked up most readily at an insonation depth of 65 to 70 mm. The PCA can then be tracked to the

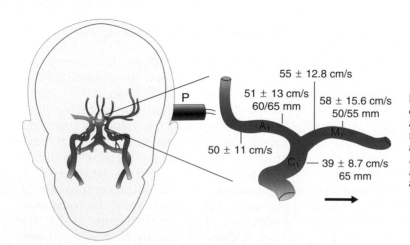

FIGURE **12–8.** Typical transtemporal distances and velocities for the anterior cerebral artery and the middle cerebral artery. *A,* The beam axis is in line with the C_1, M_1, and A_1 segments of the cerebral vessels. *B,* Representative insonation depths and flow velocities are illustrated.

BA (75 mm) and from there to the contralateral PCA (80–85 mm) (see Fig. 12–4*B*). The two criteria of traceability (i.e., the display of bilateral blood flow at the junction with the BA and the change of flow direction within the contralateral PCA) are very important features for identifying the PCAs without compression tests.

After the completion of the examination from *both* temporal windows, additional information may be obtained through the orbital, suboccipital, or mandibular pathways. The vessels that are accessible from these sites, as well as the techniques for identifying these vessels, were described previously. A protocol for TCD examination is presented in Table 12–1.

TCCS Examination

Transcranial color-coded duplex sonography is now a well-established diagnostic method, allowing noninvasive imaging of intracranial vascular structures.[3,19] This

visual approach provides for more rapid and reliable vessel identification, permitting exact localization of the Doppler sample volume, and shortening the examination time.[19,20] This technique has evolved rapidly over the past several years and includes not only vascular imaging but also imaging of the brain parenchyma. Usually, the transtemporal and suboccipital approaches are used for TCCS examinations. No systematic data exist for the submandibular and transorbital approach. For transtemporal insonation, the probe is positioned axially along the orbitomeatal line and the hypoechoic, butterfly-shaped midbrain is visualized as an anatomic landmark at a depth of 6 to 8 cm. From this perspective, the circle of Willis can then easily be depicted (Fig. 12–9). For the suboccipital approach, the hypoechoic foramen magnum and the hyperechoic clivus serve as the anatomic landmarks, with both VAs located at their lateral edges (Fig. 12–10). The origin of the BA can also visually be identified in most cases at a depths of 75 to

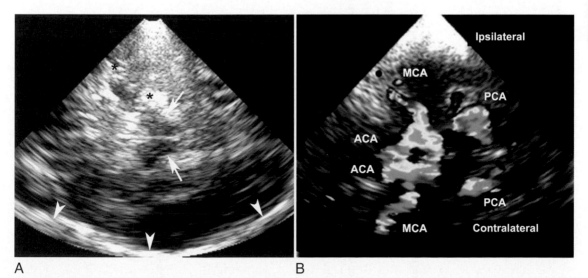

FIGURE 12–9. Illustration of a typical transtemporal TCCS examination. *A*, For initial spatial orientation, the examination is started with a large-scale, B-mode cranial view, which is usually achieved at a depth of 14 to 17 cm. Visualization of the hyperechoic contralateral skull (*arrowheads*) proves the presence of adequate transcranial ultrasound penetration. If the hypoechoic, butterfly-shaped midbrain (*arrows*) and the hyperechoic sphenoid bone (*asterisks*) can be visualized, then the correct insonation plane has been achieved. *B*, For the color-mode examination, the insonation depth is reduced to 8 to 10 cm; the pre- (p1) and post-communicating (p2) segments of the posterior cerebral artery (PCA) can be visualized as they follow the edge of the midbrain. More anteriorly, the sphenoidal (M1) and the insular (M2) parts of the middle cerebral artery (MCA), and the pre-communicating (A1) part of the anterior cerebral artery (ACA) can be depicted. In rare cases, and with excellent bone insonation conditions (as illustrated), the entire circle of Willis can be displayed. The distal part of the internal carotid artery (ICA) is also assessable with the probe tilted downwards.

Table 12–1. Transcranial Doppler Protocol: Identification Criteria and Normal Flow Velocities

Position of Probe	Arterial Segment	Insonation Depth		Normal Flow Velocity (Mean ± SD) (cm/sec)	Main Features for Identification of Vessel Segment
		Range (mm)	Reference Depth (mm)		
Transtemporal	MCA	30–60	50	55 ± 12	M_1; Insonation depth 50 mm; traceability forward and backward; flow toward probe; slightly anterior angulation of beam
	M_1	45–60	50	55 ± 12	Insonation depth; flow away from probe; traceability slightly anterior angulation of beam; for clear-cut differentiation from carotid siphon
	ACA	60–75	70	50 ± 11	
	C_1 (C_2) (carotid siphon transtemporal approach)	60–70	65	39 ± 9	Insonation depth; relatively low flow velocity compared to M_1 segment; slightly anterior and caudal angulation of beam; flow toward probe
	P_1 (posterior cerebral artery)	60 (55)–75	70	39 ± 10	Insonation depth; flow toward probe (ipsilateral P_1); traceability to top of basilar and contralateral P_1; slightly posterior and caudal angulation of beam; relatively low flow velocity compared with M_1 segment
	P_1 and P_1' (top of basilar)	70–80	75	40 ± 10	Insonation depth; bidirectional flow; traceability backward and forward; angulation of beam
	P_2 (PCA)	60–65	65	40 ± 10	Flow away from probe; placement of probe; posterior angulation of probe; modulation by opening and closing eyes

Window	Artery				Instructions
Suboccipital	Extradural distal vertebral artery	40–55	50	34 ± 8	Suboccipital placement of probe; insonation depth; strongly lateral angulation of beam; flow toward probe
	Intradural distal vertebral artery	60–95 (100)	70	38 ± 10	Insonation depth
	Basilar trunk	70 (65)–115 (120)	95 (100, if possible)	41 ± 10	Beam aimed at bridge of nose or slightly laterally; traceability forward and backward; Insonation depth; flow away from probe; often slight increase of flow velocity compared to vertebral artery; traceability of vertebrobasilar axis
Ophthalmic	C_2 (carotid siphon, transorbital approach)	65–80	70	41 ± 11	Sagittal or slightly oblique angulation of beam; flow away from beam; flow away from probe; insonation depth
	C_3 (carotid siphon, transorbital approach)	65 (60)	65 (bidirectional, not measured)	—	Bidirectional signal; sagittal angulation of beam; insonation depth
	C_4 and distal part of C_5 (carotid siphon, transorbital approach)	65–80 (85)	70	47 ± 14	Sagittal or slightly oblique and caudal angulation of beam; flow toward probe; insonation depth
	Ophthalmic artery	35–55	45	21 ± 5	Insonation depth; flow toward probe
	Contralateral A1 (ACA; transorbital approach, ancillary approach if lack of temporal window)	75–80	Not defined	Measurements in a few cases only	Strongly oblique angulation of beam through optic canal; flow toward probe; compression test necessary for differentiation from carotid siphon and MCA
Submandibular	C_6 and retromandibular segment of ICA extradural ICA (submandibular)	35–80 (85)	60	30 ± 9	Flow away from probe; medial angulation of beam; insonation depth

ACA, anterior cerebral artery; ICA, internal cerebral artery; MCA, middle cerebral artery; PCA, posterior cerebral artery.

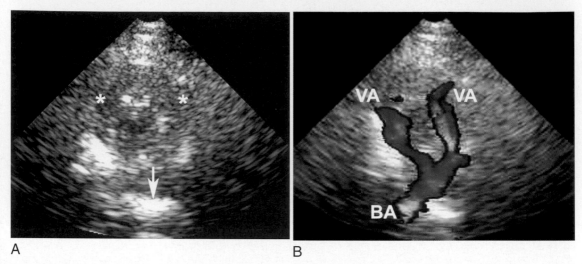

A   B

FIGURE 12–10. Illustration of a typical suboccipital (or transforaminal) TCCS examination. *A,* For initial spatial orientation, the examination is started with a large-scale, B-mode cranial view, which is usually achieved at a depth of 11 to 13 cm. Visualization of the hypoechoic foramen magnum (*asterisks*) and the hyperechoic clivus (*arrow*) proves the adequacy of transcranial ultrasound penetration. *B,* For the color-mode examination, the insonation depth is usually reduced to 8 to 11 cm, visualizing segments (V4) of both vertebral arteries (VAs) as they follow the edges of the foramen magnum. The Y-shaped conjunction of the VAs with the basilar artery (BA) is usually located close to the clivus. Note, however, that the origin of the BA is highly variable and all three arteries are not always visible within the same insonation plane.

95 mm. Generally, the reference depths of the target vessels are identical to the values given previously for TCD examination. TCCS also allows for the examination of cerebral venous sinus and large basal veins,[21] although this has not become part of the clinical routine.

Vessel Identification

The primary TCD parameters for identifying the cerebral arteries are the following:
1. Insonation depth
2. Direction of blood flow at insonation depth
3. Flow velocity (mean flow velocity and systolic or diastolic peak flow velocity)
4. Probe position (e.g., temporal, orbital, suboccipital, submandibular)
5. Direction of the ultrasonic beam (e.g., posterior, anterior, caudad, cephalad)
6. Traceability of vessels

Compression of the extracranial carotid arteries, as a means for intracranial vessel identification, has gradually been excluded from the clinical routine due to the low, but present, risk of cerebral embolism.[22,23] This is especially the case since the advent of TCCS used in conjunction with ultrasound contrast agents, as the identification of the major cerebral arteries and their collateral pathways is possible, for the most part, without compression maneuvers. In patients with extracranial atheromatous disease, carotid compression definitely should be avoided.

Flow Velocity Measurements

The mean flow velocities of various vessel segments, and their age dependency, are shown in Tables 12–2 and 12–3.[24] Normal flow velocity values in adults show little variation among different investigators.[14,25–27] The highest velocities are almost always found in the MCA or the ACA. The PCAs and BAs have lower Doppler shifts than the MCA in normal subjects. The same pattern has not been noted, however, in cerebral blood flow studies, in which flow is measured in cubic centimeters per second. Two explanations have been offered for this discrepancy between velocity and volume

Table 12–2. Normal Values of Mean Blood Velocity for Arteries* (Transtemporal Approach)

Age (yr)	Mean Blood Velocity (cm/sec)		
	MCA (M_1)	ACA (A_1)	PCA (P_1)
10–29	70 ± 16.4	61 ± 14.7	55 ± 9.0
30–49	57 ± 11.2	48 ± 7.1	42 ± 8.9
50–59	51 ± 9.7	46 ± 9.4	9 ± 9.9
60–70	41 ± 7.0	38 ± 5.6	36 ± 7.9
Insonated depth (mm)	50–55	60–65	60–65

*Measurements for the middle (MCA), anterior (ACA), and posterior (PCA) cerebral arteries according to age.

Table 12–3. Normal Values of Mean Blood Velocity for Arteries* (Suboccipital Approach)

Age (yr)	Mean Blood Velocity (cm/sec)		
	PCA (P_1)	BA	VA
10–29	54 ± 8.0	46 ± 11	45 ± 9.8
30–49	40 ± 8.5	38 ± 8.6	34 ± 8.2
50–59	39 ± 10.1	32 ± 7.0	37 ± 10.0
60–70	35 ± 11.1	32 ± 6.7	35 ± 7.0
Insonated depth (mm)	60–65	85–90	60–65

*Measurements for the posterior cerebral (PCA), basilar (BA), and vertebral (VA) arteries according to age.

flow: (1) The measurement sites may be different[28] or (2) more probably, different velocities occur as a compensatory mechanism to keep volume flow constant in vessels of different size.[25] Thus, velocities are slower in large vessels and faster in small vessels. Normal, angle-corrected blood flow velocity values using TCCS have likewise been established and are only slightly higher than those obtained with TCD.[20,29] The TCD documentation of decreasing flow velocities with increasing age[20,27] correlates well with age-related changes in cerebral blood flow[28] and underlines the validity and sensitivity of TCD and TCCS data as a semi-quantitative estimate of cerebral blood flow.

Functional Reserve Testing

Transcranial Doppler is an ideal functional test for detecting rapid changes in cerebral perfusion, because the technique provides excellent resolution of flow velocity changes occurring over time. Functional tests are predominantly aimed at the evaluation of the reserve mechanism of the cerebral vasculature, using various stimuli such as hypocapnia or hypercapnia, increased or reduced systemic arterial pressure, and hypoxia.[25] The CO_2 (carbon dioxide) dilatory effect is mainly restricted to the peripheral arterial vascular bed, particularly the small cortical vessels.[28] With changing CO_2

concentrations, the relationship between flow velocity and volume flow within a large cerebral artery is linear,[30] provided that the CO_2 level does not directly affect the diameter of the large proximal arterial segment.[31] Velocities measured from the MCA with changing CO_2 concentrations show a biasymptotic, S-shaped curve (Fig. 12–11).

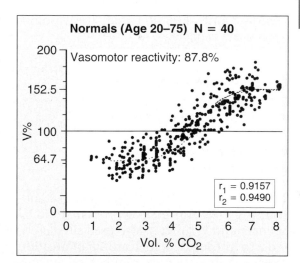

FIGURE 12–11. Vasomotor reactivity in 40 normal individuals (ages 20–75 yr). Blood flow velocity changes are shown during carbon dioxide (CO_2)-induced hypercapnia (*upper curve*) and hypocapnia (*lower curve*). The average change was 87.8% (52.5% and 35.3% hypercapnia and hypocapnia, respectively). (From Ringelstein EB, Sievers C, Ecker S, et al: Noninvasive assessment of CO_2-induced cerebral vasomotor response in normal individuals and patients with internal carotid artery occlusions. Stroke 19:964, 1988. Copyright © American Heart Association.)

A "preserved" vasomotor reserve implies that a drop in perfusion pressure can be counterbalanced by vasodilatation of cortical arterioles to maintain sufficient cortical blood supply. The vasomotor reserve may become exhausted if the resistance vessels in brain areas with low perfusion pressure are already maximally dilated.[30–33] In this state, the resistance vessels are refractory to any further vasodilatory stimuli, and hypercapnia cannot increase blood flow. This condition may be critical, because ischemic brain injury can occur if the perfusion pressure is further reduced for any reason. Measurements of the vasomotor reserve capacity are useful in evaluating the hemodynamic impact of extracranial occlusive carotid disease.

The pulsatility index, as defined by Gosling (see Chapter 3), reflects the resistance in the peripheral vascular bed and has been suggested as a sensitive index of diastolic runoff—that is, with increased peripheral vasodilatation, diastolic runoff is expected to increase and the pulsatility index to decrease.[34] However, in a large series of patients with carotid artery occlusion, the pulsatility index appeared to be much poorer for predicting the intracranial hemodynamic situation than the vasomotor reserve capacity.[35]

DIAGNOSTIC PARAMETERS FOR SPECIFIC CLINICAL APPLICATIONS

Intracranial Stenosis and Occlusion

The detection of carotid siphon (CS) stenosis using TCD was first reported in 1986 by Spencer and Whisler,[13] who used similar criteria to those used for carotid bifurcation disease. Since then, a number of authors have reported similar findings for the CS and have extended TCD applications to other brain arteries.[36–39] The most obvious clinical advantage of ultrasound is the rapid screening of the acute stroke patient for intracranial vessel obstruction. Normal TCD findings in stroke patients have considerable clinical impact.

Definition of Stenosis With TCD

The following are typical TCD features of circumscribed stenosis of a large basal cerebral artery (Fig. 12–12): (1) increased flow velocity; (2) disturbed flow (spectral broadening and enhanced systolic and low-frequency echo components); and (3) covibration phenomena (vibration of vessel wall and surrounding soft tissue).[25,35] It is unclear whether the peak systolic velocity (>120–160 cm/sec) or the mean systolic velocity (>80–120 cm/sec) should be used as a threshold value.[39] With a mean velocity value of 100 cm/sec, a sensitivity of 100% and a specificity of 97.9%, as well as positive and negative predictive values of 88.8% and 94.9%, were reported in detecting intracranial stenoses with a diameter of 50% or more.[38] For the vertebrobasilar system, a threshold of more than 2 kHz peak systolic Doppler shift showed a sensitivity of 80% and a specificity of 97% in detecting stenoses of 50% or more.[37] Most authors agree that, in comparison with the contralateral vessel segment, a relative increase in peak systolic velocity of more than 30% is suspicious for hemodynamically significant stenosis, and a relative increase of more than 50% indicates a definite intracranial artery stenosis.

Definition of Occlusion With TCD

Basal cerebral artery occlusion can be detected by three observations: (1) the absence of arterial signals at an expected depth; (2) the presence of signals in vessels that communicate with the occluded artery; and (3) altered flow in communicating vessels, indicating collateralization. For example, occlusion of the MCA is diagnosed from the lack of an MCA signal in the presence of flow signals from other vessels (i.e., the PCA, the ACA, or the distal CS). This combination of findings also confirms that the temporal window is satisfactory. In a recent study, TCD showed a sensitivity of 83% and a specificity of 94.4%, with an overall accuracy of 91.6%, in the detection of intracranial vessel occlusion.[40] In accordance with the well-established, angiography-based Thrombolysis in Myocardial

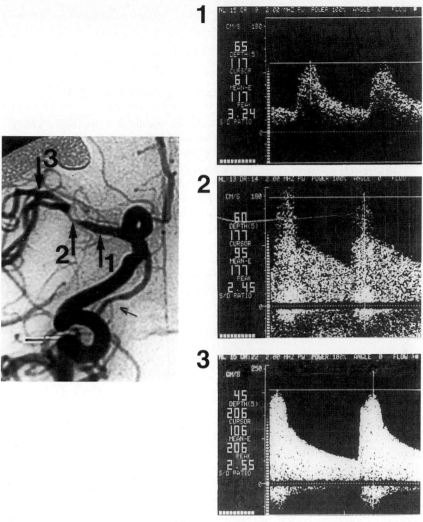

FIGURE 12–12. Middle cerebral artery stenosis and associated transcranial Doppler (TCD) changes: (*1*) normal proximal flow; (*2*) increased systolic and diastolic peak velocity and spectral broadening (turbulent flow) at the center of the stenosis; (*3*) distal turbulent flow.

Infarction (TIMI) criteria in cardiology, Demchuk and colleagues[41] have proposed the so-called TIBI (Thombolysis in Brain Ischemia) criteria for the TCD-based classification of the MCA status during and after thrombolysis. The TIBI scale, ranging from 0 (MCA occlusion) to 5 (normal MCA), is given in Table 12–4. In 109 acute stroke patients undergoing thrombolytic therapy, the TIBI criteria were found to be accurate in the prediction of the clinical outcome.

Pitfalls and Diagnostic Accuracy

Noninvasive demonstration of intracranial arterial stenosis and occlusion is a valuable clinical tool, but various errors can occur: (1) lack of flow signal due to an inadequate temporal window; (2) misinterpretation of hyperdynamic collateral channels[34] or AVM feeders[25,42] as stenosis; (3) displacement of arteries because of a space-occupying lesion; (4) misinterpretation of physiologic variables in the circle of Willis[25]; (5) misdiagnosis of vasospasm as stenosis[43]; and (6) misinterpretation of reactive hyperemia following spontaneous recanalization as stenosis.[44] In most of these situations, however, the velocity increases are generally seen *throughout* the course of the involved arteries, which distinguishes these conditions from the typically *localized* areas of increased velocity resulting from stenosis.

Table 12–4. TIBI Criteria for TCD Monitoring of the MCA Recanalization During and After Thrombolytic Therapy[41]

TIBI Score	Status of the MCA Flow	TCD Criteria
0	Occlusion	• No flow signal
1	Near occlusion or minimal residual flow	• Early systolic low-flow signal • No diastolic flow signal
2	Strongly reduced	• Reduced systolic and diastolic velocity • Flattened early systolic increment • Pulsatility index <1.2
3	Moderately reduced	• Normal systolic increment • Pulsatility index >1.2 • Relative reduction of blood flow velocity of >30% as compared with the contralateral side
4	Stenotic signal	• Mean blood flow velocity >80 cm/sec or relative increase of velocity >30% as compared with the contralateral side • Detection of turbulent flow
5	Normal signal	• Side-to-side difference of blood flow velocity <30% • Comparable values of pulsatility index

MCA, middle cerebral artery; TCD, transcranial Doppler; TIBI, Thombolysis in Brain Ischemia.

Diagnostic accuracy of TCD in the VA-BA system remains a particular problem. Difficulties with VA-BA diagnosis result from the following: (1) The normal flow and the size of the vessels are highly variable; (2) the location and course of the arteries are unpredictable; (3) often the junction of the VAs cannot reliably be identified; (4) absence of the VA flow signal on one side may not represent disease (e.g., so-called PICA*-ending anomaly in severe VA hypoplasia); and (5) occlusion of one VA or a "top of the basilar" occlusion does not necessarily lead to relevant flow abnormalities.[45]

Detection of Intracranial Stenosis and Occlusion With TCCS

For TCCS, usually the angle-corrected peak systolic velocity is used as the main parameter for the definition of intracranial stenosis. In 1999, Baumgartner and coworkers[46] published the results of the largest TCCS validation study yet on the detection of intracranial stenosis. Table 12–5 gives the cutoff values of PSV for the different intracranial vessels. These values show excellent accuracy for the identification of stenoses of 50% or greater diameter. Cutoff

Table 12–5. Threshold Values of Angle-Corrected Peak Systolic Velocity (PSV) for the Detection of Intracranial Stenoses of ≥50% With TCCS[46]

Vessel	PSV Cutoff (cm/sec)	Sensitivity	Specificity	Positive Predictive Value	Negative Predictive Value
MCA	≥220	100	100	100	100
ACA	≥155	100	100	100	100
PCA	≥145	100	100	100	91
BA	≥140	100	100	100	100
VA	≥120	100	100	100	100

ACA, anterior cerebral artery; BA, basilar artery; MCA, middle cerebral artery; PCA, posterior cerebral artery; VA, vertebral artery.

*posterior inferior cerebellar artery

values ranged from 220 cm/sec for the MCA to 120 cm/sec for the VA. The TCCS accuracy in the detection of stenoses between 30% and 50% (diameter) showed a high negative predictive value (100%) but only a moderate positive predictive value, ranging from 73% to 100%. The latter results can be explained by the weak hemodynamic effects of low-grade stenosis. Others have used much lower cutoff values of 120 cm/sec or more PSV, or a side-to-side difference of more than 30 cm/sec, for the definition of TCCS-based intracranial stenosis.[47]

Transcranial color-coded duplex sonography diagnosis of an intracranial artery occlusion is based on the absence of flow signals using both the color and the spectral Doppler modes (Fig. 12-13). In some cases, the occluded vascular segment appears slightly hyperechoic on B-mode imaging. In contrast to the TCD technique, the use of the correct insonation site and the presence of an adequate insonation window can be easily confirmed with TCCS. Diagnostic confidence of TCCS for intracranial vessel occlusion is up to 100%[48,49] and can be further supported by the use of ultrasound contrast agents.[50,51] In a multicenter trial, the feasibility and validity of TCCS, in conjunction with ultrasound contrast agents, for the detection of intracranial steno-occlusive disease has been convincingly shown.[47]

Assessment of the Effects of Extracranial Occlusive Disease

In addition to directly assessing the basilar cerebral arteries, an additional important clinical application of TCD is evaluation of the hemodynamic effects of *extracranial* vascular disease on the *intracranial* circulation.

Carotid Stenosis or Occlusion

Significant changes occur in the intracranial circulation because of the reduced perfusion pressure caused by extracranial flow-limiting disease. With ICA obstruction of 80% or more, the ipsilateral MCA velocity and the pulsatility index generally decrease as a result of vasodilatation in the distal arterial circulation ipsilateral to the obstruction.[30,35] Increased velocities and turbulence are encountered and usually indicate collateralization. The identification of collateral flow in patients with extracranial carotid

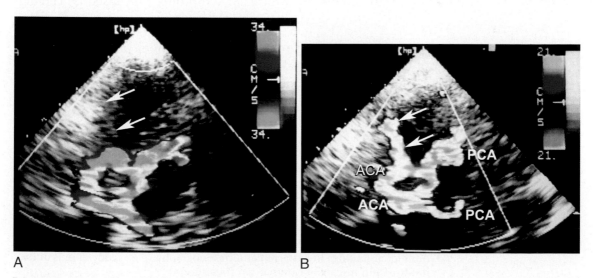

A   B

FIGURE 12–13. Middle cerebral artery (MCA) occlusion and recanalization detected with transcranial color-coded duplex sonograph (TCCS). *A*, Typical finding of a proximal MCA occlusion, with echocontrast-enhanced TCCS (Levovist[R]) in an acute stroke patient. Note the excellent visualization of both posterior cerebral arteries (PCAs) around the midbrain and both anterior cerebral arteries (ACAs) as well. No flow is present within the presumed course of the MCA using both the color mode (*arrows*) and the Doppler spectral mode (not shown). Compare this image with Figure 7B). *B*, Several days later, spontaneous MCA recanalization has occurred, with the entire MCA (*arrows*) depicted with contrast-enhanced TCCS.

disease is possible with TCD[12,14,52] and TCCS.[53] Four main collateral pathways can be distinguished: (1) via the anterior communicating artery (ACoA), (2) via the posterior communicating artery (PCoA), (3) via the ophthalmic artery, and (4) via ipsilateral leptomeningeal arteries. Because the small communicating arteries are not always visible with TCCS,[53] indirect hemodynamic signs of the involved arteries are of considerable importance for identifying and localizing collateralization. Sonographic criteria for intracranial collateralization are given in Table 12–6. In general, the more sonographic criteria that are present, the more confident is the TCCS diagnosis of collateralization.

Evaluation of hemodynamic disturbances within the carotid artery–MCA pathway is of particular interest in patients with subtotal ICA obstruction, both unilateral and bilateral. Although the predominant mechanism of stroke is thromboembolism, rather than a low-flow effect, a small subgroup of patients experience transient ischemic attacks, permanent stroke, or progressive ischemic eye disease caused by critically reduced blood flow.[54,55] This subgroup of patients may benefit from recanalization surgery, including external carotid–internal carotid bypass. The identification of these individuals is based on the detection of an exhausted cerebral vascular reserve, which can be done through TCD assessment of the CO_2 responsiveness of the cerebral arteries.[30]

Vertebrobasilar System

The subclavian steal mechanism is the classic paradigm for studying hemodynamic disturbances in the human vertebrobasilar system. Rapid flow changes caused by any type of VA blood flow restriction can be measured directly within the BA. Under resting conditions, blood flow within the BA is almost never critically impaired, even if the subclavian steal is continuous. If the contralateral feeding VA is also diseased (or hypoplastic), however, BA blood flow may become reduced, may demonstrate a to-and-fro pattern, or may even be reversed. During hyperemia testing of the stealing arm, flow velocity and direction of flow within the basilar trunk may become more or less affected (Fig. 12–14). BA blood flow is very resistant to any critical changes resulting from the subclavian steal mechanism. Actually, the subclavian steal, as such, is a benign condition, and even in symptomatic patients, most vertebrobasilar symptoms are caused by cerebral

Table 12–6. Sonographic Criteria for TCD and TCCS for the Detection of Intracranial Collateralization in Case of Severe Extracranial Artery Disease[53]

Collateral Pathway	TCD/TCCS Criteria
ACoA	• Retrograde and increased flow in ACA$_{ipsilateral}$ • Orthograde and increased flow in ACA$_{contralateral}$ • Strong turbulences in the region of the AcoA (mostly with TCCS)
PCoA	• Direct visualization of the PCoA (TCCS) • Increased velocity in P1 segment of the PCA$_{ipsilateral}$ • Velocity ratio of P1/P2 segment of the PCA$_{ipsilateral}$ >1.5 • Velocity ratio of P1$_{ipsilateral}$/P1$_{contralateral}$ >1.5 • Increased velocity within the BA (and sometimes VAs)
Ophthalmic artery	• Retrograde flow in ipsilateral ophthalmic artery • Additional findings in extracranial ultrasonography (e.g., reduced pulsatility index within ipsilateral external carotid artery)
Leptomeningeals	• Increased velocity in the entire ipsilateral PCA (P1$_{ipsilateral}$ = P2$_{ipsilateral}$) • Increased velocity in ACA$_{contralateral}$ without retrograde flow within ACA$_{ipsilateral}$

ACA, anterior cerebral artery; ACoA, anterior communicating artery; BA, basilar artery; PCA, posterior cerebral artery; PCoA, posterior communicating artery; TCCS, transcranial color-coded duplex sonography; TCD, transcranial Doppler; VA, vertebral artery.

FIGURE 12–14. Schematic representation of flow conditions in various vertebrobasilar vessel segments in patients with the subclavian steal mechanism. With latent steal, flow in the feeding (contralateral) vertebral artery (F) is increased during brachial hyperemia and is normal in the basilar artery trunk (B). By contrast, the blood column shows an alternating flow direction in the stealing vertebral artery (S). During manifest steal, blood flow in the stealing vertebral artery (VA; S) is continuously reversed. This either has no effect on basilar artery blood flow or causes alternating or reverse flow within the basilar artery trunk (B). During transcranial Doppler examination, each of the three vessel segments can be clearly differentiated by means of their characteristic flow changes during brachial hyperemia.

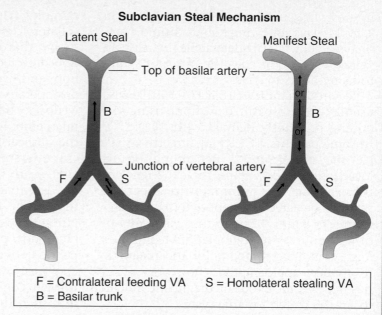

Subclavian Steal Mechanism

Latent Steal

Manifest Steal

Top of basilar artery

Junction of vertebral artery

F = Contralateral feeding VA   S = Homolateral stealing VA
B = Basilar trunk

microangiopathy rather than large artery flow disturbances.[12] Subclavian artery disease, however, is a strong indicator of coexisting coronary artery disease.

Monitoring of Cerebral Vasospasm

Monitoring of vasospasm using TCD is a well-recognized tool in the clinical management of patients suffering from subarachnoid hemorrhage.[14,43] There is a close correlation between increased flow velocities within the spastic basal arteries (MCA, PCA, ACA) and the severity of the subarachnoid hemorrhage.[56,57] This correlation

is valid with respect to the size and extent of the subarachnoid clot, the clinical state of the patient, and the angiographically documented severity of spasm (if the Doppler shift is greater than 3 kHz or 120 cm/sec). The side with the more severe flow changes on TCD examination corresponds to the predominant location of the blood clot and the presumed site of the aneurysm. A steep increase in flow velocity (>20 cm/sec/day) within the first few days after the bleed is associated with a poor prognosis. Usually, an MCA velocity exceeding 200 cm/sec in patients with vasospasm is associated with a critical reduction in cerebral blood flow (Table 12–7). The time course of the development of vasospasm is also of clinical

Table 12–7. Clinical Relevance of Increased Middle Cerebral Artery Flow Velocities After Subarachnoid Hemorrhage

Middle Cerebral Artery Flow Velocity	Time-Averaged Peak Velocity (mean; cm/sec)	Clinical Consequences
Normal or nonspecifically increased	≤80	Should be observed further
Subcritically accelerated	>80–120	Moderate vasospasm; preventive therapy indicated
Critically accelerated	>120–140	Severe vasospasm; consequent treatment necessary
Highly critical flow acceleration	>140	Severe vasospasm; delayed ischemic deficit highly probable

Modified from Harders A: Neurosurgical Applications of Transcranial Doppler Sonography. New York, Springer-Verlag, 1986.

interest. In general, vasospasm occurs from 4 to 14 days following subarachnoid hemorrhage, but a TCD-detectable increase in velocity often precedes the onset of symptoms by hours to days.

Recent data indicate that TCCS is likewise useful for vasospasm detection, using the criteria previously defined with TCD.[19,58,59] In some patients, TCCS may directly visualize the aneurysm,[59–61] depending on its localization and size and the experience of the examiner. The minimum-size aneurysm that can be detected is reported to be greater than 6 to 8 mm.[60] Due to the availability of other noninvasive angiographic techniques (e.g., computed tomography and magnetic resonance angiography), however, TCCS has not become a routine diagnostic modality in the search for aneurysms.

Intraoperative Monitoring

Another evolving, and ostensibly important, application of TCD is intraoperative monitoring. The unique advantages of TCD, in comparison with other relative cerebral blood flow measurement techniques, are its complete noninvasiveness and its potential for detecting rapid alterations of blood supply on a real-time basis. TCD monitoring delivers direct, immediate information regarding cerebral perfusion, thus anticipating potential hazards or permitting rapid modification of therapy. TCD monitoring has been used during carotid endarterectomy, open heart surgery with cardiopulmonary bypass, and intensive care therapy.[12,62] In most studies, the M_1 segment of the MCA is insonated at a depth of 50 to 55 mm. TCD monitoring can be performed either with repeated examinations at extremely short intervals or continuously, using a headband to hold the transducer in place.

Most experience with TCD monitoring has been accumulated during *carotid endarterectomy*.[63–65] It has been shown that MCA flow is affected far less during intraoperative clamping of the carotid artery than expected, raising the possibility that shunts are inserted too often. An MCA velocity of more than 10 cm/sec during clamping has been associated with adequate collateral circulation.[65] It has further been shown that the amount of microembolization detected with TCD during the dissection and wound closure is predictive of postoperative stroke.[65] This on-line acoustic feedback from TCD, indicating cerebral microembolism, had a direct influence on the surgical technique.[66]

Transcranial Doppler monitoring during *open heart surgery* has revealed a number of disturbances in cerebral blood flow that result from extracorporeal bypass (a pumping technique that severely alters blood flow physiology).[62] Brain damage and perioperative stroke may occur during extracorporeal bypass. TCD measurements have thrown considerable doubt on the theory that such injury is caused by critical *hypoperfusion*. On the contrary, accidental cerebral *hyperperfusion* may play a more decisive role, as well as air microemboli and loss of cerebral autoregulation. In addition, the frequency of cerebral microemboli detected with TCD during open heart surgery correlates with the degree of neuropsychological deficit.[67,68]

Intensive Care Unit Monitoring

Transcranial Doppler is a useful technique for monitoring critically ill patients in the intensive care unit.[69] Eligible patients are predominantly those with raised intracranial pressure (e.g., after head injury) and those with severe cerebrovascular disease.[70] Monitoring may also be informative, and possibly beneficial, for the patient's outcome in high- and low-pressure hydrocephalus, and in low-flow states associated with extracranial occlusive disease, myocardial failure, or valvular disease, as well as impending brain death. TCD monitoring may provide further information about the pathophysiology of various abnormal conditions that affect intensive care patients, and ultimately may be helpful for therapy. In a recent multicenter study, the use of TCD modified the diagnostic and therapeutic management in 36% of critically ill patients.[71] Although Aaslid and Lindegaard[72] have proposed certain parameters of the TCD profile that are likely to reflect the cerebral perfusion pressure, and thus also the intracranial pressure, these parameters have not yet been validated. Only a few TCCS studies have been conducted concerning critical care applications.[73]

Brain Death

The accurate diagnosis of brain death has become more important in view of the ethical issues that surround the transplantation field. Determination of brain death was for a long time based on three parameters: (1) clinical criteria, (2) electroencephalographic criteria, and (3) angiographic demonstration of absent intracranial circulation.[74] The arrest of intracranial flow results in a characteristic reflux phenomenon in the basal cerebral arteries during late systole. This to-and-fro movement is easily noted in the TCD flow velocity waveform[72] (Fig. 12–15). In several large clinical studies, TCD findings correlated perfectly with ancillary diagnostic tests to confirm brain death, with neither false-positive nor false-negative findings.[75,76] Therefore, besides angiography, scintigraphy, and electroencephalography, TCD constitutes an accepted noninvasive diagnostic test to confirm brain death.[77]

Arteriovenous Malformations and Fistulae

Although an arteriovenous malformation (AVM) is a developmental abnormality, the arteries and veins involved in supplying blood to the AVM are essentially normal and are the usual arteries supplying the region of the brain where the AVM is located. These arteries, which exclusively or partially feed AVMs, can unequivocally be identified with TCD by means of their significant flow abnormalities—that is, increased flow velocity, reduced pulsatility, and reduced responsiveness to CO_2.[78] In a consecutive series, more than 80% of large- to medium-sized AVMs were detected, but more than 60% of smaller AVMs were missed with TCD.[79] TCCS, additionally, allows the direct visualization of the AVM.[19,60] For TCCS, a similar diagnostic sensitivity of 80% in the identification of AVMs was reported.[80] In addition to AVMs, other types of intracranial arteriovenous shunts can be detected with TCD and TCCS, such as carotid siphon–cavernous sinus fistulae or dural fistulae.[19]

Cerebral Venous Thrombosis and Intracerebral Hemorrhage

Studies on healthy volunteers indicate that cerebral sinus and veins can be visualized in 50% to 90% of cases, depending on the vessel segment examined.[81] Preliminary data suggest that cerebral venous thrombosis can be diagnosed using TCCS.[82] Ultrasonographic criteria are (1) abnormal elevation of blood flow velocities within intracranial sinus and veins and (2) direct visualization of cerebral sinus with decreased or absent flow. In a recent study in patients suffering from thrombosis of cerebral sinus and veins, monitoring of

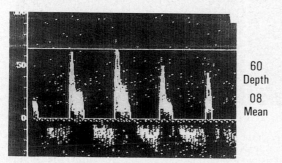

60 Depth

08 Mean

Middle Cerebral Artery

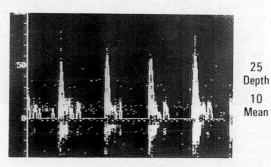

25 Depth

10 Mean

Common Carotid Artery

FIGURE 12–15. Brain death. Transcranial Doppler (TCD) changes are noted in the left middle cerebral and extracranial common carotid arteries. The characteristic reflux phenomenon seen during late systole is demonstrated.

venous hemodynamics was a significant predictor of the long-term outcome.[83] Direct visualization of the intracranial sinus, however, requires significant expertise and, generally, the use of ultrasound contrast agents.

TCCS studies have shown that a sharply demarcated, hyperechogenic area within the brain tissue in stroke patients is indicative of intracerebral hemorrhage.[19,84] Although sensitivity and specificity values were as high as 94% and 95% in 133 consecutive stroke patients with sufficient temporal bone windows,[85] TCCS still cannot replace computed tomographic or magnetic resonance brain imaging in this cohort of patients.

NEW DEVELOPMENTS

Microembolic Signals

The first reports on *gaseous* microemboli detected with ultrasound were published by Spencer and colleagues in 1969 and were associated with decompression sickness and open-heart surgery.[86] More than 20 years later, the technique entered the focus of clinical interest when the same group detected microembolic signals (MES, also termed HITS, or high-intensity transient signals) for the first time with TCD in a

patient undergoing carotid endarterectomy.[87] Surprisingly, MES occurred during the preparation time, before the artery was opened, indicating that the MES represented *solid* emboli arising from the arteriosclerotic plaque. Since then, numerous experimental and clinical studies have been published concerning MES, including two consensus statements.[10,88] The latter provide internationally accepted definitions of MES and cover major issues involving TCD instrumentation and software systems. The consensus opinions state that a microembolic TCD signal must: (1) be short in duration (<300 ms), (2) be at least 3 dB above the background signal, (3) be mainly unidirectional within the Doppler spectrum, and (4) produce a characteristic sound ("chirp," "snap," "moan"). Typical MESs detected with TCD are illustrated in Figure 12–16. It has been shown that MESs are usually too small to elicit clinical symptoms. Nevertheless, there is now overwhelming evidence that MESs possess clinical relevance and, on an individual basis, permit the assessment of the actual thromboembolic risk. They also permit the monitoring of treatment efficacy.[89] The recent introduction of sophisticated MES detection software has considerably improved the monitoring procedure and its diagnostic confidence. MES detection represents a useful tool for improving the stratification of individuals prone to

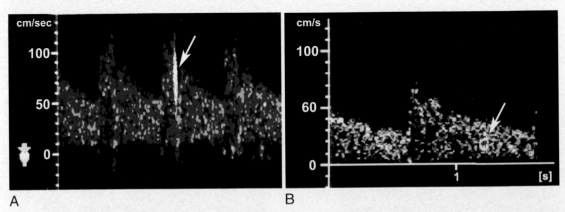

FIGURE 12–16. Illustrative examples of typical microembolic signals (MESs), detected with TCD, in a patient with artificial heart valves. These appear randomly within the systolic *(A)* or the diastolic *(B)* phase of the Doppler spectrum *(arrows)*. The origin of the MES and the maximum intensity elevation are always located within the Doppler spectrum; however, with strong MES intensity gradients (mostly seen with systolic MES), the upper edges—and, rarely, also the lower edges—of the signal may run off the flow spectrum. Note that the intensity of the background transcranial Doppler (TCD) signal has to be decreased for MES monitoring (as seen) to allow for effective MES identification.

thromboembolism and for evaluating new primary and secondary prevention strategies with high sensitivity.

Ultrasound Perfusion Imaging

The introduction of ultrasound contrast agents presented the possibility for ultrasound-based measurement of tissue perfusion, based on fundamental indicator-dilution principles.[90] This made it possible to monitor the tissue perfusion of the brain in patients suffering from cerebrovascular disease almost noninvasively and at the bedside. With the use of harmonic imaging techniques, it recently has been shown that contrast enhancement is visible using transcranial B-mode ultrasound imaging, permitting transtemporal brain perfusion mapping.[9] In the first clinical series reported on acute stroke patients, a positive correlation was found between the TCCS-derived brain perfusion maps and the later occurrence of brain infarction.[91,92] A major limitation of the *bolus-tracking appoach* with ultrasound contrast agents is the destruction of the microbubbles (i.e., the indicator) by ultrasound, limiting one of the prerequisites for perfusion measurements based on indicator-dilution principles.[93] Therefore, an alternative approach, using refill kinetics, based on a *constant infusion* of an ultrasound contrast agent, was proposed and has already proved to be useful for brain perfusion measurements.[94] A general limitation of ultrasound-based brain perfusion measurements is the low spatial resolution of current TCCS systems, which may be overcome in the future. At present, this technique is still within the early clinical stage, and upcoming studies will show which of the two techniques (bolus approach versus refill kinetics) is superior in generating reproducible perfusion maps of the brain.

Sonothrombolysis

In 1942, Lynn and coworkers[95] showed for the first time that focused, in vivo ultrasound can induce selective tissue damage without affecting the surrounding areas. It is now well known that tissue insonation may lead to various physiochemical tissue reactions, such as heating and denaturation, microstreaming effects, release of free radicals, and alterations of blood cells and coagulation, that are already being used in clinical medicine.[11] The ability of ultrasound to augment the dissolution of thrombus was first reported in 1989 by Kodo and coworkers.[96] This capability has been verified in numerous experimental studies using in vitro and animal models.[97] It has been shown that the insonation of thrombus alone[98] or in combination with fibrinolytic agents[99] significantly accelerates the thrombolytic process. This effect has been termed *ultrasound-assisted thrombolysis* or *sonothrombolysis*. Using a variety of ultrasound frequencies (20 kHz–3 MHz) and intensities (3 mW–8 W/cm^2), a clear dose relationship of this phenomenon has been demonstrated.[100] It is now believed that not *macrostructural* (e.g., clot disruption) but rather *microstructural* alterations (e.g., dysconfiguration of fibrin molecules) are mainly responsible for the sonothrombolytic effect, via a microcavitation process. In addition to several clinical studies in patients suffering from acute coronary syndromes, the first reports on successful sonothrombolysis in acute stroke patients have appeared.[101,102] Sonothrombolysis is a very exciting, novel tool that may increase the efficacy of the purely pharmacologic approach of thrombolysis in acute stroke. Acceleration of intracranial vessel recanalization could reduce the final infarction size and therefore improve the long-term outcome[102] of stroke patients. Establishing this bedside technique as a *therapeutic* tool could revolutionize the entire field of acute stroke treatment.

CONCLUSIONS

Through continuous refinements and technical innovations during the past two decades, transcranial ultrasound is no longer limited to the sonographic measurement of blood flow velocities. Today, transcranial ultrasonound means multimodal,

Table 12–8. Main Indications for Vascular TCD and TCCS in Clinical and Experimental Settings

1. Detection of intracranial stenoses and occlusions in the major basal arteries
2. Evaluation of intracranial hemodynamic effects and collateral flow of extracranial occlusive disease (e.g., occlusions, subclavian steal)
3. Monitoring of intracranial vessel recanalization in acute stroke
4. Monitoring of intracranial cerebral hemodynamics
   a. After subarachnoid hemorrhage (e.g., presence and severity of vasospasms)
   b. In patients with increased intracranial pressure (e.g., on the intensive care unit)
   c. During and after extracranial revascularization procedures (e.g., carotid endarterectomy, carotid angioplasty)
   d. Before and during neuroradiologic interventions (e.g., balloon occlusion) for presence of collateral pathways
   e. During open heart surgery
   f. In evolution of brain death
5. Detection and quantification of cerebral circulating microemboli
6. Detection and quantification of right-to-left shunts
7. Functional tests
   a. Stimulation of intracranial arterioles with carbon dioxide or other vasoactive drugs (e.g., assessing vasomotor reserve capacity)
   b. Language lateralization (e.g., before neurosurgery)
   c. External stimulation of visual cortex
8. Still in the developmental stage
   a. Brain perfusion imaging
   b. Ultrasound-assisted thrombolysis

high-resolution, and real-time imaging of the brain's structure and vasculature. Using modern equipment and a variety of ultrasound modalities, information can be acquired about anatomy, hemodynamic status, and function of the central nervous system and its supplying arteries and veins (Table 12–8). Nevertheless, TCD and TCCS remain portable, easy-to-access, dynamic, highly reliable, and reproducible techniques in clinical medicine that support various therapeutic decisions. Noninvasiveness further advocates the use of TCD as a monitoring tool, particularly during surgical or neurointerventional procedures. Overall, transcranial ultrasound with TCD and TCCS has revolutionized our understanding of cerebrovascular disease, and these modalities now are key in the diagnostic workup of cerebrovascular disorders. In most countries, TCD and TCCS are in the hands of physicians and technicians with neurologic background who deal appropriately, and carefully, with its capabilities and limitations. However, we must be aware that all these methods require *sufficient knowledge, practical skills,* and *technical expertise.* In other words, we have to ensure continuous

education and adequate training in the fascinating field called *neurosonology.*

References

1. Miyazaki M, Kato K: Measurement of cerebral blood flow by ultrasonic Doppler technique. Jpn Circ J 29:375, 1965.
2. Aaslid R, Markwalder T-M, Norris H: Noninvasive transcranial Doppler ultrasound recording of flow velocity in basal cerebral arteries. J Neurosurg 57:769, 1982.
3. Bogdahn U, Becker G, Winkler J, et al: Transcranial color-coded real-time sonography in adults. Stroke 21:1680, 1990.
4. Bude RO, Rubin JM, Adler RS: Power versus conventional color Doppler sonography: Comparison in the depiction of normal intrarenal vasculature. Radiology 192:777, 1994.
5. Klötzsch C, Bozzato A, Lammers G, et al: Contrast-enhanced three-dimensional transcranial color-coded sonography of intracranial stenoses. Am J Neuroradiol 23:208, 2002.
6. Otis S, Rush M, Boyajian R: Contrast-enhanced transcranial imaging. Results of an American phase-two study. Stroke 26:203, 1995.
7. Nabavi DG, Droste DW, Schulte-Altedorneburg G, et al: Diagnostic benefit of echocontrast enhancement for the insufficient

transtemporal bone window. J Neuroimaging 9:102, 1999.

8. Jauss M, Zanette E: Detection of right-to-left shunt with ultrasound contrast agent and transcranial Doppler sonography. Cerebrovasc Dis 10:490, 2000.

9. Wiesmann M, Seidel G: Ultrasound perfusion imaging of the human brain. Stroke 31:2421, 2000.

10. Ringelstein EB, Droste DW, Babikian VL, et al: Consensus on microembolus detection by TCD. International Consensus Group on Microembolus Detection. Stroke 29:725, 1998.

11. Francis CW, Behrens S: Ultrasonic thrombolysis. In Hennerici M, Meairs S (eds): Cerebrovascular Ultrasound. Theory, Practice and Future Developments. Cambridge, UK, Cambridge University Press, 2001.

12. Ringelstein EB: A practical guide to transcranial Doppler sonography. In Weinberger J (ed): Noninvasive Imaging of Cerebral Vascular Disease. New York, AR Liss, 1989, p 75.

13. Spencer MP, Whisler D: Transorbital Doppler diagnosis of intracranial arterial stenosis. Stroke 17:916, 1986.

14. Aaslid R, Markwalder TM, Nornes H: Noninvasive transcranial Doppler ultrasound recording of flow velocity in the basal cerebral arteries. J Neurosurg 57:769, 1982.

15. Arnolds B, von Reutern GM: Transcranial Doppler sonography: Examination technique and normal reference values. Ultrasound Med Biol 12:115, 1986.

16. White DN, Curry GR, Stevenson RJ: The acoustic characteristics of the skull. Ultrasound Med Biol 4:225, 1978.

17. Grolimund P: Transmission of ultrasound through the temporal bone. In Aaslid R (ed): Transcranial Doppler Sonography. New York, Springer-Verlag, 1986, p 10.

18. Aaslid R (ed): Transcranial Doppler Sonography. New York, Springer-Verlag, 1986, p 39.

19. Baumgartner RW: Transcranial color duplex sonography in cerebrovascular disease: A systematic review. Cerebrovasc Dis 16:4, 2003.

20. Schöning M, Buchholz R, Walter J: Comparative study of transcranial color duplex sonography and transcranial Doppler sonography in adults. J Neurosurg 78:776–784, 1993.

21. Baumgartner RW, Gonner F, Arnold M, Muri RM: Transtemporal power- and frequency-based color-coded duplex sonography of cerebral veins and sinuses. Am J Neuroradiol 18:1771, 1997.

22. Mast H, Ecker S, Marx P: Cerebral ischemia induced by compression tests during transcranial Doppler sonography. Clin Investig 71:46, 1993.

23. Khaffaf N, Karnik R, Winkler WB, et al: Embolic stroke by compression maneuver during transcranial Doppler sonography. Stroke 25:1056, 1994.

24. Otis S, Ringelstein EB: Transcranial Doppler sonography. In Bernstein ED (ed): Noninvasive Diagnostic Techniques in Vascular Disease. St. Louis, CV Mosby, 1990, p 59.

25. Ringelstein EB, Otis SM, Kahlscheuer B, et al: Transcranial Doppler sonography. Anatomical landmarks and normal velocity values. Ultrasound Med Biol 16:745–761, 1990.

26. Hennerici M, Rautenberg W, Sitzer G, et al: Transcranial Doppler ultrasound for the assessment of intracranial arterial flow velocity— Part I. Examination technique and normal values. Surg Neurol 27:439, 1987.

27. Grolimund P, Seiler RW: Age dependence of the flow velocity in the basal arteries—a transcranial Doppler ultrasound study. Ultrasound Med Biol 14:191, 1988.

28. Frackowiak RSJ, Lenzi GL, Jones T: Quantitative measurements of cerebral blood flow and oxygen metabolism in man using 15-oxygen and positron emission tomography. Theory, procedure and normal values. J Comput Assist Tomogr 4:727, 1980.

29. Baumgartner RW, Mathis J, Sturzenegger M, Mattle HP: A validation study on the intraobserver reproducibility of transcranial color-coded duplex sonography velocity measurements. Ultrasound Med Biol 20:233, 1994.

30. Ringelstein EB, Sievers C, Ecker S, et al: Noninvasive assessment of CO_2-induced cerebral vasomotor response in normal individuals and patients with internal carotid artery occlusions. Stroke 19:963, 1988.

31. Huber P, Handa J: Effect of contrast material, hypercapnia, hyperventilation, hypertonic glucose and papaverine on the diameter of the cerebral arteries—angiographic determination in man. Invest Radiol 2:17, 1987.

32. Markwalder TM, Grolimund P, Seiler RW, et al: Dependency of blood flow velocity in the middle cerebral artery on end-tidal carbon dioxide partial pressure—a transcranial ultrasound Doppler study. J Cereb Blood Flow Metab 4:368, 1984.

33. Ringelstein EB, Otis SM, Schneider PA: Noninvasive assessment of CO_2-induced cerebral vasomotor reactivity. Comparison with rCBF findings during 133-xenon inhalation measurement. J Cereb Blood Flow Metab 1:161, 1989.

34. Gosling RG, King DH: Processing arterial Doppler signals for clinical data. In De Vlieger M (ed): Handbook of Clinical Ultrasound. New York, John Wiley & Sons, 1978.

35. Ley-Pozo J, Willmes K, Ringelstein EB: Relationship between pulsatility indices of Doppler flow signals and CO_2-reactivity

within the middle cerebral artery in extracranial occlusive disease. Ultrasound Med Biol 16:763, 1990.

36. Niederkorn R, Neumayer K: Transcranial Doppler sonography: A new approach in the noninvasive diagnosis of intracranial brain artery disease. Eur Neurol 26:65, 1987.

37. de Bray JM, Missoum A, Dubas F, et al: Detection of vertebrobasilar intracranial stenoses: Transcranial Doppler sonography versus angiography. J Ultrasound Med 16:213, 1997.

38. Felberg RA, Christou I, Demchuk AM, et al: Screening for intracranial stenosis with transcranial Doppler: Tthe accuracy of mean flow velocity thresholds. J Neuroimaging 12:9, 2002.

39. Rorick MB, Nichols FT, Adams RJ: Transcranial Doppler correlation with angiography in detection of intracranial stenosis. Stroke 25:1931, 1994.

40. Demchuk AM, Christou I, Wein TH, et al: Accuracy and criteria for localizing arterial occlusion with transcranial Doppler. J Neuroimaging 10:1, 2000.

41. Demchuk AM, Burgin WS, Christou I, et al: Thrombolysis in brain ischemia (TIBI) transcranial flow grades predict clinical severity, early recovery, and mortality in patients treated with intravenous tissue plasminogen activator. Stroke 32:89, 2001.

42. Schwartz A, Hennerici M: Noninvasive transcranial Doppler ultrasound in intracranial angiomas. Neurology 36:626, 1986.

43. Aaslid R, Huber P, Nornes H: Evaluation of cerebrovascular spasm with transcranial Doppler ultrasound. J Neurosurg 60:37, 1984.

44. Ringelstein EB, Biniek R, Weiller C, et al: Type and extent of hemispheric brain infarctions and clinical outcome in early and delayed middle cerebral artery recanalization. Neurology 42:289, 1992.

45. Brandt T, Knauth M, Wildermuth S, et al: CT angiography and Doppler sonography for emergency assessment in acute basilar artery ischemia. Stroke 30:606, 1999.

46. Baumgartner RW, Mattle HP, Schroth G: Assessment of ≥50% and <50% intracranial stenoses by transcranial color-coded duplex sonography. Stroke 30:87, 1999

47. Gerriets T, Postert T, Goertler M, et al: DIAS I: Duplex-sonographic assessment of the cerebrovascular status in acute stroke. A useful tool for future stroke trials. Stroke 31:2342, 2000.

48. Seidel G, Kaps M, Gerriets T: Potential and limitations of transcranial color-coded sonography in stroke patients. Stroke 26:2061, 1995.

49. Kenton AR, Martin PJ, Abbott RJ, Moody AR: Comparison of transcranial color-coded sonography and magnetic resonance angiography in acute stroke. Stroke 28:1601, 1997.

50. Nabavi DG, Droste DW, Kemeny V, et al: Potential and limitations of echocontrast-enhanced ultrasonography in acute stroke patients: A pilot study. Stroke 29:949, 1998.

51. Postert T, Federlein J, Braun B, et al:. Contrast-enhanced transcranial color-coded real-time sonography: A reliable tool for the diagnosis of middle cerebral artery trunk occlusion in patients with insufficient temporal bone window. Stroke 29:1070, 1998.

52. Anzola GP, Gasparotti R, Magoni M, Prandini F: Transcranial Doppler sonography and magnetic resonance angiography in the assessment of collateral hemispheric flow in patients with carotid artery disease. Stroke 26:214, 1995.

53. Baumgartner RW, Baumgartner I, Mattle HP, Schroth G: Transcranial color-coded duplex sonography in the evaluation of collateral flow through the circle of Willis. Am J Neuroradiol 18:127, 1997.

54. Caplan LR, Sergay S: Positional cerebral ischemia. J Neurol Neurosurg Psychiatry 39:385, 1976.

55. Ringelstein EB, Zeumer H, Angelou D: The pathogenesis of strokes from internal carotid artery occlusion: Diagnostic and therapeutic implications. Stroke 14:867, 1983.

56. Harders A, Gilsbach JM: Time course of blood velocity changes related to vasospasm in the circle of Willis measured by transcranial Doppler ultrasound. J Neurosurg 66:718, 1987.

57. Seiler RW, Grolimund P, Aaslid R, et al: Cerebral vasospasm evaluated by transcranial ultrasound correlated with clinical grade and CT-visualized subarachnoid hemorrhage. J Neurosurg 64:594, 1986.

58. Proust F, Callonec F, Clavier E, et al: Usefulness of transcranial color-coded sonography in the diagnosis of cerebral vasospasm. Stroke 30:1091, 1999.

59. Becker G, Greiner K, Kaune B, et al: Diagnosis and monitoring of subarachnoid hemorrhage by transcranial color-coded real-time sonography. Neurosurgery 28:814, 1991.

60. Martin PJ, Gaunt ME, Naylor AR, et al: Intracranial aneurysms and arteriovenous malformations: Transcranial colour-coded sonography as a diagnostic aid. Ultrasound Med Biol 20:689, 1994.

61. Wardlaw JM, Cannon JC, Sellar RJ: Use of color power transcranial Doppler sonography to monitor aneurysmal coiling. Am J Neuroradiol 17:864, 1996.

62. von Reutern GM, Hetzel A, Birnbaum D, et al: Transcranial Doppler ultrasonography during cardiopulmonary bypass in patients with

severe carotid stenosis or occlusion. Stroke 19:674, 1989.

63. Schneider PA, Rossman ME, Otis SM, et al: Transcranial Doppler monitoring during carotid arterial surgery. Surg Forum 38:333, 1987.

64. Padayachee TS, Gosling RG, Bishop CC, et al: Monitoring middle cerebral artery blood velocity during carotid endarterectomy. Br J Surg 73:98, 1986.

65. Ackerstaff RG, Moons KG, van de Vlasakker CJ, et al: Association of intraoperative transcranial Doppler monitoring variables with stroke from carotid endarterectomy. Stroke 31:1817, 2000.

66. Jansen C, Vriens EM, Eikelboom BC, et al: Carotid endarterectomy with transcranial Doppler and electroencephalographic monitoring: A prospective study in 130 operations. Stroke 24:665, 1993.

67. Barbut D, Yao FS, Lo YW, et al: Determination of size of aortic emboli and embolic load during coronary artery bypass grafting. Ann Thorac Surg 63:1262, 1997.

68. Braekken SK, Reinvang I, Russell D, et al: Association between intraoperative cerebral microembolic signals and postoperative neuropsychological deficit: Comparison between patients with cardiac valve replacement and patients with coronary artery bypass grafting. J Neurol Neurosurg Psychiatry 65:573, 1998.

69. Alvarez del Castillo M. Monitoring neurologic patients in intensive care. Curr Opin Crit Care 7:49, 2001.

70. Babikian VL, Pochay V, Burdette DE, Brass ML: Transcranial Doppler sonographic monitoring in the intensive care unit. J Intensive Care Med 6:36, 1991.

71. Grupo de Trabajo de Neurointensivismo y Trauma de la Sociedad Espanola de Medicina Intensiva, Critica y Unidades Coronarias (SEMICYUC); Grupo de Trabajode Neurologia Critica de la Societat Catalana de Medicina Intensiva i Critics (SOCMIC): Clinical use of transcranial Doppler in critical neurological patients. Results of a multicenter study. Med Clin (Barc) 120:241, 2003.

72. Aaslid R, Lindegaard KF: Cerebral hemodynamics. In Aaslid R (ed): Transcranial Doppler Sonography. New York, Springer-Verlag, 1986, p 60.

73. Shiogai T, Nagayama K, Damrinjap G, et al: Morphological and hemodynamic evaluations by means of transcranial power Doppler imaging in patients with severe head injury. Acta Neurochir Suppl (Wien) 71:94, 1998.

74. Black PM: Brain death. Medical progress. N Engl J Med 299:338, 1978.

75. Ducrocq X, Braun M, Debouverie M, et al: Brain death and transcranial Doppler: Experience in 130 cases of brain dead patients. J Neurol Sci 160:41, 1998.

76. Zurynski Y, Dorsch N, Pearson I, Choong R: Transcranial Doppler ultrasound in brain death: Experience in 140 patients. Neurol Res 13:248, 1991.

77. Wijdicks EF: The diagnosis of brain death. N Engl J Med 344:1215, 2001.

78. Diehl RR, Henkes H, Nahser HC, et al: Blood flow velocity and vasomotor reactivity in patients with arteriovenous malformations: A transcranial Doppler study. Stroke 25:1574, 1994.

79. Mast H, Mohr JP, Thompson JL, et al: Transcranial Doppler ultrasonography in cerebral arteriovenous malformations. Diagnostic sensitivity and association of flow velocity with spontaneous hemorrhage and focal neurological deficit. Stroke 26:1024, 1995.

80. el-Saden SM, Grant EG, Sayre J, et al: Transcranial color Doppler imaging of brain arteriovenous malformations in adults. J Ultrasound Med 16:327, 1997.

81. Stolz E, Kaps M, Kern A, et al: Transcranial color-coded duplex sonography of intracranial veins and sinuses in adults. Reference data from 130 volunteers. Stroke 30:1070, 1999a.

82. Stolz E, Kaps M, Dorndorf W: Assessment of intracranial venous hemodynamics in normal individuals and patients with cerebral venous thrombosis. Stroke 30:70, 1999b.

83. Stolz E, Gerriets T, Bodeker RH, et al: Intracranial venous hemodynamics is a factor related to a favorable outcome in cerebral venous thrombosis. Stroke 33:1645, 2002.

84. Seidel G, Kaps M, Dorndorf W: Transcranial color-coded duplex sonography of intracerebral hematomas in adults. Stroke 24:1519, 1993.

85. Maurer M, Shambal S, Berg D, et al: Differentiation between intracerebral hemorrhage and ischemic stroke by transcranial color-coded duplex-sonography. Stroke 29:2563, 1998.

86. Spencer MP, Lawrence GH, Thomas GI, Sauvage LR: The use of ultrasonics in the determination of arterial aeroembolism during open-heart surgery. Ann Thorac Surg 8:489, 1969.

87. Spencer MP, Thomas GI, Nicholls SC, Sauvage LR: Detection of middle cerebral artery emboli during carotid endarterectomy using transcranial Doppler ultrasonography. Stroke 21:415, 1990.

88. Consensus Committee of the Ninth International Cerebral Hemodynamic Symposium. Basic identification criteria of Doppler microembolic signals. Stroke 26:1123, 1995.

89. Mess W, Hennerici M: High intensity transient signals. In Hennerici M, Meairs S: Cerebrovascular ultrasound. Theory, practice and future

developments. Cambridge University Press, Cambridge, UK, 2001.

90. Meier P, Zierler KL: On the theory of the indicator-dilution method for measurement of blood flow and volume. J Appl Physiol 6:731, 1954.

91. Federlein J, Postert T, Meves S, et al: Ultrasound evaluation of pathological brain perfusion in acute stroke using second harmonic imaging. J Neurol Neurosurg Psychiatry 69:616, 2002.

92. Meyer K, Wiesmann M, Albers T, Seidel G: Harmonic imaging in acute stroke: Detection of a cerebral perfusion deficit with ultrasound and perfusion MRI. J Neuroimaging 13:166, 2003.

93. Lassen NA, Perl W: Tracer kinetic methods in medical physiology. New York, Raven Press, 1979.

94. Rim SJ, Leong-Poi H, Lindner JR, et al: Quantification of cerebral perfusion with "Real-Time" contrast-enhanced ultrasound. Circulation 20:2582, 2001.

95. Lynn JG, Zwemer RL, Chick AJ, et al: A new method for the generation and use of focused ultrasound in experimental biology. J Gen Physiol 26:179, 1942.

96. Kudo S: Thrombolysis with ultrasound effect. Tokyo Med J 104:1005, 1989.

97. Ishibashi T, Akiyama M, Onoue H, et al: Can transcranial ultrasonication increase recanalization flow with tissue plasminogen activator? Stroke 33:1399, 2002.

98. Rosenschein U, Furman V, Kerner E, et al: Ultrasound imaging-guided noninvasive ultrasound—thrombolysis: Preclinical results. Circulation 102:238, 2000.

99. Lauer CG, Burge R, Tang DV, et al: Effect of ultrasound on tissue-type plasminogen activator-induced thrombolysis. Circulation 86:1257, 1992.

100. Ishibashi T, Akiyama M, Onoue H, et al: Can transcranial ultrasonication increase recanalization flow with tissue plasminogen activator? Stroke 33:1399, 2002.

101. Alexandrov AV, Demchuk AM, Felberg RA, et al: High rate of complete recanalization and dramatic clinical recovery during tPA infusion when continuously monitored with 2-MHz transcranial Doppler monitoring. Stroke 31:610, 2000.

102. Eggers J, Koch B, Meyer K, et al: Effect of ultrasound on thrombolysis of middle cerebral artery occlusion. Ann Neurol 53:797, 2003.

SECTION III
EXTREMITY ARTERIES

Ao

CIA

The Role of Noninvasive Procedures in the Management of Extremity Arterial Disease

J. Dennis Baker, MD

The common denominator of most conditions involving the arterial circulation in the extremities is the reduction or limitation of blood flow. In the majority of situations, the perfusion available depends not only on the condition of the main artery but also on the extent to which collateral branches provide an alternate route. The clinical presentation is determined by the net decrease in flow. In the case of limited occlusive disease, there is no perfusion deficit at rest and symptoms are only manifested when there is an increased demand, such as occurs with exercise. Occlusive lesions develop gradually, as in the case of an atherosclerotic plaque, so there is time for parallel improvement in the function of the collaterals, and the patient may have no symptoms until there is advanced stenosis. Even progression to occlusion may produce only mild symptoms. On the other hand, an acute occlusion, such as that produced by an arterial embolus, will result in much more severe symptoms because initially there is only limited contribution by collateral pathways.

Extremity arterial disease can occur at a single level or at multiple levels. The location of different stenoses will determine the distribution and severity of symptoms. For example, a person with both iliac and superficial femoral artery lesions may have moderate proximal leg symptoms and severe calf symptoms. The proximal muscle groups only suffer the hemodynamic effect of the iliac stenosis while the calf is affected by the combination of the two lesions, thus producing a greater drop in perfusing pressure in the calf.

Patients with arterial disease present with a wide range of signs and symptoms. Obtaining optimal results from noninvasive vascular testing requires knowledge of normal anatomy and anatomic variants, as well as the different types of arterial pathology that may be encountered.

CHRONIC OCCLUSIVE PATHOLOGY

Arteries throughout the body have a similar structure. The intima is the innermost layer and is normally very thin. It consists of a monolayer of endothelial cells separated from the internal elastic lamina by a thin layer of mixed cells. Although the endothelium is a thin structure, it plays an important role. Its functions include (1) prevention of platelet aggregation and thrombosis, (2) regulation of smooth muscle tone in the deeper layer, (3) modulation of smooth muscle cell growth and migration, and (4) control of entry of lipoproteins into the vessel wall. The media extends from the inner portion of the internal elastic lamina to the adventitia. Within the media, there are discrete bundles of smooth muscle cells, elastic fibers, and collagen. The muscle component is responsible for variations in the tone of the wall, responding to both local factors interacting with the endothelium and central factors initiated by nerve control. The elastic lamellae determine the elasticity. The aorta and its primary branches have the greatest proportion of elastic fibers and the greatest elasticity. The more peripheral branches have a greater proportion of smooth muscle cells and so are less elastic but have a greater range of muscular tone. The outer layer, the adventitia, is primarily fibrocellular and provides a major portion of the tensile strength of the vessel. The vasa vasora and small nerves course through this layer.

Atherosclerosis is by far the most common cause of arterial occlusive disease in the western hemisphere. This condition is primarily a disease of the intima. In the earliest stages, there is slow thickening of the intima. Subsequently, there is gradual deposition in the intima of foam cells, white blood cells that have taken up lipids. Areas of initial lipid accumulation are called fatty streaks. Not all of these progress to atherosclerotic plaques. By definition, the development of atherosclerosis is heralded by the appearance of the early fibrous plaque. Such plaques are usually focal lesions, rather than involving a diffuse surface of the artery. Histologic examination reveals a low-profile, homogeneous lesion with a well-organized structure of connective tissue fibers and smooth muscle cells. The endothelium covering the early plaque is intact. The plaque initially increases in thickness while maintaining a homogeneous appearance, but gradually there is a transition to a complex plaque. Necrosis in the deeper portions results in an increasingly heterogeneous appearance. These areas contain liquid and crystalline lipid and cellular debris. There are varying degrees of inflammatory reaction, characterized by the presence of monocytes around the necrotic regions. Progression can lead to breakdown of the covering endothelium, exposing subendothelial tissues that can trigger the formation of thrombus or platelet aggregates. Further deterioration can result in breakdown of the fibrous cap covering the necrotic core, producing an ulcer. This change can lead to acute symptoms due to distal embolization of plaque contents or of thrombi formed in the ulcer. Many plaques, both large and small, develop calcium deposits. Recent studies suggest that deposition of calcium may be related to the degree of inflammatory reaction within the developing plaque. Some plaques can have focal hemorrhage, often resulting in an acute increase in the degree of stenosis.

Atherosclerotic plaques, whether early or advanced, are asymmetric in cross-section. The orientation of the main mass of the plaque varies in different parts of the arterial tree. In the carotid bifurcation, the bulk of the plaque is in the outer portion of the bulb, away from the flow divider. On the other hand, iliac artery plaques are predominantly in the posterior portion of the cross-section. The marked asymmetry is the main reason why imaging studies, such as contrast arteriography, must be obtained in multiple planes to provide an accurate estimate of severity of stenosis.

Atherosclerosis is a diffuse disease, affecting different parts of the arterial tree. Nevertheless, the plaques tend to be focal, rather than involving long arterial segments diffusely. Typically, lesions develop at bifurcations, sparing long, straight sections. It is this focal characteristic that permits interventions, such as endarterectomy or bypass grafting. In the peripheral arteries, the most frequent site for significant atherosclerotic narrowing is in the distal superficial femoral artery. Plaques also preferentially develop at the level of the adductor canal (Hunter's canal) in the distal thigh. (This location is an exception to the rule that disease occurs primarily at bifurcations. The tight tethering of the artery in the canal is thought to cause focal disease at this level.) The second most common site is the aorto-iliac segment. Disease at this level involves the terminal abdominal aorta and the common iliac arteries. Although some patients may have advanced plaque in the internal or external iliac arteries, these locations are less frequent than the common iliac location. Diabetic patients also have significant plaque formation in the deep femoral artery and in the crural arteries in the calf. These additional sites result in more severe symptoms and higher risk of limb loss. A problem in the diabetic is diffuse calcification of the media of the branches in the calf, making operation on these vessels challenging.

Symptomatic atherosclerotic occlusive disease is much less common in the upper extremities. The subclavian arteries are the most common locations, and unilateral subclavian disease is common. Plaques in these vessels are often asymptomatic but may produce arm claudication or posterior cerebral symptoms as the result of a vertebral artery steal.

Nonatherosclerotic occlusive peripheral arterial problems represent a small portion of the referrals to most vascular laboratories. Table 13–1 lists the variety of conditions that may require evaluation. The large vessel conditions usually present with symptom patterns similar to atherosclerosis and are assessed in the same fashion. In some situations, it may be possible to suspect nonatherosclerotic pathologies, because these conditions are often more diffuse or have a different distribution. The small vessel diseases usually involve just the hands or the feet, and normal vessels may be present down to the wrist or ankle level. Since the usual noninvasive tests focus primarily on the more proximal arteries, different protocols are needed for patients with these disorders. Duplex scanning is of little use, and examination must focus on digital pressures and plethysmographic techniques. Vasospastic conditions present an additional diagnostic challenge, since the occlusive component is not fixed but is brought on by a triggering stimulus such as cold exposure. Although digital plethysmography may suggest the presence of vasospastic disease, an adequate diagnostic evaluation requires the use of a provocative test. The best test is the measure of digital systolic pressure before and after a standardized cold exposure.

ACUTE OCCLUSIVE PATHOLOGY

The most common cause of acute arterial occlusive disease is the arterial embolus. The embolus can consist of a piece of thrombus that formed in the arterial system (including the heart) or can be a piece of an atherosclerotic plaque. The embolus travels through the arterial tree until it reaches a branch that is small enough to prevent its passage, and there it becomes wedged. The stasis of blood produced by the sudden blockage results in propagation of thrombus proximally and distally along the branch, so that the resulting occlusion is much more extensive than the embolus itself. Cardiogenic emboli can originate in the left atrial appendage of patients with atrial fibrillation or on the damaged endocardial surface after myocardial infarction. These emboli are usually large and occlude major branches, such as the axillary, brachial, femoral or popliteal arteries. Atheroembolism can originate from ulceration of plaque in any part of the body. These lesions are small and block small branches, producing small regions of necrosis. It is not uncommon to have a shower of multiple particles at one time.

Arterial dissection can cause acute changes in the peripheral circulation. A dissection is produced by a tear in the intima into the media, with a splitting of the arterial wall to create a false lumen. The process can extend either up or down the vessel. A dissection most commonly originates in the thoracic aorta and may extend into major branch vessels, such as the subclavian, iliac, or visceral arteries. These branches may have decreased flow via the false lumen or may become

Table 13–1. Nonatherosclerotic Peripheral Arterial Conditions

Large Vessels

Inflammatory
  Systemic giant cell arteritis
  Radiation-induced arteritis
Noninflammatory
  Popliteal entrapment
  Adventitial cystic disease

Small Vessels

Inflammatory
  Vasculitis of connective tissue disease
    Systemic sclerosis (scleroderma)
    Rheumatoid vasculitis
    Systemic lupus erythematosus
  Buerger's disease (thromboangiitis obliterans)
Vasospastic
  Raynaud's syndrome

occluded. An acute dissection may have much the same presentation as a large cardiac embolus, and differentiating between these two etiologies is important for clinical management.

NONOCCLUSIVE PATHOLOGY

An aneurysm is a focal dilation of an artery involving all layers of the wall. Peripheral aneurysms are most frequent in the popliteal artery but can also be found in other branches. As the dilation increases, there is a gradual accumulation of layered thrombus, so that the lumen may be close to the size of the normal portion of the vessel. Unlike abdominal aortic aneurysm, the most common complication of peripheral arterial aneurysms is acute ischemia from thrombosis or embolization, rather than rupture. Symptoms may also be produced by compression of adjacent nerves and veins.

A false aneurysm usually forms following a focal breakdown of the arterial wall, with contained extravasation of blood to form a hematoma adjacent to the artery. Local trauma, including catheter placement for invasive procedures, is a common cause. Disruption of a bypass anastomosis, due to either infection or mechanical problems, is another common etiology. In many cases, the break in the arterial defect heals and the hematoma is reabsorbed. If not, there is an ongoing communication between the artery and the hematoma. With time, a fibrous capsule forms around the pulsating hematoma. Some small pseudoaneurysms resolve by spontaneous thrombosis, but others may gradually expand. Pseudoaneurysms can rupture or produce symptoms by local compression.

Arteriovenous communications result from developmental abnormalities or trauma. The embryologic arteriovenous malformations present with many small communications within a tissue mass. Traumatic arteriovenous fistulas most commonly have a single connection. As the amount of blood passing directly to the venous circulation increases, a partial compensation occurs with dilation of the proximal arterial system. In some cases, the feeding vessel can reach twice normal size. Chronic vascular insufficiency can occur if the proximal arterial enlargement is insufficient and the volume of blood shunted away from the extremity is great enough to limit perfusion distal to the communication. A special case of arteriovenous fistula can occur as a complication of invasive arterial procedures in the femoral artery. Placement of a large-bore device through both the artery and the vein can initiate the problem. It is possible to have a combination of a fistula and a pseudoaneurysm in the same groin.

SIGNS AND SYMPTOMS

Atherosclerosis develops slowly, and a low-profile plaque does not have a significant effect on flow. Reduction of blood flow does not occur until the plaque reduces the lumen diameter about 50%. Such a limited lesion only exerts effects during the elevated flow requirements of maximal exercise. Symptoms occur at periods when the flow demand of the muscle beyond the stenosis exceeds the supply. During the periods of inadequate perfusion, a cramping or aching sensation occurs in the muscles. Simply standing in place reduces the demand, and all symptoms disappear. The term *intermittent claudication* is used for this symptom pattern. Most commonly, the patient initially experiences pain limited to the muscles of the lower leg (calf). As the occlusive disease worsens, there is further limitation of flow and the patient walks shorter and shorter distances before stopping to rest. With more severe disease, symptoms may appear in both the calf and the thigh. Commonly, the calf symptoms are more severe than those in the thigh, as the more distal bed has more severe flow limitation. Atypical distribution of occlusion may present unusual pain patterns. For example, isolated hypogastric artery disease can produce buttock claudication without symptoms in the thigh or calf. Patients with claudication only have arterial insufficiency during exercise. As a result, there may be pulses that are palpable at rest, but these cannot be found immediately after exercise. This phenomenon is often called the *disappearing pulse*. The extremity skin and temperature are unaffected.

A more serious clinical picture occurs when the occlusive disease reaches the point that there is reduced flow at rest. This condition usually occurs when there are significant plaques at two or more levels. The net effect at the distal-most part is the sum of the effects of the stenoses at each level. The chronic, severe ischemia results in *rest pain*, with which the worst symptoms occur in the toes and the forefoot. Patients often complain that the pain is most bothersome at night, frequently awakening them from sleep. Relief can be obtained by dangling the foot over the side of the bed or walking a few steps. There is no muscular pain in the calf or the thigh at rest, but claudication will come on at a very short walking distance. Any injury to the foot or the toes may not heal due to inadequate skin perfusion. These patients are categorized as being in a *limb threat* situation, as loss of limb is highly probable unless the circulation can be improved. Physical examination shows chronic changes in the appearance of the foot and lower leg, including a temperature gradient in the lower leg, thinning of the skin, loss of hair, atrophy of sweat follicles with loss of sweating, and poor healing of ulcers or lacerations. There is delayed capillary filling, causing pallor on elevation of the extremity and dependent rubor. It is important not to consider night muscle cramps or painful diabetic neuropathy as symptoms of ischemic rest pain.

Most of the inflammatory and vasospastic conditions involve primarily the hands or the feet, sparing the proximal vessels in the arms or the legs. The involved vessels are the palmar or pedal arches and the distal branches. As a result, these patients do not present with claudication but only with distal ischemic symptoms, including severe pain, skin and intrinsic muscle atrophy, and digital ulceration. Buerger's disease is an exception, with occlusive lesions in both the medium- and small-size arteries in the extremity. As a result, the presentation of Buerger's disease can include both claudica-tion and advanced ischemic symptoms in the foot. Unlike the fixed lesions of vasculitis, vasospasm is intermittent and usually is triggered by a specific stimulus, such as cold exposure. During the episodes of spasm, there can be pain, but this improves as the episode ends. Between episodes, the extremity may appear normal and the patient reports no symptoms. Although vasospasm can be very symptomatic, it does not have the same poor prognosis as vasculitis, which can include problems of chronic ulceration and possible digit loss.

An arterial embolus or a dissection involving peripheral arterial branches presents with a sudden onset of ischemic symptoms, including severe pain, pallor, coolness, weakness, and numbness. The extremity is most symptomatic initially, with gradual improvement over the ensuing hours to days, as collateral branches compensate for the flow deficit. There can also be deterioration from the initial presentation, resulting from extension of the thrombosis distal to the initial obstruction.

CLINICAL ISSUES FOR THE VASCULAR LABORATORY

The initial evaluation of the patient with vascular disease comes from the history and the physical examination. There are, however, limitations of this clinical assessment. Early degrees of arterial pathology may not be detected, and gradual progression is difficult to determine. In addition, findings by different examiners may result in different interpretations. Noninvasive testing serves to refine the evaluation by providing objective measurements of anatomic and physiologic parameters. These studies can be repeated at intervals to provide documentation of changes in the patient's status. The choice of the appropriate examination requires knowledge of the possible disease processes and an understanding of the different techniques, including applicability and limitations. In some situations, a simple physiologic test provides the answer, whereas in others, an extensive duplex ultrasound scan is required.

Establishing the Diagnosis

Most patients present with some symptoms, but the etiology is not always clear. The claudication of arterial disease may not always fit the typical description, and on the other hand, other leg pain patterns may be difficult to distinguish. Diagnostic possibilities include degenerative joint disease, chronic venous insufficiency, and neurogenic pain patterns. The latter are often called *pseudoclaudication* or *neurogenic claudication*. These symptoms are caused by nerve compression or irritation associated with degenerative spine changes, disc disease, or spinal stenosis. Objective measurements with noninvasive tests may help to define the presence or absence of arterial occlusive disease. Simple physiologic tests, such as the ankle pressure index or distal plethysmographic measurements, when abnormal, can confirm that interference with blood flow is the cause of symptoms. A normal result does not exclude the diagnosis of arterial obstruction. Moderately advanced atherosclerosis may not alter blood flow at rest sufficiently to be detected by the different physiologic tests. Only when increased blood flow is induced by exercise of distal muscles is there an alteration of the recorded parameters. The exercise test is frequently used to detect early disease. Ankle pressures are measured before and after a standardized treadmill walking protocol. The test uses a low level of exercise, so that it is well tolerated by most patients. The ankle pressure in subjects without occlusive disease does not drop following exercise. A normal exercise test rules out significant occlusive disease and prompts exploration of other explanations for the symptoms. Patients with arterial disease have a decrease in extremity pressure following exercise. The magnitude of the decrease and the duration of the recovery time are related to the severity of arterial insufficiency.

Small-vessel occlusive disease can be confirmed in a similar way. Pressures and waveforms (Doppler velocity tracings or plethysmographic recordings) obtained from the digits are abnormal with significant occlusive disease. The diagnosis of vasospastic conditions is more difficult,

because the abnormality is intermittent. As with the case of early claudication, a stress test is required to induce the abnormality, with the diagnosis based upon the extent of changes observed. The most common method is to attempt to induce vasospasm with cold exposure. One simple protocol uses immersion of the whole hand in cold water, whereas a more sophisticated technique cools individual fingers. Digital waveforms or pressure measurements obtained before and after cold exposure are used to determine whether there is a significant change.

Nonocclusive arterial pathology, such as aneurysm, is usually diagnosed with a duplex ultrasound scan. Not all pulsatile extremity masses are aneurysms. Demonstration of arterial flow within the mass confirms the vascular nature of the lesion, distinguishing an aneurysm from a cystic mass adjacent to an artery. It sometimes may be difficult to distinguish a true from a false aneurysm, but the pattern of circulation within the mass aids in identification of the pathology. With a true aneurysm, the flow is from the proximal artery directly into the widening aneurysm neck. On the other hand, a pseudoaneurysm often fills from the arterial communicating tract into the mid-portion of the mass. Most communications are small, so there is a high-velocity jet going into the sac.

Duplex scanning is also used in the diagnosis of arteriovenous fistulas and malformations. These present with elevated velocities and a low-resistance waveform in the artery and continuous flow with an arterial pulsation in the vein. With an arteriovenous fistula, a high-velocity jet through the communication can be found, while with a malformation a distinct jet is not usually detected, due to the presence of many smaller communications.

Severity of Disease

Determination of the severity of arterial disease is important, both in the initial workup and in follow-up. Traditionally, physicians have used the patient's description of how far they can walk as an index of disability. The information is usually expressed in distances, such as yards or number of city blocks. Unfortunately, the patient-reported initial claudication distance, or the maximal claudication distance, is affected by a variety of factors, the most important of which is how fast the patient tries to walk. A common approach is to use the ankle/brachial pressure index at rest to reflect severity of disease. Although there is only a moderate correlation between the pressure index and maximal walking distance, the parameter provides a simple clinical measurement. Reproducibility studies have shown that the index must change by 0.15 to be considered significant. Changes are associated with clinical improvement with treatment or deterioration caused by disease progression. An important limitation of extremity pressures is that an artifactual elevation can be caused by stiff vessels. In an attempt to reduce errors, the pressure results should only be used when they correlate with Doppler or pulse volume recorder tracings. This limitation occurs most frequently in diabetic patients. Depending on the referral pattern, a laboratory may have between 5% and 20% of patients for whom pressure values cannot be used.

A standardized treadmill walking protocol is the best way to determine the functional severity of lower-extremity arterial disease. Both the initial claudication distance (the point at which symptoms first appear) and the maximum claudication distance can be determined, but the latter appears to be a better endpoint. The advantage of a walking challenge is that it addresses the specific symptom of claudication. The test can also identify other causes of ambulatory limitation, such as shortness of breath. Other methods of increasing blood flow to maximize the effects of a stenosis have been tried. These include more limited exercise with toe-rises, unilateral exercise with a pedal ergometer, and reactive hyperemia induced by 3 to 5 minutes of thigh compression with a pneumatic cuff. None of these alternatives have gained widespread use.

Another reason for determining the severity of arterial insufficiency is the assessment of wound healing potential. This is usually a concern in patients who have severe claudication and face either minor or major amputation. Routine segmental pressures have not proven to be very predictive, for a large proportion of these patients have advanced diabetes with stiff arteries. Systolic toe pressure measurements can help, as there is less calcification in the foot arteries. A number of vascular laboratories measure skin oxygenation with a transcutaneous oximeter. Values above 30 mm Hg at the level of surgery predict a high likelihood of healing. A major drawback of this method is the length of the examination. More recently, investigators have described the measurement of skin perfusion pressures to predict skin healing. A laser Doppler probe is used to detect arterial pulsation in the skin. The probe is built into a pneumatic cuff that is inflated above systolic pressure, eliminating the detection of pulsatile flow. During deflation, the cuff pressure at which a pulsatile signal returns defines the systolic endpoint of the skin. Studies have shown good correlation between transcutaneous oximetry and skin perfusion pressure. The latter technique is simpler and faster to perform.

Location of Disease

In the initial patient assessment, an overall diagnosis and an estimate of disease severity are adequate. On the other hand, when it comes time to select intervention options, it is necessary to know as accurately as possible the level or levels of occlusive lesions. For many years, segmental pressures and waveforms were the only techniques available. Detection of either a pressure gradient of more than 30 mm Hg or a qualitative change in a waveform from one segment to another defined the level of severe disease. The greatest limitation with this approach was the error that occurred in separating aortoiliac disease from disease in the thigh. Accurate thigh pressure measurement is problematic, especially in large legs. A variety of quantitative waveform analysis parameters have been tried, but none have gained popularity. The introduction of duplex ultrasound scanning has greatly enhanced our ability to locate the specific obstructive plaque. It is possible to distinguish a tight stenosis from an occlusion and to measure the length of the occlusion. These parameters are particularly important in the selection of interventional procedures. The quality of duplex studies improves continually, and we are now at the point that an increasing number of operations are planned without preliminary contrast angiography.

Follow-up

The earliest follow-up examination is the completion study in the operating room at the end of an operation. Many vascular surgeons use objective methods to verify the adequacy of a repair, especially where technical excellence is most important, such as with carotid endarterectomy or distal bypass grafts. For many years, the standard was a contrast angiogram, usually performed as a single-shot study. Increasingly, ultrasound techniques have been adopted in the operating room to reduce the need for expensive equipment and the injection of angiographic contrast. Initially, simple continuous-wave Doppler detectors were used in the operating room to detect stenoses by the increase in the audible frequency or by abnormal waveforms seen on signal processors. The introduction of the duplex scanner into the operating room greatly increased the quality and specificity of studies. Not only could a tight stenosis be detected, but nonstenotic lesions, such as dissections, intimal flaps or retained venous valves, could be seen.

Serial follow-up examination after vein bypasses in the leg and after carotid endarterectomy has been shown to yield clinical benefit. In some patients, leg symptoms will reappear if a reconstruction is deteriorating due to stenosis; however, others progress to occlusion before the patient notes that anything is wrong. Waiting until thrombosis occurs greatly reduces the possibility of long-term success with secondary repair. Physiologic tests, such as extremity pressures and waveform recording, have been done to monitor the health of vein bypasses; however, studies have demonstrated that a subset of graft patients may progress to thrombosis without significant change in the pressure index. Duplex scanning has become the method of choice to study vein grafts. Detection of an advanced stenosis allows for repair before thrombosis occurs, greatly improving long-term patency. There has been limited experience reported with surveillance of transcatheter interventions (balloon dilation, stenting). It remains to be shown whether follow-up of these interventions will have a clinical benefit regarding further intervention.

Intervention

The vascular laboratory has long been considered to have a purely diagnostic function. Recently, the ultrasound service has taken on a role in treating femoral artery false aneurysms, most frequently those resulting from catheter-based interventions. After a few reports of the success with inducing thrombosis with ultrasound-guided compression, the technique gained considerable acceptance. The duplex scanner provides real-time visualization of the filling of the aneurysm. Pressure is applied with the scan head until flow into the sac is stopped. Although successful, this technique is uncomfortable for the patient and is time consuming. The active treatment of pseudoaneurysm was substantially improved with ultrasound-guided injection of thrombin directly into the open portion of the pseudoaneurysm sac. In most cases, there is almost immediate thrombosis. Inadvertent injection of thrombin into the main artery can lead to major thrombosis in the leg, with immediate ischemia. This problem can be avoided by careful placement of the needle and by the use of a small volume of fluid for the injection.

Chapter 14

Arterial Anatomy of the Extremities

GREGORY M. KECK, MD, AND WILLIAM J. ZWIEBEL, MD

The evaluation of arterial disease of the extremities requires knowledge of vascular anatomy. This chapter provides this basic information for the upper and lower extremities. Normal anatomy, common variants, and major collateral routes[1-6] are illustrated, primarily by representative arteriograms. The chapter is formatted as a series of captioned illustrations, with the bulk of the instructional material contained within the figure captions.

It is increasingly common for arterial anatomy and pathology to be depicted non-invasively in a clinical setting with computed tomography or magnetic resonance imaging. Generally speaking, however, image quality with these modalities is not up to that of catheter angiography. We have chosen, therefore, to again use angiographic images in this chapter, as they best depict anatomic detail.

The following terms are used to describe extremity anatomy in this chapter. The *arm* is the portion of the upper extremity between the shoulder and elbow. The *forearm* is the portion between the elbow and wrist. The *thigh* is the portion of the lower extremity between the hip and knee, and the *leg* is the portion between the knee and ankle.

UPPER EXTREMITY

Normal Features

The normal arterial anatomy of the upper extremity is depicted graphically in Figure 14–1. Figures 14–2 through 14–5 are detailed arteriographic views of specific regions of the upper extremity arterial tree, beginning at the aorta and extending to the digits. These figures should be reviewed carefully, because their legends provide the instructional content.

Anatomic Variants

Many anatomic variants can occur in the arterial tree of the upper extremities. The more commonly encountered variants are presented in Table 14–1.[1-3] Familiarity with these variants can prevent confusion and error during duplex examination. An example of an upper extremity anatomic variant is presented in Figure 14–6.

Collateral Routes

Many of the tributaries seen in Figures 14–1 through 14–6 may serve as collaterals when the main arterial trunks of the upper extremity are blocked.

The following is a summary of the more common collateral routes.[2]
1. Obstruction of the proximal subclavian or brachiocephalic arteries
    a. Collateral flow from cranial and/or neck arteries to the subclavian artery distal to the obstruction (e.g., subclavian steal phenomenon)
    b. Collateral flow from pelvic, abdominal wall, and thoracic wall arteries to the subclavian artery distal to the obstruction
2. Obstruction of the distal subclavian or axillary arteries

a. Collateral flow from the thoracic wall or shoulder region to the axillary artery distal to the obstruction

3. Obstruction of the brachial artery or its branch vessels
    a. Collateral flow from the distal arm to the proximal forearm

b. Collateral flow from the mid-arm to the distal arm and/or forearm
c. Retrograde flow filling the palmar arches of the hand

Figure 14–7 shows an example of collateralization in response to radial artery occlusion.

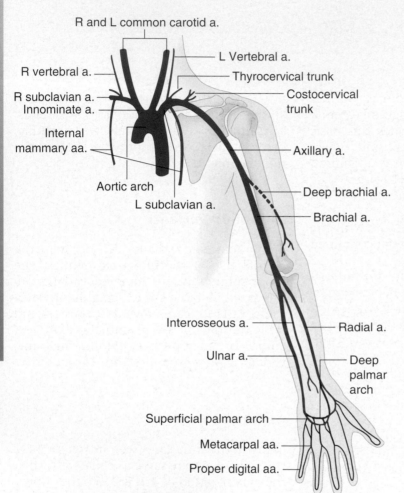

FIGURE 14–1. Arterial anatomy of the upper extremity. Note that the internal mammary arteries, which are tributaries of the subclavian arteries, are used commonly for coronary artery bypass. The deep palmar arch arises from the radial artery, and the superficial palmar arch arises from the ulnar artery. These arches may or may not communicate with each other.

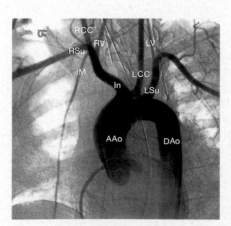

FIGURE 14–2. The aortic arch connects the ascending aorta (AAo) with the descending aorta (DAo). Three great vessels originate from the aortic arch; the innominate artery (In) originates on the right side of the arch, followed by the left common carotid artery (LCC) and the left subclavian artery (LSu). The innominate artery divides into the right common carotid artery (RCC) and the right subclavian artery (RSu). The right and left vertebral arteries (RV, LV) originate from the subclavian arteries, even though this is not apparent on the right side of this illustration. The internal mammary artery (IM) also arises from the subclavian artery.

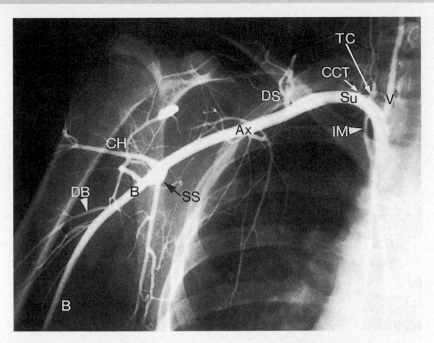

FIGURE 14–3. The subclavian artery (Su) becomes the axillary artery (Ax) at the lateral margin of the first rib. The axillary artery, in turn, becomes the brachial artery (B) after crossing the inferolateral margin of the teres major muscle.[3] The thyrocervical (TC) and costocervical (CCT) trunks are noteworthy branches of the subclavian artery, because they may be mistaken for the vertebral artery (V) during duplex examination. The multiple branches that supply the scapular musculature serve as collaterals when the subclavian or innominate arteries are obstructed. CH, circumflex humeral artery; DB, deep brachial artery; DS, dorsal scapular artery; IM, internal mammary artery; SS, subscapular artery.

FIGURE 14–4. Arterial anatomy (A) and osseous landmarks (B) at the elbow. The brachial artery (B) divides at the elbow, forming the radial (R) and ulnar (U) arteries. The interosseous artery (I) is a branch of the ulnar artery, which in some individuals continues to the wrist. RR, recurrent radial artery; UR, ulnar recurrent artery.

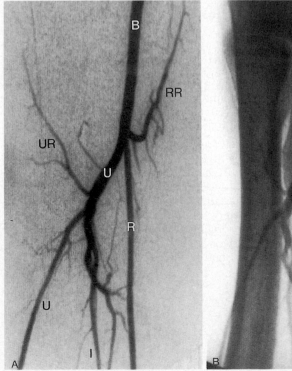
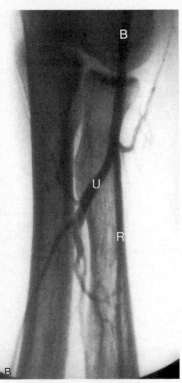

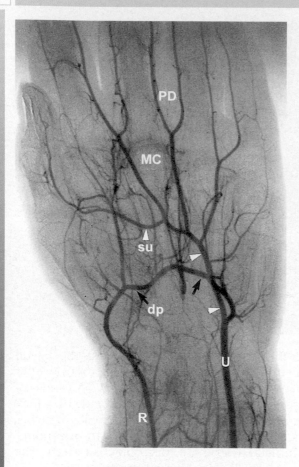

FIGURE 14–5. The radial artery (R) terminates in the deep palmar arch (dp, *black arrows*). The ulnar artery (U) terminates in the superficial palmar arch (su, *white arrowheads*). Communicating vessels usually connect the deep and superficial arches, as shown here. The metacarpal (MC; also called the common palmar digital artery or dorsal metacarpal artery) and proper palmar digital (PD) arteries are branches of the superficial and deep arches.

Table 14–1. Arterial Variants of the Upper Extremity

Structure	Variant	Frequency of Occurrence in the Population (%)
Aortic arch and great vessels	Common origin of the right brachiocephalic and left common carotid arteries	22
	Left vertebral artery origin directly from the aorta	4–6
	Common origin of both common carotid arteries	<1
Arm and forearm	Radial artery origin from the axillary artery	1–3

	Early division of the brachial artery:
	  1. High origin of the radial artery (Fig. 14–6)
	  2. Accessory (duplicated) brachial artery
		19

	Ulnar artery origin from the brachial or axillary artery	2–3
	Low origin (5–7 cm below elbow joint) of ulnar artery	<1
	Persistent median artery	2–4

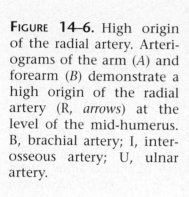

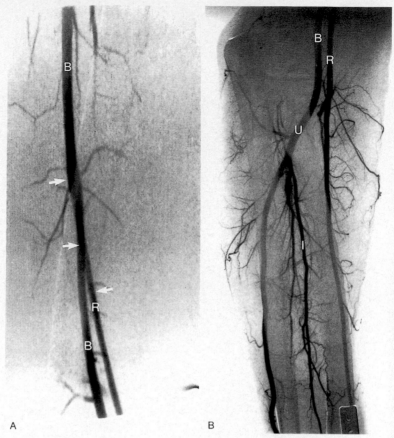

FIGURE 14–6. High origin of the radial artery. Arteriograms of the arm (*A*) and forearm (*B*) demonstrate a high origin of the radial artery (R, *arrows*) at the level of the mid-humerus. B, brachial artery; I, interosseous artery; U, ulnar artery.

A

B

LOWER EXTREMITY

Normal Anatomy

The lower extremity arterial tree begins at the aortic bifurcation, and this portion of the vasculature is included in this chapter. For details concerning abdominal vascular anatomy, see Chapter 28. The major arteries of the lower extremity are illustrated graphically in Figure 14–8. Figures 14–9 through 14–13 are angiographic depictions of the regional arterial anatomy of the lower extremity.

Anatomic Variants

The arterial anatomy of the lower extremity is fairly constant. Anatomic variations that may be encountered occasionally are presented in Table 14–2.[4] The relative infrequency of these variations is also cited in this table.

Collateral Routes

Multiple variations are possible in the collateral routes that circumvent lower extremity arterial obstruction. The following is an outline of the more common collateral pathways.[4,5] It is important for vascular laboratory personnel to be familiar, in general terms, with the more commonly seen collateral pathways, as illustrated in Figures 14–14 through 14–18:

1. Distal aorta or bilateral common iliac artery obstruction
   a. Collateral flow from thoracic and abdominal wall arteries to pelvic arteries distal to the obstruction
   b. Collateral flow from arteries of the bowel to pelvic arteries distal to the obstruction
   c. Collateral flow from lumbar arteries to pelvic arteries distal to the obstruction

Text continued on p. 273

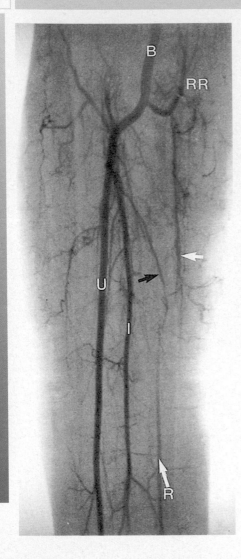

FIGURE 14–7. Collateral circulation in radial artery occlusion. The distal portion of the radial artery (R, *large arrow*) is primarily filled in a retrograde manner from the superficial and deep palmar arches (not shown). Antegrade collateral supply also is provided by the recurrent radial artery (RR, *small white arrow*) and by the interosseous artery (I, *small black arrow*). B, brachial artery; U, ulnar artery.

Table 14–2. Arterial Variants of the Lower Extremity

Variant	Frequency of Occurrence in the Population (%)
Duplication of the superficial femoral artery	Rare
High bifurcation of the popliteal artery	~4
High bifurcation of the popliteal artery, with the peroneal arising from the anterior tibial artery	~2
Normal level bifurcation of the popliteal artery, with the peroneal arising from the anterior tibial artery	Rare
Absent posterior tibial artery; may have distal reconstitution at the level of the ankle by way of the peroneal artery	1–5
Hypoplasia or aplasia of the anterior tibial artery with resultant absence of dorsalis pedis pulse	4–12
Anomalous location of the dorsalis pedis artery	8

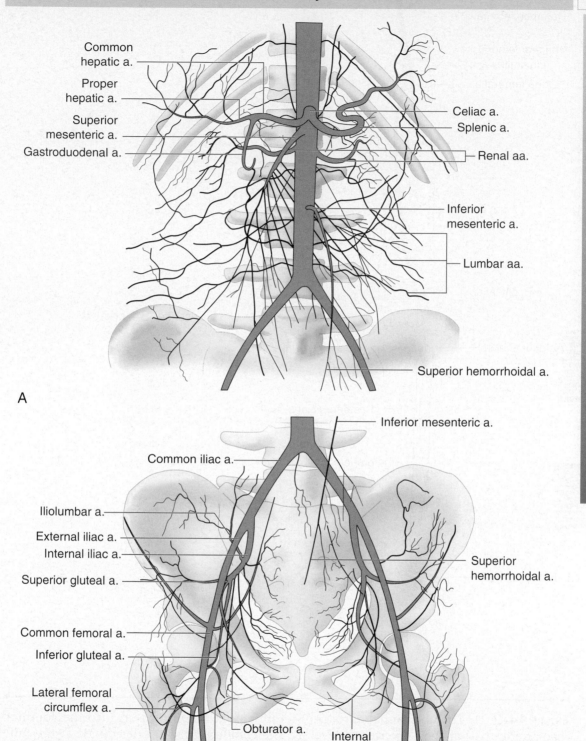

FIGURE 14–8. Arterial anatomy of the abdomen (*A*), pelvis (*B*), and lower extremity (*C*).

Continued

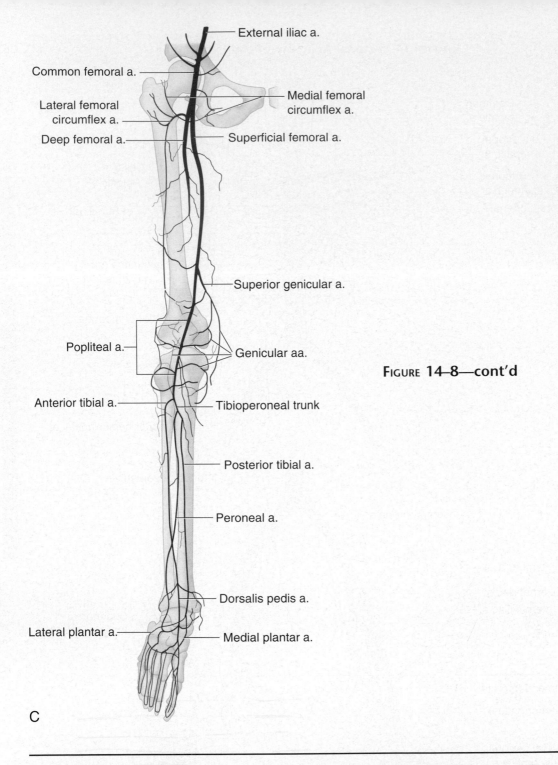

External iliac a.

Common femoral a.

Lateral femoral
circumflex a.

Deep femoral a.

Medial femoral
circumflex a.

Superficial femoral a.

Superior genicular a.

Popliteal a.

Genicular aa.

Anterior tibial a.

Tibioperoneal trunk

Posterior tibial a.

Peroneal a.

Dorsalis pedis a.

Lateral plantar a.

Medial plantar a.

C

FIGURE 14–8—cont'd

FIGURE 14–9. *A*, The abdominal aorta (Ao) terminates at its bifurcation into the common iliac arteries (CI) at the L4 vertebral level. *B*, The common iliac arteries divide at the lumbosacral junction into the internal (II) and external iliac (EI) arteries. The internal iliac artery (also called the hypogastric artery) supplies the pelvic viscera and musculature. The branches of this artery become important collateral routes, as seen in other figures. The external iliac artery is continuous with the common femoral artery at the inguinal ligament, as shown in Figure 14–10. *C*, Three-dimensional, shaded surface display of the aorta and iliofemoral arterial segment. The anatomy is dramatically illustrated by three-dimensional reconstruction methods, as well as by other methods for illustrating vascular anatomy noninvasively. C, celiac artery; H, hepatic artery; IMA, inferior mesenteric artery; R, left renal artery; rRH, replaced right hepatic artery; S, splenic artery; SMA, superior mesenteric artery.

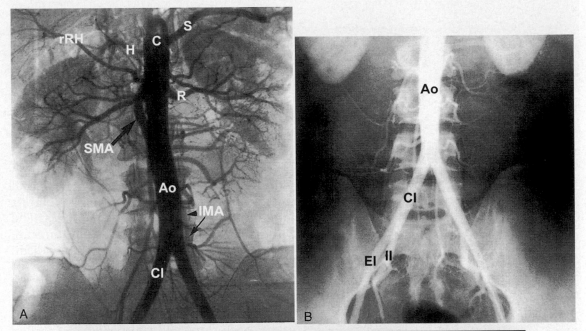

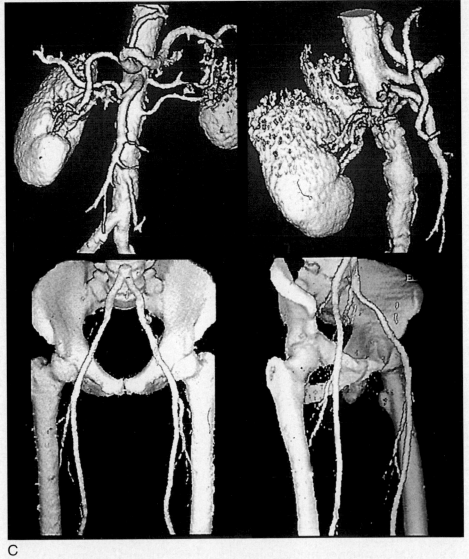

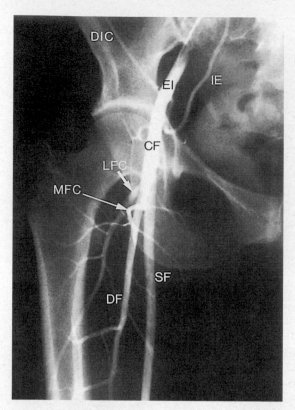

FIGURE 14-10. The external iliac artery (EI) is continuous with the common femoral artery (CF), which is a short segment (about 4 cm long). The common femoral artery bifurcates, forming the superficial (SF) and deep (DF) femoral arteries. A prominent branch, called the lateral femoral circumflex artery (LFC), arises dorsally, just before the common femoral artery divides. The superficial femoral artery continues throughout the thigh without major branches. The deep femoral artery, also called the profunda femoris artery, has multiple muscular branches. The proximal muscular branches communicate with the pelvic arteries, and the distal branches communicate with tributaries of the popliteal artery at the knee. Thus, the deep femoral artery is an important collateral route, for both iliac and superficial femoral artery occlusion. DIC, deep iliac circumflex artery; IE, inferior epigastric artery; MFC, medial femoral circumflex artery.

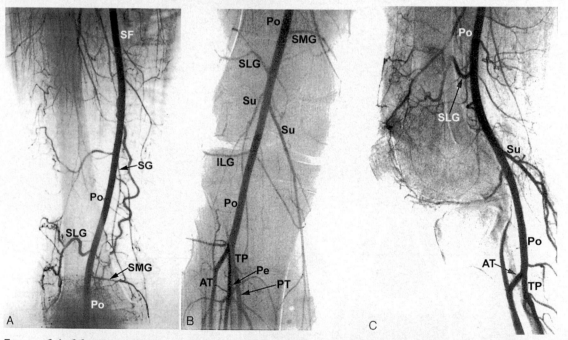

FIGURE 14-11. Anteroposterior (*A*, *B*) and lateral (*C*) views of the superficial femoral and popliteal arteries. In the distal portion of the thigh, the superficial femoral artery (SF) enters the adductor canal and becomes the popliteal artery (Po). This junction is also marked by the supreme genicular artery (SG). The popliteal artery passes behind the knee and ends, in most individuals, by bifurcating into the anterior tibial artery (AT) and the tibioperoneal trunk (TP). The genicular and sural arteries are important collateral routes for both superficial femoral and popliteal arterial obstruction. ILG, inferior lateral genicular artery; Pe, peroneal artery; PT, posterior tibial artery; SG, supreme genicular artery; SLG, superior lateral genicular artery; SMG, superior medial genicular artery; Su, sural artery.

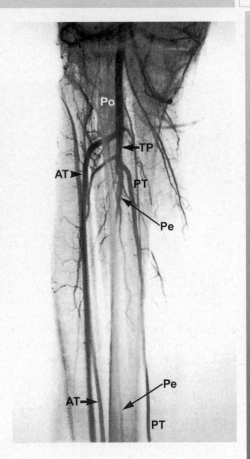

FIGURE 14–12. The anterior tibial artery (AT) courses anterolaterally from its origin and passes through the interosseous membrane. It then courses along the anterolateral aspect of the leg to the foot. The tibioperoneal trunk (TP) is of variable length and usually bifurcates into the peroneal (Pe) and posterior tibial (PT) arteries. The peroneal artery, also seen in Figure 14–11B, extends down the leg to just above the ankle. The posterior tibial artery continues along a posteromedial course to the foot. Po, popliteal artery.

FIGURE 14–13. Oblique view of the right foot. The anterior tibial artery (AT) courses onto the dorsum of the foot, where it becomes the dorsalis pedis artery (DP). The posterior tibial artery (PT) passes behind the medial malleolus and shortly thereafter bifurcates, forming the medial plantar (MP) and lateral plantar (LP) arteries. The plantar arch of the foot is formed by the union of the lateral plantar artery with the plantar metatarsal branch (not shown) of the dorsalis pedis artery. The plantar arch gives rise to the metatarsal and digital branches.

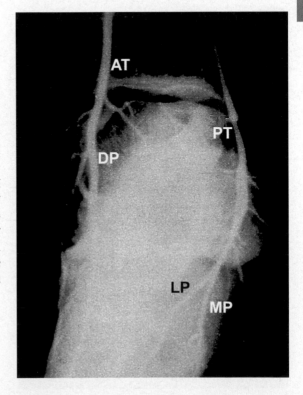

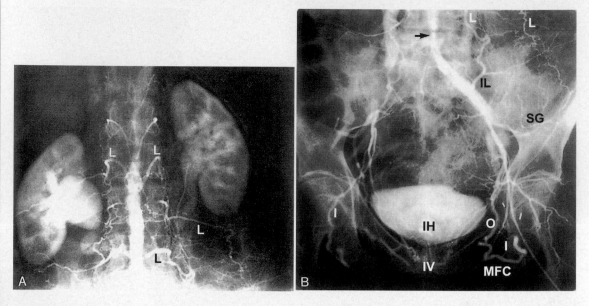

FIGURE 14–14. Aortic and iliac obstruction—superior (*A*) and inferior (*B*) segments. The site of a severe aortic stenosis is indicated by the *black arrow* in *B*. The right common iliac artery is occluded, and the left external iliac artery is severely stenotic. The following collateral routes are apparent: (1) lumbar arteries (L) → to the iliolumbar (IL) and superior gluteal (SG) arteries; (2) obturator internis artery (O) → to the median femoral circumflex artery (MFC), circumventing the left external iliac obstruction; (3) inferior hemorrhoidal (IH) and inferior vesicle (IV) branches across the pelvis from the left to the right internal iliac system (circumventing the right common iliac occlusion).

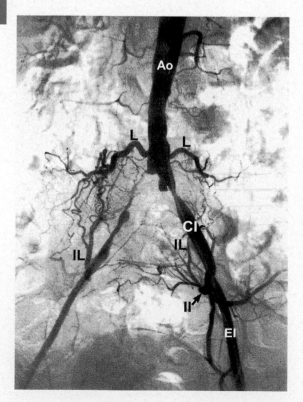

FIGURE 14–15. Right common iliac artery occlusion and left common iliac artery (CI) stenosis are circumvented by lumbar (L) collaterals, which communicate with iliolumbar (IL) branches of the internal iliac artery (II). The internal iliac artery, in turn, restores flow to the external iliac (EI) artery. Ao, aorta.

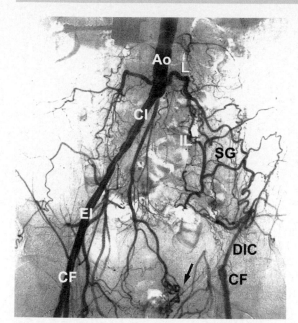

FIGURE 14–16. Hemorrhoidal collaterals (*arrow*) are of particular interest in this illustration. These branches of the inferior mesenteric artery illustrate the potential for collateralization from arteries that supply the gut. Prominent lumbar (L) → to gluteal (IL, SG) collaterals are evident on the left side. Ao, aorta; CF, common femoral artery; CI, common iliac artery; DIC, deep iliac circumflex artery; EI, external iliac artery; IL, iliolumbar artery; SG, superior gluteal artery.

2. Unilateral common iliac artery obstruction
    a. Collateral flow from contralateral iliac and/or femoral arteries to arteries of the pelvis or thigh distal to the obstruction
    b. Collateral pathways as just mentioned, with supply to the ipsilateral pelvic arteries
3. External iliac and common femoral artery obstruction
    a. Collaterals arising primarily from ipsilateral pelvic arteries or contralateral pelvic and/or femoral arteries to supply arteries of the proximal thigh distal to the obstruction
    b. Previously mentioned pathways also possibly involved to varying degrees
4. Deep femoral artery obstruction
    a. Collateral flow from proximal ipsilateral pelvic arteries, contralateral pelvic arteries, and/or contralateral femoral arteries to the deep femoral artery distal to the obstruction
    b. Collateral flow from the distal superficial femoral or popliteal arteries to the distal deep femoral artery
5. Superficial femoral or popliteal artery obstruction
    a. Collateral flow from the deep femoral artery to the distal superficial femoral artery or to the popliteal artery
    b. Collateral flow from the distal superficial femoral artery to the popliteal artery or to the proximal trifurcation vessels in the calf

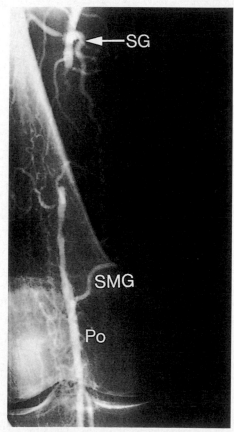

FIGURE 14–17. Occlusion of the proximal popliteal artery (Po) is circumvented by genicular collaterals (supreme genicular, SG → to superior medial genicular, SMG).

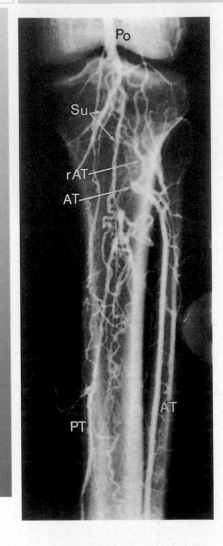

FIGURE 14–18. Distal popliteal (Po) artery occlusion is circumvented as follows: 1) sural (Su) and small muscular branches → to the recurrent anterior tibial artery (rAT), which supplies the anterior tibial artery (AT); 2) sural (Su) and small muscular branches → to the posterior tibial artery (PT).

   c. Collateral flow from the proximal to distal popliteal artery and/or popliteal artery to trifurcation vessels

6. Obstruction of trifurcation arteries

   a. Collateral flow from patent proximal calf branches to distal arteries in the lower leg or ankle

   b. Collateral flow from distal peroneal branches to distal anterior or posterior tibial arteries

References

1. Kadir S: Arteriography of the thoracic aorta. In Kadir S (ed): Diagnostic Angiography. Philadelphia, WB Saunders, 1986, pp 124–171.

2. Kadir S: Arteriography of the upper extremities. In Kadir S (ed): Diagnostic Angiography. Philadelphia, WB Saunders, 1986, pp 172–206.

3. Rose SC, Kadir S: Arterial anatomy of the upper extremity. In Kadir S (ed): Atlas of Normal and Variant Angiographic Anatomy. Philadelphia, WB Saunders, 1991, pp 55–95.

4. Kadir S: Arteriography of the lower extremities. In Kadir S (ed): Diagnostic Angiography. Philadelphia, WB Saunders, 1986, pp 254–307.

5. Stieghorst MF, Crummy AB: Lower extremity arterial anatomy and collateral routs. In Zwiebel WJ (ed): Introduction to Vascular Ultrasonography, 2nd ed. Orlando, FL, Grune & Stratton, 1986, pp 278–303.

6. Muller RF, Figley MM, Rogoff SM, DeWeese JA: Arteries of the Abdomen, Pelvis and Lower Extremity. Rochester, NY, Eastman Kodak.

Chapter 15

Nonimaging Physiologic Tests for Assessment of Lower Extremity Arterial Occlusive Disease

R. Eugene Zierler, MD

The basic purpose of lower extremity noninvasive testing is to document both the presence and severity of arterial disease. The importance of such documentation has been underscored by the study of Marinelli and colleagues,[1] in which 458 diabetic patients were evaluated prospectively for lower extremity arterial insufficiency. Arterial occlusive disease was documented by objective testing in 31% of patients who gave no history of claudication and in 21% with a normal physical examination.

Digital subtraction arteriography may also be used to document lower extremity arterial disease. This technique has been the standard method for preoperative assessment, and the precise anatomic information provided may be essential in planning reconstructive arterial operations. Arteriography has certain limitations, however, particularly in estimating the hemodynamic significance of stenoses. Single-plane views may underestimate the severity of disease whenever plaques do not produce concentric narrowing. The addition of multiple views may improve accuracy to some extent, but even then, the problem of interpretation is considerable.[2–5] Three-dimensional magnetic resonance angiography or computed tomographic angiography ameliorates the problems of single-plane angiography, but currently, these methods are not widely used for extremity arteriography. Finally, the presence of occlusive disease at multiple levels may make it difficult to predict angiographically which

segment is most responsible for ischemic symptoms.[6,7]

The limitations of arteriography, together with the inherent invasiveness of this procedure, were the stimulus for development of noninvasive physiologic methods for studying the arterial circulation of the lower extremities. Among the many devices and techniques that have been described,[8] those that employ Doppler ultrasound have been most widely applied and thoroughly evaluated. This chapter reviews Doppler and plethysmographic approaches to the evaluation of lower extremity arterial disease. The techniques described do not produce images of the arteries; hence, they are described as nonimaging or indirect methods. These techniques should not be confused with duplex sonography, which produces images of blood vessels using B-mode ultrasound. Duplex sonography of the lower extremities is discussed in Chapter 18.

INSTRUMENTATION

Doppler Flowmeters

The transmitting frequency of Doppler instruments used for peripheral arterial examinations is in the range of 2 to 10 MHz. Because the depth in tissue to which the ultrasound beam penetrates is inversely proportional to the transmitting frequency, lower frequencies are best suited for examining deeply located vessels, such as those in the thigh. As noted in Chapter 2, the

Doppler effect refers to the shift in frequency that occurs when sound is reflected from a moving object. The Doppler shift in vascular diagnosis varies from a few hundred to several thousand cycles per second, and this signal can be amplified to provide an audible signal with a frequency (or pitch) that is directly proportional to blood velocity.

The simplest Doppler instruments used in peripheral vascular diagnosis are pocket-sized units with the audio output presented through earphones or a loudspeaker. These are satisfactory for a rapid bedside arterial or venous examination. For more elaborate studies, a direction-sensing Doppler flowmeter (directional Doppler) is necessary to separate the forward- and reverse-flow components normally present in peripheral arteries.[9] The direction of flow may be indicated through stereo headphones, by deflections on a pair of meters, or as an analogue waveform on a strip chart recorder.

Pocket-sized Doppler devices and many directional instruments operate in the continuous-wave mode. Because these instruments provide no information regarding depth in tissue or distance from the ultrasound source, Doppler shifts resulting from blood flow in superimposed vessels are summed in the audible or analogue output. However, arterial and venous signals are easily distinguished by their different flow characteristics: Venous flow produces low-frequency signals that vary with respiration, whereas arterial flow is associated with relatively high-frequency signals having pulsatile components that correspond to the cardiac cycle. Failure to obtain a Doppler signal from an artery usually indicates occlusion; however, extremely low flow rates (<2 cm/sec) do not produce a detectable Doppler shift.[10]

With pulsed-wave ultrasound, it is possible to detect flow at discrete points along the sound beam.[11] This technique eliminates the problem of superimposed signals and permits characterization of flow patterns at specific sites in tissue. Pulsed-wave Doppler is employed in the duplex scanner, which combines B-mode imaging and Doppler flow detection.[12–14] Duplex scanning with spectral analysis of pulsed Doppler signals is used widely to assess cerebral, abdominal, and extremity arteries.[15–19] A more detailed discussion of basic principles and instrumentation in Doppler ultrasound is given in Chapters 2 and 3.

Plethysmographs

Plethysmographic techniques all rely on the measurement of volume changes in the extremities. Because these changes are primarily a result of alterations in blood volume, plethysmographic measurements can be used to assess blood flow parameters such as arterial pulsations and limb blood pressure. Most plethysmographs used in the noninvasive vascular laboratory measure volume indirectly, based on changes in limb circumference, electrical impedance, or reflectivity of infrared light.

The air-filled plethysmograph uses pneumatic cuffs that are placed around the limb being studied and inflated to a pressure in the range of 10 to 65 mm Hg.[20] This instrument is considered to be "segmental" because it measures only those volume changes in the limb segments surrounded by the cuffs. Enlargement of the enclosed limb segment with each arterial pulse compresses the air in the cuff, and the resulting increase in cuff pressure is recorded by a pressure transducer. Although the frequency response of air-filled plethysmographs is low (8 to 20 Hz), this method generally provides accurate volume pulse waveforms.

Strain-gauge plethysmography uses small silicone rubber tubes filled with mercury or a liquid-metal alloy.[21] This gauge is wrapped around the limb being studied and, as the encircled segment expands or contracts, the length of the strain gauge changes. Because the electric resistance of the liquid-metal alloy in the gauge is proportional to its length, changes in limb circumference result in corresponding changes in the voltage drop across the gauge. Assuming that the limb resembles a cylinder, changes in limb circumference can be used to calculate changes in limb volume.[22] Thus, changes in gauge length or resistance are related to variations in volume. The high-frequency response of strain-gauge plethysmographs (up to 100 Hz) makes them particularly well suited for accurate recording of volume pulses in the limbs.[23] However, because they are also more sensitive and difficult to use in the clinical setting, this approach has not been used as widely as the other plethysmographic techniques.

Impedance plethysmography is based on the principle that the resistive impedance of a body segment is inversely proportional to its total fluid content. Therefore, changes in the blood volume of a limb are reflected by changes in electric impedance.[23] The instrumentation usually includes four electrodes: an outer pair to send a weak current through the limb and an inner pair to sense the voltage drop. Impedance plethysmographs are relatively simple to operate, and the results are easy to interpret. Impedance plethysmography has been one of the most popular indirect methods for the noninvasive diagnosis of lower extremity deep vein thrombosis.

The sensor of the photoelectric plethysmograph contains an infrared light–emitting diode and a phototransistor. When this sensor is placed on the limb, the infrared light is transmitted into the superficial layers of the skin and the reflected portion is received by the phototransistor. The resulting signal is proportional to the quantity of red blood cells in the cutaneous circulation.[23] Although the photoelectric method does not measure actual volume changes and is therefore not a true plethysmographic technique, the pulse waveforms obtained closely resemble those acquired with strain-gauge instruments. Photoelectric plethysmographs are frequently used in the vascular laboratory to detect blood flow when the application of Doppler or other plethysmographic techniques is especially difficult. For example, this technique can be used to detect arterial pulsations in the terminal portions of the digits.

Recording Devices

The nonimaging or indirect lower extremity arterial evaluation is based primarily on the noninvasive measurement of systolic blood pressures, the audible characteristics of arterial Doppler signals, and analogue waveforms derived from the Doppler signal. Although it is not usually necessary, the Doppler signals may be recorded on audiotape for subsequent analysis and review.

A simple device for generating an analogue waveform on a strip chart recorder is the zero crossing detector. Although this instrument is subject to errors and artifacts related to signal-to-noise ratio, amplitude dependency, and transient response,[24] it provides a graphic representation of the Doppler signal suitable for qualitative interpretation. Spectral analysis and color flow imaging, as discussed in Chapter 3, are alternative methods for Doppler signal processing that overcome the inherent limitations of the analogue waveform. These techniques are usually considered part of duplex scanning.

Equipment for Indirect Arterial Testing

The following is a description of the commonly used equipment for indirect lower extremity testing:

1. The qualitative assessment of arterial flow patterns requires a direction-sensing continuous-wave Doppler device and a strip chart recorder coupled with a zero crossing detector.
2. The measurement of segmental systolic blood pressures in the extremities requires pneumatic cuffs of appropriate size, a manometer to measure cuff pressure, and a means for detecting distal flow. Any continuous-wave Doppler or plethysmographic device can be used as a flow detector. The photoelectric plethysmograph is particularly valuable in situations in which low flow velocities or arterial wall calcification makes Doppler flow detection difficult.

A standard mercury or aneroid manometer is used to measure cuff pressure. Although cuff inflation can be accomplished manually, the examination is facilitated by using a rapid cuff inflator with a built-in manometer and an external air source.

Cuff width is an important consideration in measurement of limb blood pressure.[25] To minimize cuff artifact, the cuff width should be at least 50% greater than the diameter of the limb in which pressure is being measured. The use of smaller cuffs results in the recording of falsely high pressures. Some laboratories use large cuffs, 18 to 20 cm wide, for the thigh and smaller, 12-cm-wide cuffs around the calf and ankle. The large thigh cuff allows only a single pressure measurement above the knee. An alternative method uses four 11-cm-wide cuffs placed at high-thigh (HT), above-knee (AK), below-knee (BK), and ankle levels. If the cuff artifact is properly accounted for, this technique can provide useful information on the distribution of occlusive arterial lesions in the lower extremity.[10,26]

3. An electronic treadmill is required for exercise testing of patients with symptoms of lower limb claudication. One standard protocol uses a speed of 2 mph on a 12% grade; however, the speed and grade can be varied according to the individual limitations of each patient.[27]

4. The vascular laboratory should be kept warm enough to ensure the comfort of patients who must lie or walk with their limbs exposed during noninvasive testing. Cold-induced vasospasm may make arterial flow signals difficult to detect in patients with arterial occlusive disease. To avoid this problem, electric blankets are useful for keeping patients warm on the examining table.

METHODS AND PHYSIOLOGIC BASIS FOR INDIRECT ARTERIAL TESTING

Measurement of Arterial Pressure

In the arterial circulation, peak systolic pressure is amplified as the pulse wave progresses down the lower limb.[28] This amplification is a result of reflected waves originating from the relatively high peripheral resistance and differences in compliance between the central and peripheral arteries. Thus, the systolic pressure measured at the ankle is normally higher than that in the upper arm. However, the diastolic and mean pressures gradually decrease as the pulse wave moves distally.

Diastolic pressure in the lower limb is reduced only in the presence of severe proximal stenosis, but the peak systolic pressure decreases with lesser degrees of disease.[29] Therefore, determination of systolic blood pressure is the most reliable pressure parameter for diagnosis of arterial narrowing. Normally, the mean pressure drop along the main arteries of the limb is minimal. The term *critical stenosis* has been used to describe the degree of narrowing that produces a significant drop in distal pressure or flow.[30] In the resting state, distal pressure is reduced by stenoses that decrease luminal diameter by about 50% or more. Because the critical stenosis value is flow dependent, lesser degrees of narrowing may be detected by increasing flow with exercise or reactive hyperemia.

It should be emphasized that blood pressure and flow are not necessarily altered to the same extent by arterial occlusive disease. Resting calf blood flow in patients with intermittent claudication seldom differs significantly from that measured in normal individuals.[31] Normal flow can be maintained distal to arterial stenoses by a compensatory decrease in peripheral resistance, which results in a lowered peripheral pressure.

Ankle Pressure

The systolic pressure at any level of the lower extremity can be measured by positioning a pneumatic cuff at the desired site. Any patent artery distal to the cuff that is accessible to Doppler ultrasound can be used for flow detection, but the posterior tibial (PT) and dorsalis pedis (DP) arteries are usually most convenient. When the cuff is inflated to above systolic pressure, the arterial flow signal disappears. As cuff pressure is gradually lowered to slightly below systolic pressure, the flow signal reappears, and the pressure at which flow resumes is recorded as the systolic pressure. It is important to recognize that the level of pressure measurement is determined by cuff position and not by the site of Doppler flow detection.

In general, measurement of ankle systolic pressure is the most valuable physiologic test for assessing the arterial circulation in the lower limb. If the pressure measured by a cuff placed just above the malleoli is less than that of the upper arm, proximal occlusive disease in the arteries to the lower limb is invariably present.[21,32,33] In addition, the degree of reduction in ankle systolic pressure is proportional to the severity of arterial obstruction.[33] Patients with severe arterial occlusive disease and ischemic rest pain usually have ankle systolic pressures below 40 mm Hg. Occlusive lesions in the small arteries distal to the ankle cannot be detected by this method.

Ankle-Brachial Index

Because the ankle systolic pressure varies with the central aortic pressure, it is desirable to compare each ankle pressure measurement with the simultaneous aortic pressure. The brachial systolic pressure measured by an upper arm cuff is essentially equal to central aortic pressure, assuming the subclavian and axillary arteries are not obstructed. The ratio of ankle systolic pressure to brachial systolic pressure is called the ankle-brachial index or ABI. (Alternative but equivalent terms are *ankle-pressure index* and *ankle-arm index*.) The use of this index compensates for variation in central perfusion pressure and allows for direct comparison of serial tests.[32]

In the absence of proximal arterial occlusive disease, the ankle-brachial index is greater than 1.0, with a mean value of 1.11 ± 0.10.[34] However, because of variability related to this pressure measurement technique, values greater than 0.90 are typically interpreted as normal. Although the ankle-brachial index does not discriminate among occlusions at various levels, in general, limbs with single-level occlusions have

indexes greater than 0.5, and limbs with lesions at multiple levels have indexes less than 0.5.[33]

The ankle-brachial index provides a general guide to the degree of functional disability in the lower extremity. In limbs with intermittent claudication, the ankle-brachial index ranges from about 0.2 to 1.0, with a mean value of 0.59 ± 0.15.[34] This rather wide range is explained by differing levels of physical activity and pain tolerance among individuals. The ankle-brachial index in limbs with ischemic rest pain ranges from 0 to 0.65, with a mean of 0.26 ± 0.13. Limbs with impending gangrene tend to have the lowest ankle pressures, with a mean ankle-brachial index of 0.05 ± 0.08. Many limbs with impending gangrene or ischemic ulceration have absent Doppler flow signals at the ankle level. Although the ankle-brachial index reflects the overall severity of arterial occlusive disease in the lower extremity, it is clear that there is considerable overlap among values from patients with different clinical presentations. Therefore, the ankle pressure index must be combined with other clinical information to determine the functional status of each patient.

Segmental Pressures in the Lower Extremity

The ankle-brachial index cannot determine the location of proximal arterial lesions, nor does it indicate the relative significance of lesions at multiple levels. Some of this information may be obtained by measuring the systolic pressure at various levels in limbs exhibiting an abnormal ankle pressure.[21] In the procedure described here, four pneumatic cuffs, 83 cm long and 11 cm wide, with 41-cm-long inflatable bladders, are used on each leg. The cuffs are applied at HT, AK, BK, and ankle levels. Systolic pressure is determined at each level using the Doppler technique outlined previously. The Doppler probe can be placed over the PT or DP arteries for all measurements (Fig. 15–1).

The systolic pressure in the proximal thigh, as measured by the four cuff method, normally exceeds brachial systolic pressure

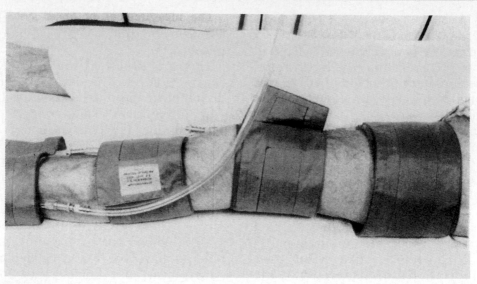

FIGURE 15–1. Cuffs are applied at high-thigh, above-knee, below-knee, and ankle levels for measurement of segmental pressures.

by 30 to 40 mm Hg. Direct intra-arterial pressure measurements have shown that the actual pressures in the brachial and common femoral arteries are identical in normal individuals;[35] however, the use of a relatively small cuff on the thigh results in a significant cuff artifact. The ratio of HT systolic pressure to brachial systolic pressure (thigh-brachial index) is normally greater than 1.2.[36] An index between 0.8 and 1.2 suggests aortoiliac stenosis, whereas an index less than 0.8 is consistent with complete iliac occlusion. Although the thigh-brachial index usually reflects iliac inflow to the common femoral artery, the combination of superficial femoral occlusion and profunda femoris stenosis also may result in reduced HT pressure.

The difference in systolic pressure between any two adjacent levels in the same leg should be less than 20 mm Hg in normal individuals.[21] Gradients in excess of 20 mm Hg usually indicate hemodynamically significant occlusive disease in the intervening arterial segment: An HT-AK gradient reflects superficial femoral disease; an AK-BK gradient reflects popliteal disease; and a BK-ankle gradient reflects disease in the tibial and peroneal arteries.[10] In addition to vertical gradients down a single leg, the horizontal gradients between corresponding segments of the two legs may also suggest the pres-

ence of occlusive lesions. The systolic pressures measured at the same level in both legs normally should not differ by more than 20 mm Hg.

Although measurement of segmental pressure gradients is still performed in many vascular laboratories, it provides only general information about the location and hemodynamic significance of arterial occlusive lesions. If more specific anatomic detail is required for clinical decision-making, direct imaging techniques such as duplex scanning must be used.

Toe Pressure

Measurement of toe pressure can be used to identify obstructive disease involving the pedal arch and digital arteries that does not produce changes in the ankle systolic pressure. Toe pressure is also valuable when the ankle pressure is found to be spuriously high because of arterial calcification. Because of the smaller size and lower flow rates of digital arteries, flow detection by Doppler methods is usually difficult. In this situation, a photoelectric plethysmograph is especially useful.

The ratio of toe systolic pressure to brachial systolic pressure (toe-brachial index) ranges from 0.80 to 0.90 in normal individuals.[37] The mean toe-brachial index is 0.35 ± 0.15 in patients with intermittent claudication and 0.11 ± 0.10 in patients with rest pain or ischemic ulceration.[38] There appears to be no significant difference in mean toe-brachial indexes between diabetic and nondiabetic patients.

Exercise and Reactive Hyperemia Testing

Lower extremity exercise and reactive hyperemia both increase limb blood flow by causing vasodilatation of peripheral resistance vessels. In limbs with normal arteries, this increased flow occurs with little or no decrease in ankle systolic pressure. When occlusive lesions are present in the main lower limb arteries, blood is diverted through high-resistance collateral pathways. Although the collateral circulation may provide adequate flow to the resting extremity with only a modest reduction in ankle pressure, the capability of collateral vessels to increase flow during exercise is limited. Pressure gradients, which are minimal at rest, may be accentuated when flow rates are increased by exercise. Thus, stress testing provides a method for detecting less severe degrees of arterial disease.

Treadmill Exercise

Standard treadmill walking exercise at 2 mph on a 12% grade is a simple way to stress the lower limb circulation.[27] Treadmill testing is advantageous because it simulates the activity that produces the patient's symptoms and determines the degree of disability under controlled physiologic conditions. It also permits an assessment of nonvascular factors that may affect performance, such as musculoskeletal or cardiopulmonary disease. The ability to perform treadmill exercise is limited, however, by patient effort, motivation, and pain tolerance.

Walking on the treadmill is continued for 5 minutes or until symptoms occur and the patient is forced to stop. The walking time and nature of any symptoms are recorded, and the ankle and arm systolic pressures are measured before and immediately after exercise. Two components of the response to exercise are evaluated: (1) the magnitude of the immediate decrease in ankle systolic pressure; and (2) the time for recovery to resting pressure. Changes in both these parameters are proportional to the severity of arterial occlusive disease.

A normal response to treadmill exercise is a slight increase or no change in the ankle systolic pressure compared with the resting value (Fig. 15–2). If the ankle pressure is decreased immediately after exercise, the test is considered positive and repeated measurements are taken at 1- to 2-minute intervals for up to 10 minutes or until the pressure returns to pre-exercise levels. When a patient is forced to stop walking because of symptomatic arterial occlusive disease, the ankle systolic pressure in the affected limb is usually less than 60 mm Hg. If symptoms occur without a significant fall in the ankle pressure, a nonvascular cause of leg pain must be considered.

The postexercise ankle pressure changes in patients with symptomatic arterial disease can be divided into three groups.[33] Ankle pressures that fall to low or unrecordable levels immediately after exercise and then rise toward resting values in 2 to 6 minutes suggest occlusion or stenosis at a single level, such as the superficial femoral artery. When ankle pressures remain decreased or unrecordable for up to 12 minutes, lesions involving multiple arterial levels are almost always present. Rarely, this pattern may occur with an isolated iliac artery occlusion. In patients with ischemic rest pain, postexercise ankle pressures may remain unrecordable for 15 minutes or more.

Reactive Hyperemia Testing

Reactive hyperemia testing is an alternate method for stressing the peripheral circulation.[39] Inflating a pneumatic cuff at thigh level to suprasystolic pressure for 3 to 5 minutes produces ischemia and vasodilatation distal to the cuff. The changes in ankle

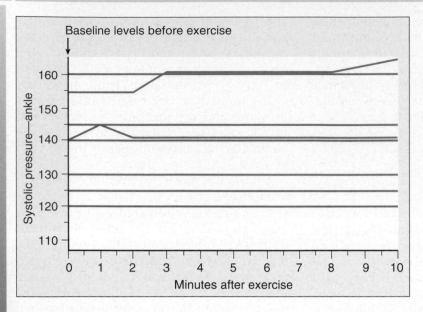

FIGURE 15–2. Ankle systolic pressure values are shown for eight normal subjects after walking on the treadmill for 5 minutes at 2 mph on a 12% grade. In each case, the ankle pressure either remained at the pre-exercise level or increased slightly. (From Strandness DE: Abnormal exercise responses after successful reconstructive arterial surgery. Surgery 59:326, 1966.)

pressure that occur on release of cuff occlusion are similar to those observed in the treadmill exercise test. However, although normal limbs do not show a drop in ankle systolic pressure after treadmill exercise, a transient drop does occur with reactive hyperemia.[40] This decrease in ankle pressure is in the range of 17% to 34%.[40] In patients with arterial disease, there is a good correlation between the maximum pressure drop with reactive hyperemia and the maximum pressure drop after treadmill exercise. However, there may be considerable overlap in the ankle pressure response to reactive hyperemia among normal subjects and patients with arterial disease.[41] Patients with single-level arterial disease show less than a 50% drop in ankle pressure with reactive hyperemia, whereas patients with multiple-level arterial disease show a pressure drop greater than 50%.[40] Reactive hyperemia testing is useful for those patients who cannot walk on the treadmill because of amputations or other physical disabilities. Treadmill exercise is generally preferred over reactive hyperemia testing, because the former produces a physiologic stress that accurately reproduces a patient's ischemic symptoms.

Doppler Signal Waveform Analysis

Qualitative analysis of the arterial flow pattern can be performed by simply listening to the Doppler audio output. An experienced examiner learns to recognize the high-pitched, harsh character and the changes in phasic components of the Doppler signal that are associated with stenoses. A graphic display of the velocity waveform permits more objective analysis. The previously described zero crossing detector is a convenient method for generating analogue waveforms on a strip chart recorder, and the output of this device closely resembles that of an electromagnetic flowmeter (Fig. 15–3).

The Arterial Analogue Waveform

The flow pattern in the main arteries of the lower extremity normally has three components or phases during each cardiac cycle. The first phase has the highest Doppler frequency and is the large, forward flow velocity peak produced by cardiac systole. This is followed by a second, brief

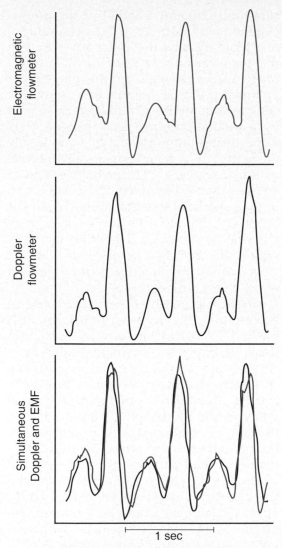

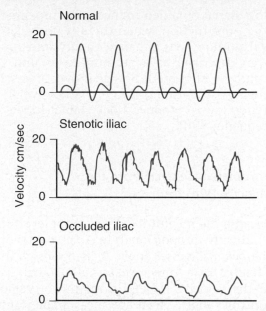

FIGURE 15–4. Velocity patterns obtained with a directional Doppler flowmeter from the femoral artery of a normal subject, a patient with a stenotic external iliac artery, and a patient with an occluded common iliac artery. The triphasic pattern in the normal artery includes a brief phase of flow reversal. Flow velocity is proportional to Doppler frequency. (From Strandness DE, Sumner DS: Hemodynamics for Surgeons. New York, Grune & Stratton, 1975, p 257.)

FIGURE 15–3. Comparison of electromagnetic and Doppler flow tracings obtained from the carotid artery of a dog shows their similarity. (From Strandness DE, Sumner DS: Hemodynamics for Surgeons. New York, Grune & Stratton, 1975, p 41.)

phase of flow reversal in early diastole and a third, low-frequency phase of forward flow in late diastole (Fig. 15–4). This triphasic flow pattern is modified by various factors, one of the most important being peripheral vascular resistance. For example, body heating, which causes vasodilation and decreased resistance, abolishes the second phase of flow reversal; the opposite occurs with vasoconstriction on exposure to cold.

When a waveform is obtained from an arterial site *distal* to a stenosis or occlusion, a single, forward velocity component is observed, with flow remaining above the zero baseline throughout the cardiac cycle. The peak systolic frequency is lower than normal, and the waveform becomes flat and rounded (see Fig. 15–4). These changes result from decreased velocity of flow and from the compensatory fall in peripheral resistance that occurs in limbs with arterial occlusive disease.

If the Doppler probe is placed *directly over* a stenotic lesion, the signal has an abnormally high peak systolic frequency. This reflects the increased flow velocity in the stenotic segment. The character of Doppler signals obtained *proximal* to an arterial obstruction depends on the capability of the collateral circulation. If there are well-developed collaterals between the Doppler probe and the point of obstruction, the waveform may be relatively normal. The flow signal obtained immediately proximal to an obstruction, when there is no collateral outflow, has a harsh quality and has been described as a "thumping" sound.[42] Failure to obtain a flow signal over a vessel indicates occlusion or, rarely, a flow velocity too low to produce a detectable Doppler frequency shift.

Parameters Derived from the Velocity Waveform

Because the magnitude of the Doppler shift is directly proportional to the cosine of the beam-to-vessel angle, θ, as discussed in Chapter 3, a direct quantitative analysis of the velocity waveform requires a value for this angle. Accurate measurement of the beam-to-vessel angle is difficult with simple, hand-held Doppler equipment; however, quantitative data can still be obtained by using ratios of Doppler shifts that are independent of the beam-to-vessel angle.

One such ratio is the pulsatility index (PI), which is calculated by dividing the peak-to-peak frequency difference by the mean frequency. Measurements for calculating PI can be based on either analogue waveforms or the output of a spectrum analyzer. The use of analogue waveforms has been criticized on the grounds that they may contain errors and artifacts.[24] Nonetheless, there is a close correlation between reduction in PI and the severity of arterial occlusive disease as assessed by arteriography and ankle pres-

sure measurement.[43] The PI of the normal common femoral artery has a mean value of 6.7. More distally, the PI increases to 8 in the popliteal and 14.1 in the PT artery.[44] These values decrease in the presence of proximal occlusive lesions. In a study that compared common femoral artery PI with intra-arterial pressure measurement, a PI value greater than or equal to 4 was highly predictive of a hemodynamically normal aortoiliac segment.[45] The predictive value of a PI less than 4 depended on the condition of the superficial femoral artery. When the superficial femoral artery was patent, a PI less than 4 indicated a hemodynamically significant aortoiliac lesion, but a low PI value with an occluded superficial femoral artery was not diagnostic.

Another approach to velocity waveform analysis is the Laplace transform (LT) method.[46,47] For LT analysis, the waveform shape is expressed mathematically by a curve-fitting technique, and a damping coefficient that indicates lumen size is calculated. A comparison of common femoral artery PI and LT damping values indicated that the LT method was more sensitive in the detection of iliac artery stenoses.[46] Furthermore, the LT damping results were not affected by the presence or absence of occlusive disease in the superficial femoral artery. Thus, LT damping would be a more useful diagnostic test than PI in patients with multiple-level arterial occlusive disease.

A summary of the measurements and indexes used in lower extremity arterial diagnosis is given in Table 15–1.

Table 15–1. Summary of Measurements and Indexes for Assessment of Lower Extremity Arterial Disease

Parameter	Interpretation
Ankle systolic pressure	Normally exceeds brachial systolic pressure by about 10%
Ankle-brachial index	Normally >1.0 (values >0.90 typically interpreted as normal)
High-thigh systolic pressure	Normally 30–40 mm Hg > brachial systolic pressure
Thigh-brachial index	Normally >1.2
Segmental pressure gradients	Normally <20 mm Hg between adjacent levels on the same leg or the same levels on the two legs
Toe systolic pressure	Normally 80%–90% of brachial systolic pressure
Treadmill exercise test	Normal walking time 5 min without symptoms or drop in ankle systolic pressure (2 mph, 12% grade)

Plethysmographic Pulse Forms

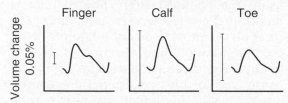

FIGURE 15–5. Normal plethysmographic volume pulses. *Vertical bars* indicate a 0.05% volume change. The dicrotic notch can be seen best on the downslope of the finger volume pulse. (From Strandness DE, Sumner DS: Hemodynamics for Surgeons. New York, Grune & Stratton, 1975, p 227.)

Plethysmographic Assessment of Arterial Flow

Pulse Plethysmography

The soft tissues of the extremities expand and contract as blood moves through them with each cardiac cycle. By using a plethysmograph, these changes can be detected as a volume pulse (Fig. 15–5). Tissue volume initially increases during systole when arterial inflow exceeds venous outflow. The volume of the part decreases during diastole as inflow diminishes and outflow predominates. There is often a brief period of retrograde flow in the peripheral arteries during early diastole, and this flow reversal produces the dicrotic notch on the downslope of the volume pulse.

Although segmental plethysmography of the limbs can be performed with either air-filled or strain-gauge instruments, the air-filled method has been most popular.[20] As shown in Figure 15–6, the normal volume pulse rises rapidly to a sharp peak during systole and falls more slowly in diastole. The downslope of the normal volume pulse is bowed toward the baseline and includes the dicrotic notch mentioned earlier. With proximal arterial occlusive disease, one of the earliest changes in the volume pulse is loss of the dicrotic notch. When the proximal disease is more severe, the systolic rise becomes slower, the peak is delayed with a flat or rounded shape, and the downslope is bowed away from the baseline (see Fig. 15–6). Because segmental pressure measurements are more easily obtained than segmental plethysmographic measurements, the latter are not widely used in the routine noninvasive evaluation of the extremities. Segmental volume pulses may be valuable, however, when pressure measurements are artifactually elevated because of medial calcification.

LOWER EXTREMITY ARTERIAL EXAMINATION

The sequence of noninvasive tests most commonly used in the routine indirect lower extremity arterial examination can be summarized as follows:

1. Measurement of bilateral ankle pressures (DP and PT) and brachial pressures at rest
2. Calculation of ankle-brachial indexes
3. Segmental pressure gradients if ankle pressures are abnormal
4. Common femoral artery velocity waveforms at rest
5. Treadmill exercise or reactive hyperemia testing with repeat common femoral artery velocity waveforms and serial ankle pressure measurements

FIGURE 15–6. Normal and abnormal lower extremity volume pulse waveforms.

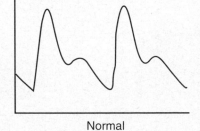

Normal

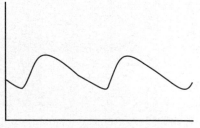

Abnormal

6. Special studies to be used in selected patients
   a. Toe pressures
   b. Plethysmography (digital or segmental)
   c. Duplex scanning

The examination begins with a brief history and physical examination emphasizing the symptoms and signs of peripheral vascular disease. The status of palpable peripheral pulses, the location of bruits, and the presence of ischemic skin lesions are noted. If a significant degree of cardiac or pulmonary disease is present, the patient's ability to perform treadmill exercise must be determined.

Any continuous-wave Doppler device is satisfactory for measuring ankle or segmental limb pressures. Initially, ankle systolic pressure should be measured in both the DP and PT arteries (Fig. 15–7). Bilateral brachial pressures are also measured using the same Doppler technique. The ankle-brachial index for each leg is calculated by dividing the highest ankle pressure by the highest brachial pressure. When the ankle-brachial index is normal, measurement of segmental pressure gradients is not necessary. In limbs with severe arterial disease and no detectable flow signals at the ankle, thigh pressures often can be obtained by using the popliteal artery flow signal. As mentioned previously, segmental limb pressures do not provide precise anatomic detail on the location and severity of arterial lesions. For those patients who are being considered for invasive arterial procedures, direct imaging by duplex scanning can be useful for planning therapy by either catheter-based interventions or open arterial surgery. This approach is discussed in Chapter 18.

Analogue waveforms are usually recorded with a direction-sensing continuous-wave Doppler and a strip chart recorder incorporating a zero crossing detector. The Doppler angle is adjusted by visual inspection of the waveform to minimize noise and artifact. Although waveforms can be obtained from any site with a Doppler signal, only the common femoral artery waveform is routinely recorded in most cases. This waveform is helpful in detecting proximal aortoiliac occlusive lesions. It is valuable to record the common femoral artery waveforms both before and immediately after treadmill exercise or reactive hyperemia testing, because some less severe lesions are apparent only at increased flow rates.

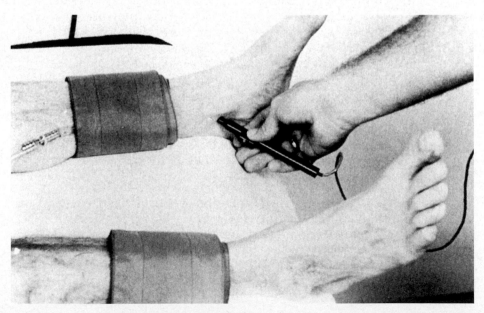

Figure 15–7. To measure ankle systolic pressures, the Doppler probe is positioned over the left posterior tibial artery.

Stress testing with treadmill exercise or reactive hyperemia can be tolerated by most patients who do not have ischemic rest pain. As previously stated, the treadmill test is preferred because it is a more physiologic form of stress. The speed and grade of the electronic treadmill can be varied to suit the individual patient, but the standard test is done at 2 mph and a 12% grade. It is convenient to have the patient wear ankle cuffs and an arm cuff while walking on the treadmill (Fig. 15–8). Immediately after cessation of exercise, the patient returns to the examining table, and ankle and arm pressures are measured. Serial ankle pressure measurements are then made at about 1-minute intervals for up to 10 minutes or until they return to pre-exercise values. An automatic cuff inflator facilitates this rapid sequence of measurements. A worksheet for recording the noninvasive test results is shown in Figure 15–9.

Additional studies, such as plethysmography or measurement of toe pressures, are of value only in selected clinical circumstances. Toe pressures can be used to detect occlusive lesions between the level of the ankle and the digital arteries. Duplex scanning is indicated when detailed information on the location and severity of lesions is desired without resorting to arteriography. Duplex methods are described in detail in Chapter 18.

SOURCES OF ERROR

Technical and Physiologic Variability

The variability in measurements of arterial pressure results from biologic and technical factors. The ankle-brachial index and other ratios that relate peripheral and central arterial pressures compensate for changes in central pressure, thus avoiding a major source of biologic variation. Because of variability related to technique, changes in ankle-brachial index must be 0.15 or greater to be considered significant.[48]

Incompressible Vessels

Accurate measurements of arterial pressure using pneumatic cuffs require that cuff pressure be transmitted through the arterial wall to the flow stream. The presence of medial calcification in the arterial wall results in varying degrees of incompressibility and recording of falsely high pressures.[21] Occasionally, it may be impossible to eliminate the distal flow signal, even with maximal cuff inflation pressures. When this situation is encountered, the main arteries are usually patent, because collateral vessels are more easily obliterated by the cuff.

Diabetic patients are particularly prone to medial calcification, and artifactual elevation of leg pressures must always be considered in this group. In approximately 5% to 10% of diabetic patients, ankle pressures cannot be measured because of incompressible vessels.[49] In these patients, toe pressure measurement is a more reliable method for assessing the severity of arterial occlusive disease because the digital vessels are not usually affected by medial calcification.

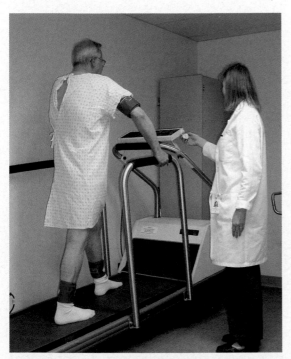

FIGURE 15–8. Ankle cuffs and one arm cuff are in place to facilitate postexercise pressure measurements in the treadmill stress test.

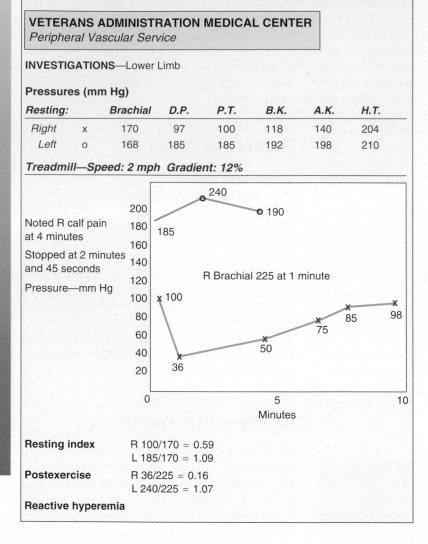

VETERANS ADMINISTRATION MEDICAL CENTER
Peripheral Vascular Service

INVESTIGATIONS—Lower Limb

Pressures (mm Hg)

Resting:		Brachial	D.P.	P.T.	B.K.	A.K.	H.T.
Right	x	170	97	100	118	140	204
Left	o	168	185	185	192	198	210

Treadmill—Speed: 2 mph Gradient: 12%

Noted R calf pain at 4 minutes

Stopped at 2 minutes and 45 seconds

Pressure—mm Hg

R Brachial 225 at 1 minute

Resting index	R 100/170 = 0.59
	L 185/170 = 1.09
Postexercise	R 36/225 = 0.16
	L 240/225 = 1.07
Reactive hyperemia	

FIGURE 15–9. Worksheet for recording test results. *D.P.* and *P.T.* refer to the ankle pressures obtained with the Doppler probe over the dorsalis pedis and posterior tibial arteries, respectively. A.K., above-knee; B.K., below-knee; H.T., high-thigh.

Cuff Artifact

As previously mentioned, cuff width should be at least 50% greater than limb diameter for accurate pressure measurement. The use of smaller cuffs results in falsely elevated pressure readings, particularly in obese patients. In most patients, the magnitude of the cuff artifact can be anticipated, and relatively narrow thigh cuffs can be successfully used to measure segmental pressure gradients.

In theory, the pressure obtained with a pneumatic cuff on the proximal thigh should reflect the status of the aortoiliac segment. When the proximal thigh pressure is measured with a relatively narrow cuff, the systolic pressure normally exceeds the brachial systolic pressure by a cuff artifact of 30 to 40 mm Hg, and the thigh-brachial index is greater than 1.2.[36] Patients with decreased thigh-brachial indexes would be expected to have significant aortoiliac disease; however, the presence of superficial femoral and profunda femoris artery disease can also result in a decreased thigh-brachial index, even when the aortoiliac segment is hemodynamically normal. The main problem with this indirect assessment of aortoiliac or inflow disease is with the practical difficulty of measuring proximal thigh pressures accurately. When this situation is suspected, other methods such as segmental plethysmography, common femoral artery Doppler waveform analysis, or duplex scanning should be used.

Other Sources of Error

In limbs with severe arterial occlusive disease and low flow rates, Doppler signals may be unobtainable, even when the arteries are patent. Plethysmographic techniques may provide useful information in these cases. When very weak Doppler signals are detected, it may be difficult to distinguish between arterial and venous flow. A direction-sensing Doppler device is useful in this situation. In addition, venous signals are augmented with distal limb compression, whereas arterial signals either remain the same or diminish.

The pressure gradients between adjacent limb segments may be increased in markedly hypertensive patients. On the other extreme, segmental pressure gradients may be decreased when cardiac output is low.[50] When the collateral vessels bypassing an arterial obstruction are unusually large and efficient, the corresponding segmental gradient may be normal. If this is the case, a significant gradient should become apparent after treadmill exercise.

Arterial occlusive lesions distal to the ankle are not detected by the routine lower extremity evaluation, because the ankle is the most distal site of pressure measurement. Lesions involving the plantar or digital arteries, such as vasculitis and microembolism, may be identified by toe pressure measurement and digital plethysmography.

CLINICAL APPLICATIONS OF NONINVASIVE ARTERIAL TESTING

The goals of the lower extremity arterial evaluation are to confirm the diagnosis of arterial occlusive disease, indicate the location of any obstructing lesions, and quantify the resulting degree of disability. Various conditions produce signs and symptoms in the legs that may be confused with arterial occlusive disease (e.g., claudication, rest pain). These include osteoarthritis (hip, knee), neurospinal disease (lumbar disk, spinal stenosis), nocturnal muscle cramps, peripheral neuropathy (diabetes mellitis), reflex sympathetic dystrophy (causalgia), deep vein thrombosis (venous claudication), cellulitis, and trauma. Furthermore, it is not unusual for a patient to have multiple causes for leg pain, and it may be difficult to determine which is most responsible for a patient's symptoms. The measurements of arterial pressure and flow patterns described in this chapter can be applied to both the initial evaluation and subsequent follow-up of patients with arterial occlusive disease.

Initial Evaluation

In the evaluation of any patient with signs or symptoms that suggest arterial occlusive disease, two questions must be answered: (1) Is arterial occlusion present? and (2) Is arterial occlusion causing the patient's symptoms? For the lower extremity, recording of ankle-brachial indexes, segmental pressure gradients, Doppler velocity waveforms, and the response to treadmill exercise or reactive hyperemia will answer these questions in most patients.

The finding of a normal ankle-brachial index at rest and a normal response to treadmill exercise essentially rules out any significant lower extremity arterial occlusive disease. Some patients have a decreased ankle-brachial index at rest and symptoms during treadmill exercise but little or no ankle pressure drop after cessation of exercise. This finding suggests that, although arterial disease is present, it is not producing the symptoms in question and another cause of leg pain should be considered. The limitations imposed by cardiac, pulmonary, and musculoskeletal conditions are directly observed during exercise testing, allowing these factors to be considered in the overall management of the patient.

For those patients who require only medical management for lower extremity arterial occlusive disease (i.e., an exercise program, risk factor management, anti-platelet agents, and drug therapy for intermittent claudication), the nonimaging physiologic tests are ideally suited for both initial evaluation and follow-up. However, those patients who will require invasive arterial procedures based on their clinical presentation and physiologic test results should be evaluated with duplex scanning (Chapter 18). The more detailed anatomic information provided by lower extremity arterial duplex scanning can be valuable in planning of interventions.

Follow-Up Testing

Noninvasive testing is a convenient and practical means for serial follow-up of patients after their initial evaluation. Evidence of disease progression or improvement may be observed, and the results of medical or surgical therapy can be documented objectively.

In patients who have had a successful arterial intervention for lower extremity occlusive disease, ankle pressures and appropriate segmental pressure gradients should be significantly improved compared with the preoperative values.[51] If a single level of disease was present preoperatively, success-

ful bypass grafting or endarterectomy should result in normal or near-normal ankle pressures. Failure of ankle pressures to improve immediately following surgery suggests either a problem related to surgical technique or the selection of an inappropriate reconstructive procedure.[52] Deterioration of noninvasive measurements later in the postoperative period may reflect either structural changes occurring in the reconstructed segment or progression of occlusive disease at other sites.[53,54] Serial postoperative follow-up is desirable, because early identification and repair of a failing arterial reconstruction results in the greatest chance of maintaining patency. This subject is discussed further in Chapter 19.

Patients whose condition is improved after intervention but whose conditions still have not returned to normal may have their status documented by noninvasive testing. For example, a patient may show a significant improvement in treadmill walking time after arterial reconstruction despite a persistent drop in ankle pressure. This observation is common in patients with arterial occlusive disease at multiple levels who have only one level corrected; the abnormal hemodynamic response then reflects the remaining untreated disease. Figure 15–10 shows

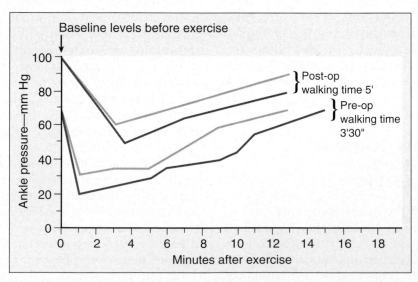

FIGURE **15–10.** Ankle pressure response to treadmill exercise before and after an aortofemoral bypass graft in a patient with bilateral superficial femoral artery stenoses. The postoperative exercise test shows some improvement in walking time but remains abnormal (*dashed lines,* left ankle; *solid lines,* right ankle). (From Strandness DE: Abnormal exercise responses after successful reconstructive arterial surgery. Surgery 59:328, 1966.)

the ankle pressure changes recorded before and after an aortofemoral bypass graft in a patient who also has stenoses in both superficial femoral arteries. Although the treadmill walking time improved, an abnormal ankle pressure response is still present.

Specific Clinical Problems

Claudication

The term *intermittent claudication* refers to a muscular ache or cramp that occurs during exercise and is relieved by rest. It results from inadequate blood flow to muscle during exercise and is a definite, reproducible symptom. Claudication usually involves the calf, but the thigh or buttock may also be affected when arterial occlusions reduce blood flow to those areas. Arteriosclerosis obliterans (atherosclerosis) is the most common cause of claudication; popliteal artery entrapment must be considered when claudication occurs in young adults or children.[55,56]

When the characteristic symptoms are produced by treadmill exercise in association with a drop in ankle pressure to less than about 60 mm Hg, the clinical impression of intermittent claudication is confirmed. The walking time documents the extent of disability and serves as a baseline for subsequent follow-up. Segmental pressure gradients or plethysmography can be used to determine the approximate location of arterial occlusive lesions. More detailed information on the location and severity of the lesions can be obtained by duplex scanning.

Rest Pain

Ischemic rest pain develops in the toes or forefoot when blood flow is insufficient to maintain normal cellular function at rest. Noninvasive tests usually show multiple-level arterial occlusive disease with an ankle systolic pressure less than 40 mm Hg and an ankle-brachial index less than 0.35. Treadmill exercise or reactive hyperemia testing is not necessary in patients with this degree of abnormality.

Healing of Ulcers and Amputations

Noninvasive pressure measurements can be used to assess the probability of achieving primary healing in the ischemic lower extremity. Ischemic foot ulcers are unlikely to heal if ankle systolic pressure is less than 55 mm Hg in nondiabetics or less than 80 mm Hg in diabetics.[49] The ankle pressures in diabetic patients may be falsely elevated because of medial calcification.

Ankle pressures have not been consistently helpful in predicting healing of BK or foot amputations.[8] A BK or calf pressure greater than 70 mm Hg correlates with primary healing of BK amputations, whereas the absence of detectable Doppler flow signals at the BK level predicts failure of healing.[57] Primary healing may still be achieved with BK pressures less than 70 mm Hg, so the choice of amputation level should not be based on this pressure measurement alone.

Because lesions in the pedal or digital arteries are not detected by ankle or calf pressure measurement, toe pressure measurement may be more reliable for predicting healing of the foot. Healing of foot ulcers, toe amputations, or transmetatarsal amputations was observed in only 5% of limbs when toe pressures were less than 30 mm Hg; however, with pressures of 30 mm Hg or greater, healing occurred in approximately 90% of limbs.[38]

The transcutaneous oxygen tension ($tcPo_2$) or amount of oxygen diffusing through the skin from the dermal capillaries can be measured with an electrode applied to the skin surface. This technique has been proposed as a method for predicting wound healing and determining the most appropriate level for amputation.[58] Clinical experience has shown that $tcPo_2$ measurements are valuable for predicting healing at a particular level of the limb; however, this approach is less reliable for identifying those sites that fail to heal. In one study, successful healing of BK amputations occurred in 96% of patients with a calf

$tcPo_2$ greater than 20 mm Hg but only in 50% of patients with a calf $tcPo_2$ less than 20 mm Hg.[59] Refinements of this technique, such as use of a critical Po_2 index (calf/brachial $tcPo_2$ ratio, foot/chest $tcPo_2$ ratio) or breathing supplemental oxygen, may improve the overall predictive value.[59–61] Estimation of skin blood flow by $tcPo_2$ may be more sensitive than ankle pressure measurements in the assessment of severe limb ischemia. In general, critical ischemia must be suspected whenever forefoot $tcPo_2$ is less than 40 mm Hg.[62,63]

Predicting the Results of Arterial Surgery

Noninvasive measurements of lower extremity blood pressure have been used to predict the functional results of arterial reconstruction in terms of symptom relief and graft patency. In patients undergoing aortofemoral bypass procedures, a preoperative thigh-brachial index of 0.85 or less is a reliable predictor of a good postoperative result; however, improvement also may occur in many patients with a thigh-brachial index greater than 0.85.[64] The presence of occlusive disease limited to the aortoiliac arteries, as demonstrated by normal segmental pressure gradients in the leg, is also predictive of a good result after aortofemoral bypass grafting. A comparison of ankle-brachial indexes before and after aortofemoral bypass showed that an increase of 0.1 or more during the first 12 hours after operation correlated highly with subsequent symptomatic improvement.[64] The preoperative ankle-brachial index alone also has some predictive value.[65] When the ankle-brachial index is greater than 0.8, 94% of patients obtain significant symptom relief after aortofemoral bypass, whereas only 64% of patients show the same degree of improvement if the ankle-brachial index is less than 0.4. These observations indicate the aortofemoral bypass grafting is most successful in these patients with significant aortoiliac occlusive disease and normal distal arteries.

The predictive value of noninvasive pressure measurements in femoropopliteal bypass procedures has not been firmly established. An early study suggested that an ankle-brachial index of greater than 0.4 predicts a high graft patency rate, whereas an ankle-brachial index of less than 0.2 is associated with early graft failure.[66] Later reports have not confirmed these observations, however, and very low ankle pressures should not be regarded as a contraindication for femoropopliteal bypass.[52]

Predicting the Results of Sympathectomy

The role of sympathectomy in the management of patients with arterial disease has been controversial. Lumbar sympathectomy is sometimes considered for patients with impending limb loss caused by severe, unreconstructable occlusive disease. In this situation, ankle pressure measurements provide a means for selecting those patients most likely to benefit from the procedure.[67] An ankle-brachial index greater than 0.35 predicts a favorable clinical response to sympathectomy; an index less than 0.2 correlates highly with sympathectomy failure and subsequent limb loss. The value of lumbar sympathectomy depends on the adequacy of collateral circulation in the leg, and the ankle-brachial index provides an indirect assessment of the potential for increasing flow through the collateral vessels.

In addition to adequate collateral flow, the success of sympathectomy depends on the capability of the peripheral arterioles to vasodilate and on the presence of sympathetic activity in the extremity. Vasodilation can be assessed by performing a reactive hyperemia test while monitoring a plethysmographic digit volume pulse. In normal extremities, the excursion of the volume pulse at least doubles during hyperemia, usually within the first few seconds after flow is restored. Failure of the volume pulse to increase suggests that further vasodilation is not possible. The presence of intact sympathetic tone can be demonstrated plethysmographically by observing the response of the digit volume pulse to a deep breath. If vasodilation or sympathetic tone is absent, sympathectomy is not beneficial.[68]

References

1. Marinelli MR, Beach KW, Glass MJ, et al: Noninvasive testing vs. clinical evaluation of arterial disease. JAMA 241:2031–2034, 1979.
2. Beales JSM, Adcock FA, Frawley JE, et al: The radiological assessment of disease at the profunda femoris artery. Br J Radiol 44:854–857, 1971.
3. Crummy AB, Rankin RS, Turnipseed WD, et al: Biplane arteriography in ischemia of the lower extremity. Radiology 126:111–115, 1978.
4. Sethi GR, Scott SM, Takaro T: Multiple-plane angiography for more precise evaluation of aortoiliac disease. Surgery 78:154–159, 1975.
5. Thomas M, Andrews MR: Value of oblique projections in translumbar aortography. Am J Roentgenol 116:187–193, 1973.
6. Castenada-Zuniga W, Knight L, Formanek A, et al: Hemodynamic assessment of obstructive aortoiliac disease. Am J Roentgenol 127:559–561, 1976.
7. Karayannacus PE, Talukder N, Nerem RM, et al: The role of multiple noncritical arterial stenoses in the pathogenesis of ischemia. J Thorac Cardiovasc Surg 73:458–469, 1977.
8. Kempczinski RF, Rutheford RB: Current status of the vascular diagnostic laboratory. Adv Surg 12:1–52, 1978.
9. Nippa JH, Hokanson DE, Lee DR, et al: Phase rotation for separating forward and reverse blood velocity signals. IEEE Trans Sonics Ultrasonics 22:340–346, 1975.
10. Blackshear WM: Surgical indications for lower extremity arterial occlusive disease. Part I. Curr Probl Cardiol 6:22–32, 1981.
11. Baker DW: Pulsed ultrasonic Doppler blood flow sensing. IEEE Trans Sonics Ultrasonics 17:170–185, 1970.
12. Mozersky DJ, Hokanson DE, Sumner DS, et al: Ultrasonic visualization of the arterial lumen. Surgery 72:253–259, 1972.
13. Zierler RE: Carotid artery evaluation by duplex scanning. Semin Vasc Surg 1:9–16, 1988.
14. Strandness DE Jr: Vascular Studies: Past and Present. In Strandness DE (ed): Duplex Scanning in Vascular Disorders, 3rd ed. Philadelphia, Lippincott Williams & Wilkins, 2002, pp 3–19.
15. Blackshear WM, Phillips DJ, Strandness DE: Pulsed Doppler assessment of normal human femoral artery velocity patterns. J Surg Res 27:73–83, 1979.
16. Moneta GL, Yeager RA, Lee RW, et al: Noninvasive localization of arterial occlusive disease: A comparison of segmental Doppler pressures and arterial duplex mapping. J Vasc Surg 17:578–582, 1993.
17. Kohler TR, Nance DR, Cramer MM, et al: Duplex scanning for diagnosis of aortoiliac and femoropopliteal disease: A prospective study. Circulation 76:1074–1080, 1987.
18. Hoffman U, Edwards JM, Carter S, et al: Role of duplex scanning for the detection of atherosclerotic renal artery disease. Kid Int 39:1232–1239, 1991.
19. Zwolak RM, Fillinger MF, Walsh DB, et al: Mesenteric duplex scanning: A validation study. J Vasc Surg 27:1078–1088, 1998.
20. Darling RC, Raines JK, Brener BJ, et al: Quantitative segmental pulse volume recorder: A clinical tool. Surgery 72:873–887, 1973.
21. Strandness DE Jr, Bell JW: Peripheral vascular disease: Diagnosis and objective evaluation using a mercury strain gauge. Ann Surg 161(Suppl):1–35, 1965.
22. Hokanson DE, Sumner DS, Strandness DE Jr: An electrically calibrated plethysmograph for direct measurement of limb blood flow. IEEE Trans Biomed Eng 22:25–29, 1975.
23. Sumner DS: Volume plethysmography in vascular disease: An overview. In Bernstein EF (ed): Noninvasive Diagnostic Techniques in Vascular Disease, 3rd ed. St. Louis, CV Mosby, 1985, pp 97–118.
24. Johnston KW, Marozzo BC, Cobbold RSC: Errors and artifacts of Doppler flowmeters and their solution. Arch Surg 112:1335–1342, 1977.
25. Strandness DE, Sumner DS: Hemodynamics for Surgeons. New York, Grune & Stratton, 1975, p 29.
26. Knox RA, Strandness DE: Ultrasound techniques for evaluation of lower extremity arterial occlusion. Semin Ultrasound 2:264–275, 1981.
27. Strandness DE Jr, Zierler RE: Exercise ankle pressure measurements in arterial disease. In Bernstein EF (ed): Noninvasive Diagnostic Techniques in Vascular Disease, 3rd ed. St. Louis, CV Mosby, 1985, pp 575–583.
28. Strandness DE, Sumner DS: Hemodynamics for Surgeons. New York, Grune & Stratton, 1975, p 21.
29. Carter SA: Clinical measurements of systolic pressures in limbs with arterial occlusive disease. JAMA 207:1869–1874, 1969.
30. May AG, Van de Berg L, De Weese JA, et al: Clinical arterial stenosis. Surgery 54:250–259, 1963.
31. Strandness DE, Sumner DS: Hemodynamics for Surgeons. New York, Grune & Stratton, 1975, p 233.
32. Yao JST, Hobbs JT, Irvine WT: Ankle systolic pressure measurements in arterial diseases

affecting the lower extremities. Br J Surg 56:676–679, 1969.

33. Sumner DS, Strandness DE: The relationship between calf blood flow and ankle blood pressure in patients with intermittent claudication. Surgery 65:763–771, 1969.

34. Yao JST: Hemodynamic studies in peripheral arterial disease. Br J Surg 57:761–766, 1970.

35. Pascarelli EF, Bertrand CA: Comparison of blood pressures in the arms and legs. N Engl J Med 270:693–698, 1964.

36. Cutajar CL, Marston A, Newcombe JF: Value of cuff occlusion pressures in assessment of peripheral vascular disease. Br J Med 2:392–395, 1973.

37. Carter SA, Lezack JD: Digital systolic pressures in the lower limbs in arterial disease. Circulation 43:905–914, 1971.

38. Ramsey DE, Manke DA, Sumner DS: Toe blood pressure—A valuable adjunct to ankle pressure measurement for assessing peripheral arterial disease. J Cardiovasc Surg 24:43–48, 1983.

39. Fronek A, Johanson K, Dilley RB, et al: Ultrasonically monitored postocclusive reactive hyperemia in the diagnosis of peripheral arterial occlusive disease. Circulation 48:149–152, 1973.

40. Hummel BW, Hummel BA, Mowbry A, et al: Reactive hyperemia vs treadmill exercise testing in arterial disease. Arch Surg 113:95–98, 1978.

41. Keagy BA, Pharr WF, Thomas D, et al: Comparison of reactive hyperemia and treadmill tests in the evaluation of peripheral vascular disease. Am J Surg 142:158–161, 1981.

42. Strandness DE, Schultz RD, Sumner DS, et al: Ultrasonic flow detection: A useful technique in the evaluation of peripheral vascular disease. Am J Surg 113:311–320, 1967.

43. Johnston KW, Taraschuk I: Validation of the role of pulsatility index in quantitation of the severity of peripheral arterial occlusive disease. Am J Surg 131:295–297, 1976.

44. Gosling RG, Dunbar G, King DH, et al: The quantitative analysis of occlusive peripheral arterial disease by a noninvasive ultrasonic technique. Angiology 22:52–55, 1971.

45. Thiele BL, Bandyk DF, Zierler RE, et al: A systematic approach to the assessment of aortoiliac disease. Arch Surg 118:477–481, 1983.

46. Baird RN, Bird DR, Clifford PC, et al: Upstream stenosis—its diagnosis by Doppler signals from the femoral artery. Arch Surg 115:1316–1322, 1980.

47. Campbell WB, Baird RN, Cole SEA, et al: Physiological interpretation of Doppler shift waveforms—the femorodistal segment in combined disease. Ultrasound Med Bio 9:265–269, 1983.

48. Baker JD, Dix D: Variability of Doppler ankle pressures with arterial occlusive disease: An evaluation of ankle index and brachial-ankle pressure gradient. Surgery 89:134–137, 1981.

49. Raines JK, Darling RC, Both K, et al: Vascular laboratory criteria for the management of peripheral vascular disease of the lower extremities. Surgery 79:21–29, 1976.

50. Winsor T: Influence of arterial disease on the systolic blood pressure gradients of the extremity. Am J Med Sci 220:117–126, 1950.

51. Strandness DE, Bell JW: Ankle pressure responses after reconstructive arterial surgery. Surgery 59:514–516, 1966.

52. Corson JD, Johnson WC, LoGerfo RS, et al: Doppler ankle systolic blood pressure: Prognostic value in vein bypass grafts of the lower extremity. Arch Surg 113:932–935, 1976.

53. Blackshear WM, Thiele BL, Strandness DE: Natural history of above- and below-knee femoropopliteal grafts. Am J Surg 140:234–241, 1980.

54. Strandness DE: Abnormal exercise responses after successful reconstructive arterial surgery. Surgery 59:325–333, 1966.

55. Insua JA, Young JR, Humphries AW: Popliteal artery entrapment syndrome. Arch Surg 101:771–775, 1970.

56. Rich NM, Collins GJ, McDonald PT, et al: Popliteal vascular entrapment: Its increasing interest. Arch Surg 114:1377–1384, 1979.

57. Barnes RW, Shanik GD, Slaymaker EE: An index of healing in below-knee amputation: Leg blood pressure by Doppler ultrasound. Surgery 79:13–20, 1976.

58. Wyss CR, Robertson C, Love SJ, et al: Relationship between transcutaneous oxygen tension, ankle blood pressure, and clinical outcome of vascular surgery in diabetic and nondiabetic patients. Surgery 101:56–62, 1987.

59. Kram HB, Appel OL, Shoemaker WC: Multisensor transcutaneous oximetric mapping to predict below-knee amputation wound healing: Use of a critical P_{O_2}. J Vasc Surg 9:796–800, 1989.

60. Harward TRS, Volny J, Golbranson F, et al: Oxygen inhalation-induced transcutaneous P_{O_2} changes as a predictor of amputation level. J Vasc Surg 2:220–227, 1985.

61. Lalka SG, Malone JM, Anderson GG, et al: Transcutaneous oxygen and carbon dioxide pressure monitoring to determine severity of limb ischemia and to predict surgical outcome. J Vasc Surg 7:507–514, 1988.

62. Karanfilian RG, Lynch TG, Zirul VT, et al: The value of laser Doppler velocimetry and transcutaneous oxygen tension determination in predicting healing of ischemic forefoot ulcerations and amputations in diabetic and nondiabetic patients. J Vasc Surg 4:511–516, 1986.

63. Larsen JF, Jensen BV, Christensen KS, et al: Forefoot transcutaneous oxygen tension at

different leg positions in patients with peripheral vascular disease. Eur J Vasc Surg 4:185–189, 1990.

64. Bone GE, Hayes AC, Slaymaker EE, et al: Value of segmental limb blood pressures in predicting results of aortofemoral bypass. Am J Surg 132:733–738, 1976.

65. Bernstein EF, Stuart SH, Fronek A: The predictive value of noninvasive testing in peripheral vascular disease. In Bernstein EF (ed): Noninvasive Diagnostic Techniques in Vascular Disease. St. Louis, CV Mosby, 1982, pp 396–403.

66. Dean RH, Yao JST, Stanton PE, et al: Prognostic indicators in femoropopliteal reconstruction. Arch Surg 110:1287–1293, 1975.

67. Yao JST, Bergan JJ: Predictability of vascular reactivity relative to sympathetic ablation. Arch Surg 107:676–680, 1973.

68. Strandness DE Jr: Long-term value of lumbar sympathectomy. Geriatrics 21:144–155, 1966.

Chapter 16

Assessment of Upper Extremity Arterial Occlusive Disease

STEVEN R. TALBOT, RVT, FSVU, AND WILLIAM J. ZWIEBEL, MD

The unique structure and function of the upper extremity create challenges for the diagnosis of vascular abnormalities. Unlike the lower extremity, where atherosclerosis or thrombi are almost always the cause of symptomatic disease, upper extremity vascular problems can be more complex. Mechanical compression occurring in the troublesome thoracic outlet region, vasospasm in digital arteries, trauma-related thrombi in the hand and wrist, and embolic thrombi from the heart or from proximal arm aneurysms all must be considered when troubleshooting in the upper extremity. Hand arterial anatomy is confusing and variable and therefore requires a high level of technical expertise. Specialized probes that are capable of resolving small vessels, and displaying flow within them, are required for optimal studies. Finally, physicians and sonographers are generally out of their comfort zone when working in the arm, because arterial disease occurs less commonly in the upper extremity than in the lower extremity. Only about 5% of arterial cases involve the upper extremities.[1]

This chapter provides the basics of upper extremity arterial assessment, including
1. What to look for clinically
2. What questions to ask before getting started with testing
3. The basic anatomy of the arm and hand arteries that require examination
4. What types of noninvasive tests should be used, and in what order
5. How each examination is performed and interpreted
6. How to know when you have answered the clinical question at hand

DIAGNOSTIC WORKUP

The first steps in solving the diagnostic puzzle of hand and arm problems are to take a careful history and closely examine the fingers, hand, and arm. Both arms should be examined side by side, with attention to the following findings: Are any fingers discolored? Is there a temperature difference from one hand or finger compared with another? Are there ulcers on fingertips? Is there pain, and if so, how long has it been present? Did the pain or discomfort come on suddenly or slowly? Is the pain constant or transient? What makes the pain or discomfort better or worse? Does exposure to cold or stressful situations bring on or intensify symptoms?

CHOOSING THE RIGHT DIAGNOSTIC TOOL

Observations and historical information affect the types of tests that should be done to pinpoint the problem. Common basic noninvasive tools to investigate upper extremity arterial problems include the following:
1. Continuous-wave Doppler (with a recording device to display arterial waveforms)
2. Nonimaging physiologic tests (pulse volume recordings and segmental pressures)
3. Photoplethysmographic (PPG) sensors to detect flow in the digits
4. Color Doppler imaging to directly visualize the vessels and the flow within

them, and also to identify the type of pathology that is present.

One or all of these tools may be needed to diagnose a given problem. For instance, if fingers are cool and discolored with exposure to cold but fine otherwise, the examination will focus on the question of whether this is a vasospastic disorder versus a situation in which digital thrombus is present, or a combination of the two. Extensive diagnostic work will have to be done, with close attention to each finger (usually with PPG) and then some kind of cold challenge to provoke symptoms. If cold does not seem to be a factor, the cold challenge may be omitted. If the problem is positional, a baseline plethysmographic study should be done, followed by monitoring of flow in as many different arm positions as possible. Finally, if Doppler and plethysmographic information suggest obstruction, duplex imaging should be done to identify the cause.

Once the examiner has in mind the nature of the problem he/she is looking for, a plan of action can be formulated for that individual. This plan may change as new information becomes available during the examination. For example, a patient with no positional symptoms turns out to have thrombus in a distal radial artery. Extra attention should then be given to the subclavian and axillary arteries, using duplex ultrasound to check for an embolic source, such as an aneurysm or atherosclerosis. It would also be wise to have the patient go through different arm positions, with the plethysmographic cuffs attached, to check for thoracic outlet impingement.

START WITH THE BASICS

For almost every situation where arterial disease is suspected in the upper extremity, the standard noninvasive starting point is the pulse volume recording (PVR) of arm waveforms, combined with segmental pressure measurements (Fig. 16–1). Continuous-wave Doppler signal assessment of the sublcavian, axillary, brachial, radial, and ulnar arteries (Fig. 16–2) is complementary to the segmental pressures and PVR infor-

mation. If the fingers are symptomatic, PPGs (see Fig. 16–1*B*) of all digits should be obtained as well. With this simple group of tests, one can answer the basic clinical question: Is hemodynamically significant arterial obstruction present in a major arm artery?

The PVR and Doppler examination is conducted as follows. Blood pressure cuffs are placed about the midportion of the arm and the forearm, and PVR waveforms are taken at both levels. Then, the systolic blood pressure is measured at both levels, using the audible Doppler signal as an indication of systolic pressure. The measured blood pressures should be similar side to side, as well as from one level to the other (see Fig. 16–1*A*). A side-to-side blood pressure difference of more than 20 mm Hg or between levels, accompanied by an abnormal pulse volume recording (Fig. 16–3), may indicate a hemodynamically significant lesion on the side/level with the lower pressure. This finding requires additional testing to determine the cause, usually with direct ultrasound imaging of the vessel(s) in question, as described later in this chapter.

If pressures and waveforms are normal, one can assume there is no hemodynamically significant obstruction in the arteries of the upper extremity. This observation may be an appropriate stopping point, especially if the referring physician only needs to rule out major, limb-threatening disease. It must be understood, however, that normal results of these indirect tests cannot rule out nonobstructive plaque or thrombus, aneurysm, transient mechanical compression of vessels, vasospasm, or other pathologies (such as arteritis). If any of these problems are suspected, additional testing may be required.

IS THERE A PROBLEM AT THE THORACIC OUTLET?

When a patient presents with an upper extremity circulatory problem, such as a cold, painful, or numb extremity that varies with limb positioning, a potential cause that should be identified or eliminated from the equation early on is mechanical vascular

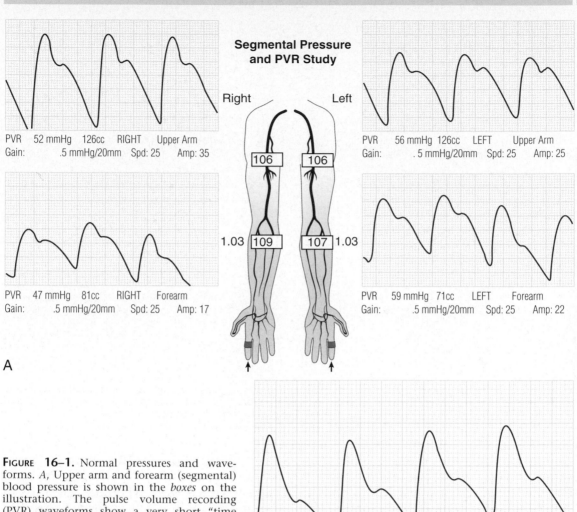

Segmental Pressure and PVR Study

Right   Left

PVR   52 mmHg   126cc   RIGHT   Upper Arm
Gain: .5 mmHg/20mm   Spd: 25   Amp: 35

PVR   56 mmHg   126cc   LEFT   Upper Arm
Gain: . 5 mmHg/20mm   Spd: 25   Amp: 25

PVR   47 mmHg   81cc   RIGHT   Forearm
Gain: .5 mmHg/20mm   Spd: 25   Amp: 17

PVR   59 mmHg   71cc   LEFT   Forearm
Gain: .5 mmHg/20mm   Spd: 25   Amp: 22

106   106
1.03 109   107 1.03

A

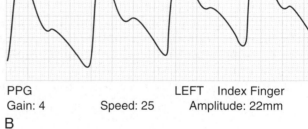

PPG   LEFT   Index Finger
Gain: 4   Speed: 25   Amplitude: 22mm

B

FIGURE 16–1. Normal pressures and waveforms. *A,* Upper arm and forearm (segmental) blood pressure is shown in the *boxes* on the illustration. The pulse volume recording (PVR) waveforms show a very short "time to peak" (from end diastole to peak systole), and a prominent dicrotic notch is present in the descending portion of the waveform. *B,* Normal *digital* photoplethysmographic (PPG) waveform shows the same features as the pneumatic, volume-based waveforms seen in *part A.*

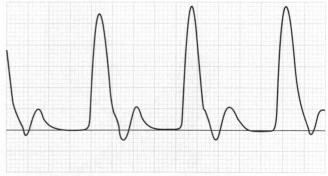

FIGURE 16–2. Normal continuous-wave Doppler waveforms have a high-impedance, triphasic shape characteristic of extremity arteries (with the limb at rest). Note that time to peak is very short, the systolic peak is narrow, and flow is absent in late diastole.

Doppler 8Mhz   RIGHT Axillary
Gain: 48 Hz/mm   Speed: 25

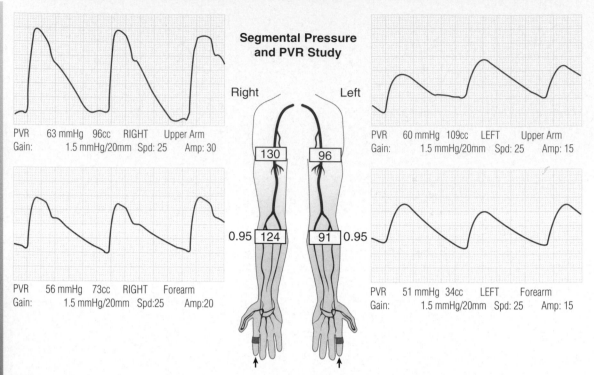

Segmental Pressure and PVR Study

	Right	Left	
	130	96	
0.95	124	91	0.95

PVR   63 mmHg   96cc   RIGHT   Upper Arm
Gain: 1.5 mmHg/20mm Spd: 25   Amp: 30

PVR   60 mmHg   109cc   LEFT   Upper Arm
Gain: 1.5 mmHg/20mm Spd: 25   Amp: 15

PVR   56 mmHg   73cc   RIGHT   Forearm
Gain: 1.5 mmHg/20mm Spd:25   Amp:20

PVR   51 mmHg   34cc   LEFT   Forearm
Gain: 1.5 mmHg/20mm Spd: 25   Amp: 15

Figure 16–3. Subclavian occlusive disease. The right arm shows normal pressures and pulse volume recording (PVR) waveforms. On the left, the pressure measurement are more than 20 mm Hg lower than on the right, and the PVR waveforms are damped (slowed time to peak, broad waveform, absent dicrotic notch).

compression at the thoracic outlet. As shown in Figure 16–4, the thoracic outlet is bounded by the clavicle, the first rib, and the scalene muscles. The thoracic outlet syndrome is a common problem, caused by impingement of the subclavian vessels and/or the brachial plexus as they leave the chest. Restriction at the thoracic outlet causes the vessels to be partially or completely compressed when the arm is in certain positions. The repeated vascular irritation over time may injure the artery or vein, leading to intimal damage or thrombus formation. Arterial emboli from

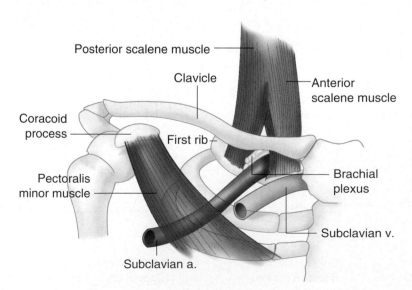

Posterior scalene muscle

Clavicle

Anterior scalene muscle

Coracoid process

First rib

Brachial plexus

Pectoralis minor muscle

Subclavian v.

Subclavian a.

Figure 16–4. Thoracic outlet anatomy. The subclavian artery, brachial plexus, and subclavian vein pass through a narrow opening framed by the anterior and posterior scalene muscles, the clavicle, and the first rib.

thrombus formed in this area may travel distally to other parts of the upper extremity. Therefore, whenever emboli are found, one should consider that they might have originated in the subclavian or axillary arteries.

Most patients with uncomplicated thoracic outlet syndrome (without thrombus, plaque, or aneurysm) have no arm complaints unless the arm is in a certain position. The discomfort the patient experiences is likely, at least originally, to result from nerve compression, rather than transient loss of blood flow from arterial impingement. The patient describes pain or numbness and loss of sensation when the upper extremity is in a predictable and reproducible position, such as occurs with hair brushing or driving a car (with the hands in a constant position on the steering wheel). The symptoms go away soon after the arm is repositioned.

If the examiner is presented with symptoms suggesting thoracic outlet problems, the upper extremity examination should begin routinely with resting pulse volume recordings and segmental pressures, as described previously, but this assessment should be supplemented with a check for the thoracic outlet syndrome, using the following technique. The examiner has the patient sit very straight and, using continuous-wave Doppler to monitor radial or ulnar artery flow, guides the patient through maneuvers that begin with the arm abducted and externally rotated. The blood pressure cuffs are left on the arms to monitor the pulse volume waveforms during the position changes, providing the examiner with two independent indicators of the quality of blood flow in the arm as the patient moves through the provocative position changes. This can be a clumsy operation for one examiner, so two examiners should be present during this procedure, if possible. One of the examiners is positioned behind the patient and maintains gentle pressure on the patient's back with the left hand, to keep the back straight, while holding the Doppler probe used to monitor the radial or ulnar artery in the right hand. The other examiner operates the pulse volume recording device and monitors the PVR waveforms during the arm position changes. (Note: A PPG sensor attached to a finger may be used instead of continuous-wave Doppler, if desired.)

Once a good-quality Doppler signal is acquired at the radial or ulnar artery and the pulse volume recording device is adequately registering PVR waveform, the examiner holding the Doppler probe guides the patient through the arm maneuvers. We usually start with the arm maximally abducted and externally rotated, with the shoulders pulled back as far as possible. The arm is then directed through every conceivable position, while the operators watch the PVR waveform tracing for diminished amplitude or total flattening of the waveform, accompanied by dampening or total loss of the Doppler signal. If a position is identified where such changes occur (Fig. 16–5), with recovery of the signals when the arm is moved out of the position, the test is positive and indicates thoracic outlet impingement. This arm position should be repeated, however, and the findings should be the same every time the arm is moved into the obstructing position. Care should be taken to make sure the examiner did not simply move the Doppler probe off of the monitored artery during positioning, as this can be a potential source of false-positive results. If the Doppler signal disappears, yet

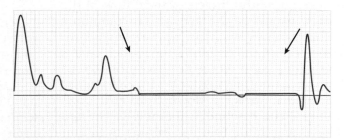

FIGURE 16–5. Thoracic outlet impingement. The Doppler signal at the radial artery goes flat (*small arrow*), as the arm is positioned such that the subclavian artery is compressed. The signal resumes (*large arrow*) when the arm is repositioned.

the pulse volume recording continues to be robust, recheck the Doppler probe orientation and repeat the maneuver.

A positive result, as described previously, suggests the presence of the thoracic outlet syndrome, but many patients without symptoms may test positive when an arm is in an extreme position, such as that used for this test. This fact contributes to the controversy surrounding the use of this test alone in making the diagnosis of thoracic outlet syndrome. The diagnosis is much more solid, however, if sublcavian artery stenosis is visualized with duplex imaging with the arm in the position that causes abnormal Doppler and PVR findings, or if an aneurysm is demonstrated with duplex ultrasound. The latter finding proves the occurrence of significant and repeated arterial impingement.

If Doppler signals and PVR waveforms do not diminish with various arm positions, these positions should be repeated with the head in a neutral position, with the head turned to the left, with the head to the right, with the head tilted up, and finally, with the chin on the chest. Only after every conceivable position has been tested can the examination be terminated. If all of these maneuvers fail to identify a position where flow is diminished, the test is determined to be negative for thoracic outlet impingement. This does not necessarily mean that the condition does not exist in the given patient, only that this test has been unable to identify it.

PHOTOPLETHYSMOGRAPHY OF DIGITAL FLOW EVALUATION

After flow in the arms has been checked, attention is next turned to the digits. If there are any problems such as cold, discolored, or painful fingers, arterial flow in the digits should be checked. This is commonly done with PPG sensors that are applied to the pads of the fingers. Double-stick tape is usually used to secure the PPG probe to the fingers. A normal digital PPG waveform has a rapid upstroke, a downstroke that bows toward the baseline, a dicrotic notch, and good amplitude (see Fig. 16–1*B*). A person with normal digital arteries may have small, abnormal-looking waveforms if the extremity is cold, so care must be taken to ensure that the examination room is sufficiently warm. If there is any question of the PPG waveforms' being adversely affected by cold temperature, have the patient warm the hands with a warming blanket before testing. If good-quality, normal waveforms are present in all of the digits, the examination is complete. If the waveforms are blunted, rounded, or absent, additional testing is required.

Check for Digital Artery Thrombus

One of the main questions that must be answered in the event of abnormal digital PPG waveforms is whether the vessels are obstructed with thrombus, as opposed to a vasospasm problem, or whether the etiology is a combination of both. Sometimes the digital arteries are filled with intraluminal thrombus that will have originated, most likely, from a proximal artery (usually the subclavian/axillary segment) or from the heart. When the digital arteries are occluded, waveforms will be rounded (Fig. 16–6*A*), flat, or nearly flat. No amount of warming will restore the waveform contour to normal, although slight improvement may sometimes occur. Likewise, nerve block induced with local anesthesia will have little or no effect. When thrombus is suspected in the digital arteries, the palmar arches, or the arteries of the arm, duplex imaging, as described later in this chapter, may be appropriate to verify the presence and exact location of the thrombus.

Check for Raynaud's Disease

When digits display signs of intermittent pallor, cyanosis, and rubor that is caused solely by digital arterial spasm, the condition is called Raynaud's disease (as opposed to a more serious condition called Raynaud's phenomenon, to be discussed later). Raynaud's disease usually represents an overreaction of vasomotor responses to cold

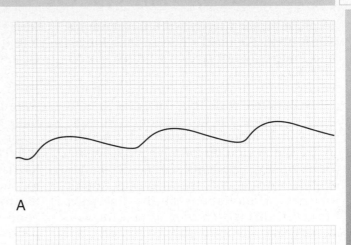

A

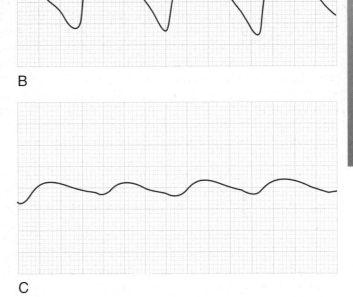

B

FIGURE 16–6. Abnormal digital photople-thysmographic waveforms. *A*, Proximal arte-rial obstruction—the photoplethysmographic waveforms are severely damped (widened, flat-tened). *B*, Raynaud's disease—mildly damped waveforms with unusually high dicrotic notch. *C*, Raynaud's phenomenon—severely damped waveforms.

C

or stress stimuli. Symptoms include fingers of both hands becoming virtually white as the arteries and arterioles undergo intense spasm in response to cold or stress.[2] Digital PPG waveforms may be normal or nearly normal at rest but flatten or become severely damped in response to cold stimuli or stress. The typical PPG waveform seen in this condition displays a somewhat slower upstroke than normal, along with a sharp anacrotic notch and a dicrotic notch that is located unusually high on the downslope of

the waveform (see Fig. 16–6B). However, a normal waveform may be seen in a patient with mild Raynaud's disease when vaso-spasm is aborted by warming the hand.

A cold challenge test may be helpful in identifying Raynaud's disease. This test is performed as follows. Baseline digital PPG waveforms are obtained, and the hands are immersed in ice water for 3 to 5 min. Wave-forms are again obtained, and their return to preimmersion appearance is timed. Indi-viduals with normal circulation will return to preimmersion levels within 10 minutes. Those with Raynaud's disease take longer, and some may not recover within a reasonable observation time unless the cycle of vasospasm is broken by warming the hand. Most patients with this condition merely need to protect the fingers from cold exposure a little more than other individuals to avoid the symptoms of Raynaud's disease. Occasionally, patients with Raynaud's disease worsen and they develop trophic changes or ulcerations at the fingertips. However, this is seen only in patients who do not take adequate steps to protect their hands from cold exposure.

Check for Raynaud's Phenomenon

The presence of cold sensitivity complicated by fixed arterial obstruction is referred to as secondary Raynaud's phenomenon. This is a much more serious condition than Raynaud's disease, because there is vasospasm mixed with intraluminal obstruction of some kind. The fact that these two conditions are given similar names creates confusion, even among experienced examiners. *Raynaud's disease*, *Raynaud's phenomenon*, *Raynaud's syndrome*, *primary Raynaud's*, and *secondary Raynaud's* are all terms used—and misused—to describe these two conditions. In this chapter, we use the term *Raynaud's disease* to describe the vasospastic disorder *without intraluminal occlusion* and *Raynaud's phenomenon* to describe vasospastic disease *accompanied by* fixed arterial obstruction.[3] Regardless of the terms used, the major diagnostic challenge is to differentiate between those patients who have only vasospasm and those who have arterial obstruction as well.

Photoplethysmographic waveforms in a patient with Raynaud's phenomenon are more rounded in appearance than those in a patient with Raynaud's disease and may also be low in amplitude (see Fig. 16–6C). The waveform shape is similar to that seen with proximal arterial occlusion, and it is important to differentiate between these two etiologies with segmental pressure and Doppler, as discussed previously. When severe digital waveform abnormalities are found in the proper clinical setting, it is clear that the condition is Raynaud's phenomenon, and further assessment with hand cooling is not necessary. However, warming the hand may be useful to determine if flow to the fingers can be improved.

For those who insist on performing a cold challenge on patients with findings of Raynaud's phenomenon, it is advisable to follow the cold challenge with a sympathectomy, as follows. The baseline study is done first, followed by immersion of the hands in ice water for 3 to 5 min. The waveforms typically go flat in response to the cold challenge. Then the sympathectomy is performed. In such cases, a physician injects a small amount of a local anesthetic into a nerve, plexus, or ganglion to temporarily inactivate its effect on sympathetic tone. Once the sympathectomy has been set up properly, the PPG waveforms are taken again. Major waveform improvement, above baseline levels, suggests that sympathectomy or vasodilator therapy may be helpful. If vasospasm is a major component of the problem, the hand and fingers may become very warm and the PPG waveforms may go off scale (Fig. 16–7A). The hand is then reimmersed in the cold water. If the waveforms survive reimmersion (see Fig. 16–7B), this is an especially hopeful sign that some degree of improvement can be expected with therapy. It is not advisable to do the cold immersion test in patients with severe Raynaud's phenomenon without follow-up sympathectomy, as a severe vasospastic response may occur that is hard to reverse.

As noted previously, Raynaud's phenomenon represents a combination of vasospasm and arterial occlusion. Therefore, there may be a role for duplex ultrasound assessment of digital and palmar arterial patency, as discussed later.

WHEN TO ADD DUPLEX IMAGING

The decision as to whether duplex ultrasound imaging is necessary in the course of an upper extremity arterial examination

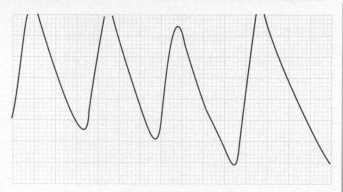

A

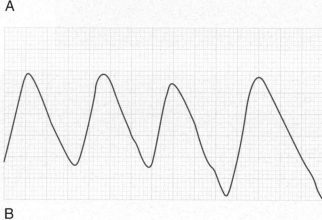

B

FIGURE 16–7. Vasospastic disease. *A,* The photoplethysmographic waveform of a digit is off scale after cold immersion, followed by nerve block to reopen the digital arteries. *B,* Waveform amplitude decreases after reimmersion in ice water, but the amplitude remains quite high.

depends on whether the indirect studies already performed have answered the clinical question at hand. If the answer is no, then duplex imaging should be performed. For example, duplex is necessary whenever the indirect tests suggest arterial obstruction. In this situation, the arm arteries are scanned to identify the exact location and severity of stenosis or occlusion. Duplex imaging can also be used to see if the problem identified by indirect tests is caused by atherosclerotic plaque or thrombus. Arterial thrombus may be treated with anticoagulants, thrombolytics, or even thrombectomy, whereas plaque is treated differently.

Duplex imaging is also used to detect an arterial aneurysm. This is an important piece of information, as an aneurysm may be the source of distal arterial thromboembolization. The subclavian and axillary arteries are the most likely areas for aneurysm formation in the arm. Repeated injury to these arteries, due to impingement at the thoracic outlet, can lead to thrombus formation, plaque formation, and even aneurysmal dilation.

For this reason, whenever there is thrombus anywhere in the arm or hand, even when there is no indication of proximal stenosis on indirect tests, the subclavian/axillary artery region should be scanned.

Duplex Imaging Technique and Diagnostic Criteria

Duplex examination of the arm arteries is similar to duplex imaging of the lower extremity. Typically, a vessel is imaged first with short-axis views to get the examiner oriented, and then the transducer is turned 90 degrees to obtain long-axis views, which are used to follow the vessels (Fig. 16–8). The entire course of each major artery is imaged, including the subclavian, axillary, brachial, radial, ulnar, deep palmar arch, superficial palmar arch, and digital arteries.

Because the arm arteries are mostly superficial, high-frequency transducers can be used. Most, or sometimes all, of the arteries in the arm can be imaged with frequencies between 8 and 15 MHz. However, some

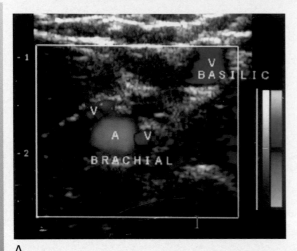

A

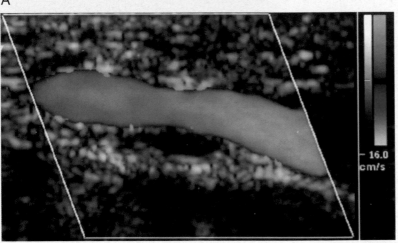

B

FIGURE 16–8. Typical duplex ultrasound transducer positions. *A,* The short-axis view shows the vessel in cross-section. The brachial artery (A) is seen in this color flow image, accompanied by the brachial and basilic veins (V). *B,* The long-axis view shows vessels, such as this axillary artery, along their length.

areas near the clavicle may require the use of a 3- to 8-MHz transducer. Imaging of hand arteries requires very high frequencies, because these vessels are extremely small. Transducers designed for use in surgery work quite well for imaging the digital arteries, since they have a small footprint and operate at frequencies between 10 and 15 MHz.

Color flow ultrasound is used to identify blood flow within the vessels and to give the examiner an idea of the velocity and direction of flow. Pulsed-wave Doppler signals and spectral analysis are used to determine the velocity of flow at key points within the vessel (Fig. 16–9). Normal, angle-corrected peak systolic velocities within the larger arm arteries, such as the subclavian and axillary arteries, generally run between 70 and 120 cm/sec. Brachial artery peak systolic

velocities range from 50 to 100 cm/sec. Velocities in normal radial and ulnar arteries run between 40 and 90 cm/sec, while velocities within the palmar arches and digits are lower. Normal upper extremity Doppler waveforms are triphasic, but changes in temperature, or even maneuvers such as clenching of the fist, may dramatically change the characteristics of upper extremity waveforms, especially in and near the hand (Fig. 16–10). The large arteries of the upper arm and forearm are relatively easy to identify and evaluate with ultrasound. Imaging the small arteries of the hand is very challenging for several reasons. Not only are the vessels small, but, in addition, there are numerous anatomic variations. Furthermore, the vascular anatomy of the hand described herein is a simplified version of the actual anatomy, which

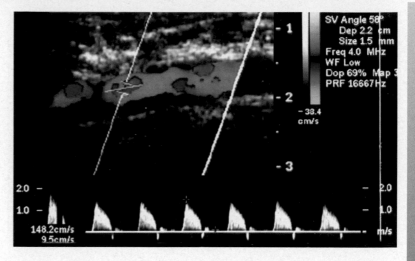

FIGURE 16–9. Pulsed-wave Doppler example. The axillary artery (AX ART) is seen in long axis with color and pulsed wave Doppler. Note that the angle-corrected velocity must be obtained with the cursor lined up with the vessel wall, and the Doppler angle must be 60 degrees or less.

includes arterial pathways beyond the scope of this chapter.[4] That having been said, knowledge of the anatomy shown herein is adequate to answer most of the clinical questions that are raised.

A patterned approach is required for accurate duplex ultrasound evaluation of upper extremity arteries. The ultrasound imaging protocol used in our department, as well as the relevant arterial anatomy, is illustrated in detail in Figures 16–11 through 16–19. This material is not repeated in the text; therefore, readers who are unfamiliar with upper extremity arterial ultrasound should review these figures before proceeding.

Text continued on p. 315

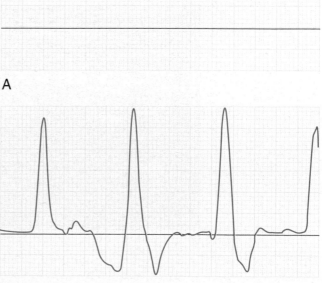

FIGURE 16–10. Environmental and muscular effects. *A*, This continuous-wave Doppler waveform was obtained from the radial artery with the hand very warm and relaxed. Note that the waveform is entirely above the baseline and it is difficult to make judgments about its triphasic pattern. *B*, This continuous-wave Doppler waveform was taken from the same vessel as in *part A*, but now the patient has his fist clenched, causing increased flow resistance. Note the dramatic change in the Doppler waveform. The triphasic, high-resistance pattern now is easily identified.

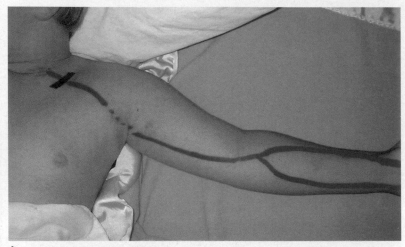

A

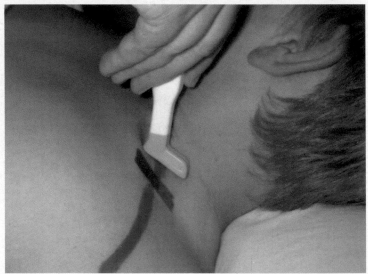

B

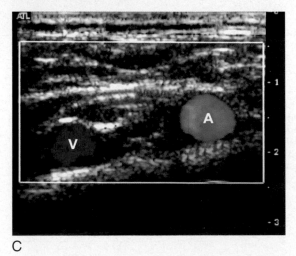

C

FIGURE 16–11. Subclavian segment examination. *A*, Anatomic location of the major upper extremity arteries. *B*, Duplex ultrasound imaging begins with short-axis views of the subclavian artery obtained *above* the clavicle. *C*, In the short-axis view, the artery (A) and vein (V) are identified side by side. Compression with the transducer can be used to identify the artery and vein, since the vein is more easily compressed than the artery. Visualization of the subclavian artery is difficult, at best, because of interference from the clavicle, which limits the space for the transducer and often restricts above-clavicle imaging to short-axis views.

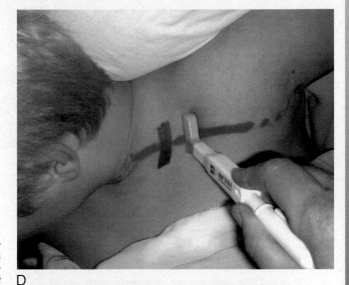

D

FIGURE 16–11—cont'd. *D* and *E*, An alternative approach is to visualize the subclavian artery from an *infraclavicular* transducer position, with which the artery (A) and vein (V) are seen through the pectoral muscles, in either short- or long-axis views.

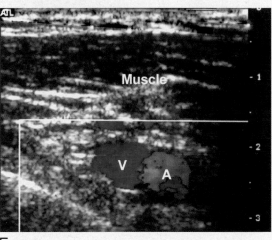

E

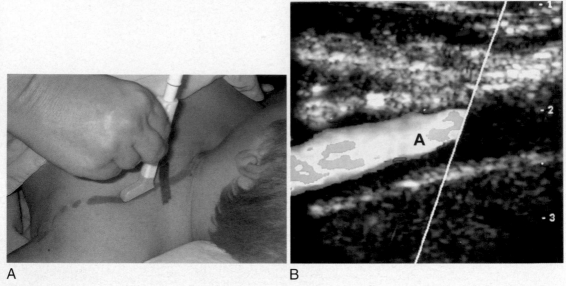

A   B

FIGURE 16–12. Long-axis subclavian examination. *A*, Once the subclavian artery is identified, rotate the transducer to visualize the artery (A) in long axis as shown in part *B*. The artery should be examined proximally and distally as far as possible for the presence of plaque, thrombus, or aneurysm. Frequently, a short segment of the proximal subclavian artery is hidden under the clavicle and cannot be examined directly.

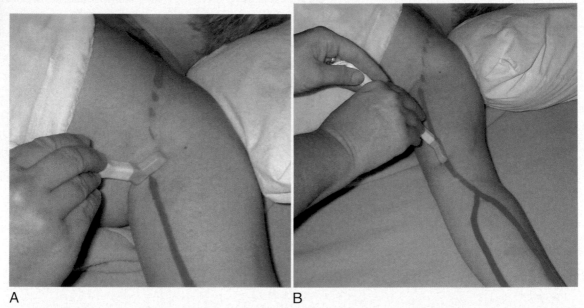

A   B

FIGURE 16–13. Axillary and brachial segment examination. At its distal end, the subclavian artery dives deeply, and at this point, the arm is raised and the probe is repositioned in the axilla to examine the axillary artery. *A*, Begin high in the axilla, with the tranducer positioned for a short-axis view, and get oriented. *B*, After identifying the axillary artery, switch to a long-axis view and follow the axillary and brachial arteries down the medial side of the upper arm in the groove between the biceps and triceps muscles. The axillary artery becomes the brachial artery where it crosses the lower margin of the tendon of the teres major muscle, but this landmark is not readily identified sonographically.

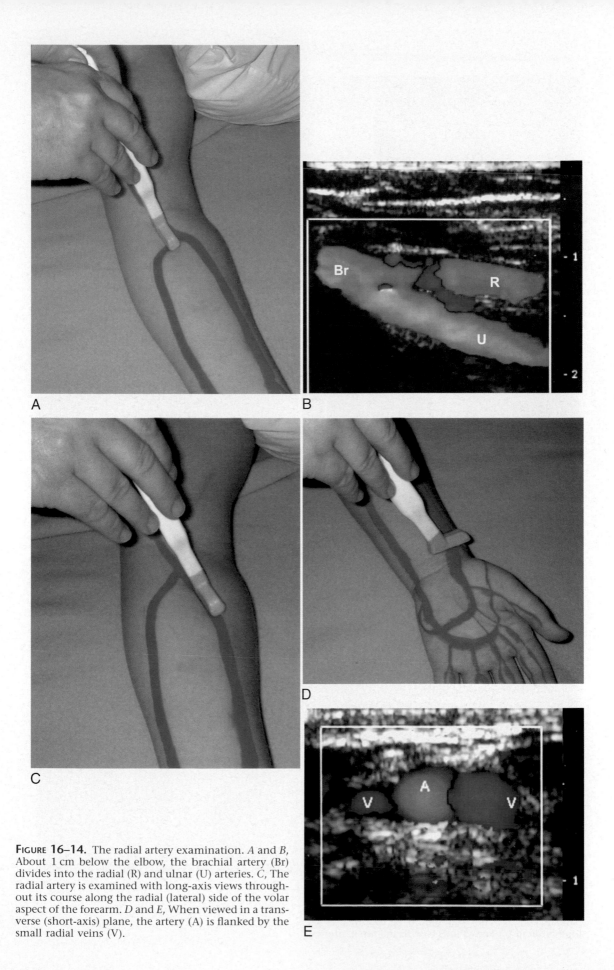

FIGURE 16–14. The radial artery examination. *A* and *B*, About 1 cm below the elbow, the brachial artery (Br) divides into the radial (R) and ulnar (U) arteries. *C*, The radial artery is examined with long-axis views throughout its course along the radial (lateral) side of the volar aspect of the forearm. *D* and *E*, When viewed in a transverse (short-axis) plane, the artery (A) is flanked by the small radial veins (V).

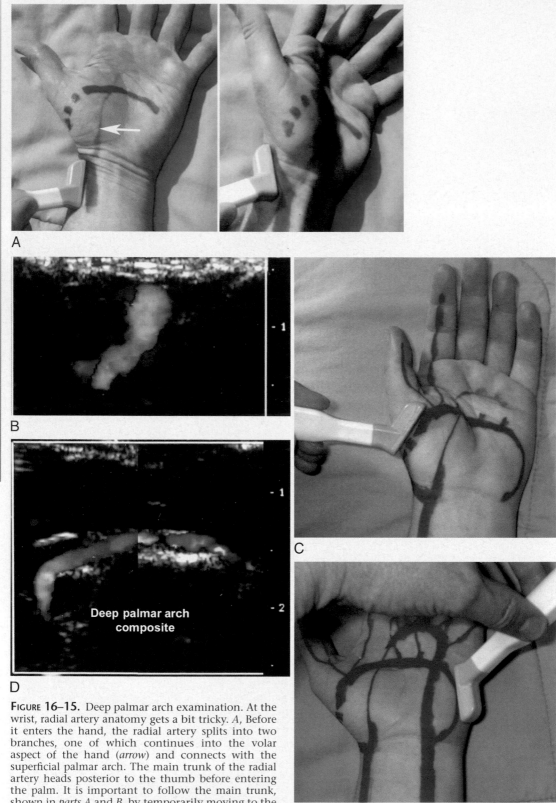

A

B

C

D

Deep palmar arch
composite

E

FIGURE 16–15. Deep palmar arch examination. At the
wrist, radial artery anatomy gets a bit tricky. *A*, Before
it enters the hand, the radial artery splits into two
branches, one of which continues into the volar
aspect of the hand (*arrow*) and connects with the
superficial palmar arch. The main trunk of the radial
artery heads posterior to the thumb before entering
the palm. It is important to follow the main trunk,
shown in *parts A* and *B*, by temporarily moving to the
dorsal aspect of the hand. *C*, The sonographer then
returns to the volar surface and follows the main
trunk into the palm, where it becomes the deep
palmar arch. *D*, The arch should be followed as it
loops around (*E*) and connects with the ulnar artery.

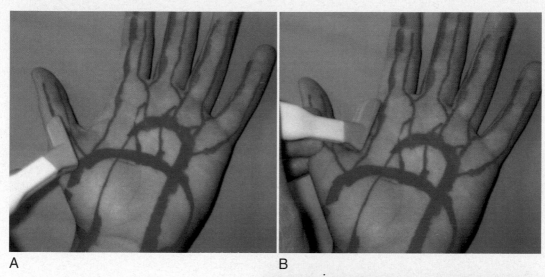

A

B

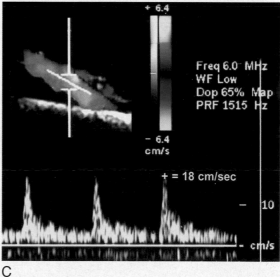

FIGURE 16–16. Examining branches of the deep palmar arch. Two branches of the deep palmar arch are commonly visualized in normal individuals. *A,* Beginning at the radial side, the first branch is the princeps pollicis, which supplies the thumb. *B,* This is followed by another small branch called the radialis indicis, which travels up the radial side of the index finger. These two vessels sometimes share a common trunk. *C,* Doppler signals in these small vessels typically are quite weak and show flow features that differ from the radial and ulnar arteries. Note that while the pattern is one of moderate resistance, flow is present through diastole. Three other small digital arteries (not shown), called the palmar metacarpals, may be seen branching from the deep palmar arch, and these eventually join the common digital arteries to supply the fingers. These arteries are usually difficult to see and follow with ultrasound.

C

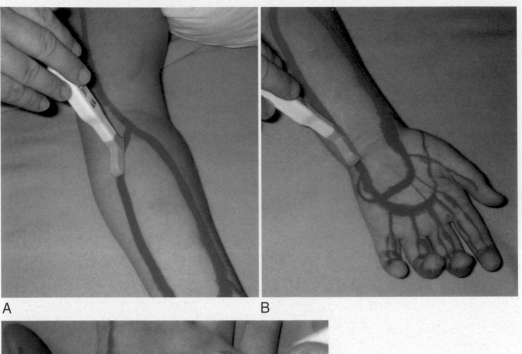

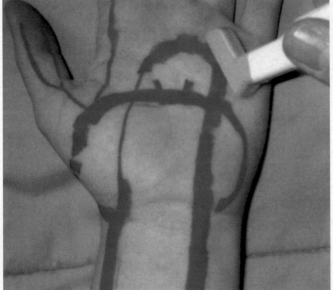

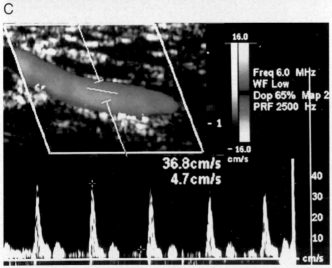

A

B

C

D

FIGURE 16–17. The ulnar artery and superficial palmar arch examination. After evaluating the radial artery and deep palmar arch, the examiner returns to the antecubital fossa to inspect the ulnar artery. *A*, After traveling deeply in the flexor muscles, the ulnar artery runs more superficially, along the volar aspect of the ulnar (medial) side of the forearm. *B*, It can be followed into the palm as a single large trunk, where it curves laterally to form the superficial palmar arch. *C*, When followed, the superficial plamar arch is seen to connect with the smaller branch of the radial artery shown in Figure 16–15A. *D*, Doppler signals in the superficial palmar arch have relatively high resistance, but flow throughout diastole, similar to the deep arch.

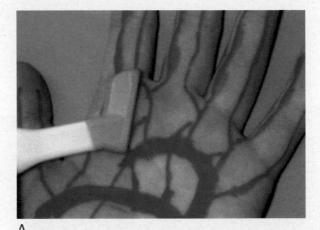

A

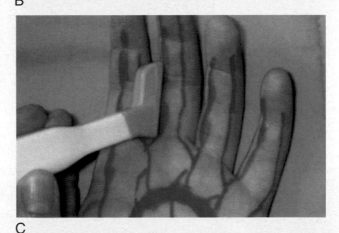

B

FIGURE 16–18. Digital artery examination. *A* and *B*, The principal arterial supply to digits three, four, and five is via the common digital arteries (CDA), which arise from the superficial palmar arch (SPA). *C* and *D*, These can be followed into the fingers, where each branches to form the proper digital arteries that lie on either side of the fingers. Relatively low flow resistance is evident in these vessels.

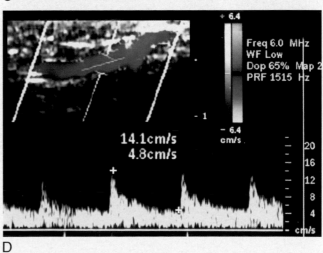

C

D

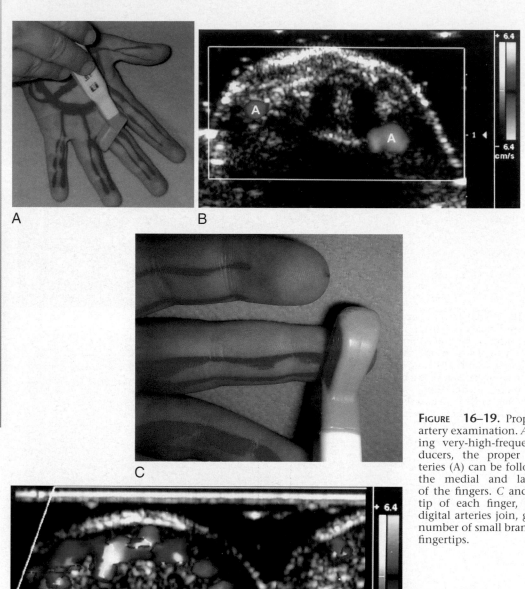

FIGURE 16–19. Proper digital artery examination. *A* and *B*, Using very-high-frequency transducers, the proper digital arteries (A) can be followed along the medial and lateral sides of the fingers. *C* and *D*, At the tip of each finger, the proper digital arteries join, giving off a number of small branches at the fingertips.

Duplex Ultrasound–Detected Pathology

Atherosclerotic plaque forms commonly in the subclavian and axillary arteries. The principal effect is blood flow reduction due to stenosis or occlusion that can result in arm ischemia. Atherosclerotic obstruction of more distal arteries, such as the radial and ulnar arteries, is less common; nevertheless, distal vessels may undergo thrombosis secondary to low-flow states or atherosclerosis-related embolization.

Although stenosis of larger upper extremity arteries is most often caused by atherosclerosis, it may also be caused by vasculitis, trauma, or thoracic outlet compression. Stenosis of smaller arteries usually results from vasospastic disease or vasculitis. In the extremities, stenoses that reduce the lumenal diameter by 50% or greater are flow reducing, or hemodynamically significant. Such stenoses are identified by increased velocity, post-stenotic turbulence, and waveforms that are damped distal to the level of the stenosis, as shown in Figure 16–20. In addition, high-grade arterial stenosis or occlusion causes overall reduced flow velocity proximal to the point of obstruction. There are no universally accepted velocities that determine the severity of a stenosis in the arm arteries; however, when a stenosis causes the peak systolic velocity to double (compared with the prestenotic velocity), it is considered hemodynamically significant. Tighter stenoses increase systolic and diastolic velocities to obvious extremes.

Color flow imaging shows narrowing of the arterial lumen as well as altered colors in the stenotic region consistent with elevated flow velocity and a post-stenotic mosaic pattern that results from turbulent flow. With arterial occlusion, no flow is detected in the vessel lumen with color or spectral Doppler, and a damped, monophasic Doppler signal is seen distal to the area of obstruction (Fig. 16–21). When occlusion is detected, it is important to determine the extent of the occluded segment and where in the arterial tree flow is reconstituted by collaterals.

Arterial thrombosis may occur distal to a critical stenosis or may result from embolization, trauma, or thoracic outlet compression. The result may be occlusion or partial occlusion. Thrombus filling a vessel may be visualized directly with gray-scale imaging, but color or power Doppler imaging is useful to determine if the vessel is patent and to assess the degree of vessel recanalization with thrombolysis (Fig. 16–22). Whenever thrombus is thought to be seen in an artery, the examiner should attempt to compress the artery using transducer pressure. If the artery is truly filled with thrombus, compression will *not* cause the artery to collapse. This is important because artifacts may be present that look like thrombus in an artery. If the artery collapses in response to compression (Fig. 16–23), the suspected "thrombus" can be accurately determined to be artifactual.

Arterial aneurysms in the upper extremity are rare, but the most likely place for their occurrence is in the subclavian/axillary area. They usually occur as a result of chronic trauma, as is the case with thoracic outlet impingement, or they may occur on an idiopathic basis. Because laminated thrombus commonly forms in aneurysms, they become a likely source of emboli to the radial, ulnar, or hand arteries. For this reason, whenever thrombus is found in distal arteries, the subclavian/axillary arteries should be checked carefully for the presence of an aneurysm. A vessel is said to be aneurysmal when the diameter at the point of interest is at least one and a half times the size of the artery above and below it. Most aneurysms in the arm are fusiform, as seen in Figure 16–24, rather than saccular, and for that reason, they tend to be more subtle than aneurysms in other parts of the arterial system.

CHECK FOR VERTEBRAL-TO-SUBCLAVIAN STEAL

If a patient has a significant difference in arm blood pressure (20 mm Hg, as observed during the segmental pressure/PVR portion of the study), the duplex imaging examination should be expanded to check for the

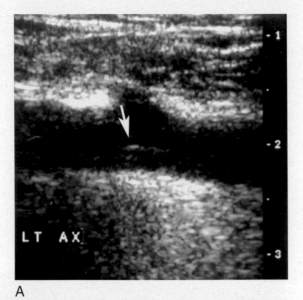

A

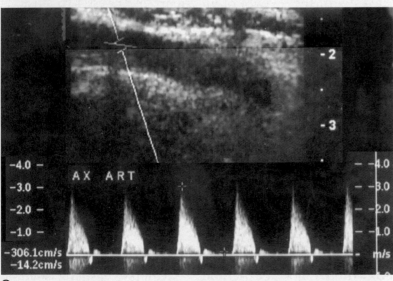

B

C

FIGURE 16–20. Hemodynamically significant stenosis. *A*, Plaque is seen in the axillary (LT AX) artery with B-mode imaging. *B*, Color is added to reveal the contour of the plaque and its flow effects. *C*, Pulsed Doppler is used to display the markedly increased flow velocity (306 cm/sec) in the stenosis. AX ART, axillary artery.

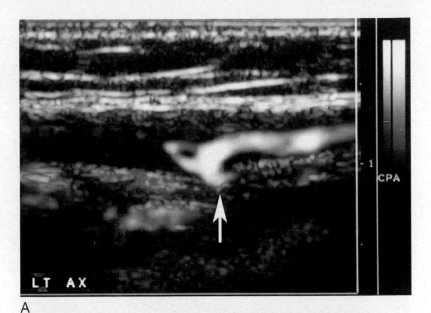

A

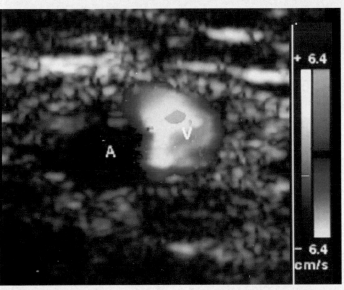

FIGURE 16–21. Arterial occlusion. *A* and *B*, Long- and short-axis color flow views show occlusion of an axillary artery (A). V, axillary vein. Note in *part A* that flow is reconstituted below the occlusion by a collateral (*arrow*). *C*, Below the occlusion, in the ulnar artery, Doppler waveforms are damped—monophasic, delayed time to peak, broad systolic peak, continuous diastolic flow.

B

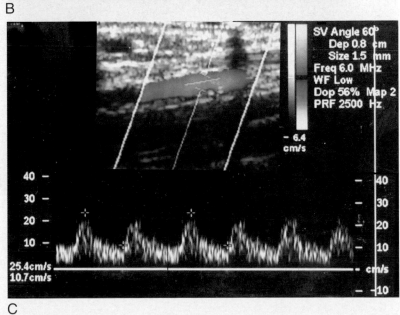

C

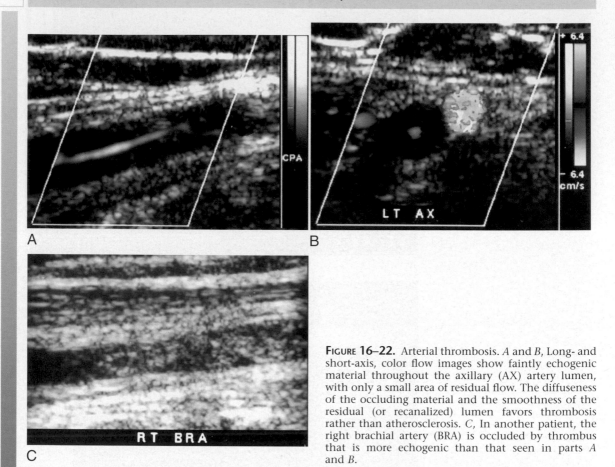

A

B

C

FIGURE 16–22. Arterial thrombosis. *A* and *B*, Long- and short-axis, color flow images show faintly echogenic material throughout the axillary (AX) artery lumen, with only a small area of residual flow. The diffuseness of the occluding material and the smoothness of the residual (or recanalized) lumen favors thrombosis rather than atherosclerosis. *C*, In another patient, the right brachial artery (BRA) is occluded by thrombus that is more echogenic than that seen in parts *A* and *B*.

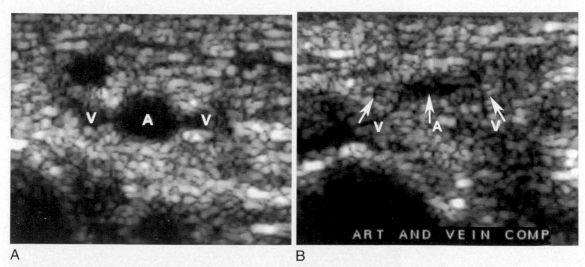

A

B

FIGURE 16–23. Artifact versus thrombus. Whenever it appears that thrombus is present in an artery (*A*), the vessel should be viewed in a transverse plane (*A*) and compressed with the transducer (*arrows*, part *B*). If the artery truly is thrombosed, the intraluminal thrombus will prevent it from collapsing in response to compression. However, if the artery compresses fully (*B*), the examiner knows the "thrombus" was actually artifactual. V, vein.

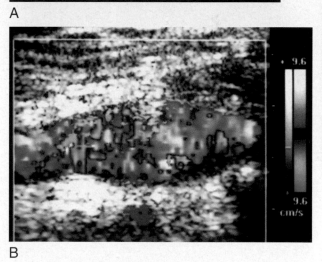

FIGURE 16–24. Aneurysm. *A* and *B*, B-mode and color flow views show a typical, fusiform aneurysm (approximately 9-mm diameter) in the subclavian/axillary segment. No thrombus is visible in this aneurysm, but aneurysms may contain thrombus that can embolize to distal vessels.

+ = 9.3 mm
x = 4.1 mm
Rt. Subclavian

A

B

vertebral-to-subclavian steal. This is a situation in which a tight stenosis or occlusion is present in the portion of the subclavian artery proximal to the ipsilateral vertebral artery. Insufficient blood flow through the obstruction causes the subclavian artery to steal blood from the contralateral vertebral artery. Vertebral-to-subclavian steal rarely causes severe neurologic symptoms, but it may cause arterial insufficiency in the affected arm that may be clinically important. For details concerning the pathophysiology of this condition and its clinical consequences, please see Chapter 11.

Whenever vertebral-to-subclavian steal is suspected, the examiner should check the direction of the flow in the ipsilateral vertebral artery. If flow is retrograde or undulating (to and fro), vertebral-to-subclavian steal is likely. This finding, combined with a blood pressure in the ipsilateral arm 20 mm or more lower than the opposite arm, makes a compelling case for subclavian steal. To make the case even stronger, the examiner can compare the axillary Doppler waveforms, noting that the waveforms on the side of the obstruction are more rounded and of lower overall velocity, and

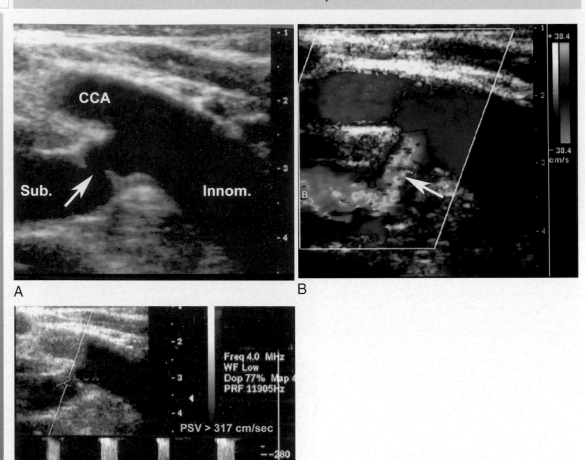

FIGURE 16–25. Subclavian stenosis. *A*, Gray-scale sonography provides a rare direct view of a stenosis at the origin of the subclavian artery (*arrows*). Sub, subclavian; CCA, common carotid artery; Innom, innominate artery. *B*, Color Doppler shows turbulent flow in the stenotic segment (*arrow*). *C*, Pulsed Doppler signals reveal markedly elevated flow velocity within the stenosis that cannot be measured as it exceeds the maximum velocity/frequency scale. Peak systolic velocity (PSV) exceeds 317 cm/sec.

they may be monophasic. The vertebral and subclavian Doppler findings are presented in detail in Chapter 11.

With diligence, the examiner can sometimes see the stenotic area of the subclavian artery directly and document the presence of stenosis, rather than occlusion. This requires angulation of the ultrasound beam deeply beneath the medial end of the clavicle. The usual features of arterial stenosis are seen (Fig. 16–25). The lumen is visibly narrowed on the color flow image, with a color shift indicating elevated flow velocity. Spectral Doppler shows high-velocity systolic and diastolic flow levels in the stenotic region and turbulence distal to the stenosis. Even if the stenosis itself cannot be seen, it may be possible to detect the severe post-stenotic turbulence that is invariably associated with a high-grade arterial stenosis.

Direct subclavian stenosis visualization is much more likely to be possible on the right side, as shown in Figure 16–25, than on the left, because the right subclavian artery is a branch of the innominate artery, which makes the area of stenosis much more superficial. On the right, the stenosis is generally seen in the most proximal segment of the subclavian artery, just beyond the bifurcation of the innominate artery into the common carotid and subclavian branches.

Seeing a stenosis on the left side is much more difficult, as the subclavian artery comes off the aorta at an angle that is difficult to image and at a depth that causes imaging problems. This is unfortunate, considering that 85% of vertebral-to-subclavian steal cases occur on the left side.

CONCLUSIONS: ANSWERING THE CLINICAL QUESTION

This chapter is a compilation of the common physiologic and Doppler tests used to assess upper extremity arteries. Only the more frequently encountered arterial disorders affecting the upper extremities could be included. It is important to consider that any combination of the methods described herein can be used at the discretion of the ordering physician, or the examiner, to answer the clinical question at hand. Knowledge of the value of a given test in a given situation is required to ensure that everything is done diagnostically that can be done. The proper combination of tests is the key to shedding light on a difficult diagnosis.

References

1. Zwiebel, WJ: Introduction to Vascular Ultrasonography, 4th ed. Philadelphia, Saunders, 2000.
2. Robbins, SL: Basic Pathology. Philadelphia, Saunders, 1981.
3. Hershey FB, Barnes RW, Sumner DS: Noninvasive Diagnosis of Vascular Disease. Pasadena, Appleton Davies, 1984.
4. Crafts RC: Textbook of Human Anatomy, 2nd ed. New York, John Wiley and Sons, 1979.

Chapter 17

Ultrasound Evaluation Before and After Hemodialysis Access

MICHELLE L. ROBBIN, MD, MS, AND MARK E. LOCKHART, MD, MPH

Ultrasound can be extremely useful in the evaluation of the many problems facing the hemodialysis patient. It is a noninvasive technique that can show more vascular detail than physical examination, without the risk of phlebitis or contrast reaction from conventional venography. Current Dialysis Outcome Quality Initiative guidelines encourage the placement of arteriovenous fistulas (AVFs) rather than grafts, because of their greater longevity and decreased incidence of infection.[1,2] Detailed evaluation of arterial and venous anatomy prior to hemodialysis access can increase the visualization of veins that may be suitable for native AVF placement, particularly in the patient with a history of prior failed access and/or central lines.

Vascular mapping prior to hemodialysis access also may change surgical management, with an increase in the number of AVFs versus grafts placed. Additionally, there is an increased likelihood of selecting the most functional vessels preoperatively, with a subsequent decrease in unsuccessful surgical explorations.[3] Vascular mapping has doubled the proportion of patients dialyzing with a fistula in our patient population.[4]

Despite preoperative vascular mapping, a substantial number of AVFs still fail to mature adequately to support hemodialysis. In these patients, ultrasound can determine the potential cause of an immature AVF. It can also determine whether the AVF would be best treated by the angiographer (angioplasty of a stenosis) or surgeon (revision or accessory vein ligation). Ultrasound is also useful in the evaluation of the patient with a hemodialysis graft, to assess for stenosis and determine the cause of perigraft palpable masses (hematoma versus pseudoaneurysm).

This chapter details hemodialysis access anatomy and the preferred order of access placement. It describes current protocols for the sonographic vascular evaluation of the end-stage renal patient, both before and after hemodialysis access placement.

BASIC CONCEPTS OF HEMODIALYSIS ACCESS

Hemodialysis is the lifeline by which the patient with end-stage renal disease eliminates excess fluid and decreases the level of various undesirable substances in the blood. The central circulation is accessed, and the blood is cleansed by diffusion across a semipermeable membrane, termed the *dialyzer*. Direct access to the circulation is accomplished by an AVF, a graft, or a central venous catheter. A native AVF is a surgically created, direct anastomosis between an artery and a vein, placed in either the forearm or upper arm. When AVF creation is not possible, an artificial graft may be tunneled in the superficial soft tissues of the forearm, upper arm, or upper thigh, with arterial and venous anastomoses. Two 15-gauge needles are placed into the AVF or graft, with the more distal needle carrying blood from the patient to the dialyzer. The second needle is placed more proximally in the AVF or graft and returns the blood to the patient's circulation. Artery/vein configurations for the various types of AVFs and grafts

Table 17–1. AVF and Graft Artery/Vein Anastomoses

AVF Types	Artery	Vein
Forearm cephalic vein	Radial	Cephalic
Forearm vein transposition	Radial	Ulnar, dorsal or volar vein transposition
Upper arm cephalic vein	Brachial	Cephalic
Basilic vein transposition	Brachial	Basilic
Graft Types	**Artery**	**Vein**
Forearm loop	Brachial	Antecubital
Upper arm straight	Brachial	Basilic
Upper arm loop	Axillary	Axillary
Thigh graft	Common femoral/superficial femoral	Greater saphenous/common femoral

AVF, arteriovenous fistula.

are shown in Table 17–1. Figure 17–1 shows anatomic drawings of the three most common AVFs and four most common graft configurations.

Surgeons prefer to create a hemodialysis access in the nondominant arm, as the activities of daily living can be carried out with the dominant arm while the nondominant arm is healing after surgical access placement. However, most will put an AVF in the dominant arm before a graft is considered. An AVF is placed first in the forearm, if the patient has suitable anatomy, and the upper arm is then "saved" for a future access. Likewise, if an AVF cannot be placed, a forearm graft is preferred to placement of an upper arm graft. If no upper extremity graft options are available, a thigh graft is preferable to dialyzing with an indwelling venous catheter.[5] A list of the preferred order of access placement is given in Table 17–2. In general, an AVF or graft will provide higher dialysis flow rates than a tunneled catheter,[6] with a lower infection rate.[7]

DESCRIPTIVE TERMINOLOGY

The conventional way to describe vascular anatomy employs the terms *proximal* and *distal*, meaning closer and farther from the heart, respectively. We find that these terms can be confusing when used in describing dialysis access anatomy. In some circumstances, therefore, we prefer the terms *cranial* and *caudal*, meaning toward the head and toward the lower end of the body.

We will use these terms in selected locations throughout this chapter, realizing that the more conventional terms are used elsewhere in this text.

VASCULAR MAPPING PRIOR TO HEMODIALYSIS ACCESS PLACEMENT

General Principles

The protocol for vascular mapping prior to hemodialysis access placement has been previously described,[3,8] A high-resolution linear ultrasound transducer is used to evaluate the arm vessels (generally 7 MHz or higher). The transverse plane is used to identify vessels (artery and vein) and evaluate their diameter and wall thickness. Sequential vein compression is used to assess for compressibility. The depth from the skin surface of the anterior wall of the cephalic vein is measured. Color and spectral Doppler waveforms are obtained in the longitudinal plane of vessels selected for potential vascular access.

The forearm veins and arteries are assessed to determine whether the patient is a candidate for a forearm AVF, the most desirable initial type of hemodialysis access. If vascular anatomy suitable for forearm fistula creation is not found, the upper arm vessels should be mapped. Arteries should be assessed for intimal thickening and stenosis. The presence of significant concentric calcification should be noted, as the

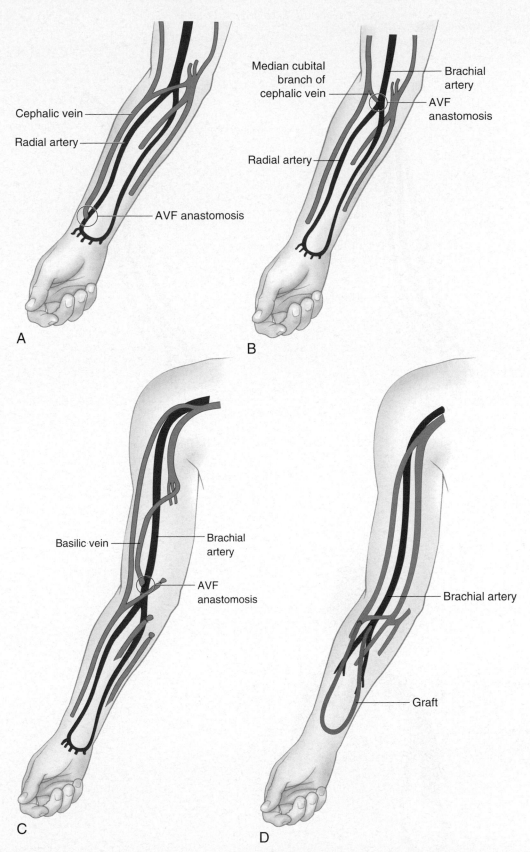

Figure 17-1. Anatomic drawings of the most common hemodialysis accesses. The three most common arteriovenous fistulas are (A) radiocephalic fistula at the wrist, (B) brachiocephalic fistula at the antecubital fossa, and (C) brachiobasilic vein transposition. The four most common grafts include (D) forearm loop graft, (E) upper arm straight graft, (F) axillary loop graft, and (G) thigh graft. AVF, arteriovenous fistula. *Continued*

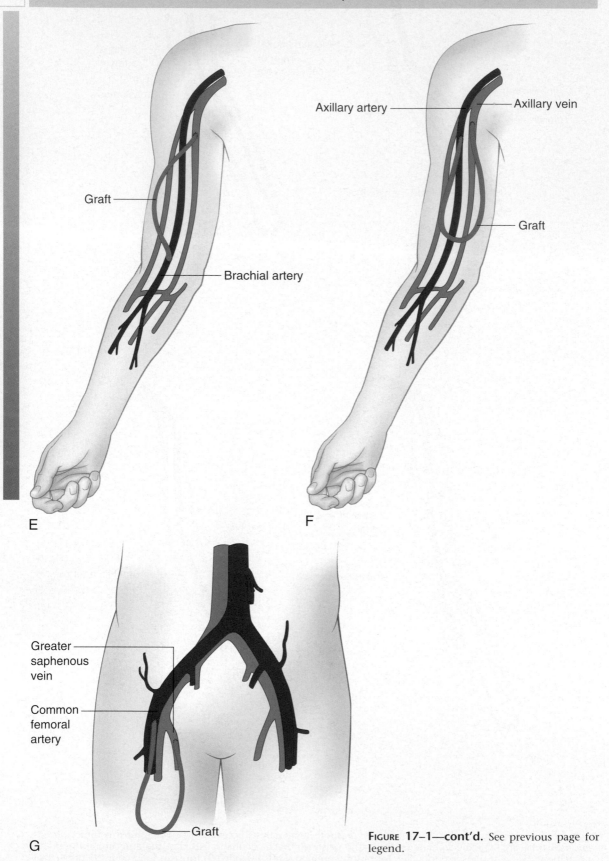

Axillary artery

Axillary vein

Graft

Brachial artery

Graft

E

F

Greater
saphenous
vein

Common
femoral
artery

Graft

G

FIGURE 17–1—cont'd. See previous page for legend.

Table 17-2. Preferred Order of Access Placement

Order of Access Placement	Type of Placement
1	Nondominant forearm cephalic vein fistula
2	Dominant forearm cephalic vein fistula
3	Nondominant or dominant upper arm cephalic vein fistula
4	Nondominant or dominant upper arm basilic vein transposition fistula
5	Forearm loop graft
6	Upper arm straight graft
7	Upper arm loop graft (axillary artery to axillary vein)

From Allon M, Robbin ML: Increasing arteriovenous fistulas in hemodialysis patients: Problems and solutions. Kidney Int 62:1109–1124, 2002.

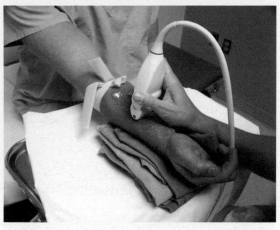

FIGURE 17-2. Proper position of arm on instrument stand for imaging of the vessels for hemodialysis planning.

artery may be too calcified for successful surgical access creation. An important aspect of planning for AVF and graft creation is vessel size assessment. Minimum artery and vein diameters are shown in Table 17–3.

Forearm Assessment

The nondominant forearm is assessed first. The patient's arm is placed in a comfortable position on towels on top of a procedure

Table 17-3. Minimum Diameter Criteria for AVF and Graft Creation

Vessel	Minimum Diameter (cm)
AVF vein	0.25
Graft vein	0.40
Artery (graft or AVF)	0.20

AVF, arteriovenous fistula.
From Silva MB, Hobson RW, Pappas PJ, et al: A strategy for increasing use of autogenous hemodialysis access procedures: Impact of preoperative noninvasive evaluation. J Vasc Surg 27(2):307–308, 1998.

stand (Fig. 17–2). The internal diameter of the radial artery at the wrist must measure at least 2 mm (Fig. 17–3). If the radial artery internal diameter is not satisfactory within several centimeters of the wrist, the internal diameter of the ulnar artery at the wrist is measured. If the diameter of the ulnar or radial artery is not at least 2 mm in the lower third of the forearm, the forearm radial and ulnar arteries are assessed on the dominant side. If no forearm artery is satisfactory, the patient is not a candidate for a forearm AVF.

If the radial or ulnar artery at the wrist meets size criteria, the next vessel to evaluate is the cephalic vein. A tourniquet is placed fairly tightly, slightly lower than mid-forearm. The entire distal forearm is percussed, similar to starting an intravenous line, for approximately 3 minutes. All wrist veins that measure greater than 2 mm after the 3-minute tapping are evaluated. Veins smaller than 2 mm will probably not dilate up to an adequate size. However, veins greater than 2 mm may dilate to greater than 2.5 mm with more focused tapping and/or a warm compress. Special attention is given to the cephalic vein, as this is the preferred venous outflow conduit. The cephalic vein area is assessed for the presence of a continuous vein up to the tourniquet with a diameter of at least 2.5 mm (Fig. 17–4). Venous patency is demonstrated with spectral Doppler interrogation, augmenting

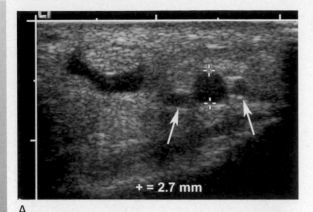

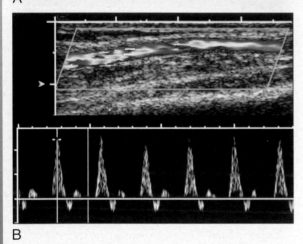

FIGURE 17–3. Normal radial artery at the wrist. *A,* Transverse gray-scale view of the radial artery shows adequate arterial diameter measuring 2.7 mm (*cursors*). Note the small paired radial veins (*arrows*). *B,* Color and spectral longitudinal views of the artery demonstrates normal triphasic flow and absence of turbulent flow or aliasing.

flow by having the patient flex his or her fingers, or by compression.

If the forearm portion of the cephalic vein is adequate, a tourniquet is placed at the elbow and the vein is followed in a cephalad direction to the elbow. If the vein is discontinuous or stenotic, it is not satisfactory for fistula creation. A search for another adequate forearm vein should be performed. Branch points should be assessed carefully, as vein narrowing below 2.5 mm may occur at branch points. Following examination of the forearm, the tourniquet is moved sequentially in stages to the axilla, and the vein of interest is followed centrally to ensure that it empties into the deep venous system. The tourniquet must be removed to evaluate the cephalic vein insertion into the subclavian vein. Occasionally, overlying muscle may give the appearance of a stenosis at the insertion of the cephalic vein into the subclavian vein. Placing the patient's arm by his or her side (rather than abducted) may alleviate an apparent cephalic vein stenosis.

If the cephalic vein is not adequate, the basilic vein in the forearm is assessed. If the basilic vein is not adequate, the volar surface of the forearm, followed by the dorsal surface of the forearm is assessed for a suitable vein. If no vein is sufficient in the forearm, a frequent finding in the end-stage renal patient, the same protocol should be followed in the dominant arm.

Upper Arm Assessment

If a forearm fistula is not possible, the upper arm should be assessed for anatomy suitable for a fistula. A tourniquet is placed at the axilla. The brachial artery is measured above its bifurcation into the radial and ulnar

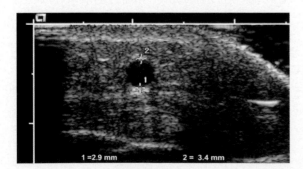

FIGURE 17–4. Normal cephalic vein at the wrist. The cephalic vein has a normal diameter measuring 2.9 mm (*cursors*) and normal depth of 3.4 mm.

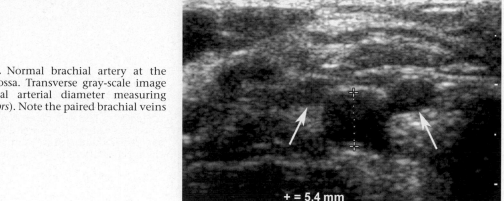

FIGURE 17–5. Normal brachial artery at the antecubital fossa. Transverse gray-scale image shows normal arterial diameter measuring 5.4 mm (*cursors*). Note the paired brachial veins (*arrows*).

arteries. Satisfactory internal diameter should be 2 mm or greater (Fig. 17–5).

The cephalic vein diameter is then measured at the elbow. For a brachiocephalic fistula, it should measure at least 2.5 mm and extend approximately 2 cm below the antecubital fossa. Several centimeters of vein are needed to make the anastomosis with the brachial artery near the antecubital fossa. Alternatively, the surgeons may use a median cubital branch of the cephalic vein as it travels close to the brachial artery; therefore, this branch should also be evaluated.

If an adequate cephalic vein is not found (Fig. 17–6), the basilic vein (Fig. 17–7) is assessed for a basilic vein transposition or graft and the brachial veins are measured (for a possible graft). A basilic vein suitable for a basilic vein transposition must extend at least 2 cm caudal to the antecubital fossa to provide a suitable length to loop around and connect with the brachial artery. If the basilic vein does not extend 2 cm into the forearm, it may still be of adequate diameter for a graft (4 mm).

If a suitable vein is found, its continuity with the deep venous system must be confirmed. To this end, the vein is followed cephalad to ensure that it is continuous and of adequate size along its entire course, until it empties into the deep venous system. The diameter of the deep system venous drainage is also evaluated to the point at which it empties into the subclavian vein. If no anatomy suitable for an AVF, forearm loop, or upper arm straight graft is found, the axillary vein and axillary artery diameters are measured for a possible upper arm loop graft.

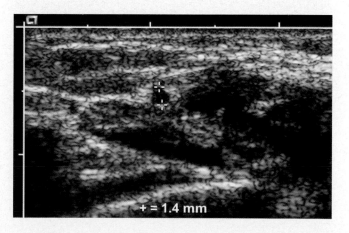

FIGURE 17–6. Small cephalic vein in the caudal upper arm. Transverse gray-scale image shows a small cephalic vein measuring 1.4 mm that does not meet 2-mm minimum diameter (*cursors*).

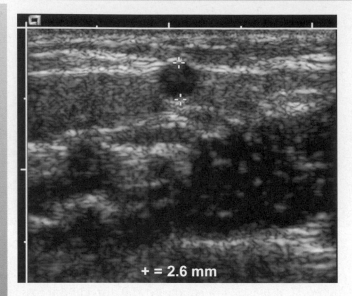

+ = 2.6 mm

FIGURE 17–7. Normal basilic vein in upper arm. Transverse gray-scale image shows a normal basilic vein measuring 2.6 mm diameter (*cursors*). The vein depth is not considered, since the vein will be surgically isolated and superficially tunneled within the upper arm to the brachial artery for anastomosis.

Subclavian, Internal Jugular, and Central Vein Assessment

The subclavian and internal jugular (IJ) veins are evaluated directly for stenosis and thrombus, from either a prior central line or venous thrombosis. Spectral waveforms should be assessed in the medial portion of the subclavian vein, and the caudal portion of the IJ, for respiratory phasicity and transmitted cardiac pulsatility (Fig. 17–8). If these flow features are absent (monophasic flow is demonstrated), central venous stenosis or obstruction is inferred. The contralateral subclavian and IJ should then be examined. If the flow abnormality is unilateral, brachiocephalic vein stenosis is likely. If bilateral, a superior vena cava (SVC) stenosis or occlusion is likely. Figure 17–9 shows abnormal unilateral respiratory phasicity and transmitted cardiac pulsatility in the left subclavian vein, consistent with a brachiocephalic vein stenosis or occlusion. Occasionally, the brachiocephalic veins and SVC can be directly visualized with ultrasound. In such cases, they are best seen with a small footprint transducer placed above the medial clavicle or in the sternal notch, using central angulation.

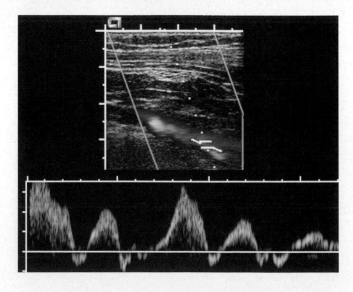

FIGURE 17–8. Normal subclavian vein. Longitudinal duplex Doppler image demonstrates color flow filling the vein and a normal spectral waveform with phasic temporary reversal of flow during respiration.

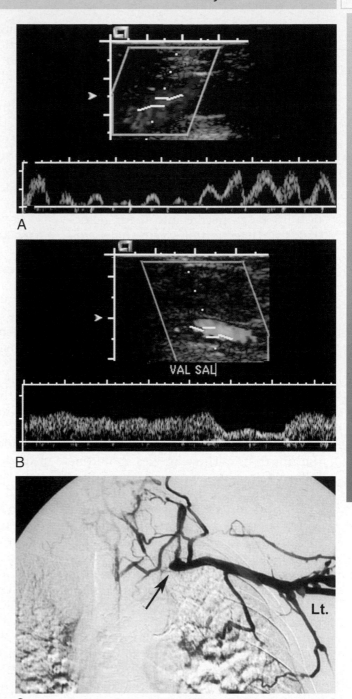

FIGURE 17–9. Abnormal subclavian vein waveform. *A*, Longitudinal duplex Doppler shows normal phasic flow within the right subclavian vein. *B*, Duplex Doppler of the left subclavian vein depicts abnormal monophasic venous waveforms. *C*, Subsequent venogram confirms occlusion of the left brachiocephalic vein (*arrow*).

KEY POINTS REGARDING PREOPERATIVE MAPPING

1. It may be possible to create a forearm cephalic vein AVF, even if the cephalic vein in the upper arm is small or occluded by thrombus. If the cephalic vein in the forearm drains into the brachial or basilic veins via an adequately sized median cubital or other branch vein, it is suitable for AVF creation.

2. It is important to carefully assess vein branch points, as areas of focal stenosis may occur at accessory vein take-offs. These stenoses may significantly

limit flow in a subsequently created access.

3. The cephalic vein may meet diameter criteria for AVF creation yet may be too deep to access easily at hemodialysis once the AVF is mature. Therefore, the depth of the cephalic vein from the skin surface should be measured during the ultrasound mapping procedure. If the vein is greater than 0.5 cm in depth, it will likely be difficult to palpate the vein with sufficient confidence to permit the insertion of a 15-gauge needle into it for hemodialysis.[9] Detection of a vein that is too deep but otherwise suitable for an AVF allows the surgeon to inform the patient preoperatively about the potential need for a second procedure to "superficialize" the vein in the subcutaneous tissues. This discussion allows the patient to decide whether to accept the procedure.

4. A high radial artery takeoff from the brachial or even axillary artery in the upper arm is a common anatomic variant. The presence of this variant can be suspected when two arteries with accompanying paired veins are seen in the upper arm. These arteries should be followed into the forearm, where they assume the respective positions of the radial and ulnar arteries. Hemodialysis access surgeons are reluctant to place a forearm graft or upper arm straight graft in a patient with a high radial artery takeoff, as the chance for arterial steal is increased. Infrequently, a prominent arterial branch that courses posteriorly toward the elbow can mimic a high radial artery takeoff. Following the course of the artery more distally allows differentiation.

5. It is important to analyze the spectral waveform of the brachial and radial arteries to detect either proximal or distal arterial obstruction. With proximal obstruction, the waveforms are monophasic and dampened. With distal obstruction, the waveforms have a normal triphasic pattern, but the velocity may be reduced because of diminished outflow. Malovrh[10] noted a higher success rate in forearm fistulas in patients who converted from triphasic to monophasic

flow after release of a clenched fist. In his series, no radial artery diameter threshold was applied. However, we did not find an arterial peak systolic velocity (PSV) cutoff or change in resistive index with a clenched fist maneuver that is predictive of subsequent AVF maturation, assuming the standard minimum diameter criteria of 2 mm is met,[11] and do not recommend the use of PSV or resistive index criteria.

AVF MATURITY ASSESSMENT

General Principles

A frequently used definition of a mature AVF in the United States is a fistula that is usable for hemodialysis at a flow of 350 cc/min at six dialysis sessions in one month.[12] Practitioners in other countries, particularly in Europe, accept lower AVF flows with subsequently longer dialysis times.[1,2] A mature AVF can be identified clinically as one that has a large, easily palpable vein that can provide access for two 15-gauge needles.[13] Experienced dialysis nurses were found to have an 80% accuracy rate in determining whether an AVF was mature enough to successfully undergo hemodialysis.[9] For the obviously mature AVF, clinical examination by an experienced nephrologist or dialysis nurse is sufficient. However, if AVF maturity is in doubt, ultrasound is a useful noninvasive modality for determining if the AVF is adequate. If not, ultrasound findings serve a triage function, directing the patient to either the interventional radiologist or surgeon. Sonographic evaluation can address multiple anatomic features of the AVF, including the presence of stenosis, minimum vein diameter, and the maximum vein depth from the skin surface.

Sonographic Evaluation of AVF Maturity

The protocol for ultrasound evaluation of an AVF for maturity has been previously described,[9] as well as associated diagnostic pitfalls.[14] The evaluation of the AVF is a more focused sonographic examination than vascular mapping prior to hemodialysis access placement. It is important to note that a tourniquet is not used during the routine AVF examination. A high-resolution (7-MHz or higher) linear ultrasound probe is used to evaluate the AVF feeding artery and draining vein or veins. The transverse plane is used to identify and evaluate vessel diameter, wall thickness, and compressibility. Spectral and color Doppler examination are conducted in the longitudinal plane of the AVF feeding artery and draining vein and at any visualized stenosis.

The arm is placed in a comfortable position on towels on a procedure stand. Using minimal pressure and abundant ultrasound gel, the feeding artery, arteriovenous anastomosis, and draining vein are evaluated. The diameter of the draining vein is measured routinely in the caudal, mid-, and cranial portions of the forearm, and similarly in the upper arm when a forearm AVF is evaluated. The entire draining vein should be scanned, and the minimum diameter should be measured, even if it occurs at a location not routinely measured. The depth of the anterior wall of the AVF from the skin surface is also measured.

The AVF feeding artery, anastomosis, and draining vein are analyzed, using spectral and color Doppler. Peak systolic velocity is measured at the anastomosis and 2 cm cephalad to the anastomosis in the feeding artery. A PSV ratio is then calculated by dividing the PSV at the anastomosis by the PSV obtained 2 cm cranial to the anastomosis (Fig. 17–10). We generally begin to be concerned about stenosis at the arteriovenous anastomosis when the PSV ratio reaches 3.0.[14] Visual confirmation of a stenosis at the arteriovenous anastomosis is useful, as the PSV in the draining vein may be significantly elevated merely because of the acute angulation of the draining vein at the anastomosis.

If the draining vein is visibly narrowed, peak systolic velocities are measured at the stenosis and 2 cm caudal to the stenosis. A PSV ratio is calculated as follows: The PSV at the stenosis is divided by the PSV obtained 2 cm caudal to the stenosis. If the

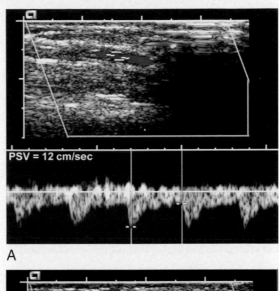

PSV = 12 cm/sec

A

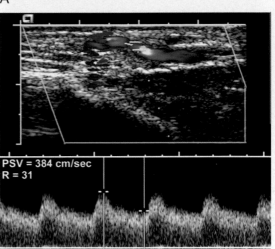

PSV = 384 cm/sec
R = 31

B

FIGURE 17–10. Anastomotic stenosis of arteriovenous fistula. *A*, Longitudinal color and spectral Doppler of the feeding artery 2 cm upstream from the arteriovenous anastomosis shows normal arterial waveform with PSV 12 cm/sec. *B*, Color and spectral Doppler at the anastomosis shows elevated PSV 384 cm/sec yielding a ratio much greater than 3.1, consistent with AVF stenosis.

PSV ratio is 2 or more, it is classified as a ≥50% diameter stenosis. Both arteriovenous and draining vein stenoses may be treated with angioplasty or surgical revision. The most frequent location of AVF stenoses is perianastomotic.[16]

The depth of the anterior wall of the draining vein from the skin surface is measured in the forearm for a forearm AVF and in the upper arm for an upper arm AVF. If the depth of the vein is greater than 0.5 cm, it will be too deep for easy access with a 15-

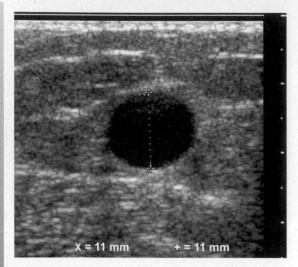

FIGURE 17–11. Deep draining vein. Transverse gray-scale image of draining cephalic vein (*cursors*) of an upper arm brachiocephalic fistula shows normal diameter of a mature fistula measuring 11 mm. However, the depth of the vein, 11 mm, may limit palpation and cannulation with dialysis needles.

gauge needle[9] (Fig. 17–11). Blood flow is measured in the AVF in mL/min, using the volume flow measurement function off the duplex instrument. If the blood flow equals or exceeds 500 mL/min, the likelihood of fistula adequacy is nearly twice as great as with lower flow rates. We found that combining venous diameter and volume flow measurement increased our ability to predict fistula adequacy. A venous diameter of 4 mm or greater and flow volume equaling or exceeding 500 mL/min confirmed AVF maturity in 95% of cases, versus a maturity rate of only 33% when neither criterion is met.[9]

KEY ADDITIONAL POINTS REGARDING AVF EVALUATION

1. Look for the presence of large vein branches involving the first 10 cm of the draining vein (Fig. 17–12). These accessory branches may divert a significant amount of flow from the primary draining vein with resultant decrease in flow to below functional levels. Such flow diversion is a frequent reason for AVF immaturity.[16] These branches can be surgically ligated, thereby increasing the likelihood that the AVF will mature.[17]

2. Occasionally, a patient with an AVF may present for evaluation of arm swelling. Respiratory phasicity and transmitted cardiac pulsatility should be evaluated in the subclavian and internal jugular veins, to assess for the possibility of a central venous stenosis (Fig. 17–13). The brachial veins should also be evaluated for the presence of deep venous thrombosis.

3. Infrequently, a patient will have symptoms of arterial steal with an AVF, such as hand pain and numbness, particularly during dialysis. Flow direction of the distal radial artery is evaluated using spectral and color Doppler. Arterial steal is diagnosed when the flow in the radial artery is reversed.[14] It is important to recognize that asymptomatic arterial steal can be present in AVFs and is of no clinical significance.

GRAFT EVALUATION

General Principles

Compared with AVFs, grafts are generally considered a less desirable method for permanent hemodialysis access because of

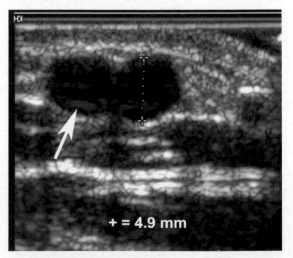

FIGURE 17–12. Large draining vein branch within 10 cm of the anastomosis. Transverse gray-scale image shows a large venous branch (*cursors*) measuring 4.9 mm, which is similar in size to the draining cephalic vein (*arrow*). A large draining vein may sump away flow from the draining vein and hinder fistula maturation.

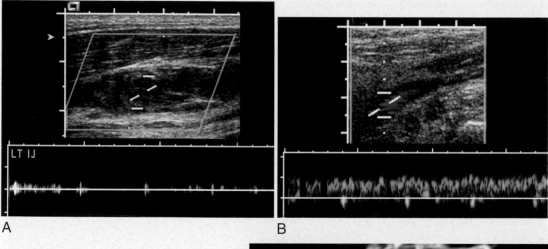

A   B

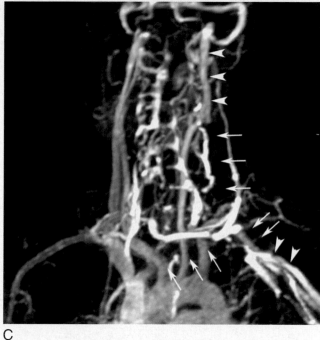

FIGURE 17–13. Central venous thrombosis. *A*, Longitudinal color Doppler of left internal jugular vein demonstrates heterogeneous clot within the vessel, which has no visible flow. *B*, Monophasic flow in the left lateral aspect of the subclavian vein (*arrows*) on spectral Doppler suggests thrombosis or stenosis of the brachiocephalic vein. Note that normal venous waveforms in the right internal jugular and subclavian veins (not shown) excluded superior vena cava location of the obstruction. *C*, Magnetic resonance venography of the chest and neck shows flow within the cranial left internal jugular vein and lateral subclavian vein (*arrowheads*). There is no flow in the expected course of the left brachiocephalic vein, caudal internal jugular vein, and medial subclavian vein (*arrows*).

C

their higher rates of stenosis, infection, and pseudoaneurysms.[1,2] Graft stenosis occurs because of intimal hyperplasia, most commonly located at the venous anastomosis.[18] Many surveillance methods for the detection of graft stenosis have been suggested, including physical examination, various laboratory measurements, static and dynamic pressure measurements performed during hemodialysis, duplex ultrasound, and ultrasound dye dilution.[1,2] Although it is widely agreed that surveillance may increase graft patency rates, no definite consensus has been established regarding the best surveillance method at the time of this writing. Research in this important area continues, however, as all of the surveillance methods described here are less invasive than routine angiography.

The clinically symptomatic graft should be referred to angiography for diagnosis and potential treatment of any stenosis found. Ultrasound graft assessment is reserved for patients with a palpable focal mass in the vicinity of the graft and those in whom there is an intermediate likelihood of graft stenosis. In the evaluation of the focal mass, it is important to differentiate a hematoma

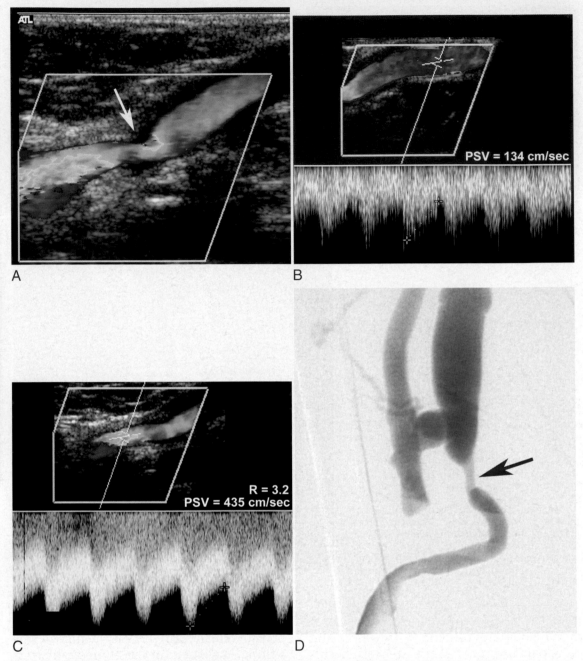

FIGURE 17–14. Stenosis of upper arm straight graft venous anastomosis. *A,* Color Doppler of the venous anastomosis (*arrows*) shows color aliasing of flow at the stenosis. *B,* Duplex Doppler within the graft 2 cm upstream from the venous anastomosis has normal flow, with PSV 134 cm/sec. *C,* Spectral Doppler at the venous anastomosis shows turbulent flow with PSV 435 cm/sec, which yields a PSV ratio of 3.2, consistent with stenosis. *D,* Angiography of the graft demonstrates a focal venous anastomotic stenosis with greater than 50% narrowing (*arrow*). The stenosis was successfully treated with balloon angioplasty (not shown).

from a pseudoaneurysm. An area of graft with a relatively larger diameter because of graft degeneration is another potential cause of a palpable mass. Additional indications for graft ultrasound include the evaluation of clinically significant arterial steal,[14] resulting in arterial insufficiency to the hand.

Sonographic Evaluation of Grafts

The protocol for evaluation of dialysis access grafts for stenosis and perigraft findings has been previously described,[15] as well as a discussion of diagnostic pitfalls.[14] A tourniquet is not used during examination of a graft. A high-resolution linear ultrasound probe, generally 7 MHz or greater, is used to evaluate the artery feeding the graft, the arterial anastomosis, the graft body, the venous anastomosis, and the draining vein or veins. The transverse plane is used to identify graft anatomy and to evaluate graft and vessel diameters. Spectral and color Doppler are assessed in the longitudinal plane of the anastomoses, within the graft, and at any visualized stenosis.

The arm is placed in a comfortable position on towels on a procedure stand. The feeding artery, graft, arterial and venous graft anastomoses, and draining vein are evaluated in both the transverse and longitudinal planes, using gentle pressure with the transducer. The graft is readily identified sonographically by the presence of two echogenic parallel lines representing the graft wall. It is useful to familiarize oneself with the particular anatomy present in the patient before attempting analysis for the presence or absence of stenosis. For example, identification of the direction of blood flow in a loop graft is useful, allowing identification and labeling of the arterial limb (the side of the loop graft closest to the arterial anastomosis) and the venous limb (the side of the loop graft closest to the venous anastomosis).

Peak systolic velocities are assessed 2 cm cranial to the arterial anastomosis (within the feeding artery), 2 cm caudal to the venous anastomosis (within the graft), at the arterial and venous anastomoses, and mid-graft. A PSV ratio is calculated at the anastomoses (as described previously for AVFs) and at any visible stenosis. A stenosis with a PSV ratio of 2.0 or greater is classified as equaling or exceeding 50% diameter reduction. A stenosis with a PSV ratio of 3.0 or greater indicates a stenosis of 75% or greater.[15] We use a PSV equaling or exceeding 3.0, as well as visual confirmation of stenosis, for the arterial anastomosis, as abrupt angulation there typically causes an increase in PSV. Figure 17–14 shows a significant stenosis at the graft venous anastomosis, with angiographic confirmation and treatment. When the PSV is close to 2.0, a significant stenosis is likely, although visual confirmation of narrowing is useful. The same PSV criteria are used for evaluating draining vein stenoses.

KEY ADDITIONAL POINTS REGARDING GRAFT EVALUATION

1. The internal jugular and subclavian veins should be evaluated routinely for respiratory phasicity and transmitted cardiac pulsatility. However, particularly in the presence of an upper arm graft, monophasic flow may be seen in the subclavian vein, in the absence of a central stenosis.
2. Graft arterial steal occurs when the venous outflow from the graft exceeds the capacity of the inflow artery. This causes the graft to "steal" blood from more caudal portions of the extremity, which can cause symptoms of arterial insufficiency, particularly during dialysis. To assess for arterial steal, a spectral waveform is obtained in the radial artery distal (caudal) to the graft insertion, usually at the wrist. If the direction of flow is reversed caudal to the graft, the diagnosis of a complete arterial steal can be made. If the spectral waveform is biphasic, a partial steal is present. Gentle, brief compression of the graft returns the abnormally reversed arterial flow direction to normal, confirming the existence of the steal phenomenon. Asymptomatic

steal is relatively common and of no clinical significance. However, severely symptomatic patients may require graft ligation to correct the steal.

Acknowledgments. We acknowledge the invaluable time and dedication of the sonographers at the University of Alabama at Birmingham and The Kirklin Clinic (particularly Michael Clements, BS, RDMS, RVT) and our hemodialysis access program. We also thank Trish Thurman for her assistance with manuscript preparation.

References

1. Allon M, Robbin ML: Increasing arteriovenous fistulas in hemodialysis patients: Problems and solutions. Kidney Int 62:1109–1124, 2002.

2. National Kidney Foundation: K/DOQI Clinical Practice Guidelines for Vascular Access, 2000. Am J Kidney Dis 37(Suppl 1):S137–S181, 2001.

3. Robbin ML, Gallichio MH, Deierhoi MH, et al: US vascular mapping before hemodialysis access placement. Radiology 217:83–88, 2000.

4. Allon M, Lockhart ME, Lilly RZ, et al: Effect of preoperative sonographic mapping on vascular access outcomes in hemodialysis patients. Kidney Int 60(5):2013–2020, 2001.

5. Miller CD, Robbin ML, Barker J, et al: Comparison of arteriovenous grafts in the thigh and upper extremities in hemodialysis patients. J Am Society Nephrol 14(11):2942–2947, 2003.

6. Moss AH, Vasilakis C, Holley JL, et al: Use of a silicone dual-lumen catheter with a Dacron cuff as a long-term vascular access for hemodialysis patients. Am J Kidney Dis 16(3):211–215, 1990.

7. Fan PY, Schwab SJ: Vascular access: Concepts for the 1990s. J Am Soc Nephrol 3(1):1–11, 1992.

8. Silva MB, Hobson RW, Pappas PJ, et al: A strategy for increasing use of autogenous hemodialysis access procedures: Impact of preoperative noninvasive evaluation. J Vasc Surg 27(2):307–308, 1998.

9. Robbin ML, Chamberlain NE, Lockhart ME, et al: Hemodialysis arteriovenous fistula maturity: US evaluation. Radiology 225(1):59–64, 2002.

10. Malovrh M: Non-invasive evaluation of vessels by duplex sonography prior to construction of arteriovenous fistulas for haemodialysis. Nephrol Dial Transplant 13(1):125–129, 1998.

11. Lockhart ME, Robbin ML, Allon M: Preoperative sonographic radial artery evaluation and correlation with subsequent radiocephalic fistula outcome. J Ultrasound Med 33:161–168, 2004.

12. Miller PE, Tolwani A, Luscy CP, et al: Predictors of adequacy of arteriovenous fistulas in hemodialysis patients. Kidney Int 56(1):275–280, 1999.

13. Beathard GA: Physical examination of the dialysis vascular access. Semin Dial 11:231–236, 1998.

14. Lockhart ME, Robbin ML: Hemodialysis access ultrasound. Ultrasound Q 17(3):157–167, 2001.

15. Robbin ML, Oser RF, Allon M, et al: Hemodialysis access graft stenosis: US detection. Radiology 208:655–661, 1998.

16. Beathard GA: Aggressive treatment of early fistula failure. Kidney Int 64(4):1487–1494, 2003.

17. Miller CD, Robbin ML, Allon M: Gender differences in outcomes of arteriovenous fistulas in hemodialysis patients. Kidney Int 63(1):346–352, 2003.

18. Swedberg SH: Intimal fibromuscular hyperplasia at the venous anastomosis of PTFE grafts in hemodialysis patients. Circulation 80(6):1726–1736, 1989.

Chapter 18

Ultrasound Assessment of Lower Extremity Arteries

R. EUGENE ZIERLER, MD

The purpose of noninvasive testing for lower extremity arterial disease is to provide objective information that can be combined with the clinical history and physical examination to form the basis for decisions regarding further evaluation and treatment. One of the most critical decisions relates to whether a patient is a candidate for therapeutic intervention and should undergo further imaging studies. Contrast arteriography has generally been regarded as the definitive examination for lower extremity arterial disease, but this approach is invasive, expensive, and poorly suited for screening or long-term follow-up testing. In addition, arteriography provides anatomic rather than physiologic information, and it is subject to significant variability at the time of interpretation.[1,2] The most valid physiologic method for detecting hemodynamically significant lesions is direct, intra-arterial pressure measurement, but this method is also impractical in many clinical situations.

As discussed in Chapter 15, the nonimaging or indirect noninvasive tests of the lower extremity arteries, including the measurement of ankle systolic blood pressure and segmental limb pressures, provide valuable physiologic information, but these tests provide relatively little anatomic detail.[3] Duplex scanning extends the capabilities of indirect testing by obtaining anatomic and physiologic information directly from sites of arterial disease. The initial application of duplex scanning concentrated on the clinically important problem of extracranial carotid artery disease. The focal nature of carotid athero-sclerosis and the relatively superficial location of the carotid bifurcation contributed to the success of these early studies.[4] Continued clinical experience and advances in technology, particularly the availability of lower-frequency duplex transducers, have made it possible to obtain image and flow information from more deeply located vessels. Therefore, it is now feasible to evaluate the abdominal and lower extremity arteries with duplex ultrasound. This chapter reviews the current status of duplex scanning for the initial evaluation of lower extremity arterial disease. The more specialized applications of intraoperative assessment and follow-up after arterial interventions are covered in Chapter 19.

INSTRUMENTATION

The commercially available duplex ultrasound instruments consist of a two-dimensional B-mode imaging system, a pulsed Doppler flow detector, and a spectrum analyzer. Transducer frequencies of approximately 3 MHz are most suitable for evaluating the abdominal vessels in average-size adults, whereas a 5-MHz transducer can be used for thin individuals. Examination of the more distal, superficially located arteries in the legs can be performed with 5-, 7.5-, or 10-MHz transducers. In general, the highest-frequency scan head that provides adequate depth penetration should be used.

Most duplex instruments also offer a color flow and power Doppler display. Color flow imaging offers several advantages over

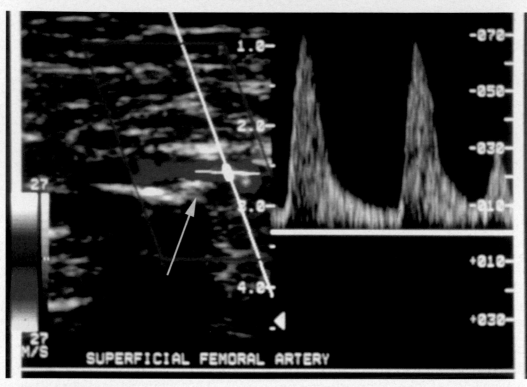

Figure 18–1. Moderate superficial femoral artery stenosis. Color Doppler image shows a posterior plaque (*arrow*) and a localized, high-velocity jet. The spectral waveform from the site of stenosis indicates a 20% to 49% diameter-reducing lesion. (From Zierler RE, Zierler BK: Duplex sonography of lower extremity arteries. Semin Ultrasound CT MR 18:39–56, 1997.)

spectral waveforms for the assessment of lower extremity arteries. The color flow image helps identify vessels and flow abnormalities caused by arterial lesions (Figs. 18–1 and 18–2). The ability to visualize flow throughout a vessel improves the precision of Doppler sample volume placement for obtaining spectral waveforms. Thus, color flow imaging has the potential for reducing examination time and improving overall accuracy. Power Doppler is an alternative method for displaying flow information that may be more sensitive to low flow rates than color flow imaging, and it is less dependent on the direction of flow and the angle of the ultrasound beam. Therefore, it tends to produce a more "arteriogram-like" vessel image. It must be emphasized, however, that color flow and power Doppler imaging are not replacements for conventional duplex techniques. In particular, spectral waveform analysis remains the primary method for classifying the severity of disease.[5]

Duplex instruments are equipped with specific combinations of ultrasound parameters for imaging and flow detection that can be selected by the examiner for a particular application. These preset combinations can be helpful, especially during the learning process, but the parameter combinations supplied with an instrument may not be adequate for all patient examinations. A complete understanding of the ultrasound parameters that are under the examiner's control is essential for producing optimal arterial duplex scans.

DUPLEX ASSESSMENT OF LOWER EXTREMITY ARTERIES

Technique

As for the other arterial applications of duplex scanning, the lower extremity assessment relies on the B-mode image to identify the artery of interest and facilitate

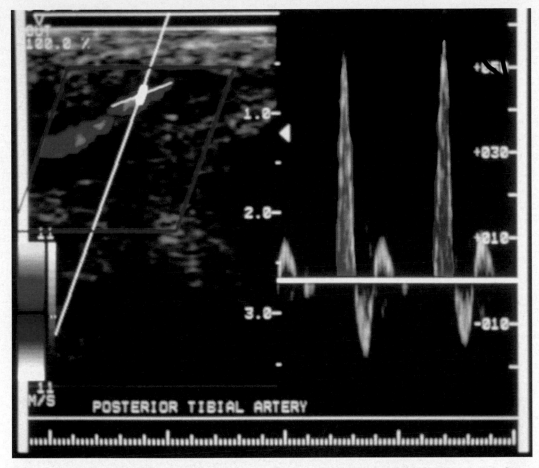

FIGURE 18–2. Color Doppler image of a posterior tibial artery showing a small vessel with relatively low flow velocities. The corresponding normal spectral waveform is triphasic. (From Zierler RE, Zierler BK: Duplex sonography of lower extremity arteries. Semin Ultrasound CT MR 18:39–56, 1997.)

precise placement of the Doppler sample volume for spectral waveform analysis.[6] Both color flow and power Doppler imaging can supplement the B-mode and spectral waveform information. The two-dimensional tissue image is valuable for recognizing anatomic variations and for identifying arterial disease by showing plaque or calcification. It has not been possible, however, to determine the degree of arterial narrowing from the image alone. Therefore, the classification of disease severity is based primarily on interpretation of the pulsed Doppler spectral waveforms.

When examining an arterial segment, it is essential to evaluate the flow pattern at closely spaced intervals. This is necessary because the flow disturbances produced by arterial lesions are only propagated along the vessel for a short distance. Experimental work has shown that the high-velocity

jets and turbulence associated with arterial stenoses are damped out over a distance of only a few vessel diameters.[7] Consequently, failure to identify localized flow abnormalities could lead to underestimation of disease severity. Because local flow disturbances are usually apparent with color flow imaging (see Fig. 18–1), pulsed Doppler flow samples may be obtained at more widely spaced intervals when color Doppler is used. Nonetheless, it is advisable to assess the flow characteristics with spectral waveform analysis at frequent intervals in extensively diseased vessels.

Lengths of occluded arterial segments can be measured with a combination of B-mode, color flow, and power Doppler imaging by visualizing the point of occlusion proximally and the site where flow is reconstituted by collateral vessels distally. Because flow velocities distal to an occluded segment may be low, it is important to adjust the imaging parameters of the instrument to detect low flow rates.

For examination of the aorta and iliac arteries, patients should be fasting for about 12 hours to reduce interference by bowel gas. Satisfactory aortoiliac Doppler signals can be obtained from approximately 90% of individuals who have been prepared in this way. It is usually most convenient to examine patients early in the morning, after an overnight fast. The patient is initially positioned supine with the hips rotated externally. A left lateral decubitus position may also be advantageous for the abdominal portion of the examination. An electric blanket placed over the patient prevents vasoconstriction caused by low room temperatures.

For a complete lower extremity arterial evaluation, scanning begins with the upper portion of the abdominal aorta. An anterior midline approach to the aorta is used, with the transducer placed just below the xyphoid process. Both ultrasound images and Doppler signals are best obtained in the longitudinal plane of the aorta, but transverse views are occasionally useful to define anatomic relationships. If specifically indicated, the mesenteric and renal vessels can be examined at this time, although these do not need to be examined routinely when evaluating the lower extremity arteries. The aorta is followed distally to its bifurcation (Fig. 18–3), and the iliac arteries are examined separately to the level of the groin.

Each lower extremity is examined in turn, beginning with the common femoral artery and working distally. After the femoral arteries are scanned throughout the thighs, it is often helpful to turn the patient to the prone position to examine the popliteal arteries. However, some examiners prefer to image the popliteal segment with the

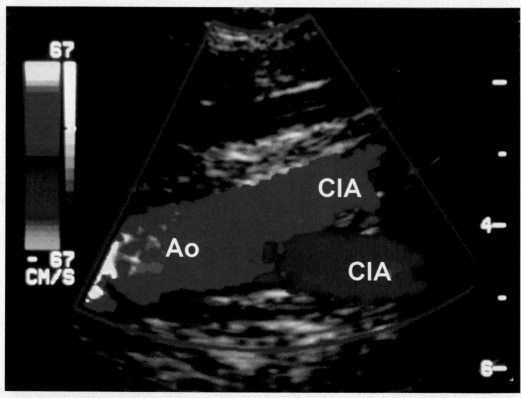

FIGURE 18–3. Color Doppler image of the aortic bifurcation. The difference in color between the common iliac branches is the result of different flow directions with respect to the transducer. Ao, aorta; CIA, common iliac artery. (From Zierler RE, Zierler BK: Duplex sonography of lower extremity arteries. Semin Ultrasound CT MR 18:39–56, 1997.)

patient supine and the leg externally rotated and flexed at the knee. The tibial and peroneal arteries can be difficult to examine completely, but they can usually be imaged with color flow or power Doppler. These vessels are best evaluated either by identifying their origins from the distal popliteal artery and scanning distally or by finding the arteries at the ankle and working proximally. Several large branches can often be seen originating from the distal superficial femoral and popliteal segments. These are readily visualized with color flow or power Doppler imaging and represent the genicular and sural arteries.

Pulsed Doppler spectral waveforms are recorded from any areas in which increased velocities or other flow disturbances are noted with color flow imaging. Recordings should also be made at the following standard locations: (1) the proximal and distal abdominal aorta; (2) the common, internal, and external iliac arteries; (3) the common and deep femoral arteries; (4) the proximal, middle, and distal superficial femoral arteries; (5) the popliteal arteries; and (6) the tibial/peroneal arteries at their origins and at the level of the ankle. A complete examination of the aortoiliac system and both lower extremities may require up to 2 hours, but a single leg can usually be evaluated in less than 1 hour. An example of a worksheet for lower extremity arterial duplex scanning is shown in Figure 18–4.

Normal Arterial Flow Characteristics

Jager and colleagues[8] have determined standard values for arterial diameter and peak systolic flow velocity in the lower extremity arteries of 55 healthy subjects (30 males, 25 females) ranging in age from 20 to 80 years (Table 18–1). Although women had smaller arteries than men, peak systolic velocities did not differ significantly between men and women in this study. However, the peak systolic velocities decreased steadily from the iliac to the popliteal arteries.

Duplex scans of normal lower extremity arteries show the characteristic triphasic velocity waveform that is associated with peripheral artery flow (Fig. 18–5). This flow pattern can be shown by both spectral waveforms and color flow imaging.[9,10] The initial high-velocity, forward flow phase that results from cardiac systole is followed by a brief phase of reverse flow in early diastole and a final low-velocity, forward flow phase later in diastole. The reverse flow component is a consequence of the relatively high peripheral vascular resistance in the normal lower extremity arterial circulation. Reverse flow becomes less prominent when peripheral resistance decreases. This loss of flow reversal typically occurs in normal limbs with the vasodilatation that accompanies reactive hyperemia or limb warming. The reverse flow component is also absent distal to severe occlusive lesions.

The normal lower extremity center stream arterial flow pattern is relatively uniform, with the red blood cells all having nearly the same velocity. Therefore, the flow is laminar, and the corresponding spectral waveform contains a narrow band of frequencies with a clear area under the systolic peak (Fig. 18–6). Arterial lesions disrupt this normal laminar flow pattern and give rise to characteristic velocity changes that produce a widening of the frequency band; this is referred to as *spectral broadening*.

Abnormal Arterial Flow Patterns

Based on the established normal and abnormal features of spectral waveforms, a set of criteria for classifying diseased lower extremity arterial segments has been developed.[6,8] These criteria are summarized in Table 18–2 and Figure 18–6. Minimal disease (1%–19% diameter reduction) is indicated by a slight increase in spectral width (spectral broadening), without a significant increase in peak systolic velocity. This minimal spectral broadening is usually found in late systole and early diastole. Moderate stenosis (20%–49% diameter reduction) is characterized by more prominent spectral broadening and by some

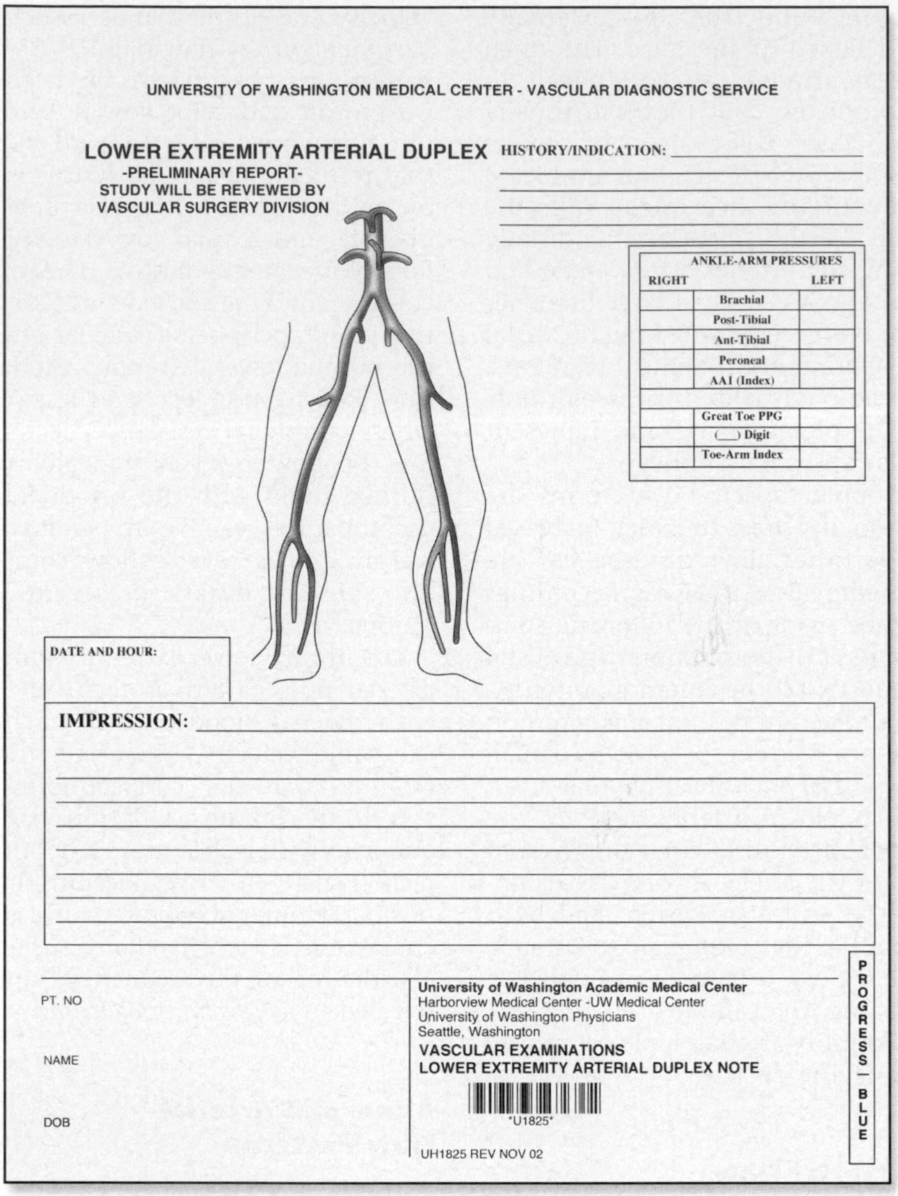

UNIVERSITY OF WASHINGTON MEDICAL CENTER - VASCULAR DIAGNOSTIC SERVICE

LOWER EXTREMITY ARTERIAL DUPLEX
-PRELIMINARY REPORT-
STUDY WILL BE REVIEWED BY
VASCULAR SURGERY DIVISION

HISTORY/INDICATION:

ANKLE-ARM PRESSURES		
RIGHT		LEFT
	Brachial	
	Post-Tibial	
	Ant-Tibial	
	Peroneal	
	AAI (Index)	
	Great Toe PPG	
	(__) Digit	
	Toe-Arm Index	

DATE AND HOUR:

IMPRESSION:

PT. NO

NAME

DOB

University of Washington Academic Medical Center
Harborview Medical Center -UW Medical Center
University of Washington Physicians
Seattle, Washington
VASCULAR EXAMINATIONS
LOWER EXTREMITY ARTERIAL DUPLEX NOTE

U1825

UH1825 REV NOV 02

PROGRESS — BLUE

FIGURE 18–4. Example of a vascular laboratory worksheet used for the lower extremity arterial assessment. (Courtesy of University of Washington Academic Medical Center, Seattle, WA)

Table 18–1. Mean Arterial Diameters and Peak Systolic Flow Velocities*

Artery	Diameter ± SD (cm)	Velocity ± SD (cm/sec)
External iliac	0.79 ± 0.13	119.3 ± 21.7
Common femoral	0.82 ± 0.14	114.1 ± 24.9
Superficial femoral (proximal)	0.60 ± 0.12	90.8 ± 13.6
Superficial femoral (distal)	0.54 ± 0.11	93.6 ± 14.1
Popliteal	0.52 ± 0.11	68.8 ± 13.5

*Measurements by duplex scanning in 55 healthy subjects.
SD, standard deviation.
Adapted from Zierler RE, Zierler BK: Duplex sonography of lower extremity arteries. Semin Ultrasound CT MR 18:42, 1997.

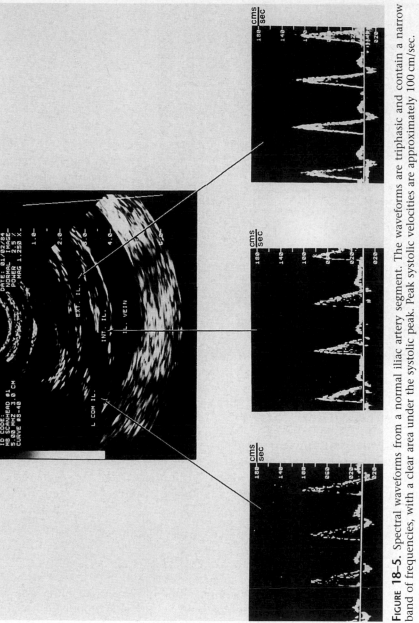

FIGURE 18–5. Spectral waveforms from a normal iliac artery segment. The waveforms are triphasic and contain a narrow band of frequencies, with a clear area under the systolic peak. Peak systolic velocities are approximately 100 cm/sec.

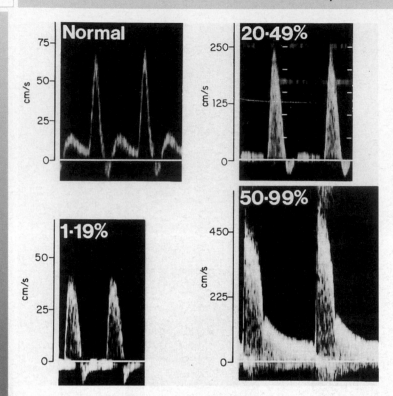

FIGURE 18–6. Lower extremity spectral waveforms. These are typical waveforms for each of the stenosis categories described in Table 18–2.

increase in peak systolic velocities. High-grade stenosis (50%–99% diameter reduction) produces the most severe flow disturbance, with markedly increased peak systolic velocities, extensive spectral broadening, and loss of the reverse flow component. Occlusion of an arterial segment is documented when no Doppler flow signal can be detected in the lumen of a clearly imaged vessel. Spectral waveforms obtained distal to a high-grade stenosis or occlusion are generally monophasic, with reduced systolic velocities. The features of waveforms taken proximal to a stenotic lesion are vari-

Table 18–2. Criteria for Classifying Peripheral Artery Lesions*

Classification	Features
Normal	Triphasic waveform; no spectral broadening
1%–19% diameter reduction	Triphasic waveform with minimal spectral broadening only; peak systolic velocities increased < 30% relative to the adjacent proximal segment; proximal and distal waveforms remain normal
20%–49% diameter reduction	Triphasic waveform usually maintained, although reverse flow component may be diminished; spectral broadening is prominent, with filling in of clear area under the systolic peak; peak systolic velocity is increased from 30%–100% relative to the adjacent proximal segment; proximal and distal waveforms remain normal
50%–99% diameter reduction	Monophasic waveform with loss of reverse flow component and forward flow throughout cardiac cycle; extensive spectral broadening; peak systolic velocity is increased > 100% relative to adjacent proximal segment; distal waveform is monophasic, with reduced systolic velocity
Occlusion	No flow detected within imaged arterial segment; preocclusive "thump" may be heard just proximal to site of occlusion; distal waveforms are monophasic, with reduced systolic velocities

*Based on duplex scanning with spectral waveform analysis.
Adapted from Zierler RE, Zierler BK: Duplex sonography of lower extremity arteries. Semin Ultrasound CT MR 18:43, 1997.

able and depend primarily on the status of the intervening collateral circulation. Immediately proximal to an arterial occlusion, the spectral waveforms show extremely low peak systolic velocities and little or no flow in diastole.

An important difference between spectral waveform analysis and color flow imaging is that spectral waveforms display the entire frequency and amplitude content of the pulsed Doppler signal at a specific site, whereas the color flow image provides a single estimate of the Doppler shift frequency or flow velocity for each site within the B-mode image. Thus, spectral waveform analysis actually provides considerably more flow information from each individual site than color flow imaging. The main advantage of the color flow display is that it presents flow information throughout the B-mode image, although the actual amount of data for each site is reduced. Spectral waveforms contain a range of frequencies and amplitudes that allow determination of flow direction and parameters such as mean, mode, and peak frequency or velocity. In contrast, color assignments are based on flow direction and a single mean or average frequency estimate. Consequently, the peak or maximum Doppler frequency shifts found with spectral waveforms are generally higher than those indicated by the color flow image. Because of this difference, the color flow image may not show some high-velocity jets that are apparent on spectral waveforms.

Validation Studies

Although the criteria listed in Table 18–2 include several categories for lesions of less than 50% diameter reduction, the distinction between these categories is often subjective and rarely of clinical importance. The most useful classification for clinical purposes recognizes those lesions of less than 50% diameter reduction, 50% to 99% diameter reduction, and occlusion. More precise classification of diameter reduction within the 50% to 99% stenosis category is not currently possible based on the commonly used spectral waveform and color flow parameters.[11] Jager and associates[6] used duplex scanning to evaluate 338 arterial segments in 54 lower extremities of 30 patients and compared the severity of stenosis as classified by spectral waveform analysis to the results of independently interpreted arteriograms. For all segments, duplex scanning differentiated between normal and diseased arteries with a sensitivity of 96% and a specificity of 81%. Duplex scanning distinguished between stenoses of greater or less than 50% diameter reduction with a sensitivity of 77% and a specificity of 98%. These results compare favorably with the variability found when two different radiologists interpreted the same lower extremity arteriograms as either normal or diseased (sensitivity, 98%; specificity, 68%), or as greater or less than 50% diameter reduction (sensitivity, 87%; specificity, 94%).[2]

A second validation study was reported by Kohler and coworkers,[12] who evaluated 393 lower extremity arterial segments in 32 patients by both duplex scanning and arteriography. For correctly identifying stenoses that had a significant (measured) pressure gradient or that reduced the lumen diameter by more than 50%, duplex scanning had a sensitivity of 82%, a specificity of 92%, a positive predictive value of 80%, and a negative predictive value of 93%. The results were especially good for lesions in the iliac arteries (sensitivity, 89%; specificity, 90%). Lesions distal to very–high-grade stenoses or complete occlusions were difficult to detect because of the low flow velocities in these segments. This limitation was also observed by Allard and colleagues,[13] who found that the presence of 50% to 99% stenoses in adjacent arterial segments decreased both the sensitivity and specificity of lower extremity duplex scanning.

Moneta and associates[14] documented the accuracy of lower extremity duplex scanning in 286 limbs of 150 patients undergoing preoperative arteriography. Ninety-nine percent of arterial segments from the common iliac to the popliteal level were successfully visualized by duplex scanning, whereas 95% of the anterior and posterior tibial arteries and 83% of the peroneal arteries were adequately imaged. For arterial segments proximal to the tibial level, duplex scanning was evaluated for its ability to identify stenoses of greater than 50% diameter reduction and for its ability to distinguish between stenosis and occlusion. In the tibial and peroneal arteries, the ability of duplex scanning to predict continuous patency from the popliteal to ankle level was assessed. In the proximal arterial segments, the overall sensitivities for detecting a greater than 50% stenosis ranged from 67% in the popliteal to 89% in the iliac arteries; corresponding specificities ranged from 97% to 99%. Stenosis was successfully distinguished from occlusion in 98% of proximal arterial lesions. For the more distal arteries, overall sensitivities for predicting continuous patency ranged from 93% to 97%. Contrary to other reported experience,[13] the accuracy of lower extremity duplex scanning was not significantly affected by the presence of multiple-level disease.

CLINICAL APPLICATIONS

The clinical role of noninvasive vascular testing can be considered in three general categories: *screening*, *definitive diagnosis*, and *follow-up*. Because the purpose of screening is to detect disease in a patient population where the prevalence of disease is presumed to be relatively low, a screening test should be low in cost and must not expose the patient to any significant risk. Screening also requires that the test have a high sensitivity or low false-negative rate to minimize the possibility of failing to detect disease. False-positive test results are less problematic, because the results of screening are generally confirmed by further diagnostic tests prior to intervention. Appropriate patient selection can improve the yield of screening by increasing the pretest probability of detecting a disease.

Testing performed for definitive diagnosis is meant to provide the precise anatomic or physiologic information required for planning treatment. Ever since it was first described in 1927, contrast arteriography has served as the "gold standard" for the anatomic diagnosis of arterial disease.[15,16] However, the high cost and invasive nature of arteriography make it unsuitable for many clinical applications, such as screening or follow-up testing. Continued improvements in the accuracy of duplex scanning, together with a mandate to reduce the risks and cost of health care, have prompted many vascular surgeons to consider performing surgical procedures based on the results of noninvasive tests alone. This trend has been particularly evident in the assessment of carotid artery disease, and the planning of carotid endarterectomy based on duplex scanning alone has become a standard of practice in selected patients.[17,18] A similar trend can be seen for patients undergoing lower extremity arterial bypass procedures.[19,20]

The purpose of follow-up testing is to detect progressive or recurrent disease at a previously diagnosed or treated site. Although this is similar to screening, it typically requires serial studies over time, and the terms *follow-up* and *surveillance* are often used interchangeably. Examples of surveillance include serial duplex scanning of infrainguinal vein grafts and patients undergoing peripheral angioplasty and stent procedures. These applications are discussed in Chapter 19.

Screening Prior to Intervention

It should be emphasized that it is not necessary to obtain a complete duplex scan on every patient who requires a noninvasive lower extremity arterial evaluation. In most clinical situations, the history, physical examination, and indirect measurement of ankle systolic blood pressures are sufficient to assess the presence and severity of arterial occlusive disease. Initial therapeutic plans can often be based on this information alone. If intervention is not warranted, then more sophisticated testing is usually not necessary. However, if more detailed anatomic information is needed for clinical decision making, then duplex scanning is the preferred method. Experience has shown that duplex scanning is superior to segmental pressure measurement for localization and classification of lower extremity arterial lesions.[21]

Lower extremity duplex scanning is generally most helpful for those patients who are being considered for some form of direct intervention—either a catheter-based intervention or open surgical repair. The goal in this setting is to determine the location and extent of arterial lesions so that decisions can be made regarding the need for additional imaging studies and the most appropriate therapeutic approach. Assessment of aortoiliac disease is particularly difficult with other noninvasive methods, and duplex scanning has been especially valu-

able for that segment (Fig. 18–7). Whether a particular arterial segment is suitable for an endovascular procedure or direct surgical reconstruction depends on the specific features of the lesion. For example, focal stenoses or short occlusions in the iliac or superficial femoral arteries are often amenable to percutaneous transluminal angioplasty and stenting, whereas arterial segments with long, irregular stenotic lesions or extensive occlusions are better treated by a surgical approach with a bypass graft. The anatomic features that are

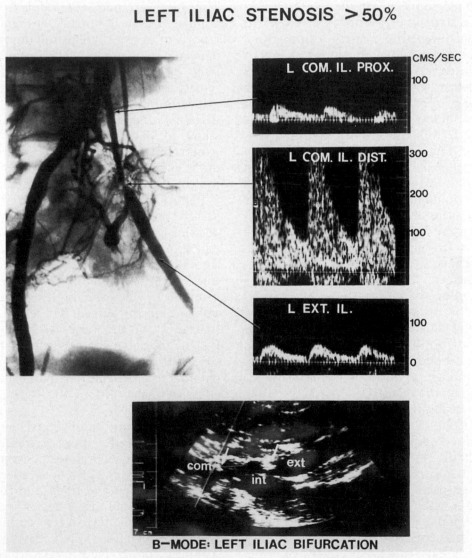

FIGURE 18–7. Left common iliac stenosis >50% detected by duplex scanning. The proximal common (com) iliac and external (ext) iliac spectral waveforms are damped and monophasic and have markedly decreased velocities. The waveform taken in the stenotic jet (LCOM IL DIST) shows high peak systolic velocities and extensive spectral broadening. int, internal iliac.

particularly important in making this determination are the site, severity, and length of the lesion. In addition, it is essential to assess the status of the inflow and the quality of the distal run-off. Duplex scanning provides a practical means for obtaining this information without resorting to contrast arteriography or other anatomic imaging techniques such as magnetic resonance or computed tomography angiography.

Edwards and coworkers[22] reported on 110 patients who underwent lower extremity duplex scanning before arteriography. Based on the duplex scan findings, 50 lesions were considered suitable for percutaneous transluminal angioplasty. Of these, the procedure was actually performed in 47 (94%). In the remaining three cases, lesions were present as predicted by the duplex scan, but angioplasty was not performed for various technical reasons. No angioplasties were performed in patients who were found not to be candidates by duplex scanning. The characterization of lesions before arteriography and angioplasty facilitates the intervention by directing attention to the appropriate arterial segment and indicating the optimal puncture site for catheter access to the lesion.[22,23] Thus, with a pre-intervention duplex scan, it should not be necessary to perform separate diagnostic and therapeutic procedures. It is often valuable to screen elderly or debilitated patients with duplex scanning. The goal in such patients is to identify lesions that can be treated by percutaneous techniques. If such lesions are not found and if open surgery is contraindicated, then further evaluation with arteriography is not necessary.

Cossman and colleagues[24] used color flow duplex scanning to examine 84 lower extremities in 61 patients undergoing evaluation for excimer laser angioplasty. There were 629 arterial sites available for comparison with contrast arteriography. The sensitivity and specificity for identifying stenoses of greater than 50% diameter reduction were 87% and 99%, respectively. Occluded arterial segments were detected with a sensitivity of 81% and a specificity of 99%. Color flow imaging correctly determined the location and length of occlusion in 44 of 51 extremities (86%). In the four

extremities in which color flow imaging underestimated occlusion length, repeat arteriography at the time of laser angioplasty showed that the original arteriogram had not visualized a patent segment of proximal superficial femoral artery and thus had overestimated the length of occlusion. Therefore, color flow imaging provided accurate information on 48 of 51 arterial occlusions (94%).

Definitive Diagnosis and Planning of Surgical Treatment

The high accuracy of duplex scanning compared with contrast arteriography and reports of cases in which the duplex results appeared to be more reliable have raised the issue of whether duplex scanning might replace arteriography in the preoperative evaluation of lower extremity arterial disease. Kohler and associates[25] performed a study to determine if vascular surgeons would choose different therapeutic procedures when provided with basic clinical information and the results of either lower extremity duplex scanning or arteriography. Relatively little disparity was found when decisions based on the two tests were compared for each individual surgeon. However, significant disagreement was noted among the clinical decisions made by various surgeons, even when the duplex scan and arteriogram reports agreed. These data suggest that most of the observed variability in patient management was caused by diversity in the clinical approach to particular patterns of disease rather than actual differences in the results of the two diagnostic tests.

The most important considerations in planning a surgical lower extremity revascularization procedure are the location and severity of arterial lesions, adequacy of inflow to the femoral level, and the identification of a distal target vessel for a bypass graft. Ligush and coworkers[19] compared the types of operations predicted by duplex scanning or conventional arteriography with the actual operations performed in 36 patients undergoing 40 infrainguinal bypass grafts for critical limb ischemia. A hemodynamically significant stenosis was defined by a twofold increase in the peak systolic velocity at the site of the lesion relative to a normal segment immediately proximal to the stenosis. The mean time required for duplex scanning was 30 minutes (range, 20–55 min). Of the actual operations performed, 83% were correctly predicted by duplex scanning, and 90% were correctly predicted by arteriography. There was no significant difference in the ability of the two preoperative imaging methods to predict operative strategy. A similar study was reported by Wain and associates,[20] who evaluated 41 patients having infrainguinal bypass grafts. The same velocity criterion was used for a hemodynamically significant stenosis, and the typical duplex scanning time was approximately 60 minutes. Duplex scanning correctly predicted whether a femoropopliteal or infrapopliteal bypass graft was required in 90% of the cases. Both anastomotic sites were correctly predicted in 90% of femoropopliteal grafts (18 of 20 patients) but only 24% of infrapopliteal grafts (5 of 21 patients). These authors concluded that duplex scanning was a reliable predictor of the distal anastomotic site for femoropopliteal bypass grafts but not for bypass grafts to the tibial or peroneal arteries.

A recent study by Grassbaugh and colleagues[26] evaluated whether preoperative duplex scanning could take the place of contrast arteriography in selecting the target vessel for distal anastomosis in patients undergoing bypass grafts to the tibial or peroneal arteries. Forty lower extremities in 38 patients were examined by both duplex scanning and arteriography, and observers blinded to the actual operation performed reviewed either the ultrasound or arteriographic results and selected the optimal target vessel. The target vessel actually used was correctly predicted by duplex scanning in 88% of patients and by contrast arteriography in 93% of patients, a difference which was not statistically significant ($P = .59$). The distal arteries used for bypass grafting had significantly higher peak systolic velocities (mean 35 cm/sec vs. 25 cm/sec; $P = .04$) and end-diastolic velocities (mean 15 cm/sec vs. 9 cm/sec; $P = .005$)

compared with those not selected as target vessels. These authors noted occasional difficulty in visualizing the peroneal artery, but they concluded that duplex scanning and arteriography typically agree when used to select the distal target vessel for a tibial or peroneal artery bypass graft.

The experience summarized above suggests that duplex scanning alone is adequate for the preoperative evaluation of selected patients who require infrainguinal bypass grafting. However, it may be necessary to combine preoperative duplex scanning with intraoperative, pre-bypass arteriography to clearly define the target vessel and anastomotic site, particularly when the distal anastomosis is to the tibial or peroneal arteries. Some investigators have found the predictive value of duplex scanning to be limited when bypass to a tibial or peroneal artery is required and multiple patent target vessels are identified.[20] Intraoperative, pre-bypass arteriography is a simple and rapid method for identifying the most suitable target vessel that still avoids the cost and risk of a formal preoperative arteriogram.

Standard preoperative arteriography is still advisable for patients who are found on duplex scanning to have significant aortoiliac occlusive disease, who do not appear to have an adequate distal target vessel for bypass, and in whom the ultrasound evaluation is limited by obesity, vessel calcification, or open wounds. This should avoid the distressing problem of taking a patient to the operating room for a bypass graft and being unable to complete the procedure. Mapping and marking of superficial veins by duplex ultrasound is also valuable to ensure that a satisfactory venous conduit is available. Magnetic resonance angiography has been advocated as an alternative method for preoperative planning of infrainguinal bypass grafts which avoids the need for arterial puncture and iodinated contrast.[27]

Evaluation of Lower Extremity Trauma

Vascular injuries in the lower extremities can produce acute arterial insufficiency or exsanguinating hemorrhage that require rapid diagnosis and treatment. In this situation, the conventional history, physical examination, and diagnostic tests are often impractical. Patients with lower extremity vascular trauma can present in two ways. Some patients have clear evidence of a vascular injury with obvious distal limb ischemia or massive hemorrhage. These patients generally undergo immediate operative exploration and repair. A second and more common presentation is when a patient has sustained blunt or penetrating trauma to an extremity but does not have specific signs or symptoms of a vascular problem. In this setting, the mechanism of trauma or location of a wound raises the clinical suspicion of an occult vascular injury.

Routine surgical exploration of vessels in proximity to traumatic wounds has been widely practiced but has a relatively low diagnostic yield. On the other extreme, the sensitivity of the physical examination alone may not be high enough to serve as a basis for treatment.[28] Consequently, arteriography has become the standard method for diagnosis of acute arterial trauma. However, in a series of 100 extremity injuries, arteriography took a mean of 2.4 hours to perform.[29] This represents an unacceptable delay in patients with major vascular injuries or multiple-system trauma who require ongoing resuscitation and immediate treatment. The use of arteriography for screening stable patients with suspected occult arterial injuries is more feasible but is associated with considerable cost and some increased risk. Furthermore, experience has shown that many post-traumatic arteriographic lesions, such as intimal flaps, pseudoaneurysms, and arteriovenous fistulae, follow a benign course and heal over time.[28]

Both indirect measurement of systolic blood pressure and duplex scanning have been used in patients with extremity trauma to avoid unnecessary arteriography and determine the need for surgical exploration. Lynch and Johansen[29] obtained Doppler pressure measurements in 100 injured limbs of 93 trauma victims who also had arteriography. An arterial pressure index (systolic pressure distal to the site of injury/brachial systolic pressure in an uninvolved arm) of greater than 0.90 was considered normal. Compared with the arteriographic findings, the arterial pressure index had a sensitivity of 87%, specificity of 97%, and overall accuracy of 95% for detecting arterial injuries. When the results of two false-positive arteriograms were excluded, the sensitivity, specificity, and accuracy increased to 95%, 98%, and 97%, respectively. The selection of trauma patients with possible occult vascular injuries for arteriography based on an arterial pressure index of less than 0.90 was prospectively evaluated in 100 limbs of 96 patients.[30] Among the 17 limbs with a decreased arterial pressure index, 16 had an abnormal arteriogram and 7 underwent arterial repair. For the 83 limbs with a normal arterial pressure index, follow-up revealed 6 minor lesions but no major injuries.

Although the arterial pressure index is a simple, rapid, and clinically valuable screening test, it has several important limitations. This approach cannot be used in cases where extensive wounds prevent placement of a pneumatic cuff on the injured extremity. In addition, it will not differentiate between an intrinsic arterial lesion, extrinsic compression, and vasospasm. Finally, distal limb pressure measurement will not detect non–flow-limiting lesions or injuries to nonaxial arteries, such as the deep femoral artery.

Duplex scanning has been applied to the diagnosis of arterial trauma in the cervicothoracic region and the extremities.[31-34] Panetta and associates[35] reported an experimental study of duplex scanning and arteriography in a canine model of arterial injury (occlusion, laceration, intimal flap, hematoma, and arteriovenous fistula). Although duplex scanning and arteriography had equivalent overall accuracy in detecting arterial injuries, duplex scanning was significantly more sensitive (90% vs. 80%) and was more accurate than arteriography in identifying arterial lacerations. This high sensitivity makes duplex scanning particularly useful as a screening test in patients with suspected arterial injuries.

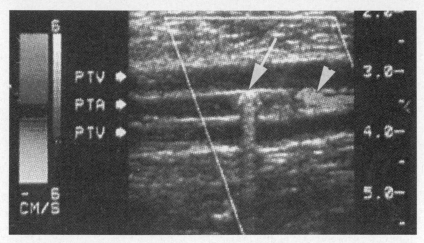

FIGURE 18-8. Color Doppler image from a patient with a lower extremity gunshot wound showing a bullet fragment (*arrow*) in the posterior tibial artery (PTA). The color flow stream stops (*arrowhead*) at the bullet, where marked acoustic shadowing is present. Two posterior tibial veins (PTV) are also visualized. (From Zierler RE, Zierler BK: Duplex sonography of lower extremity arteries. Semin Ultrasound CT MR 18:39–56, 1997.)

Meissner and coworkers[32] used duplex scanning as a screening test to evaluate 89 patients with suspected arterial trauma. Among 60 scans performed for wound proximity to adjacent vascular structures, only 4 (7%) were positive. Of the 19 scans done for specific clinical signs of arterial injury, 13 (68%) were positive (Fig. 18–8). Clinical follow-up or arteriography confirmed that no major arterial injuries were missed. A similar experience was reported by Bynoe and colleagues,[33] who prospectively evaluated 319 potential vascular injuries in 198 patients. Duplex scanning showed a sensitivity of 95%, specificity of 99%, and overall accuracy of 98% for identifying arterial injuries.

Although most of the experience with duplex scanning for lower extremity vascular injuries has been limited to a small number of trauma centers, it is clearly effective for screening and follow-up in this clinical setting. It is particularly important to follow patients with initially negative duplex scans when there is ongoing suspicion of an arterial injury, because lesions may become apparent on later examinations.[31,36] Duplex scanning is more cost-effective than either arteriography or surgical exploration as a screening test and has replaced routine arteriography in some trauma centers.[33,34] However, arteriography is still necessary in cases with technically difficult or equivocal duplex examinations.[37]

References

1. Slot HB, Strijbosch L, Greep JM: Interobserver variability in single-plane aortography. Surgery 90:497–503, 1981.
2. Thiele BL, Strandness DE Jr: Accuracy of angiographic quantification of peripheral atherosclerosis. Prog Cardiovasc Dis 26:223–236, 1983.
3. Zierler RE, Strandness DE Jr: Doppler techniques for lower extremity arterial diagnosis. In Zwiebel WJ (ed): Introduction to Vascular Ultrasonography, 2nd ed. Orlando, FL, Grune & Stratton, 1986, pp 305–331.
4. Zierler RE: Carotid artery evaluation by duplex scanning. Semin Vasc Surg 1:9–16, 1988.
5. Hatsukami TS, Primozich JF, Zierler RE, et al: Color Doppler imaging of infrainguinal arterial occlusive disease. J Vasc Surg 16:527–533, 1992.
6. Jager KA, Phillips DJ, Martin RL, et al: Noninvasive mapping of lower limb arterial lesions. Ultrasound Med Biol 11:515–521, 1985.
7. Thiele BL, Hutchinson KJ, Greene FM, et al: Pulsed Doppler waveform patterns produced by smooth stenosis in the dog thoracic aorta. In Taylor DEM, Stevens AL (eds): Blood Flow Theory and Practice. San Diego, CA, Academic Press, 1983, pp 85–104.
8. Jager KA, Ricketts HJ, Strandness DE Jr: Duplex scanning for the evaluation of lower limb arterial disease. In Bernstein EF (ed): Noninvasive Diagnostic Techniques in Vascular Disease. St Louis, Mosby, 1985, pp 619–631.

9. Blackshear WM, Phillips DJ, Strandness DE Jr: Pulsed Doppler assessment of normal human femoral artery velocity patterns. J Surg Res 27:73–83, 1979.

10. Hatsukami TS, Primozich J, Zierler RE, et al: Color Doppler characteristics in normal lower extremity arteries. Ultrasound Med Biol 18:167–171, 1992.

11. Leng GC, Whyman MR, Donnan PT, et al: Accuracy and reproducibility of duplex ultrasonography in grading femoropopliteal stenoses. J Vasc Surg 17:510–517, 1993.

12. Kohler TR, Nance DR, Cramer MM, et al: Duplex scanning for diagnosis of aortoiliac and femoropopliteal disease: A prospective study. Circulation 76:1074–1080, 1987.

13. Allard L, Cloutier G, Durand LG, et al: Limitations of ultrasonic duplex scanning for diagnosing of lower limb arterial stenoses in the presence of adjacent segment disease. J Vasc Surg 19:650–657, 1994.

14. Moneta GL, Yeager RA, Antonovic R, et al: Accuracy of lower extremity arterial duplex mapping. J Vasc Surg 15:275–284, 1992.

15. Moniz E: L'encephalographie arterielle: Son importance dans la localisation des tumeurs cerebrales. Rev Neurol 2:72–90, 1927.

16. Dos Santos R, Lamas A, Pereira CJ: L'arteriographie des membres de l'aorte et ses branches abdominales. Bull Soc Natl Chir 55:587–601, 1929.

17. Dawson DL, Zierler RE, Strandness DE Jr, et al: The role of duplex scanning and arteriography before carotid endarterectomy: A prospective study. J Vasc Surg 18:673–683, 1993.

18. Zwolak RM: Carotid endarterectomy without angiography: Are we ready? Vasc Surg 31:1–9, 1997.

19. Ligush J, Reavis SW, Preisser JS, et al: Duplex ultrasound scanning defines operative strategies for patients with limb-threatening ischemia. J Vasc Surg 28:482–491, 1998.

20. Wain RA, Berdejo GL, Delvalle WN, et al: Can duplex arterial mapping replace contrast arteriography as the test of choice before infrainguinal revascularization? J Vasc Surg 29:100–109, 1999.

21. Moneta GL, Yeager RA, Lee RW, et al: Noninvasive localization of arterial occlusive disease: A comparison of segmental Doppler pressures and arterial duplex mapping. J Vasc Surg 17:578–582, 1993.

22. Edwards JM, Coldwell DM, Goldman ML, et al: The role of duplex scanning in the selection of patients for transluminal angioplasty. J Vasc Surg 13:69–74, 1991.

23. Van Der Heijden FHWM, Legemate A, van Leeuwen MS, et al: Value of duplex scanning in the selection of patients for percutaneous transluminal angioplasty. Eur J Vasc Surg 7:71–76, 1993.

24. Cossman DV, Ellison JE, Wagner WW, et al: Comparison of dye contrast arteriography to arterial mapping with color flow duplex imaging in the lower extremities. J Vasc Surg 10:522–529, 1989.

25. Kohler T, Andros G, Porter J, et al: Can duplex scanning replace arteriography for lower extremity arterial disease? Ann Vasc Surg 4:280–287, 1990.

26. Grassbaugh JA, Nelson PR, Rzucidlo EM, et al: Blinded comparison of preoperative duplex ultrasound scanning and contrast arteriography for planning revascularization at the level of the tibia. J Vasc Surg 37:1186–1190, 2003.

27. Koelemay MJ, Lijmer JG, Stoker J, et al: Magnetic resonance angiography for the evaluation of lower extremity arterial disease. JAMA 285:1338–1345, 2001.

28. Johansen K: Evaluation of vascular trauma. In Bernstein EF (ed): Vascular Diagnosis, 4th ed. St Louis, Mosby, 1993, pp 575–578.

29. Lynch K, Johansen K: Can Doppler pressure measurement replace "exclusion" arteriography in the diagnosis of occult extremity arterial trauma? Ann Surg 241:737–741, 1991.

30. Johansen K, Lynch K, Paun M, et al: Noninvasive vascular tests reliably exclude occult arterial trauma in injured extremities. J Trauma 31:515–519, 1991.

31. Fry WR, Dort JA, Smith RS, et al: Duplex scanning replaces arteriography and operative exploration in the diagnosis of potential cervical vascular injury. Am J Surg 168:693–695, 1994.

32. Meissner M, Paun M, Johansen K: Duplex scanning for arterial trauma. Am J Surg 161:552–555, 1991.

33. Bynoe RP, Miles WS, Bell RM, et al: Noninvasive diagnosis of vascular trauma by duplex ultrasonography. J Vasc Surg 14:346–352, 1991.

34. Fry WR, Smith RS, Sayers DV, et al: The success of duplex ultrasonography scanning in diagnosis of extremity vascular proximity trauma. Arch Surg 128:1368–1372, 1993.

35. Panetta TF, Hunt JP, Buechter KJ, et al: Duplex sonography versus arteriography in the diagnosis of arterial injury: An experimental study. J Trauma 33:627–635, 1992.

36. Sorrell K, Demasi R: Delayed vascular injury: The value of follow-up color flow duplex ultrasonography. J Vasc Technol 20:93–98, 1996.

37. Bergstein JM, Blair JF, Edwards J, et al: Pitfalls in the use of color flow duplex ultrasound for screening of suspected arterial injuries in penetrated extremities. J Trauma 33:395–402, 1992.

Chapter 19

Ultrasound Assessment During and After Peripheral Intervention

Dennis F. Bandyk, MD

Duplex ultrasound assessment after peripheral arterial intervention can have a favorable impact on outcome.[1-6] When used at the time of "open" surgical bypass or percutaneous transluminal angioplasty (PTA), early patency is improved by the identification and correction of technical problems, the most frequent cause of early thrombosis. In both the operating room and angiography suite, intraprocedural duplex ultrasound contributes to cost-effective care by minimizing the incidence of early failure and secondary procedures to treat thrombosis or residual abnormalities.[7,8] Prospective studies have reported early (<30 d) failure rates of 9% to 47% after PTA and 5% to 15% after infrainguinal bypass caused by unrecognized lesions.[1,7,9] With routine ultrasound assessment, problems are found with 10% to 25% of PTA or infrainguinal/renal bypasses, yet with correction, early failure rates are low (<3%).[1,9,10] After intervention, duplex ultrasound forms the cornerstone of a vascular laboratory–based surveillance program.[3,4] Serial testing is performed to detect developing stenosis caused by myointimal hyperplasia, the most common mode of arterial repair failure, or to document the progression of atherosclerosis. Reintervention to repair duplex-detected lesions results in a higher rate of long-term patency than intervention based on clinical follow-up or in response to the recurrence of limb ischemia.[5]

INTRAPROCEDURAL DUPLEX ULTRASOUND ASSESSMENT

There is no consensus with regard to the "best" method for intraprocedural assessment of arterial interventions. Pulse palpation, continuous-wave Doppler signal analysis, arterial pressure measurements, and ultrasound flow measurements are safe and easy to perform but lack sensitivity and cannot localize intraluminal defects. Arteriography is considered the "gold standard" to identify residual stenosis and intima abnormalities but has the distinct disadvantage of being invasive, adding radiation exposure and contrast-induced toxicity, and potentially causing arterial injury.[11-13] Color duplex is preferable to arteriography because it is noninvasive and has other desirable features including availability, low cost, and the ability to evaluate an arterial repair using both real-time imaging (anatomy) and pulsed Doppler spectral analysis (physiologic testing). The intraprocedural testing method that is best suited to confirm technical adequacy depends on the arterial site, the procedure performed, and the nature of potential problems that may occur (Table 19–1). Duplex ultrasound is ideal for the assessment of surgical procedures (such as carotid, renal, visceral, and infrainguinal bypass) and infrainguinal endovascular procedures. Intraoperative ultrasound assessment can be performed within 5 to 10 min, is

Table 19–1. Diagnostic Methods and "Normal" Threshold Criteria for Commonly Used for Intraprocedural Assessments of Surgical and Endovascular Peripheral Arterial Reconstructions

Procedure	Angiogram*	Measurement of Arterial Pressure†	Duplex Ultrasound‡
"Open" Surgical Repair			
Carotid endarterectomy	Yes, <20% DR	Not used	Yes, PSV < 150 cm/sec
Renal bypass	Not used	Not used	Yes, PSV < 180 cm/sec
Mesenteric bypass	Not used	Not used	Yes, PSV < 180 cm/sec
Infrainguinal bypass	Yes, <30% DR	Not used	Yes, PSV < 180 cm/sec
Endovascular Intervention-Angioplasty (PTA)			
Carotid stent-angioplasty	Yes, <20% DR	Not used	Yes, PSV< 150 cm/sec
Renal PTA	Yes, <30% DR	Yes, <10 mm gradient	Not used
Mesenteric PTA	Yes, <30% DR	Yes, <10 mm gradient	Not used
Iliac PTA	Yes, <30% DR	Not used	Yes, PSV < 180 cm/sec
Infrainguinal PTA	Yes, <30% DR	Not used	Yes, PSV < 180 cm/sec
Vein bypass balloon PTA	Yes, <30% DR	Not used	Yes, PSV < 180 cm/sec

*Criteria for acceptable residual stenosis, expressed as diameter reduction.
†Measurement of systolic pressure gradient, expressed as mm Hg.
‡Peak systolic velocity threshold for revision of residual stenosis, used in conjunction with B-mode imaging criteria of stenosis and peak systolic velocity ratio of >2.0 at site of abnormality.
DR, diameter reduction; PSV, peak systolic velocity; PTA, percutaneous transluminal angioplasty.

more convenient than arteriography, and is associated with high (>90%) diagnostic sensitivity and negative predictive value rates.[1,2,14]

Despite careful operative technique, visual inspection, and angiographic assessment, a spectrum of lesions (stenosis, vein webs, retained valve cusps, atherosclerotic plaque dissection, focal platelet aggregation, nonoccluding thrombus) can be present following bypass grafting or peripheral angioplasty. If the residual lesion is sufficiently severe to alter hemodynamics or incite blood coagulation, complications can result, such as thrombosis, embolization, or failure to improve limb blood flow. While secondary procedures in the immediate postoperative period can often "salvage" early graft or PTA site thrombosis, procedure morbidity, patient care costs, and the incidence of subsequent failure are increased.

It is recommended that a vascular technologist participate in the duplex ultrasound evaluation, especially in the operating room, since optimizing the instrument B-mode imaging resolution and color Doppler settings is essential to obtain high-quality, interpretable studies. The technologist also archives data for the permanent medical record, including the procedure type being evaluated, the anatomic sites imaged, and whether an identified abnormality was corrected. For intraoperative assessment, a 10- to 15-MHz linear array transducer with a small footprint should be used to afford high-resolution imaging and placement within the surgical wound, directly on the repair. For transcutaneous imaging of bypass grafts, PTA sites, or arterial segments proximal and distal to the arterial repair, the use of 5- to 7-MHz linear array transducers is necessary to image the deeper-positioned vessels. By placing the transducer within a sterile plastic sleeve containing acoustic gel together with sterile gel on the prepped operative field or saline in the wound, acoustic coupling necessary for duplex imaging is achieved.

Considering the excellent diagnostic accuracy of duplex scanning for the detection of arterial occlusive lesions, it is surprising that this modality is not routinely used by vascular specialists to assess technical adequacy. A duplex-detected residual stenosis (peak systolic velocity > 150–180 cm/sec, velocity ratio > 2) has been shown to be prognostic for early PTA failure, while a normal study is associated with stenosis-free patency rates of 80% or higher.[2,5,14,15] Reluctance to use intraprocedural ultrasound has been attributed to difficulty in performing and interpreting the studies and a false belief that clinical assessment or arteriography provides equivalent assessment of the technical adequacy. When duplex scanning is used routinely, the immediate revision rate is twice that for completion arteriography, but the early (30-d) thrombosis rate is halved. Revision rates based on duplex scanning are higher for infrainguinal vein bypasses to infrageniculate arteries (17%) and when arm (27%) versus saphenous (15%) vein conduits are used.[15,16] If an infrainguinal vein bypass occludes despite a normal duplex assessment, the vein is usually of inferior quality or a coagulopathy may be present.

Infrainguinal Bypass—Testing Algorithm and Diagnostic Criteria

The algorithm for intraoperative assessment relies on real-time color Doppler imaging to identify lumen stenosis or sites of disturbed, turbulent flow.[10,17] These sites are then assessed with a high-resolution B-mode image for lumen abnormalities, and intervention is performed if significant lesions are identified or the velocity spectra criteria indicate stenosis. A lesion with a diameter reduction of more than 50% is predicted when color Doppler imaging identifies an anatomic defect in the venous conduit or an anastomosis in association with an elevated peak systolic velocity (PSV) more than 180 cm/sec and an abnormal systolic velocity ratio across the site of more than 2.5 (i.e., peak velocity in the abnormal area is > 2.5 times higher than peak velocity proximal to the abnormality). This level of hemodynamic abnormality is clinically significant and warrants correction.

The algorithm for intraoperative duplex ultrasound assessment of an infrainguinal vein bypass involves imaging the entire arterial reconstruction and classification of findings into one of four categories (Fig. 19–1). Prior to duplex scanning, papaverine hydrogen chloride (30–60 mg) is administered (via a 27-gauge needle into the vein graft) to vasodilate the runoff arterial bed and augment graft blood flow. This technique, termed *papaverine-augmented duplex scanning*, is used to improve the sensitivity of duplex scanning for the detection and grading of residual stenosis. Peripheral vasodilation is also important to confirm that the graft and runoff artery demonstrate a low peripheral vascular resistance spectra waveform (i.e., flow throughout the pulse cycle), as shown in Figure 19–2. A low peripheral vascular resistance graft flow pattern is a feature of successful bypass grafting. A high-resistance waveform (antegrade flow only during systole) in the distal graft is abnormal and when associated with a low flow velocity (PSV < 40 cm/sec) is prognostic for early failure. In these instances, a careful evaluation of the graft runoff for residual proximal or distal occlusive disease should be undertaken. Depending on the angiographic and duplex findings, procedures to augment graft flow, such as construction of a distal arteriovenous fistula or bypass to a second outflow artery, may be performed.

Scanning of the infrainguinal bypass is performed beginning at the distal graft–anastomotic segment and then proceeding proximal to include the entire venous conduit and the inflow artery–proximal graft anastomosis segment. Both longitudinal and transverse imaging planes are used as necessary to evaluate anastomoses, endarterectomized artery segments, or a vein segment with abnormal spectral Doppler findings (high PSV, spectral broadening). Recording of velocity spectra is performed at a corrected Doppler angle of 60 degrees relative to the vessel wall and with the pulsed-Doppler sample volume placed centerstream. The entire vein bypass should be imaged for anatomic and flow abnormalities, especially if the grafting technique relied on "blind" valve lysis. After in situ saphenous vein grafting, color Doppler imaging can be used to locate patent vein side-branches that require ligation. In

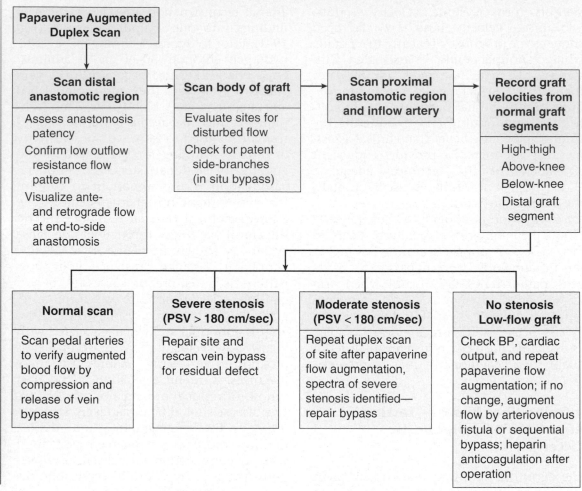

FIGURE 19–1. Algorithm for intraoperative duplex scanning of an infrainguinal vein bypass. Following duplex assessment, the study is classified into one of four categories—normal, severe stenosis identified, moderate stenosis identified, or no stenosis identified but hemodynamic assessment of graft flow demonstrates low flow velocity (peak systolic velocity [PSV] < 40 cm/sec). BP, blood pressure.

general, the assessment of prosthetic bypass grafts is limited to imaging of anastomotic sites, as grafts constructed of polytetrafluoroethylene (PTFE) are initially difficult to scan because of ultrasound attenuation by air in the graft wall.

At sites of color Doppler–detected stenosis, velocity spectra are recorded proximal to and at the site of maximum flow disturbance. Measurements of PSV are made and the velocity ratio (Vr) calculated, where Vr = $PSV_{at\ lesion}/PSV_{proximal}$. The lesion is classified into one of three stenosis categories: no stenosis, moderate stenosis, and severe stenosis (Table 19–2). Although a PSV of more than 125 cm/sec is the threshold for assigning a bypass abnormality, systolic velocity spectra in the range of 110 to 150 cm/sec may be recorded from small-diameter (<3 mm) venous conduits and should not be considered abnormal if Vr is less than 2. When duplex scanning demonstrates an anatomic defect or narrowing in the vessel lumen and velocity spectra indicating a severe or high-grade stenosis (PSV > 180 cm/sec; Vr > 2.5), immediate revision of the site is recommended (Fig. 19–3).

Intragraft platelet thrombus formation is a lesion that develops in 3% of bypass grafting procedure and has the duplex features of "high-grade" stenosis (PSV > 300 cm/sec) with mobile lumen thrombus seen on real-time B-mode imaging. This problem is best treated by replacement of the involved vein

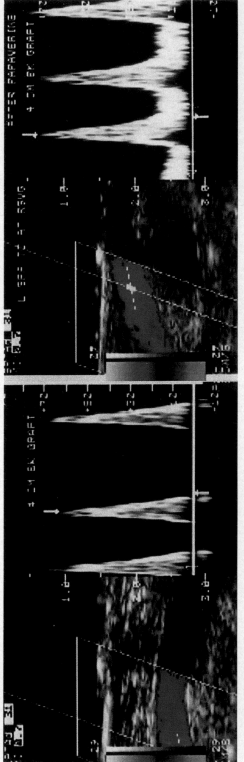

FIGURE 19–2. Velocity spectra recoded from the below-knee (BK) graft segment of an infrainguinal saphenous vein bypass prior to (*left image*) and following (*right image*) the administration of an intragraft injection of papaverine HCl (30 mg) to produce vasodilation of the graft runoff. Velocity spectra contour changes from high peripheral vascular resistance, with flow only during systole, to a low peripheral vascular resistance contour, with antegrade flow during the entire pulse cycle, indicating an increase in graft volume flow. Note that peak systolic velocity does not change appreciably.

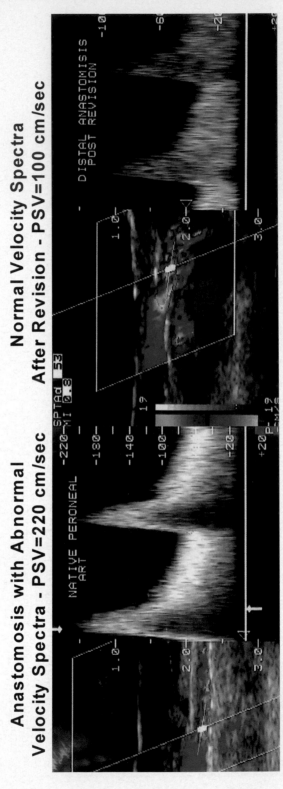

FIGURE 19–3. Intraoperative duplex scan of distal vein graft anastomosis demonstrating abnormal velocity spectra (*left image*), with peak systolic velocity (PSV) of 220 cm/sec and lumen narrowing. Following revision (*right image*), normal velocity spectra are recorded (PSV = 100 cm/sec).

Table 19–2. Interpretation and Suggested Perioperative Management of Intraoperative Duplex Ultrasound Assessment of Infrainguinal Vein Bypasses

Duplex Scan Category	Graft Flow Velocity (cm/sec)*	Peripheral Vascular Resistance	Interpretation and Perioperative Management
Normal	>40	Low	No stenosis identified and graft PSV is normal. Administer with dextran-40 (25 mL/hr, 500 mL) and oral ASA (325 mg/d)
Severe stenosis: PSV > 80 cm/sec; Vr > 2.5	<40	Low	Correct lesion and rescan graft, if no residual stenosis identified but graft PSV is low (< 40 cm/sec), administer heparin anticoagulation (weight-based) or low-molecular-weight heparin (1 mg/kg SC bid), dextran-40 (25 mL/hr), and oral ASA (325 mg/d).
Moderate stenosis, PSV < 180 cm/sec; Vr < 2.5	>40	Low	Rescan after 10 min to confirm no progression. Administer low-molecular-weight heparin (1 mg/kg SC bid), dextran-40 (25 mL/hr), and oral ASA (325 mg/d).
Low flow, no graft stenosis	<40	High	Consider an adjunctive procedure to increase graft flow (distal arteriovenous fistula, jump/sequential graft to another outflow artery); if not possible, treat as low-flow graft with antithrombotic regimen of heparin anticoagulation, dextran-40, and ASA (325 mg/d).

ASA, aspirin; PSV, peak systolic velocity; Vr, velocity ratio.

graft segment, perfusion of the distal graft, and runoff with a thrombolytic agent, followed by reimaging the entire repair for residual flow abnormality as well as the adequacy of graft flow velocity.

Graft or anastomotic sites with velocity spectra of a moderate stenosis (PSV 125–200 cm/sec; Vr 1.5–2.5) should be carefully imaged for any lumen defects (thrombus, stricture, valve cusp) using B-mode imaging. If PSV at the site increases to more than 250 cm/sec after intragraft administration of papaverine, exploration and revision is recommended. When increased velocities (PSV > 180 cm/sec) are recorded in an outflow tibial artery but the Vr is less than 2.5 compared with PSV at the distal anastomosis, spasm or hyperemic flow is likely the

cause and revision is not required. If a low-flow graft velocity or moderate stenosis is confirmed on the intraoperative study but is left unrepaired, a predischarge duplex scan is recommended to assess the graft for persistent residual stenosis and to ensure adequate graft hemodynamics.

Intraoperative assessment identifies a problem that meets threshold criteria for correction in approximately 20 percent of infrainguinal vein bypass procedures.[2,10] In a series of 626 infrainguinal vein bypasses, the most common graft abnormalities identified and corrected in descending order of frequency were vein conduit stenosis, anastomotic stenosis, platelet thrombus, and low graft flow caused by diseased tibial or isolated tibial/pedal artery runoff. The

Table 19–3. Results of Intraoperative Duplex Assessment of Infrainguinal Vein Bypass

Incidence of Graft Revision	Percent Revised
Outflow Artery	
Above-knee popliteal	13
Below-knee popliteal	16
Anterior tibial	20
Posterior tibial	12
Peroneal	15
Pedal	17
Bypass Grafting Technique	
In situ saphenous vein bypass	16
Reversed saphenous vein bypass	10
Nonreversed, translocated vein bypass	13
Arm vein bypass	27
Site of Graft Problem Repaired	**Percent of Total Lesions Repaired**
Inflow artery	8
Proximal anastomotic region	7
Venous conduit	59
Distal anastomotic region	26

incidence of graft revision is similar for the different grafting techniques and the type of outflow artery (Table 19–3). The use of arm or spliced venous conduits was associated with a higher (27%) revision rate. The incidence of "low-flow" grafts without an identified stenosis was only 3%, and a secondary procedure to increase graft flow (arteriovenous fistula, sequential graft to second runoff artery) was performed in only six limbs.

The early outcome of bypass grafting is predicted by intraoperative duplex findings. When the intraoperative duplex scan was interpreted as "normal," the incidence of early failure due to thrombosis or the need for a secondary procedure to correct a stenosis was 1% at 30 d and 1.5% from 30 to 90 d.[10] If a duplex-detected stenosis of moderate severity (PSV <180–200 cm/sec) was not repaired, the 30-d incidence of graft thrombosis was 8%, and the early (<90-d) graft revision rate was 30%. Of the 13 (2% of the total series) vein bypass grafts with low flow but no stenosis, 5 (38%) occluded within 90 d. These data indicate that residual duplex-identified defects and low graft flow are associated with subsequent graft thrombosis as well as the development of graft stenosis. With intraoperative duplex

assessment, primary patency at 90 d was similar for in situ bypass (94%), nonreversed translocated bypass (94%), and reversed (89%) saphenous vein bypass, but was lower for arm vein bypasses (82.5%, $P < 0.01$). Overall, 8% of bypasses underwent an early corrective procedure for a duplex-detected graft stenosis identified during surveillance. The application of intraoperative and postoperative duplex assessment resulted in a secondary graft patency of 99.4% at 30 d and 98.8% at 90 d. A total of eight bypasses failed. The observed 15% intraoperative revision rate, coupled with a low (2.5%) 90-d failure/revision rate, provide the rationale for routine ultrasound assessment to enhance the early outcomes after infrainguinal vein bypass.

Duplex Monitored Angioplasty

Angiographic criteria based on percent residual diameter reduction are inaccurate for predicting the clinical and hemodynamic success of PTA. In two studies, Doppler velocity elevation indicating greater than 50% stenosis was identified by duplex scanning in 20% of PTAs, despite a completion angiogram showing less than 30% stenosis.[6,14] By life-table analysis, a residual PTA site stenosis that reduces diameter by more than 50% (peak systolic velocity >180 cm/sec; velocity ratio at site > 2.5) was associated with only a 15% 1-yr clinical success rate, versus 84% success/stenosis-free patency when residual stenosis of less than 50% was verified. Intravascular ultrasound and arterial pressure measurements are useful in assessing the adequacy of PTA, but their application is better suited for monitoring aortoiliac, renal, and visceral endovascular interventions.

Duplex scanning is an efficient, cost-effective method to assess peripheral PTA site hemodynamics once an adequate anatomic result (<30% residual stenosis) is confirmed by arteriography.[15] Ideally, the lesion to be treated is scanned prior to PTA to verify its severity (PSV, velocity ratio across the stenosis) and confirm that the site can be interrogated by duplex ultrasound (Fig. 19–4). The goal of duplex-monitored angioplasty is to not terminate the procedure until normal hemodynamics are verified. Pre-PTA velocity values typically indicate high-grade, pressure-reducing stenosis, with PSV of more than 300 cm/sec and end-diastolic velocity of more than 40 cm/sec. Following successful PTA, the PSV at the site of stenosis/angioplasty should be less than 180 cm/sec and/or the Vr in the treated segment should be less than 2. After intervention by balloon dilation, stenting, or stent-graft, an angiogram of the PTA site is normal if stenosis of less than 30% is present (Fig. 19–5). If abnormal, reintervention is performed. When the PTA site angiogram is normal, "papaverine-augmented" duplex ultrasound assessment is performed, and if residual stenosis is identified (PSV > 180 cm/sec, Vr > 2), reintervention is recommended. Treatment

FIGURE 19–4. Transcutaneous use of duplex ultrasound to assess velocity spectra proximal to (A) at an occlusive lesion (B) and distal to a stenosis in the superficial femoral artery (C). PSVR, peak systolic velocity ratio.

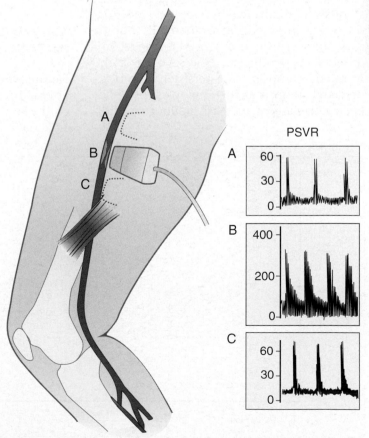

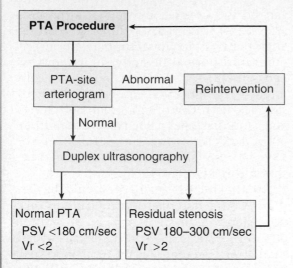

FIGURE 19–5. Algorithm of duplex-monitored angioplasty based on arteriography and duplex ultrasound findings. PSV, peak systolic velocity; PTA, percutaneous transluminal angioplasty; Vr, systolic velocity ratio.

options may include atherectomy, dilation with a larger balloon, stent placement, or prolonged balloon inflation. When a lesion is judged to be maximally dilated (e.g., for PTA of vein graft stenosis) and a persistent stenosis is identified by duplex scanning, operative intervention or frequent duplex surveillance after the procedure is recommended, depending on the severity of the residual stenosis. A persistent duplex-detected stenosis at the angioplasty site has been correlated with early failure, as indi-

cated by progression of stenosis to a velocity level similar to the primary lesion or progression to occlusion.

Our experience in using duplex-monitored PTA of femoropopliteal-tibial stenosis or infrainguinal vein bypass graft stenosis resulted in reintervention for residual duplex-detected stenosis in approximately 25% of cases (native artery lesion, 15%; vein graft lesions, 30%). Additional intervention resulted in further decrease in PSV at the lesion site (Fig. 19–6) and resulted in more than 95% of angioplasty sites having velocity values indicating stenosis of less than 50%. Thus, by using duplex-monitored angioplasty, velocity levels can reliably be normalized by balloon dilation of a focal vein graft stenosis. Confirming satisfactory flow velocity after PTA has been associated with a stenosis-free patency at 2 yr of approximately 80%, an outcome similar to bypass grafting of long segment occlusions or vein graft stenosis. PTA without duplex monitoring was associated with a lower (61%) stenosis-free patency rate at 1 yr.

SURVEILLANCE AFTER INTERVENTION

Failure within the first year after peripheral arterial intervention is commonly the result of the development of myointimal hyper-

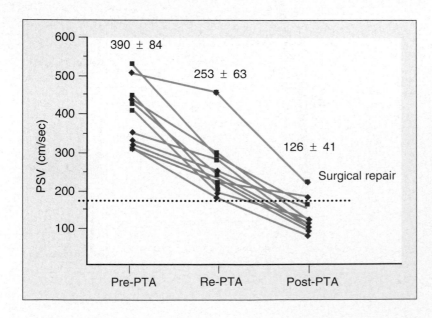

FIGURE 19–6. Peak systolic velocity (PSV) changes prior to reintervention, at the time of reintervention, and following balloon percutaneous transluminal angioplasty (PTA) of 11 vein graft stenoses with abnormal duplex scan despite an angiogram showing less than 30%-diameter-reducing stenosis. Reintervention resulted in PSV of less than 180 cm/sec in all but two procedures. Surgical repair was performed on one graft lesion with PSV of 235 cm/sec after balloon angioplasty.

plasia, and beyond that time, failure is more likely due to progression of atherosclerosis. Myointimal hyperplasia consists of smooth muscle cell proliferation and matrix formation, producing occlusive lesions at anastomotic, vein valve, PTA, or endarterectomy sites that, when progressive, reduce flow and distal perfusion pressure. Onset and progression of myointimal and atherosclerotic stenotic lesions can be monitored with duplex ultrasound. Identification of a severe progressive stenosis permits elective intervention, frequently with endovascular therapy. Duplex ultrasound surveillance after infrainguinal vein bypass is superior to clinical assessment alone.[5,15–19] An increase in arterial repair site patency also has been reported following peripheral angioplasty and carotid endarterectomy.[20–25] A randomized, prospective clinical trial conducted in Malmö, Sweden, demonstrated a 25% improvement in infrainguinal vein bypass patency at 3 yr (78% versus 53%), but no significant benefit was documented in PTFE or PTFE-vein composite graft patency.[5] Surveillance of infrainguinal prosthetic grafts was recommended by Calligaro and associates,[26] who found duplex scanning was more sensitive (81%) than ankle-brachial systolic pressure index (ABI) measurement and clinical evaluation (24%) in identifying stenoses that warrant repair. The accuracy of predicting graft failure or the need for revision was higher for femorotibial than for femoropopliteal grafts. It should be noted that, in general, thrombosis of a prosthetic graft may not be as detrimental as occlusion of a vein graft, as either catheter-directed thrombolysis or surgical thrombectomy is more effective in restoring prosthetic graft patency and can be performed several weeks after graft failure.

Timing for the initial vascular laboratory surveillance study varies with the type of procedure performed and whether an intraprocedural ultrasound study was done. If intraprocedural ultrasound assessment was normal, surveillance should be initiated within 2 to 3 wk after infrainguinal bypass, 1 mo after peripheral PTA, and 2 to 3 mo after carotid endarterectomy. Procedures with residual stenosis by arteriography or ultrasound assessment should be evaluated earlier, which may include a predischarge duplex scan. Beyond 1 yr, the incidence of failure due to myointimal hyperplasia decreases and surveillance intervals can be lengthened to 6 to 12 mo for the detection of atherosclerotic disease progression or aneurysm formation.

Infrainguinal Bypass Graft Surveillance

Duplex ultrasound is used to confirm graft patency, identify stenotic lesions, assess their risk for producing graft thrombosis, and, if not repaired, monitor stenosis progression.[17] The surveillance protocol begins with questioning the patient for symptoms of recurrent limb ischemia, performing a pulse (femoral, pedal) evaluation, and measuring the ABI. Color Doppler imaging of the entire bypass, including adjacent inflow and outflow arteries, is then performed and the hemodynamics of graft flow are characterized by duplex-derived PSV measurements along the length of the bypass, using a pulsed-Doppler beam angle of 60 degrees or less. Mean systolic graft flow velocity, calculated as the average PSV recorded from two or three nonstenotic graft sites, correlates with volume flow, and if low (<40 cm/sec), indicates a graft at increased risk for thrombosis (Fig. 19–7). Graft flow velocity may be below 40 cm/sec in large-caliber (>6-mm diameter) grafts or bypasses to a pedal or isolated tibial artery. If color Doppler imaging identifies a stenosis, measurements of PSV and Vr are obtained, as well as measurements of the lesion length and the graft/vessel diameter (Fig. 19–8). Lesions with duplex-derived velocity spectra of a high-grade stenosis (PSV > 300 cm/sec; end-diastolic velocity > 20 cm/sec, velocity ratio prestenosis/stenosis > 3.5) correlate with a stenosis with a diameter reduction of more than 70% and should be repaired. In a prospective study, the application of these threshold criteria identified all grafts at risk for thrombosis, and only one lesion with high-velocity criteria regressed.[27] Multiple investigators have observed an approximate 25% incidence of graft thrombosis in stenotic bypasses

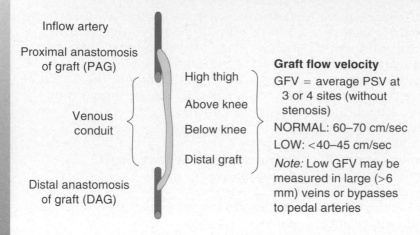

Inflow artery

Proximal anastomosis
of graft (PAG)

Venous
conduit

Distal anastomosis
of graft (DAG)

High thigh

Above knee

Below knee

Distal graft

Graft flow velocity

GFV = average PSV at
3 or 4 sites (without
stenosis)

NORMAL: 60–70 cm/sec

LOW: <40–45 cm/sec

Note: Low GFV may be
measured in large (>6
mm) veins or bypasses
to pedal arteries

FIGURE **19–7.** Calculation of
mean graft flow velocity (GFV).
PSV, peak systolic velocity.

when a policy of no intervention was followed.[3–5,8,22]

The risk of graft thrombosis is predicted by using the combination of high- and low-velocity duplex criteria discussed previously and the ABI values (Table 19–4). In the highest-risk group (Category I), the development of a pressure-reducing stenosis has produced low flow levels in the graft, which,

if it decreases below the "thrombotic threshold velocity," will result in graft thrombosis. Prompt repair of Category I lesions is recommended, while Category II lesions can be scheduled for elective repair within 1 to 2 wk. A Category III stenosis (Vp, 150 to 300 cm/sec; Vr < 3.5) is not pressure- or flow-reducing in the resting limb. Serial scans at 4- to 6-wk intervals are

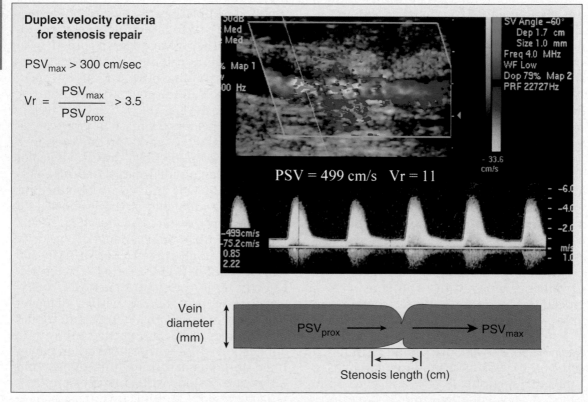

**Duplex velocity criteria
for stenosis repair**

$PSV_{max} > 300$ cm/sec

$$Vr = \frac{PSV_{max}}{PSV_{prox}} > 3.5$$

PSV = 499 cm/s   Vr = 11

Vein
diameter
(mm)

PSV_{prox} ⟶ PSV_{max}

Stenosis length (cm)

FIGURE **19–8.** Measurements recorded at site(s) of color Doppler-detected vein graft stenosis. A peak systolic velocity (PSV) of more than 300 cm/sec in conjunction with a velocity ratio (Vr) of more than 3.5 are the duplex criteria for repair.

Table 19–4. Risk Stratification for Graft Thrombosis Based on Surveillance Data

Category*	High-Velocity Criteria		Low-Velocity Criteria		ΔABI
I (highest risk)	PSV > 300 cm/sec or Vr > 3.5	*and*	GFV < 45 cm/sec	*or*	>0.15
II (high risk)	PSV > 300 cm/sec or Vr > 3.5	*and*	GFV > 45 cm/sec	*and*	<0.15
III (intermediate risk)	180 < PSV > 300 cm/sec or Vr > 2.0	*and*	GFV > 45 cm/sec	*and*	<0.15
IV (low risk)	PSV < 180 cm/sec and Vr < 2.0	*and*	GFV > 45 cm/sec	*and*	<0.15

*Category I: Prompt repair of lesion is recommended—patients are hospitalized and anticoagulated prior to repair. Category II: Lesions are repaired electively (within 2 wk). Category III: Lesions are observed with serial duplex examination at 4- to 6-wk intervals and repaired if they progress. Category IV: Lesions are at low risk for producing graft thrombosis—follow-up every 6 mo; few (<3%/yr) failures observed in this group).
ABI, Doppler-derived ankle-brachial systolic pressure index; GFV, graft flow velocity (global or distal); PSV, duplex-derived peak systolic velocity at site of flow disturbance; Vr, PSV ratio at maximum stenosis compared to proximal graft segment without disease.

recommended to determine the hemodynamic (Fig. 19–9) course of these lesions. Among graft stenoses detected within the first 3 mo of surgery, spontaneous regression of the lesion occurs in less than one third of cases, whereas 40% either remain stable or progress (40%–50% likelihood) to high-grade stenosis. In general, serial duplex scans will determine if a lesion will progress and become "graft threatening" within 4 to 6 mo of identification.[8,9,28] Important features of the "graft-threatening" stenosis are its propensity to progress in severity, reduce graft flow, and form surface thrombus,

events that ultimately will precipitate thrombosis. Using serial duplex scans, a Category III stenosis that does not progress can be distinguished from the progressive lesion that needs to be repaired.

No stenosis is identified in the majority (approximately 80%) of bypass grafts studied with ultrasound (i.e., Category IV scans). For these patients, surveillance at 6-mo intervals is generally recommended. In patients with Category IV scans but a GFV less than 40 cm/sec, signifying a "low-flow" bypass, a diligent search is conducted for additional inflow or outflow occlusive

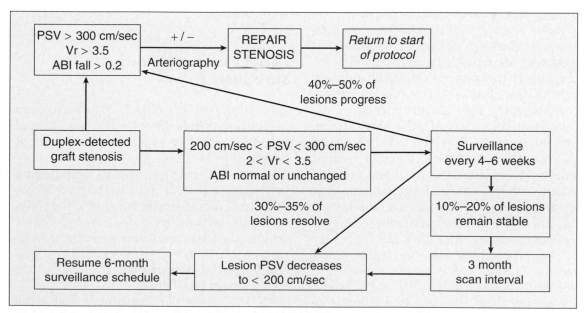

FIGURE 19–9. Duplex surveillance algorithm for detected graft stenosis. ABI, ankle-brachial index; PSV, peak systolic velocity.

lesions. If none are detected, oral anticoagulation (sodium warfarin) is prescribed to maintain the prothrombin time at an INR of 1.6 to 2.0; aspirin (325 mg/d) is also prescribed. This anticoagulation regimen is also prescribed following femorodistal PTFE bypass grafting when a peak velocity of less than 60 cm/sec is measured in the graft by duplex scanning prior to discharge. The rationale for this practice is based on the concept of the "thrombotic threshold velocity," which is lower in autologous vein grafts than in prosthetic bypasses.

Using duplex ultrasound surveillance, it can be anticipated that approximately 20% of infrainguinal vein bypasses will have a Category I or II stenosis identified within the first year after grafting. The risk of developing a graft stenosis is influenced by a number of factors, including vein caliber, the presence of venovenous anastomosis (spliced vein), the use of alternative venous conduits (arm vein, lesser saphenous vein, greater saphenous vein remnants), prior intraoperative graft revision, or early graft thrombectomy. Two thirds of lesions are focal (<2 cm in length) and may be treated by PTA. More extensive graft stenosis or early (<3-mo) appearing lesions are best treated by surgical repair. Stenosis-free patency at 2 yr was identical for surgical (63%) and endovascular intervention (63%), and overall assisted graft patency by life-table analysis was 91% at 1 yr and 80% at 3 yr. Following balloon angioplasty or open surgical repair, the graft surveillance schedule is the same as after the primary grafting procedure—1 mo, 4 mo, then every 6 mo thereafter for Category I scans.

Based on the costs of graft surveillance, the salvage of 7% to 8% of bypasses would be cost-effective. Many vascular groups believe duplex surveillance should be "part of the service" after infrainguinal vein bypass grafting. It should be emphasized that the benefit of surveillance is highly dependent on the durability and morbidity of the procedures used to repair "graft stenoses." Most series have reported a mortality of less than 0.5%, early failure rate of less than 1%, and late failure rate of less than 15% with graft revision procedures.[6]

The decision to perform confirmatory arteriography prior to graft repair depends on the location and appearance time of the stenosis. In our experience, repair based on duplex ultrasound has been possible in 80% of patients, while other vascular groups have recommended routine confirmatory arteriography to locate the lesion and aid in operative planning when duplex scanning identifies only a "low-flow" graft or multiple lesions. Arteriography also should be considered when duplex testing identifies an inflow lesion involving either the iliac arteries or the proximal anastomotic region of a graft originating from the deep or superficial femoral arteries.

In summary, routine duplex ultrasound surveillance of lower limb bypass grafts is recommended. Because the majority of graft abnormalities identified may be asymptomatic, appropriate criteria to recommend repair by either balloon angioplasty or open surgical repair should be used. The likelihood of graft revision varies with the vein bypass type and is increased when a graft stenosis is identified on a "predischarge," or early (<6-wk) duplex scan. With time, the incidence of vein graft stenosis decreases, but because of atherosclerotic disease progression in native arteries and aneurysm formation in the vein conduit, life-long surveillance (yearly after 3 yr) is recommended.[17,29]

Peripheral Angioplasty Surveillance

Late failure of peripheral angioplasty can result from restenosis caused by myointimal hyperplasia within the treated segment or progression of atherosclerosis at or remote from the PTA site. On occasion, both disease processes can occur and produce recurrent limb ischemia. Identification of a hemodynamically failing PTA does not preclude endovascular intervention by either redilation or stent placement. Repeat PTA is generally associated with a prognosis identical to a primary procedure.

Timing of initial assessment following peripheral angioplasty depends on the indications for the PTA procedure. For patients with claudication and palpable pulses after the angioplasty, lower limb duplex scanning and measurement of ABI within 2 wk of the procedure is sufficient. For critical limb ischemia, testing prior to discharge is recommended to verify diameter reduction of less than 50% at the PTA site (PSV < 180 cm/sec) and to document an increase in the ABI greater than 0.2, compared with the pre-PTA level. Subsequent surveillance of "normal" PTA sites (i.e., less than 50% stenosis) is recommended at 3 mo and then every 6 mo thereafter. If the post-PTA duplex scan identifies a stenosis with a diameter reduction of 50% to 75% but the ABI has increased appropriately, a repeat scan in 1 to 2 wk should be performed to assess for improvement or deterioration in functional patency. A progressing PTA site stenosis with a PSV of more than 300 cm/sec and a Vr of more than 3.0 should be considered for repeat endovascular therapy, depending on the anatomic characteristics/site of the lesion/arterial segment. Although the cost-benefit aspects of duplex

surveillance following PTA have not been studied, it has been shown that PTA is less expensive than surgical bypass. The ratio of hospital costs of PTA to bypass surgery was 53% for patients treated for claudication but rose to 75% for those with critical ischemia. Since angioplasty failure is expensive, efforts to improve the technical success or durability of these procedures are worthwhile. While duplex surveillance can identify PTA site stenosis, clinical symptoms and hemodynamic criteria should also be used in the decision for reintervention. Most claudicants with PTA site stenosis indicate recurrence of exertional leg pain, and because PTA has a failure mode similar to that of infrainguinal vein bypass, the cost-effectiveness and efficacy of surveillance should be comparable.

After iliac angioplasty, surveillance should include both indirect (clinical status, ABIs, toe pressures in diabetics, and femoral artery waveform analysis) and direct (aortoiliac duplex scanning) evaluation of the treated iliac system (Fig. 19–10). If the

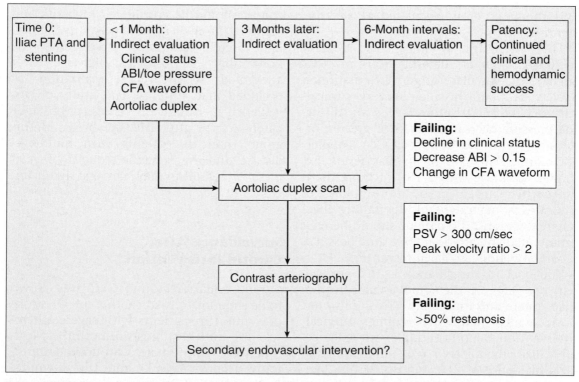

FIGURE 19–10. Algorithm for duplex surveillance after iliac angioplasty. ABI, ankle-brachial index; CFA, common femoral artery; PSV, peak systolic velocity; PTA, percutaneous transluminal angioplasty.

Doppler velocity waveform of the common femoral artery distal to the treated iliac segment is normal, duplex imaging of the iliac angioplasty is not necessary, as no significant hemodynamic lesion is present. The normal waveform is triphasic, or in the case of an occluded superficial femoral artery, the waveform is monophasic but the acceleration time is less than 200 msec. When the femoral pulse is abnormal or a damped, monophasic femoral artery waveform is identified, direct aortoiliac duplex imaging should be performed. A linear array (L4–7 MHz) transducer is used to map the external iliac artery, with deeper imaging of the common iliac and aorta in obese individuals performed using a curvilinear array (3-MHz) probe. Color Doppler imaging is performed in the infrarenal aorta, along the treated and native iliac segments, and through the common femoral artery as well as the proximal deep and superficial femoral arteries. Velocity spectra of centerstream flow are recorded at multiple sites using a Doppler-correction angle of 60 degrees or less. Peak systolic velocities within the iliac angioplasty segments are compared with velocities in the adjacent native iliac artery, and the peak Vr is calculated at sites of stenosis.

The criteria of a failing iliac system included interval deterioration of the Society of Vascular Surgery/International Society of Cardiovascular Surgery clinical category by one or more levels, an ABI or toe pressure decrease of 0.15 or greater, or development of an abnormal CFA Doppler waveform. Detection of an iliac lesion by duplex scanning with a PSV of more than 300 cm/sec and a Vr of more than 2.0 indicates a hemodynamically failing iliac angioplasty, and the patient should be recommended for arteriography and possible secondary endovascular intervention.

The goal of surveillance is to optimize patency rates in the endovascular-treated iliac system and thus avoid PTA site thrombosis, which frequently requires surgical intervention. Reports of duplex surveillance after iliac angioplasty have demonstrated a 20% incidence of PTA stenosis within 2 yr. In a prospective study, duplex surveillance resulted in reintervention in 10% of iliac

PTAs and was associated with a secondary patency of 95% at 2 yr. Four percent of the treated iliac segments thrombosed.[30]

Serial clinical evaluation, measurement of limb pressures, and Doppler waveform analysis at 6-mo intervals can reliably identify failing PTAs. Progression to occlusion is uncommon, and essentially all recurrent lesions are amenable to endovascular therapy. If limb pressures and segmental Doppler waveforms are normal or unchanged, routine duplex scanning is avoided, which reduces overall costs. The clinical usefulness of a surveillance algorithm is predicated not only on the ability to detect PTA sites at risk for failure but also on the success of reintervention and the overall rate of secondary patency. Thrombosis of an iliac PTA in a patient with multilevel disease is more likely to result in critical limb ischemia than in a patient initially presenting with claudication. Similarly, failure of the treated iliac system also may threaten patency of a downstream lower limb bypass graft and substantially increase the risk of limb loss. Angioplasty failure is more common in patients with multilevel atherosclerosis, and, thus, this cohort should be considered high risk and offered duplex ultrasound surveillance. Endovascular treatment of recurrent or de novo iliac stenosis is preferred over attempted secondary recanalization of occluded iliac systems. The utility of surveillance in claudicants is less clear, since patency rates after PTA are better in this group than in patients with multilevel disease, and the ischemic sequelae of treatment site failure may be less significant clinically.

Surveillance After Carotid Intervention

Carotid endarterectomy (CEA) was shown to be superior to medical therapy for stroke prevention in patients with severe atherosclerotic carotid stenosis in both the North American Symptomatic Carotid Endarterectomy Trial (NASCET) and the Asymptomatic Carotid Atherosclerosis Study (ACAS) and is currently being evaluated with carotid stent–assisted angioplasty (CAS) in the Carotid Revascularization Endovascular Stent Trial (CREST). The efficacy of CEA and CAS is highly dependent on completing the procedure with a low perioperative morbidity rate (<5%) and producing a durable repair with a low incidence of recurrent disease or occlusion.

Duplex ultrasound surveillance of patients after CEA and CAS procedures has demonstrated a varied (4%–22%) incidence of diameter residual of more than 50% or recurrent stenosis.[31] In the ACAS study, early restenosis (>60% reduction in diameter) was identified in 7.6% to 11.4% of cases, while late restenosis occurred in 1.9% to 4.9% of cases. When intraoperative duplex assessment of carotid surgery is applied to ensure a precise anatomic and hemodynamic result, the rate of restenosis can be decreased further (<5% early and late combined).

As seen with B-mode sonography (Fig. 19–11), the absence of the intimal-media stripe may be distinctly apparent at the postendarterectomy carotid bifurcation during the early postoperative period. Sutures used to close the arteriotomy may be visualized in the anterior wall as focal bright reflections. Later on (months to years), wall thickening (neointima) is usually apparent (Fig. 19–12) but is not of concern unless wall thickness progresses with time and is associated with an increase in peak systolic velocity. After CAS, the stent is easily seen with ultrasound (Fig. 19–13A and B). Slight lumen narrowing may persist at the ends of the stent, but such narrowing should not generate significant velocity elevation. Typically, blood flow is laminar or only slightly disturbed at both CEA and CAS sites.

Abnormal postendarterectomy findings include flow disturbances, usually caused by an intimal flap or retained plaque, stenosis, and occlusion. Intimal flaps and retained plaque are apparent in the early postoperative period and should not be encountered on a follow-up basis if intraoperative sonography is performed. Typically, intimal flaps occur at the distal end of the endarterectomy, where the cut edge of the intima is subject to dislodgement by the cephalad flow stream. The elevated intima can cause tremendous flow disturbance and may ultimately lead to restenosis. Myointimal hyperplasia (see Fig. 19–12) is a delayed complication that develops over a period of months after CEA or CAS (usually within the first 24 mo). This process can result in either focal or diffuse narrowing at the endarterectomy/angioplasty site, and is associated with elevation of flow velocity and post-stenotic flow disturbance. Velocity criteria for stenosis grading are presented below. Additional abnormal findings may be encountered post angioplasty, including malposition of the stent and separation of the stent from the vessel wall. Again, these findings would not be expected in a follow-up setting if ultrasound is employed at the time of stent deployment. The natural history of recurrent internal carotid

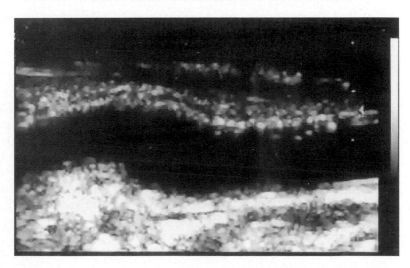

FIGURE 19–11. B-mode image of carotid endarterectomy site showing absence of intimal-media stripe in the internal and distal common carotid artery, compared with the proximal common carotid artery (*far right*). Sutures used for artery closure are seen in anterior wall of common carotid artery closure as focal, bright reflections.

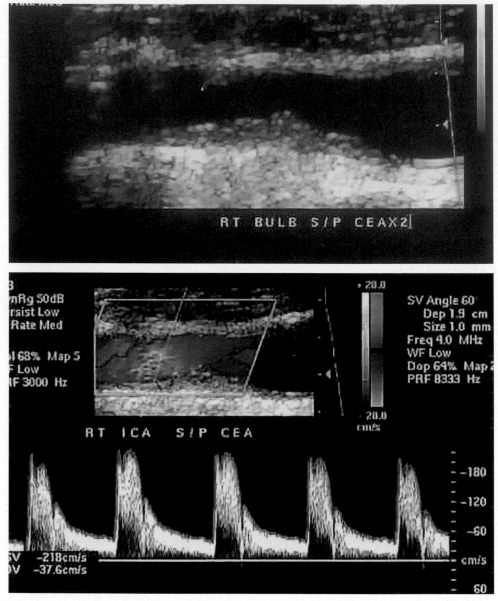

FIGURE 19–12. B-mode image (*top*) and pulsed Doppler velocity spectra (*bottom*) of the internal carotid artery (ICA) with recurrent stenosis caused by myointimal hyperplasia. A peak systolic velocity of 218 cm/sec indicates a 50%–79% diameter-reducing stenosis. CEA, carotid endarterectomy.

stenosis caused by myointimal hyperplasia is thought to be associated with a lower risk of stroke or occlusion, as compared to atherosclerosis, and some (10%) early postoperative lesions have demonstrated regression on serial duplex scans. High-grade internal carotid artery (ICA) restenosis (>75% to 80% DR; end-diastolic velocity > 150 cm/sec), may be caused by progressive myointimal hyperplasia or atherosclerosis, and such stenosis (Fig. 19–14) is associated with an increased risk of ICA thrombosis and late stroke. Restenosis within the first 3 years results from myointimal hyperplasia (smooth muscle and fibrous overgrowth of the tissue layer that replaces the intima after surgery). After 3 years, the material causing restenosis is more apt to resemble atherosclerotic plaque, with abundant collagen, foam cells, and calcium deposits. The histologic transition from early to late restenosis is a continuum,

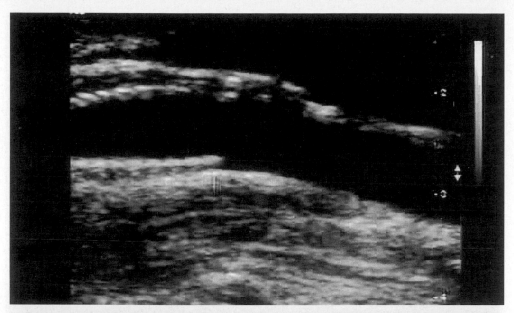

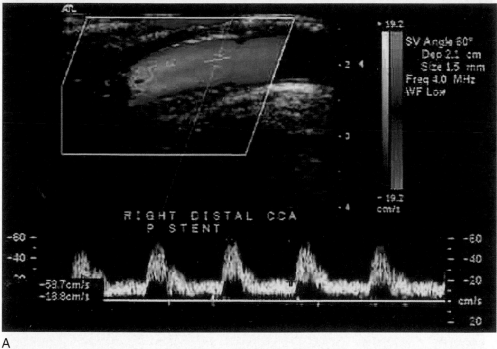

A

FIGURE 19–13. *A* and *B*, Duplex scan following carotid stent angioplasty. Stents are easily visualized. Note the close apposition of the stent to the artery wall. Velocity spectra indicate nondisturbed (laminar) flow conditions and normal carotid systolic velocity. CCA, common carotid artery. *Continued*

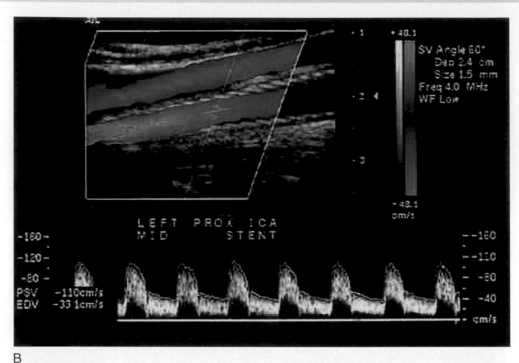

B

FIGURE 19–13—cont'd

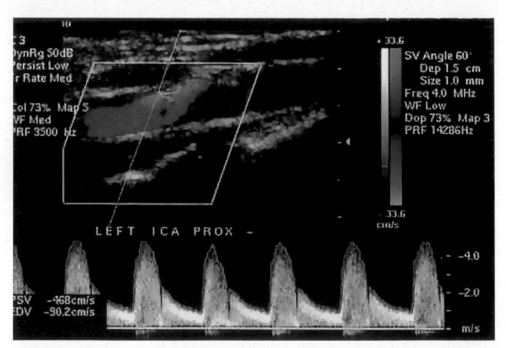

FIGURE 19–14. Duplex scan of the proximal internal carotid artery (ICA) showing a high-grade (>75%) recurrent carotid stenosis caused by myointimal hyperplasia. Peak systolic velocity, 468 cm/sec; end diastolic velocity, 90 cm/sec.

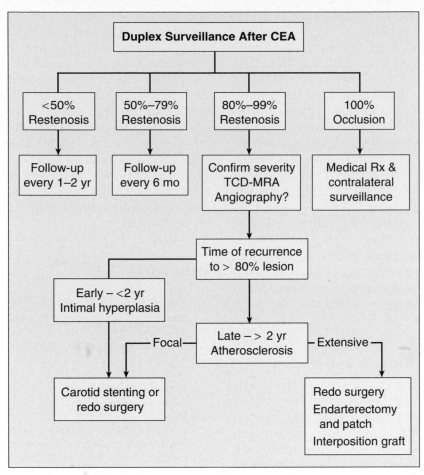

FIGURE 19–15. Algorithm for duplex surveillance after carotid endarterectomy (CEA). MRA, magnetic resonance angiography; TCD, transcranial Doppler.

however, with an early neointimal hyperplasia appearance gradually giving way to a more atherosclerotic appearance in late-occurring restenosis.

Considering the potential for recurrence of carotid stenosis, duplex surveillance after CEA or CAS is recommended (Fig. 19–15). Testing intervals of 6 mo are sufficient to detect development of restenosis and follow lesions for progression. In the majority of patients, however, the main reason for duplex surveillance is to identify progression of contralateral ICA stenosis of more than 50%, rather than to detect restenosis of the CEA or CAS site. An early duplex scan of the CEA or CAS site at 1 to 3 mo is useful to exclude residual stenosis. High-grade internal carotid artery (ICA) stenosis (peak systolic velocity > 300 cm/sec; diastolic velocity > 125 cm/sec; ICA/common carotid artery ratio > 4) should prompt consideration for reintervention, especially if the stenosis is rapidly progressing, is longer than 1 cm, or occurs following CAS. Duplex scanning every 1 to 2 yr after CEA may be adequate when no stenosis is identified within the first postoperative year and less than 50%-diameter-reducing stenosis is present in the contralateral carotid system (see Fig. 19–13). Surveillance every 6 mo is indicated in patients with residual or recurrent ipsilateral stenosis and contralateral ICA occlusion. The development of hemispheric symptoms in the presence of ICA stenosis with a diameter reduction of more than 50%, or asymptomatic disease progression to a high-grade stenosis (>75% to 80% diameter reduction; end-diastolic velocity > 150 cm/sec), should prompt a recommendation of surgical or endovascular (stent-assisted angioplasty) intervention in appropriate patients.

The yield (i.e., intervention rate for severe stenosis) of duplex surveillance after CEA (5%–7%) is less than after CAS (10%) or infrainguinal vein bypass (15%–20%).[31] Progression of contralateral disease, however, is five times more common. A policy of duplex ultrasound surveillance and reintervention for high-grade stenosis is associated with a low (<1%/yr) incidence of ipsilateral hemispheric, disabling stroke. The majority of patients after CEA or CAS have duplex scans indicating bilateral stenosis of less than 50%, and annual follow-up is appropriate. During follow-up, other CEA site abnormalities, such as mural thrombus development or aneurysmal degeneration, may be detected.

CONCLUSIONS

The patency of arterial interventions can be improved by the application of duplex ultrasound assessment. When used at the time of the procedure, duplex testing can identify residual stenosis, lumen thrombus, or other conditions that increase the likelihood of postprocedural failure. With recognition, immediate correction by surgery or endovascular intervention is possible, or additional imaging (i.e., arteriography) can be performed to further define the abnormality. The criteria for reintervention vary with the procedure type, but Doppler velocity criteria indicating arterial stenosis of more than 50% are generally used to select lesions to be corrected. An important attribute of duplex surveillance is that clinical success is predicted by a normal study, and the incidence of subsequent failure is higher if a residual stenosis is identified. The majority of arterial repairs are followed by normal duplex studies (i.e., no abnormality is detected), and these patients can be restudied less frequently than when testing indicates a "problem." Lesions that reduce flow increase the likelihood for repair failure and have Doppler velocity findings of severe stenosis—high PSV (>300 cm/sec), turbulent flow, and damped distal velocity waveform. Interventions to correct these lesions should also be monitored using duplex ultrasound, since clinical assessment and arteriography are imperfect measures of technical adequacy. All patients undergoing peripheral interventions should be enrolled in a surveillance program that includes duplex ultrasound. These surveillance programs are cost-effective by decreasing the number of failures, despite the expense of serial examinations at 3- to 6-mo intervals and the performing of secondary procedures to repair progressive, severe duplex-detected stenosis, the majority of which are asymptomatic.

References

1. Bandyk DF, Mills JL, Gahtan V, Esses GE: Intraoperative duplex scanning of arterial reconstructions: Fate of repaired and unrepaired defects. J Vasc Surg 20:426–433, 1994.
2. Bandyk DF, Johnson BL, Gupta AK, Esses GE: Nature and management of duplex abnormalities encountered during infrainguinal vein bypass grafting. J Vasc Surg 24:430–438, 1996.
3. Bandyk DF, et al: Monitoring functional patency of in situ saphenous vein bypasses: The impact of a surveillance protocol and elective revision. J Vasc Surg 9:284–296, 1989.
4. Idu MM et al: Impact of a color flow duplex surveillance program infrainguinal graft patency: A five-year experience. J Vasc Surg 17:42–53, 1992.
5. Kundell A, Linblad B, Bergqvist D, Hansen F: Femoropopliteal graft patency is improved by an intensive surveillance program: A prospective-randomized study. J Vasc Surg 21:26–34, 1995.
6. Kinney EV, Bandyk DF, Mewissen MW, et al: Monitoring functional patency of percutaneous transluminal angioplasty. Arch Surg 126:743–747, 1991.
7. Bandyk DF: Cost-effectiveness of noninvasive surveillance after arterial surgery. Semin Vasc Surg 7:261–267, 1994.
8. Wixon CL, Mills JL, Westerband A, et al: An economic appraisal of lower extremity bypass graft maintainance. J Vasc Surg 32:89–95, 2000.
9. Spijkerboer AM, Nass PC, de Valois JC, et al: Iliac artery stenoses after percutaneous transluminal angioplasty: Follow-up with duplex ultrasonography. J Vasc Surg 23:691–697, 1996.
10. Johnson BL, Bandyk DF, Back MR, et al: Intraoperative duplex monitoring of infrainguinal vein bypass procedures. J Vasc Surg 31:678–690, 2000.

11. Mills JL. Fujitani RM, Taylor SM: The contribution of routine intraoperative completion arteriography to early graft patency. Am J Surg 164:506–511, 1992.

12. Miller A, Maracaccio EJ, Tannenbaum GE, et al: Comparison of angioscopy and angiography for monitoring infrainguinal vein bypass grafts: Results of prospective randomized trial. J Vasc Surg 17:382–398, 1993.

13. Dalman RL, Harris EJ, Zarins CK: Is completion arteriography mandatory after reversed-vein bypass grafting? J Vasc Surg 23:637–644, 1996.

14. Mewissen MW, Kinney EV, Bandyk DF, et al: The role of duplex scanning versus angiography in predicting outcome after balloon angioplasty in the femoropopliteal artery. J Vasc Surg 15:860–864, 1992.

15. Johnson BL, Avino AJ, Bandyk DF: Duplex-monitored angioplasty of peripheral artery and infrainguinal vein graft stenosis. In Whittemore AD (ed): Advances in Vascular Surgery, Vol 8. St. Louis, Mosby, 2000, pp 83–95.

16. Gupta AK, Bandyk DF, Cheanvechai D, Johnson BL: Natural history of infrainguinal vein graft stenosis relative to bypass grafting technique. J Vasc Surg 25:211–225, 1997.

17. Mills JL, Bandyk DF, Gahtan V, Esses GE: The origin of infrainguinal vein graft stenosis: A prospective study based on duplex surveillance. J Vasc Surg 21:16–25, 1995.

18. Bandyk DF: Infrainguinal vein bypass graft surveillance. How to do it, when to intervene, and is it cost-effective? J Am Coll Surg 194:S40–S52, 2002.

19. Moody AP, Gould DA, Harris PL: Vein graft surveillance improves patency in femoropopliteal bypass. Eur J Vasc Surg 4:117–120, 1990.

20. Mills JL, Harris EJ, Taylor LM, Beckett WC: The importance of routine surveillance of distal bypass grafts with duplex scanning: A study of 379 reversed vein grafts. J Vasc Surg 12:379–389, 1990.

21. Roth SM, Bandyk DF: Duplex imaging of lower extremity bypasses, angioplasties, and stents. Semin Vasc Surg 12:275–284, 1999.

22. Spijkerboer AM, Nass PC, de Valois JC, et al: Evaluation of femoropopliteal arteries with duplex ultrasound after angioplasty. Can we predict results at one year? Eur J Vasc Endovasc Surg 12:418–423, 1996.

23. Tielbeek AV, Rietjens E, Buth J, et al: The value of duplex surveillance after endovascular intervention for femoropopliteal obstructive disease. Eur J Vasc Endovasc Surg 12:145–150, 1996.

24. Cluley SR, Brener BJ, Hollier L, et al: Transcutaneous ultrasonography can be used to guide and monitor balloon angioplasty. J Vasc Surg 17:23–31, 1993.

25. Ramaswami G, Al-kutoubi A, Nicolaides AN, et al: Duplex controlled angioplasty. Eur J Vasc Surg 8:457–463, 1994.

26. Calligaro KD, Musser DJ, Chen AY, et al: Duplex ultrasonography to diagnose failing arterial prosthetic grafts. Surgery 120:455–459, 1996.

27. Westerband A, Mills JL, Kistler S, et al: Prospective validation of threshold criteria for intervention in infrainguinal vein grafts undergoing duplex surveillance. Ann Vasc Surg 11:44–48, 1997.

28. Caps T, Cantwell-Gab K, Bergelin RO, Strandness DE Jr: Vein graft lesions: Time of onset and rate of progression. J Vasc Surg 22:466–475, 1995.

29. Erickson CA, Towne JB, Seabrook GR, et al: Ongoing vascular laboratory surveillance is essential to maximize long-term in situ saphenous vein bypass patency. J Vasc Surg 23:18–24, 1996.

30. Back MR, Novotney M, Roth SM, et al: Utility of duplex surveillance following iliac artery angioplasty and primary stenting. J Endovasc Ther 8:629–637, 2001.

31. Roth SM, Back MR, Bandyk DF, et al: A rational algorithm for duplex surveillance following carotid endarterectomy. J Vasc Surg 30:453–460, 1999.

Chapter 20

Ultrasound in the Diagnosis and Management of Arterial Emergencies

BRIAN J. BURKE, MD, RVT, AND STEVEN G. FRIEDMAN, MD

Vascular emergencies require a prompt diagnosis, as timely intervention is often critically important. Delays of minutes or hours in management may mean the difference between life and death, or limb preservation or loss. Ultrasound now plays an important role in the diagnosis and management of many vascular emergencies.

Since vascular emergencies often are managed nonoperatively, an accurate diagnosis is critical to appropriate patient triage. Several diagnostic modalities can be applied in such cases. In addition to duplex ultrasound, other modalities include computed tomographic angiography, magnetic resonance angiography, digital subtraction angiography, and intravascular ultrasound. The advantages of ultrasound for emergencies include ready availability, portability, speed, and high temporal and spatial resolution. A relative disadvantage is the acoustic barrier presented by bone, air in lung and bowel, and tissue edema; these limit the use of ultrasound at the skull base, in the chest, deep pelvis, and injured extremities with extensive tissue disruption. Depiction of regional arterial supply through collateral pathways around a diseased vessel is also less complete with ultrasound than with angiography. The choice of ultrasound as a diagnostic modality reflects these factors as well as the clinical information needed to direct management.

RUPTURED ABDOMINAL AORTIC ANEURYSM

An aneurysm is a localized dilation of an artery, with an increase in diameter of greater than 50% of the normal size. Abdominal aortic aneurysms (AAAs) are most commonly encountered in the infrarenal region. As the population ages, the incidence of AAAs is increasing. In the 1950s, 8.7 new aneurysms were diagnosed in the United States per 100,000 person-years, compared with 36.5 new aneurysms per 100,000 person-years during the 1970s.[1] This has also been noted in other Western countries and is the result of increased life expectancy and improved diagnostic tools. Approximately 1.5 million Americans have AAAs, and 200,000 are diagnosed each year. Nearly 50,000 aneurysmectomies are performed annually, and 15,000 deaths result from ruptured AAAs, which represents the 13th leading cause of death in our nation.[2] Most AAAs are asymptomatic and are detected during routine physical examinations or radiologic procedures for other problems. Symptomatic aneurysms may result in abdominal, flank, or back pain; embolization; thrombosis; or rupture. The latter complication is usually fatal.

The goal of treatment of AAAs is avoidance of rupture. Elective repair is reserved for subjects with AAAs of 5 to 5.5 cm in diameter, and postoperative survival is approximately

95%. The diseased portion of the aorta is replaced with a synthetic graft, or it is excluded via an endoluminal approach. Most AAAs are too small to warrant surgical treatment; however, they are prone to gradual expansion. Risk factors for expansion and rupture have been described, but there is no therapy to prevent AAA growth.[3]

A multidisciplinary research program supported by the National Heart, Lung, and Blood Institute identified four causes of AAA formation: (1) proteolytic degradation of aortic wall connective tissue, (2) inflammation and immune responses, (3) biochemical wall stress, and (4) molecular genetics.[4] In vivo models of AAA formation and studies on human aortic tissue have been used to elucidate the role of various proteases. These models suggest that matrix metalloproteinases, derived from macrophages and aortic smooth muscle cells, play an integral role in aneurysm formation. The preferential infrarenal site for AAA formation suggests that there may be differences in aortic structure, biology, and stress along its length. Increased shear and tension on the aortic wall result in collagen remodeling, and the decrease in the elastin-to-collagen ratio from the proximal to the distal aorta may also be causative. Familial clustering and a common human leukocyte antigen (HLA) subtype indicate a genetic

role in the formation of AAAs. Although no single genetic polymorphism or defect has been identified as a common denominator for AAAs, subjects with affected siblings are at increased risk for developing them.

Ultrasonography is often used as the initial procedure for diagnosis of AAAs. It is also used for screening surveys and serial measurement of AAA size. When aneurysms rupture, only 50% of patients present with the "classic" triad of abdominal or back pain, hypotension, and pulsatile abdominal mass. The clinical diagnosis may, therefore, pose a challenge, particularly in patients without a known history of AAA. An accurate imaging diagnosis of retroperitoneal hematoma in the presence of AAA enables rapid transport to the operating room.

Although noncontrast CT is also useful for this purpose, ultrasound is faster in these potentially unstable patients. Ultrasound diagnosis of an abdominal aneurysm has a sensitivity of 98% and specificity of 95% in the setting of abdominal pain and hemodynamic instability.[5] While active extravasation is never brisk enough to demonstrate by Doppler ultrasound, the resultant hematoma provides evidence of rupture (Fig. 20–1). Initially, intramural hemorrhage may be visible as an echogenic crescent within the aneurysmal wall. Following rupture, blood initially accumu-

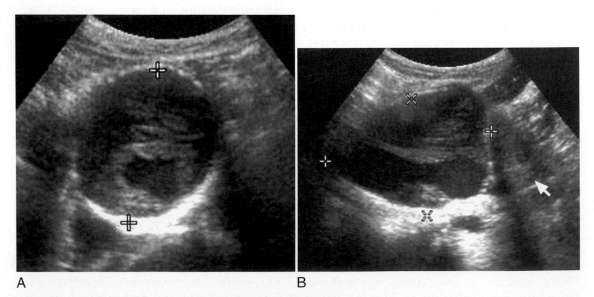

A   B

Figure 20–1. Ruptured aortic aneurysm. Transverse (A) and oblique (B) views of aortic aneurysm (cursors) with abundant mural thrombus and a small periaortic hematoma (arrow).

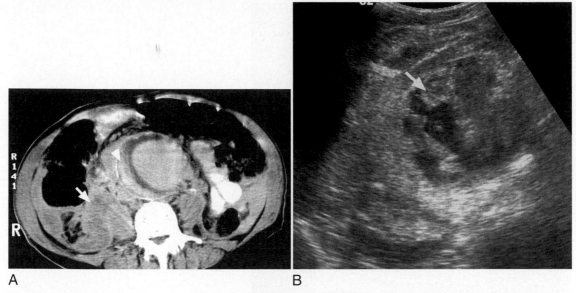

FIGURE 20–2. Retroperitoneal hematoma. *A,* Computed tomographic image shows a large abdominal aortic aneurysm with intramural (*arrowhead*) and retroperitoneal (*arrow*) hemorrhage. *B,* Ultrasound shows a large retroperitoneal hematoma in the left flank, infiltrating the psoas muscle (*arrow*) and distorting tissue planes.

lates in the para-aortic space, extending toward the flanks via the pararenal space. Hemorrhage may track along the course of the iliac arteries to the extraperitoneal spaces of the pelvis (Fig. 20–2). Anterior extension may transgress the posterior peritoneum, resulting in hemoperitoneum.

When the patient presents with abdominal pain, the operator may be reluctant to use probe pressure to visualize the aorta for fear of provoking or exacerbating rupture. Although this is rarely a practical concern, the use of a coronal approach from the left flank avoids trapping the aneurysm between the transducer and the spine. Additionally, this approach frequently provides improved visualization of the aorta by circumventing overlying bowel gas.

Aortic dissection may be encountered as an alternative diagnosis in patients with a clinical presentation suggesting aneurysm rupture. Although ultrasound is not a primary diagnostic modality, since it cannot reveal the full extent of dissection in the thorax, the characteristic intimal flap and altered blood flow pattern is readily visible and can lead to appropriate workup and treatment (Fig. 20–3). Additional details about aortic aneurysm and dissection are presented in Chapter 29.[6]

CAROTID ARTERY STENOSIS

Duplex scanning is the most popular non-invasive method for diagnosing carotid artery occlusive disease. Many surgeons use it as the sole diagnostic test prior to carotid endarterectomy. Carotid plaque morphology and the severity of carotid stenosis can be accurately determined with this technique. The combination of gray-scale and color flow imaging allows proper positioning of the Doppler sample volume and provides information about plaque morphology. Accurate quantitation of carotid stenosis is achieved by analysis of Doppler-derived spectral waveforms.

Symptomatic carotid artery stenosis is manifested by transient ischemic attacks (TIAs) or stroke (cerebrovascular accident, CVA). Neurologically unstable patients, in whom emergency carotid endarterectomy may be indicated, include those with crescendo transient ischemic attacks, stroke in evolution, fluctuating or fixed neurologic deficits caused by acute carotid artery thrombosis, and free-floating thrombus. In these cases, rapid sonographic evaluation of the carotid bifurcation can result in timely surgery to prevent stroke or death.

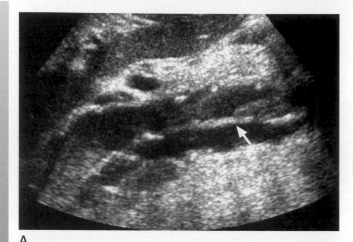

A

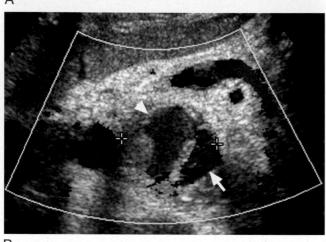

B

FIGURE 20–3. Aortic dissection. Sagittal (*A*) image of the abdominal aorta shows an echogenic intimal flap (*arrow*). Transverse color view (*B*) clearly distinguishes the patent true lumen (*arrow*) from the thrombosed false lumen (*arrowhead*).

Sonographic detection and quantification of carotid stenosis in the emergency setting (i.e., progressive neurologic deficit) is similar to the nonacute setting and is described in Chapter 9. It is important to distinguish acute carotid thrombosis from stable (chronic) carotid occlusion. Whereas revascularization of a chronic occlusion is generally contraindicated, timely intervention may avoid or limit neurologic sequelae in cases of acute thrombosis.

Acute thrombosis may occur as a complication of endarterectomy or stenting, or it may represent acute progression of carotid stenosis. The thrombus is usually heterogeneously echogenic (Fig. 20–4). The vessel lumen is of normal caliber or slightly expanded, as opposed to chronic occlusion, which may result in luminal narrowing or obliteration.[7] Pulsations may be observed in the vessel wall, which retains its normal compliance. Swirling, sludgelike flow may be observed in the carotid bulb at the interface of the thrombosed and patent lumen. Spectral waveforms assume a high impedance, hammer-like or to-and-fro configuration proximal to the thrombus. Internalization of the external carotid artery waveform is uncommonly seen with acute thrombosis due to insufficient time to develop collateral pathways.

If the thrombus is nonocclusive, its free edge may oscillate back and forth in the bloodstream; the "free-floating" thrombus has a characteristic appearance at real-time examination (Fig. 20–5).[8] The risk of

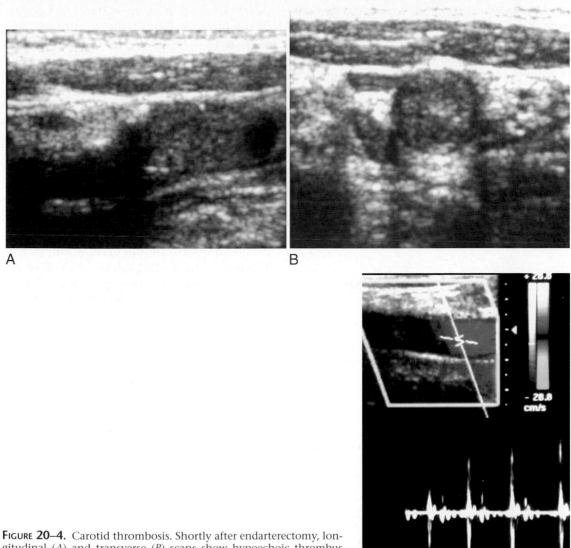

A   B

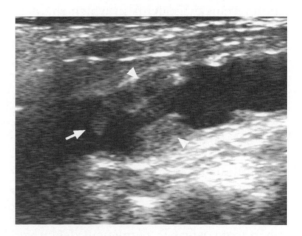

FIGURE 20–4. Carotid thrombosis. Shortly after endarterectomy, longitudinal (*A*) and transverse (*B*) scans show hypoechoic thrombus filling the common carotid artery. Duplex scan (*C*) shows "water-hammer" waveforms at the interface of the patent lumen and acute thrombus. PCCA, proximal common carotid artery.

C

FIGURE 20–5. Free-floating thrombus. Longitudinal ultrasound in the distal common carotid artery shows nonocclusive thrombi (*arrowheads*) with a nonadherent tail (*arrow*) seen to move back and forth in the bloodstream on real-time examination.

embolization is related to the extent of attachment of the base of the thrombus to the vessel wall; this can be depicted with the aid of color Doppler or B-flow.[9]

When patients with acute carotid stenosis or thrombosis undergo thrombectomy or revascularization, intraoperative ultrasound is a useful adjunctive technique. Scanning directly over the vessel in the exposed surgical field yields superb resolution of the vessel wall. It is possible to visualize small intimal flaps, ulcerative plaques, or retained thrombi, leading to immediate surgical revision, which favorably impacts patency rates.[10]

CAROTID ARTERY DISSECTION

Carotid artery dissection results from a hemorrhage within the carotid wall. The media is the most common location for hemorrhage, and this may extend into the subintimal or subadventitial layers. The former may result in thrombosis of the vessel; aneurysms may occur from the latter. Carotid dissection usually occurs in the proximal internal carotid artery and extends distally to the carotid canal in the petrous portion of the temporal bone.

Spontaneous dissections may be associated with type IV Ehler-Danlos syndrome, Marfan syndrome, fibromuscular dysplasia, and cystic medial necrosis; however, most spontaneous dissections are idiopathic. They often happen in previously healthy individuals younger than 40 yr.[11] Most traumatic carotid dissections result from motor vehicle accidents in which the neck is hyperextended, compressing the carotid artery against the atlas or second cervical vertebra. Blunt trauma, penetrating injuries, and catheter injuries during arteriography also cause traumatic dissections.[12]

In the United States, the annual incidence of symptomatic carotid artery dissection is 2.6 per 100,000. The actual incidence may be higher, since many episodes may be asymptomatic or cause only minor transient symptoms, thereby remaining undiagnosed. Morbidity from carotid artery dissection varies in severity from transient neurologic deficit to permanent deficit and death. Dissection of the intracranial portion of the internal carotid artery, although rare, is associated with a 75% mortality rate. The male-to-female ratio of carotid dissection is 1.5:1. The mean age for extracranial internal carotid artery dissection is 40 yr; intracranial dissections are more common in those 20 to 30 years old. Approximately 20% of strokes in young patients are caused by carotid artery and vertebral artery dissections in the neck, compared with 2.5% in older patients.

Patients with carotid dissection often complain of neck pain, headache, tinnitus, or a focal neurologic deficit. Horner syndrome, transient monocular blindness, neck swelling, and cranial nerve palsy may also result. The onset of symptoms may be hours to days after the dissection occurs.[13]

Duplex scanning of patients with suspected carotid dissection can be performed quickly in the emergency department to make this diagnosis. Typical findings with duplex scanning include a patent carotid bifurcation with tapering of the internal carotid artery, leading to a distal stenosis or occlusion (Fig. 20–6). Intimal flaps or membranes may be seen (Fig. 20–7), and spectral analysis reveals high-resistance waveforms with reduced flow velocity in the internal carotid artery.[14]

The false lumen may be thrombosed or patent. If acutely thrombosed, the intimal flap may bulge in convex fashion toward the true lumen. A patent false lumen usually exhibits flow characteristics differing from the true lumen, unless a second intimal tear downstream reestablishes continuity between the true and false lumen. More commonly, the false lumen demonstrates low peak flow velocity with reversal of flow during diastole.

If the site of dissection is near the skull base, it may not be visible with ultrasound. In such cases, altered hemodynamics in the ICA proximal to the dissection (reduced peak velocity, increased impedance) constitute indirect evidence for the diagnosis in a patient with a compatible clinical presentation. Magnetic resonance angiography is indicated in this situation to confirm the diagnosis and establish the extent of dissection.

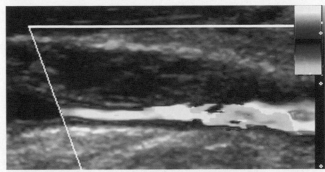

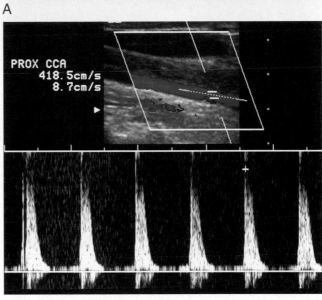

FIGURE 20–6. Common carotid artery (CCA) dissection. *A*, The true lumen tapers distally, compressed by the thrombosed false lumen. *B*, High-velocity, high-impedance flow reflects the degree of stenosis caused by the displaced intimal flap.

ACUTE LOWER EXTREMITY ISCHEMIA

Acute ischemia of the lower extremity is caused by an embolism from the heart or a more proximal arterial location, or from acute thrombosis of the affected artery. Approximately 80% of peripheral arterial emboli originate in the heart. Cardiac thrombus may develop secondary to rheumatic heart disease, myocardial infarction, endocarditis, prosthetic valve, arrhythmia, and neoplasms. An embolism can also originate from any artery outside the heart, and the abdominal aorta is the most common source of artery-to-artery emboli. Atherosclerotic plaques and small aneurysms of the aorta or iliac arteries account for approximately 70% of these emboli. More distal lower extremity arteries (e.g., superficial

femoral) account for most of the other cases of emboli of arterial origin. Duplex imaging of infrainguinal occlusive disease has become popular in elective revascularization cases, leading some practitioners to abandon angiography.[15] The same arguments supporting preferential use of ultrasonography in acute situations will undoubtedly lead to its use in cases of acute arterial thrombosis.

Detection of lower extremity aneurysms that may be the source of emboli is readily accomplished with ultrasound (Fig. 20–8). The upper limit of the normal arterial diameter is 10 mm in the common femoral artery, 8 mm in the superficial femoral artery, and 5 to 6 mm in the popliteal artery. Fusiform enlargement is often accompanied by vessel tortuosity and may be multifocal. Popliteal aneurysms are associated with

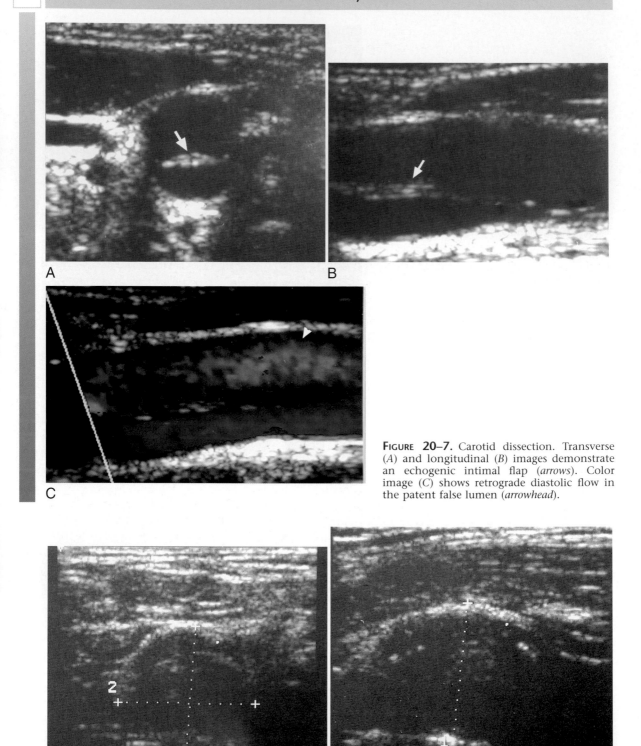

A

B

C

FIGURE 20–7. Carotid dissection. Transverse (*A*) and longitudinal (*B*) images demonstrate an echogenic intimal flap (*arrows*). Color image (*C*) shows retrograde diastolic flow in the patent false lumen (*arrowhead*).

A

B

FIGURE 20–8. Popliteal aneurysm. Transverse (*A*) and longitudinal (*B*) images of 2-cm aneurysm with irregular intimal plaque.

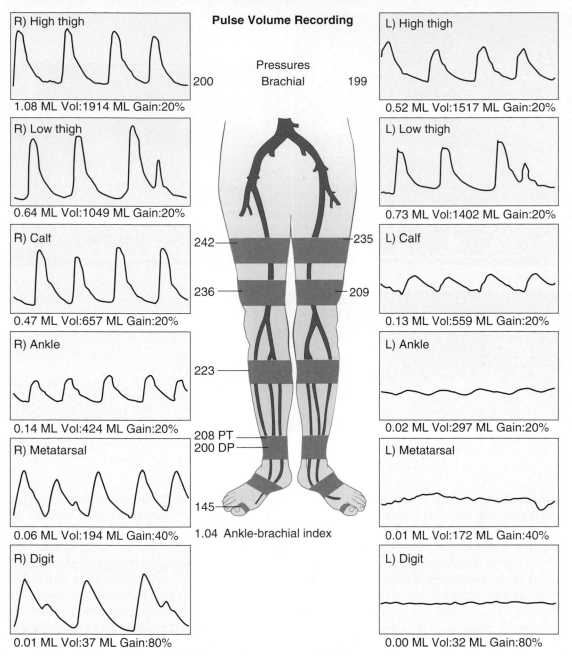

Pulse Volume Recording

R) High thigh
1.08 ML Vol:1914 ML Gain:20%
200

Pressures
Brachial
199

L) High thigh
0.52 ML Vol:1517 ML Gain:20%

R) Low thigh
0.64 ML Vol:1049 ML Gain:20%

L) Low thigh
0.73 ML Vol:1402 ML Gain:20%

R) Calf
0.47 ML Vol:657 ML Gain:20%
242

L) Calf
0.13 ML Vol:559 ML Gain:20%
235

R) Ankle
0.14 ML Vol:424 ML Gain:20%
236

L) Ankle
0.02 ML Vol:297 ML Gain:20%
209

223

R) Metatarsal
0.06 ML Vol:194 ML Gain:40%
208 PT
200 DP

L) Metatarsal
0.01 ML Vol:172 ML Gain:40%

145

1.04 Ankle-brachial index

R) Digit
0.01 ML Vol:37 ML Gain:80%

L) Digit
0.00 ML Vol:32 ML Gain:80%

FIGURE 20–9. Atheroembolic occlusion. Lower extremity arterial Doppler examination on a patient presenting with cold left foot. The ankle-brachial index is unobtainable, due to inaudible pulses in the left foot. Pulse volume recordings show progressively diminishing amplitude and pulsatility below the left knee. DP, dorsalis pedis; PT, posterior tibial.

AAA in 30% to 35% of patients. Intra-luminal plaque with an irregular luminal contour and heterogeneous echogenicity may be of higher risk for embolization than smooth, homogeneous plaque.[16]

In acute arterial thrombosis, nonduplex physiologic testing (i.e., segmental arterial pressure measurement and volume plethys-mography) is useful to confirm the pres-ence of a flow-limiting lesion, and this test can often indicate the involved vascular segment (Fig. 20–9). Duplex scanning can then be directed to the area of suspicion, and the site of embolization can be

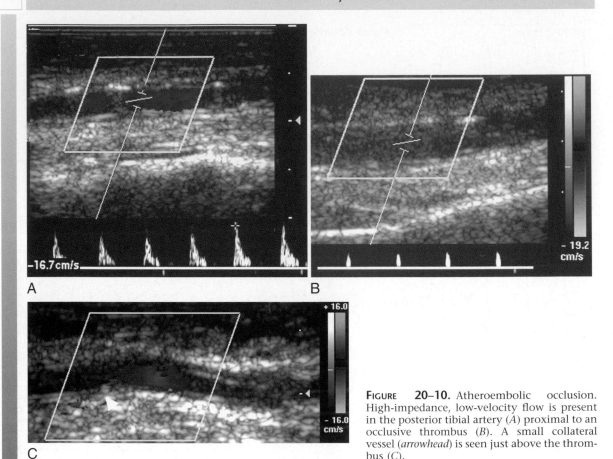

FIGURE 20–10. Atheroembolic occlusion. High-impedance, low-velocity flow is present in the posterior tibial artery (*A*) proximal to an occlusive thrombus (*B*). A small collateral vessel (*arrowhead*) is seen just above the thrombus (*C*).

identified (Fig 20–10). For example, if segmental pressure measurements demonstrate a pressure gradient across the knee, duplex scanning should begin above this level, in the mid–superior femoral artery. The examination should proceed distally to the point of obstruction. Color Doppler is essential for surveying long segments of vessel for the presence of flow and to identify the disturbed color pattern and collateral branches at the site of occlusion. Spectral Doppler sampling at intervals along the vessel may demonstrate characteristic changes in the arterial waveform. Proximal to the occlusion, the waveform shows increased impedance and may convert from triphasic to biphasic flow, with flow reversal in end-diastole. Downstream from the occlusion, waveforms are typically monophasic, with diminished peak velocities. Caution is necessary with such waveform analysis in patients with significant atherosclerosis, as serial-segment or long-segment stenoses upstream and downstream from the occlusion may exert unpredictable effects on regional hemodynamics.

After an acute embolic occlusion, the artery may undergo retrograde thrombosis to the nearest proximal branch that provides a collateral pathway around the obstruction. It is seldom feasible to track the entire course of the small, sinuous collateral vessels, but in following the thrombosed arterial trunk with color Doppler, one can often detect the point at which arterial patency is reconstituted. Tracking the thrombosed artery is complicated by the lack of color signal within its lumen, but the accompanying vein (or in the calf, paired veins) provides a useful landmark for its location. Small vessel size, as well as extensive atheromatous disease and collaterals in patients with chronic ischemia, limit the use of duplex scanning in the infrapopliteal arteries. However, the distal anterior and posterior tibial arteries are readily accessible to duplex sampling due to their constant superficial location.[17]

Failure of infrainguinal bypass grafts may present acutely with lower extremity ischemia. The cause of graft failure usually relates to stenosis within or adjacent to the graft, impairing blood flow and ultimately leading to thrombosis. The typical cause of graft failure is related to the age of the graft. In the early postoperative period (<1 mo), technical problems with vein selection or anastomosis construction are often implicated. At graft maturity (1 mo–2 yr), the development of fibrointimal hyperplasia at vein valves and anastomoses leads to stenoses. In the later period (>2 yr), graft failure is usually due to progression of atherosclerotic disease in the adjacent native circulation. A program of duplex graft surveillance is beneficial in improving graft patency by detecting asymptomatic lesions before graft thrombosis. In one study of 101 infrainguinal vein grafts, no grafts with normal duplex examinations progressed to occlusion, while 54% of grafts with abnormal duplex examinations proceeded to failure.[18] Correction of asymptomatic lesions prior to graft failure improves secondary patency rates.

When patients present with acute ischemia, duplex scanning often reveals graft thrombosis with absence of flow (Fig. 20–11). Flow being present within the graft, average peak systolic velocity of less than 45 cm/sec, and interval (compared with prior examinations) fall in ankle-brachial index of more than 0.15 are signs of impending graft failure (Fig. 20–12). Other graft complications detectable by duplex scanning include arterial-venous shunting through unligated vein branches, anastomotic pseudoaneurysm, and perigraft abscess.

FEMORAL PSEUDOANEURYSM

Thousands of diagnostic catheterization procedures are performed daily in the United States to delineate the coronary or peripheral arterial circulation. The most common entry route is the femoral artery. A pseudoaneurysm, or false aneurysm, is a confined collection of thrombus and blood associated with disruption of one or more layers of an artery wall. This occurs at the puncture site as a complication of percutaneous arterial catheterization. Pseudoaneurysms differ from true aneurysms in that the latter contain all three histologic layers of the arterial wall, whereas pseudoaneurysms contain less than three and often none of these layers.

Modern duplex imaging makes the diagnosis of femoral artery pseudoaneurysm routine.[19] The pseudoaneurysm usually arises from the superficial aspect of the artery at the site of puncture. This is most often at the level of the common femoral artery, but occasionally puncture occurs above the inguinal ligament in the external iliac artery or below the bifurcation in the superficial or deep femoral artery. The pseudoaneurysm lumen is connected to the

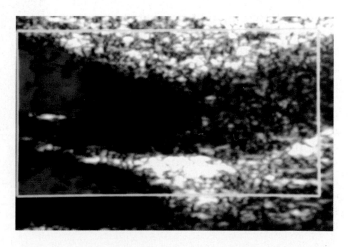

FIGURE 20–11. Bypass graft failure. Echogenic thrombus occludes all but the most proximal segment of this autogenous vein graft.

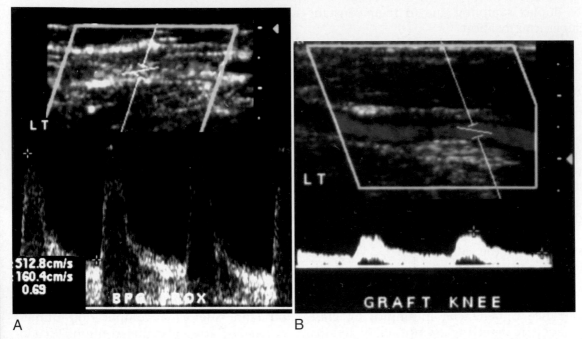

A   B

FIGURE 20–12. Impending graft failure. *A,* Disturbed color flow and high peak velocity (512.8 cm/sec) are demonstrated by duplex study at a high-grade stenosis just beyond the proximal graft anastomosis. *B,* Low-velocity flow downstream from the stenosis portends impending graft failure.

underlying artery by a cylindrical neck—variable in length and diameter—which takes the course of the needle tract. Color Doppler is useful for detection of the pseudoaneurysm and its neck. Once detected, spectral Doppler flow within the neck is diagnostic (Fig. 20–13).

The pseudoaneurysm lumen is often 1 to 3 cm in diameter, although large pseudoaneurysms can exceed 5 cm, and the presence of a string of aneurysms with multiple lumens is common (Fig. 20–14). Sometimes flow within a needle tract is detectable by color flow imaging without an associated lumen.[20] A swirling pattern of blood flow in the lumen often appears on color imaging as a characteristic "yin-yang" sign (Fig. 20–15). The lumen may be partially thrombosed at the time of diagnosis.

Because of the potential risk of growth and rupture, pseudoaneurysms should be treated at the time of diagnosis. Since initial description of the technique in 1992, ultrasound-guided compression repair has been efficacious and safe.[21] Approximately 75% of femoral pseudoaneurysms are successfully thrombosed with this method; however, it can require prolonged compression

(up to or exceeding 1 hr) to achieve success. This is tedious for the operator and painful for the patient. A certain percentage of pseudoaneurysms are not amenable to this technique, because, despite forceful

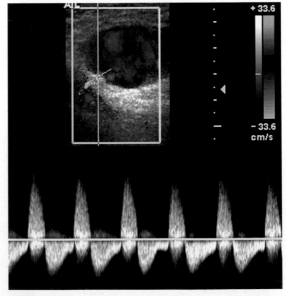

FIGURE 20–13. Femoral artery pseudoaneurysm. Duplex sampling in the pseudoaneurysm neck demonstrates characteristic to-and-fro flow.

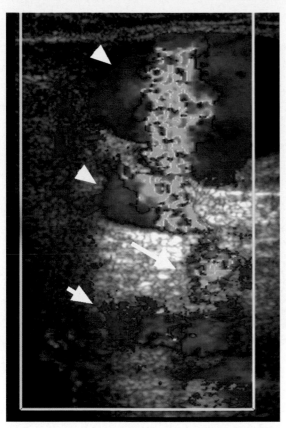

FIGURE 20–14. Multilocular pseudoaneurysm. Two distinct lumens (*arrowheads*) communicate with the common femoral artery (*short arrow*) via a single neck (*long arrow*).

drape. The transducer was covered with a sterile sleeve. A 22-gauge spinal needle was placed in a biopsy guide and advanced into the false aneurysm under direct ultrasound visualization. A radiologist performed the initial examination for diagnosis. The pseudoaneurysm was identified and characterized with color flow imaging. Pulsed Doppler was performed to demonstrate flow direction in the neck of the pseudoaneurysm. Color Doppler was turned off during placement of the needle into the false aneurysm to improve visualization of the needle tip. Color Doppler was used to assess thrombosis during thrombin injection. The injection was performed by a vascular surgeon. In all cases, once the needle tip was seen within the false aneurysm, a 1-cc syringe was used to inject 0.5 to 1 mL of a 1000-U/mL solution of bovine thrombin. The majority of cases required only 0.5 mL of thrombin to accomplish pseudoaneurysm thrombosis (Fig. 20–16). One case required a second injection. The needle tip was placed away from the pseudoaneurysm neck to avoid injection into the femoral artery. Color Doppler was performed after

compression, flow cannot be completely excluded from the aneurysm neck.

Ultrasound-guided thrombin injection is the current treatment of choice for femoral pseudoaneurysms; it may be used in elective or emergency situations.[22] We recently reported our results with thrombin injection in 40 patients with femoral pseudoaneurysms.[23] All 40 patients had initial complete thrombosis of their femoral pseudoaneurysms. In each case, except for one, the aneurysm was thrombosed on follow-up duplex ultrasound; there was one complication. The following technique was employed.

A 5-MHz linear array transducer, or a 5-2–MHz curved array transducer was used for scanning and guidance for thrombin injection. Informed consent was obtained in all cases. The skin was prepped with povidone iodine (Betadine) and covered with a sterile

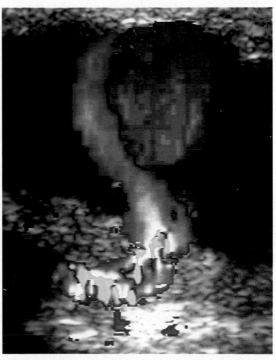

FIGURE 20–15. Femoral artery pseudoaneurysm. The lumen shows the distinctive "yin-yang" appearance.

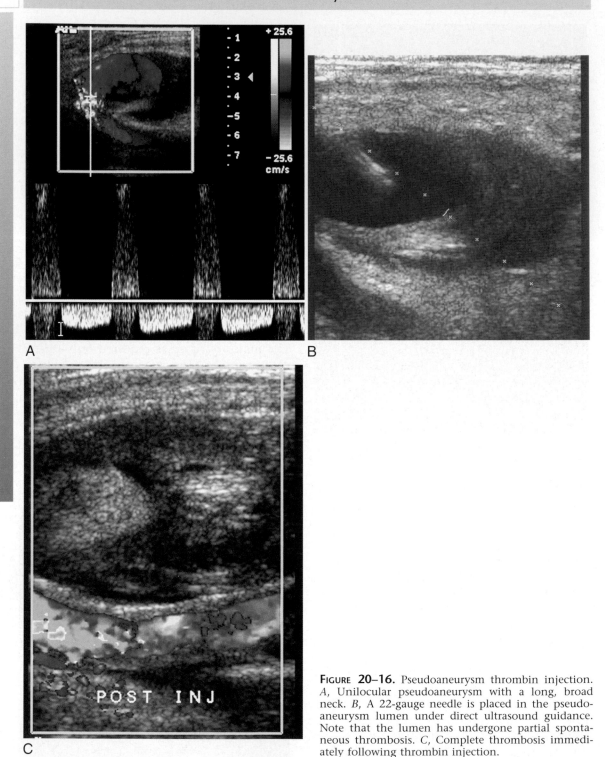

FIGURE 20–16. Pseudoaneurysm thrombin injection. *A*, Unilocular pseudoaneurysm with a long, broad neck. *B*, A 22-gauge needle is placed in the pseudoaneurysm lumen under direct ultrasound guidance. Note that the lumen has undergone partial spontaneous thrombosis. *C*, Complete thrombosis immediately following thrombin injection.

injection to assess the degree of thrombosis and to check patency of the femoral artery and vein. Distal pulses were also checked after treatment. No patients required local anesthesia or conscious sedation. After successful aneurysm thrombosis, all patients were kept on bedrest for several hours. A follow-up duplex scan was obtained the next day to assess for pseudoaneurysm recurrence.

We also reviewed 19 additional studies of more than 400 patients undergoing thrombin injection of femoral pseudo-aneurysms. The initial success rate was 99%. In most cases, aneurysm thrombosis occurred within seconds of the initial injection. Few cases required more than 15 min to complete. The complication rate with this technique was strikingly low, and no cases of limb-threatening ischemia were reported following thrombin injection of pseudoaneurysms.

PENETRATING ARTERIAL TRAUMA

Penetrating trauma is the most common cause of noniatrogenic injury to blood vessels. Age, gender, race, socioeconomic status, education, a criminal record, alcohol and drug use, and gun ownership have been associated with this type of injury.[24] The anatomic distribution of penetrating vascular injuries depends on the mechanism of injury. Nonfatal gunshot wounds usually involve abdominal vessels, followed by the lower extremities.[25] Shotgun wounds are more likely to involve extremity blood vessels, and truncal shotgun wounds are more often fatal. Stab wounds are most common in the neck, arms, and trunk.

Some patients with extremity trauma have clear evidence on examination of significant vascular injury and undergo surgical exploration without imaging. In some cases, however, a vascular injury is suspected without hemodynamic compromise, based on the location or nature of the injury. Most of these patients undergo angiography, but some centers have investigated the utility of duplex ultrasound for these cases, seeking intimal injury/thrombosis, traumatic pseudoaneurysms, and arterial-venous fistulas (Fig. 20–17).

An extremity/brachial pressure index in the affected limb of less than 0.90 has been used as a threshold to prompt duplex evaluation. Bynoe and colleagues[26] used duplex scanning in 198 patients; they achieved a sensitivity of 95%, a specificity of 99%, and an overall accuracy of 98% for identifying arterial injuries.[27] In an experimental study comparing duplex sonography and arteriography in a canine model of arterial injury, duplex scanning was significantly more accurate than angiography in identifying arterial lacerations.[28] These results, however, have been achieved in relatively few institutions, and those undertaking use of duplex scanning for the diagnosis of arterial injuries are advised to establish a mechanism of assessing results achieved in their own laboratory.

Patients undergoing duplex evaluation to assess for occult vascular injury from penetrating trauma in proximity to the vascular bundle are by definition hemodynamically stable; thus, the examination does not have to be performed immediately on admission to the trauma room. However, it should be done expeditiously to facilitate management, especially in multitrauma victims. Since the site of vessel injury is difficult to predict based on the location of entry and exit wound, the study should extend to the joints above and below the level of injury. For shotgun wounds, where the injury is often more diffuse, the examiner should be especially careful to evaluate the entire affected area. Evaluation should include veins as well as arteries to assess for traumatic arteriovenous fistulae, as well as isolated venous injuries.

Several factors can complicate performance of the duplex examination in the trauma setting. Uncooperative or combative patients may require sedation to limit motion of the extremity. Acoustic access may be limited by the presence of wound dressings, orthopedic immobilizing devices, and air or metallic foreign bodies in the soft tissues. Soft tissue hematomas increase the depth of penetration needed to visualize the vessels. Repositioning of the transducer may provide an alternative window to overcome some of these obstacles. Scanning through an open wound requires the use of a sterile probe cover and sterile gel to minimize risk of infection.

Color flow survey of the regional arteries and veins facilitates rapid assessment of the affected area. Sites of disturbed or absent color flow, or extravascular flow should prompt closer inspection. Gray-scale imaging should be performed to seek

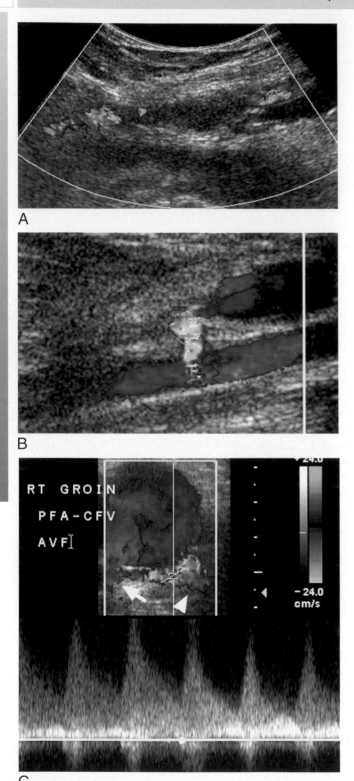

A

B

C

FIGURE 20–17. Peripheral arterial trauma. *A,* Segmental thrombosis of the common femoral artery after blunt trauma. *B,* Brachial artery extravasation due to penetrating injury. *C,* Combined pseudoaneurysm and arteriovenous fistula formation following deep femoral artery laceration. Arrow, profunda femoris artery; arrowhead, common femoral vein.

intimal irregularity or flap formation and the presence of intraluminal thrombus. Because it does not overwrite the vessel wall like color flow Doppler can, B-flow imaging can be especially useful in visualizing a vessel wall abnormality in relation to the local flow disturbance. Assessment of the degree of narrowing incurred at the site of injury requires pulsed Doppler sampling.

Arterial injuries from penetrating trauma detectable by duplex scanning include arterial stenosis or occlusion (from intramural hematoma or transmural laceration), dissection or intimal flap formation, pseudoaneurysm, and arteriovenous fistula. Venous injuries include thrombosis, extrinsic compression (from hematoma or soft tissue swelling), and fistula. Diagnostic criteria for these entities are similar to those that apply in the nontrauma setting.

Another potential role for duplex sonography in the setting of extremity trauma is the diagnosis of compartment syndrome. Compartment syndromes are caused by increased pressure within a closed tissue space, leading to impaired perfusion and tissue ischemia. Duplex analysis of venous and arterial flow proximal and distal to the involved limb segment would be expected to demonstrate changes characteristic of venous congestion and increased arterial impedance (Fig. 20–18).[29] Compartment

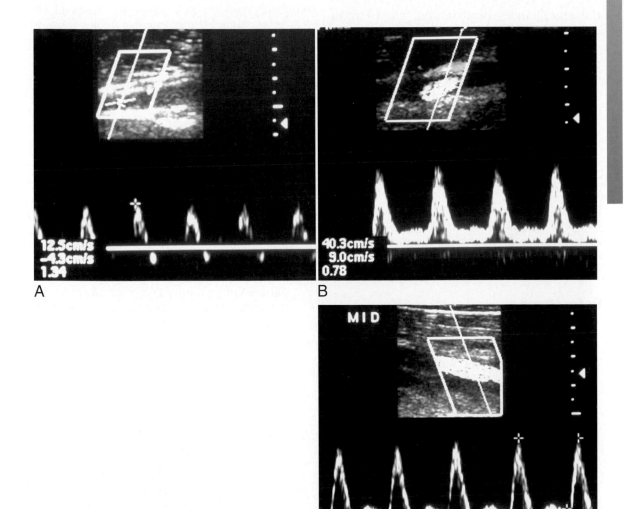

FIGURE 20–18. Compartment syndrome. Changes in impedance are seen in the posterior tibial artery waveforms obtained proximal (A) and distal (B) to the site of calf swelling. Normal triphasic flow is present in the asymptomatic contralateral posterior tibial artery (C).

pressure measurements, however, remain the most important diagnostic modality. Further investigation is necessary to confirm the clinical utility of ultrasound for this syndrome.

CONCLUSIONS

Algorithms for the diagnosis of arterial pathology are evolving with the rapidly advancing capabilities of cross-sectional imaging. The expanding therapeutic role associated with catheter angiography has made this traditional mainstay of vascular diagnosis and intervention even more valuable. In this perspective, the ultimate role of duplex sonography in the workup of arterial emergencies is unsettled. Its strengths are most clearly displayed in the acute care setting, where rapid resolution of a focused clinical question results in timely intervention in a critically ill patient. This role has led to increasing use of portable ultrasound devices in the operating room, emergency department, and intensive care unit settings, as well as in out-of-hospital environments (i.e., combat fields). If it can be shown that high rates of diagnostic accuracy achieved by experienced sonographers using high-end equipment can be achieved in these alternative settings, ultrasound will maintain a defined role in the management of these challenging problems.

References

1. Bickerstaff LK, Hollier LH, Van Peenen HJ, et al: Abdominal aortic aneurysms: The changing natural history. J Vasc Surg 1:6–12, 1984.
2. Melton LJ 3rd, Bickerstaff LK, Hollier LH, et al: Changing incidence of abdominal aortic aneurysms: A population-based study. Am J Epidemiol 120:379–386, 1984.
3. Powell JT, Brown LC: The natural history of abdominal aortic aneurysms and their risk of rupture. Adv Surg 35:173–185, 2001.
4. Wassef M, Baxter BT, Chisholm RL, et al: Pathogenesis of abdominal aortic aneurysms: A multidisciplinary research program supported by the National Heart, Lung, and Blood Institute. J Vasc Surg 34:730–738, 2001.
5. Shuman WP, Hastrup W, Kohler TR, et al: Suspected leaking abdominal aortic aneurysm: Use of sonography in the emergency room. Radiology 168:117–119, 1988.
6. Thomas EA, Dubbins PA: Duplex ultrasound of the abdominal aorta—a neglected tool in aortic dissection. Clin Radiol 42:330–334, 1991.
7. Kimura K, Yonemura K, Terasaki T, et al: Duplex carotid sonography in distinguishing acute unilateral atherothrombotic from cardioembolic carotid artery occlusion. Am J Neuroradiol 18:1447–1452, 1997.
8. Kimura K, Yasaka M, Minematsu K, et al: Oscillating thromboemboli within the extracranial internal carotid artery demonstrated by ultrasonography in patients with acute cardioembolic stroke. Ultrasound Med Biol 24:1121–1124, 1999.
9. Kemany V, Jung DK, Devuyst G: Ultrasound characteristics of adherent thrombi in the common carotid artery. Circulation 104:E24–E25, 2001.
10. Padayachee TS, McGuinness CL, Modaresi KB, et al: Value of intraoperative duplex imaging during supervised carotid endarterectomy. Br J Surg 88:389–392, 2001.
11. Schievink WI, Mokri B, Piepgras DG: Spontaneous dissections of the cervicocephalic arteries in childhood and adolescence. Neurology 44:1607–1612, 1994.
12. Sanzone AG, Torres H, Doundoulakis SH: Blunt trauma to the carotid arteries. Am J Emerg Med 13:327–330, 1995.
13. Silbert PL, Mokri B, Schievink WI: Headache and neck pain in spontaneous internal carotid and vertebral artery dissections. Neurology 45:1517–1522, 1995.
14. Sturzenegger M, Mattle H, Rivoir A: Ultrasound findings in carotid artery dissection: Analysis of 43 patients. Neurology 45:691–698, 1995.
15. Grassbaugh JA, Nelson PR, Rzucidlo EM, et al: Blinded comparison of preoperative duplex ultrasound scanning and contrast arteriography for planning revascularization at the level of the tibia. J Vasc Surg 37:1186–1190, 2003.
16. MacGowan SW, Saif MF, O'Neill G, et al: Ultrasound examination in the diagnosis of popliteal artery aneurysms. Br J Surg 72:528–529, 1985.
17. Zierler RE, Zierler BK: Duplex sonography of lower extremity arteries. Semin Ultrasound CT MRI 18:39–56, 1997.
18. Westerband A, Mills JL, Kistler S, et al: Prospective validation of threshold criteria for intervention in infrainguinal vein grafts undergoing duplex surveillance. Ann Vasc Surg 11:44–48, 1997.
19. Mitchell DG, Needleman L, Bezzi M, et al: Femoral artery pseudoaneurysm: Diagnosis with conventional duplex and color Doppler ultrasound. Radiology 165:687–690, 1987.
20. O'Malley C Jr, Paulson EK, Kliewer MA, et al: Color Doppler sonographic appearance of

patent needle tracts after femoral arterial catheterization. Radiology 197:163–165, 1995.

21. Feld R, Patton GM, Carabasi RA, et al: Treatment of iatrogenic femoral artery injuries with ultrasound-guided compression. J Vasc Surg 16:832–840, 1992.

22. Paulson EK, Sheafor DH, Kliewer MA, et al: Treatment of iatrogenic femoral artery pseudoaneurysms: Comparison of US-guided thrombin injection with compression repair. Radiology 215:403–408, 2000.

23. Friedman SG, Pellerito JS, Scher L, et al: Ultrasound-guided thrombin injection is the treatment of choice for femoral pseudoaneurysms. Arch Surg 137:462–464, 2002.

24. Grassel KM, Wintemute GJ, Wright MA, Romero MP: Association between handgun purchase and mortality from firearm injury. Inj Prev 9:48–52, 2003.

25. Mattox KL, Feliciano DV, Burch J, et al: Five thousand seven hundred sixty cardiovascular injuries in 4459 patients: Epidemiologic evolution 1958 to 1987. Ann Surg 209:698–705, 1989.

26. Bynoe RP, Miles WS, Bell RM, et al: Noninvasive diagnosis of vascular trauma by duplex ultrasonography. J Vasc Surg 14:346–352, 1991.

27. Bynoe RP, Miles WS, Bell RM, et al: Noninvasive diagnosis of vascular trauma by duplex ultrasonography. J Vasc Surg 14:346–352, 1991.

28. Panetta TF, Sales CM, Marin ML, et al: Natural history, duplex characteristics, and histopathologic correlation of arterial injuries in a canine model. J Vasc Surg 16:867–874, 1993.

29. Turnipseed WD, Hurschler C, Vanderby R Jr: The effects of elevated compartment pressure on tibial arteriovenous flow and relationship of mechanical and biochemical characteristics of fascia to genesis of chronic anterior compartment syndrome. J Vasc Surg 21:810–816, 1995.

SECTION IV
EXTREMITY VEINS

Chapter 21

The Role of Ultrasound in the Management of Extremity Venous Disease

ROBERT S. SINGH, MD, AND SPENCER W. GALT, MD

Duplex sonography can effectively diagnose any of the acute or chronic disease processes that affect extremity veins. Most commonly, duplex sonography is used when acute deep venous thrombosis is suspected. Evaluation of chronic venous pathology is a less common but nevertheless important function of this technique.

ACUTE VENOUS THROMBOEMBOLIC DISEASE

Evaluation for venous thromboembolic disease (VTE) is the most common reason that clinicians choose duplex sonography to evaluate the extremity veins. While a comprehensive review of VTE is beyond the scope of this chapter, a brief review of risk factors and conditions fostering the development of VTE is in order. *VTE* refers to deep venous thrombosis (DVT) and pulmonary embolism (PE), related aspects of the same disease process. The annual incidence of VTE in the United States is 2.5 million cases.[1] Roughly 25% of untreated patients with DVT will sustain a nonfatal PE. Moreover, without treatment, PE is associated with a mortality rate of approximately 30%.[2] The population at risk represents a myriad of clinical conditions that predispose to the triad that Virchow first described in 1865—venous stasis, endothelial damage, and hypercoagulability.

Thrombogenesis occurs through the activation of enzymatic reactions in the intrinsic and tissue factor pathways, leading to the ultimate formation of thrombin via the prothrombinase enzyme complex. The thrombomodulin–protein C system primarily limits coagulation, while the fibrinolytic system further limits fibrin deposition. This homeostatic system is continuously active and balances activation and inhibition of coagulation and fibrinolysis. Thrombosis abnormalities, and the predisposition to thrombus formation, result either from inherited or acquired prothrombotic conditions.

Inherited prothrombotic disease states have been described with increasing frequency over the past 20 years. *Antithrombin III deficiency* was the first reported congenital thrombotic condition.[3] It is transmitted in an autosomal dominant pattern with a prevalence of 1 : 5000. Isolated spontaneous thrombosis has been described with this condition; however, precipitating circumstances, such as trauma, pregnancy, and surgical procedures, seem to lower the threshold for the development of DVT. *Protein C and protein S* are vitamin K–dependent cofactors that facilitate degradation of activated factor V. Deficiencies, therefore, predispose to thrombosis. Congenital deficiencies of these factors are well described,[4] but since these proteins are synthesized in the liver, acquired deficiencies also may occur from variations in liver function as well as with dietary changes. Protein C or S deficiency confers a roughly sevenfold increased risk for developing venous thrombosis. *Resistance to activated protein C* is also known as factor V Leiden. This disorder results from a point mutation in the factor V gene, rendering activated factor V resistant to degradation by activated protein C. It is present in 12% to 33% of patients with spontaneous VTE,[5] making it the most common inherited hypercoagulable condition. *Factor II (prothrombin) G20210A* is a mutation seen in 2% to 3% of individuals, predominantly those of European descent. In a recent study, it was observed to confer a 2.8-fold increase in relative risk for VTE.[6] *Primary hyperhomocysteinemia* increases risk for VTE, along with the development of premature atherosclerosis. Serum elevation of *coagulation factors VIII, IX, and XI* have been shown to confer elevated risk for venous thrombosis in the Leiden thrombophila study.[7] Factor IX and XI levels greater than the 90th percentile confer a 2.5-fold and 2.2-fold increased risk of VTE, respectively. *Dysfibrogenemias and hypofibrinolysis* impair the steps involved in the generation, crosslinkage, and breakdown of fibrin. Bleeding diathesis, as well as VTE, has been described with this condition.

Acquired prothrombotic states are more numerous than inherited states. Table 21–1, adapted from the PIOPED* study,[8] shows clinical conditions that predispose to VTE. Several of these conditions are briefly considered. *Pregnancy* and the postpartum period confer a higher risk of developing VTE than the nonpregnant state. PE is a leading cause of maternal death after childbirth, with one fatal PE per 100,000 births.[9,10] *Oral contraceptives* and *hormone replacement therapy* affect women at the spectrum of ages. Lidegaard and colleagues[11] reported a prevalence of VTE in women receiving oral contraceptives of one to three in 10,000. Women receiving hormone replacement therapy have a 2- to 4-fold increased risk of VTE. *Antiphospholipid antibody syndrome* refers to the presence of either the lupus anticoagulant antibody or anticardiolipin antibodies. Overall, the syndrome can be identified in 1% to 5% of the population. Among those with positive titers for the lupus anticoagulant, the risk of developing VTE is 6% to 8%. Patients with anticardiolipin antibody titers greater than the 95th percentile have a 5.3-fold increased risk of developing VTE.[12]

ANTICOAGULATION AND THROMBOLYIS IN THE MANAGEMENT OF VENOUS THROMBOEMBOLIC DISEASE

Heparin anticoagulation is standard for initial management of VTE. Heparin potentiates the action of antithrombin III, thereby preventing additional thrombus formation and permitting endogenous fibrinolysis. In the absence of contraindication to anticoagulation, prompt institution of heparin therapy is indicated for patients with either confirmed VTE (through imaging techniques) or among patients in whom a moderate or high clinical suspicion of VTE exists. Either unfractionated or low-molecular-weight heparin is effective. Oral warfarin therapy is instituted once therapeutic heparin anticoagulation has been achieved. Warfarin dosing is guided by measuring the International Normalized Ratio (INR), a reflection of the inhibition of vitamin K–dependent cofactors. While the target INR will vary, depending on the clinical circumstance, it is important to understand that early elevations in the INR (1–3 days after institution of warfarin therapy) usually result from inhibition of factor VII because of its short half-life. However,

Table 21–1. Acquired Risk Factors for VTE

Immobilization
Surgery within 3 mo
Stroke, paralysis of extremities
History of VTE
Malignancy
Obesity
Cigarette smoking
Hypertension
Oral contraception, hormone replacement therapy
Preganacy and puerperium
Secondary hyperhomocysteinemia
Antiphospholipid syndrome
Congestive heart failure
Myeloproliferative disorders
Nephrotic syndrome
Inflammatory bowel disease
Sickle cell anemia
Marked leukocytosis in acute leukemia

VTE, venous thromboembolic disease.

effective anticoagulation depends on the depletion of factor II (thrombin), typically requiring about 5 days of warfarin therapy. Therefore, at least 5 days of heparin therapy is recommended[13] until an adequate and stable INR is achieved. Therapy with oral warfarin in the absence of heparin anticoagulation should be avoided, as days will pass before anticoagulation is adequate, leaving the patient unprotected against PE; moreover, warfarin therapy in the absence of heparin anticoagulation may paradoxically intensify hypercoagulability and predispose to recurrent VTE.

The necessary duration for anticoagulation varies with the clinical scenario. In general, for initial cases of uncomplicated DVT, 3 months of anticoagulation is recommended. PE, inherited and acquired procoagulant states, and cases of recurrent VTE usually require longer anticoagulation therapy. In some cases of recurrent VTE, lifelong anticoagulation is often recommended.

Thrombolysis is not commonly used among patients with VTE, but there are situations in which it should be considered. Thrombolysis can be lifesaving for patients in whom massive PE causes hemodynamic instability, but this situation is rare. More commonly, thrombolysis may be useful for patients with extensive iliofemoral venous thrombosis, where the risk of development of the post-thrombotic syndrome is high. The results of randomized trials suggest that the prevalence and severity of the post-thrombotic syndrome is decreased if complete thrombolysis is achieved.[13] However, the substantial proportion of patients with contraindications to thrombolysis and the associated increase in major bleeding severely limit the use of thrombolytic therapy.

ACUTE DEEP VENOUS THROMBOSIS OF SPECIFIC EXTREMITY VEINS

Calf Vein Thrombosis

Most lower extremity DVTs become established in the deep veins of the calf,[14,15] although acute DVT can originate anywhere in the venous system. The soleal sinuses are thought to be the most common site of origin of calf DVT,[16] which may progress into the popliteal and femoral veins. Once the popliteal or femoral vein contains thrombus, therapeutic anticoagulation or caval interruption is necessary to prevent PE. However, the clinical importance of isolated calf DVT remains uncertain. Abundant literature has been published, but much of it is contradictory. Therefore, it is not surprising that there is no consensus over the prevalence of isolated calf DVT, the propensity for it to progress, the risk of its causing PE, and the likelihood of its causing post-thrombotic syndrome.

The prevalence of isolated calf DVT in specific patient groups is difficult to establish, because many studies include mixed patient populations and a variety of diagnostic techniques. Nevertheless, in a review of 20 studies, Philbrick and Becker[17] reported a 49% prevalence of symptomatic isolated calf DVT in medical and surgical patients. Several other authors have corroborated this figure, albeit in mixed populations of medical and surgical patients. A 1996 study by Atri and colleagues[18] attempted to better separate patient populations by examining an asymptomatic postoperative high-risk group and a symptomatic ambulatory group. In the asymptomatic postoperative group, 20% of patients were found to have isolated calf DVT; in the symptomatic ambulatory group, there was a 30% prevalence. These studies indicate that although it is difficult to establish precisely, isolated calf DVT is not uncommon.

Since most DVTs arise in calf veins, calf DVT can obviously propagate to the popliteal vein and more proximally. More important, do *all* calf DVTs propagate, and can those that do so be identified? The reported frequency of calf DVT propagation varies markedly. In postoperative patients, the reported rate of propagation varies from 6% to 34%.[17,19–23] Unfortunately, it is not possible to identify those thrombi that are likely to propagate.

In symptomatic ambulatory patients, the chances of propagation are even less certain.

Equally unclear, but probably of more importance, is the risk of PE originating from isolated calf thrombi in which no propagation into the popliteal vein has occurred. Some authors[24–26] argue that few, if any, significant pulmonary emboli arise from isolated calf DVT and that anticoagulation is unnecessary in the absence of demonstrable propagation. Other investigators are less sanguine. They reported that patients with PE have calf-only thrombi about 5% of the time.[27,28] Furthermore, others have reported that approximately 15% of fatal pulmonary emboli originated from isolated calf thromboses.[16,29] These series must be interpreted with caution, because it can be difficult to be certain that PE did not originate from a more proximal source, with embolization of the entire thrombus, rendering the previously thrombosed segment normal in appearance on imaging studies.

In light of the variation in observed rates of proximal propagation and PE, it is not surprising that there is no general agreement on the management of isolated calf DVT. Lohr and associates[23] cited a high risk of propagation (32%) in their conclusion that all patients with calf DVT should be treated with anticoagulation. Others have suggested treating only those patients with symptomatic calf vein thrombi (who appear to have a greater risk of embolism), those that demonstrate proximal propagation, or those who in follow-up are found to have developed clinically apparent PE.[30] No well-controlled, prospective, randomized trial of treatment of patients with isolated calf DVT has been published; therefore, the risks and benefits of the various approaches are not established.

Currently, two approaches in the treatment of patients with isolated calf DVT seem reasonable. In the first, the patient should be maintained on therapeutic anticoagulation for 6 weeks. In the second, surveillance duplex sonography should be continued for 7 to 10 days (or longer in an immobilized patient), with institution of therapeutic anticoagulation if propagation to veins proximal to the calf is documented.

Femoropopliteal Vein Thrombosis

Deep venous thrombosis proximal to the calf is a more serious clinical problem than isolated calf DVT. The risk of PE is greater, thus mandating therapeutic anticoagulation. For patients in whom anticoagulation is contraindicated, caval filter placement or caval interruption is necessary. The clinical presentation of DVT may change appreciably as thrombus propagates more proximally. When the superficial femoral vein is involved, the calf is usually painful. Swelling and warmth are typically evident on physical examination. When thrombus extends into the common femoral or iliac vein, the patient perceives a deep leg discomfort and tightness. Swelling may be present up to the inguinal ligament, and there may be tenderness over the deep veins, particularly in the inguinal region.

Duplex sonography is now accepted as the initial diagnostic test of choice in patients suspected of having femoropopliteal DVT. Duplex sonography easily permits visualization of complete thrombotic occlusion, allowing accurate thrombus localization. Additionally, nonocclusive thrombi and free-floating thrombi that are loosely attached to the vein wall and may have a greater potential for embolization[11] can also be identified. Some clinicians also use duplex sonography to follow the progression of a thrombus in the vein as an indicator of the effectiveness of anticoagulation therapy. Duplex sonography is also a useful technique to determine both the relative age of the thrombus (acute vs. chronic) and the degree of spontaneous lysis, information that may provide clinical guidance with respect to suspected recurrence of DVT, the adequacy of anticoagulation, and the length of time anticoagulation is maintained.

Iliac Vein Thrombosis

The clinical presentation and therapeutic implications of iliac vein thrombosis are generally similar to those of femoropopliteal vein thrombosis, and the diagnostic approach is identical. The difference in the diagnostic approach is the inability of duplex sonography to directly image many iliac thrombi that lie deep within the pelvis. If iliac vein thrombi are visualized, the diagnosis of DVT is established. However, despite a convincing clinical scenario, the only evidence of proximal DVT may come from the Doppler interrogation rather than the B-mode image. Indirect Doppler evidence of proximal thrombosis includes the loss of respiratory phasicity of the signal and the inability to augment the signal with distal thigh compression, but these signs may be absent with nonocclusive thrombi. Nonocclusive thrombi, or thrombi isolated to the hypogastric vein, are likely to be missed by duplex sonography. Therefore, when the clinical scenario is compelling, further evaluation of the deep venous system is indicated, usually with venography.

EXTREMITY VEIN DUPLEX SCANNING TO DIAGNOSE PULMONARY EMBOLISM

Because duplex ultrasound has become the diagnostic test of choice in DVT evaluation and because the majority of PEs originate in lower extremity veins, some clinicians now utilize lower extremity duplex ultrasound as the first diagnostic study in the evaluation of possible PE. This approach is based on the noninvasive nature of the study, the portability of the machine, and the rapidity with which results may be obtained in institutions where technical support is readily available. The merit to this approach is supported when the diagnosis of extremity DVT is confirmed, as the diagnosis of PE may then be safely assumed in the appropriate clinical setting.

There are potential drawbacks to this insensitive but specific approach to the diagnosis of PE. Several investigators have addressed these issues, examining both the yield of positive results in those cases in which lower extremity duplex sonography has been used as a screening test for patients with suspected PE and the frequency of detection of DVT in those patients known to have suffered PE.

Beecham and colleagues[31] reviewed 225 patients who underwent both ventilation perfusion ($\dot{V}/\dot{Q}$) scans and lower extremity duplex sonography in the evaluation of suspected PE. Of 56 patients with high-probability $\dot{V}/\dot{Q}$ scans, only 36% demonstrated duplex evidence of DVT. Furthermore, of 22 patients whose $\dot{V}/\dot{Q}$ scans were indeterminate or low probability and who had no evidence of DVT by duplex scanning, 25% were found to have suffered PE detected by angiography.

Similarly, in a study by Glover and Bendick,[32] the authors reviewed the charts of 978 patients who were studied by duplex sonography to "rule out PE." In a subgroup of 38 patients with acute unilateral leg swelling, acute femoropopliteal DVT was diagnosed in 68%. A second subgroup of patients included those with minimal leg symptoms who had significant risk factors for DVT. In this group, 16% of patients were found to have acute femoropopliteal or tibial DVT. In contrast, acute femoropopliteal DVT was not detected in the remaining 433 patients who had no risk factors or acute unilateral leg swelling. Three patients were found to have tibial DVT. Similar to the previous reports cited, in patients with high-probability $\dot{V}/\dot{Q}$ scans but no risk factors for DVT or lower extremity symptoms, no DVT was detected in more than 60% of patients, again underscoring the inability of the lower extremity venous duplex examination to rule out PE. Killewich and coworkers[33] similarly documented the absence of duplex-diagnosed DVT in 60% of patients with PE confirmed by pulmonary angiography.

Like Glover and Bendick,[32] Eze and associates[34] demonstrated the usefulness of stratifying patients with suspected PE based on unilateral leg symptoms. In their series of 336 patients with clinically suspected PE, 7% demonstrated proximal DVT by duplex sonography. However, in the 25 patients with unilateral leg swelling, 40% were found to have DVT by duplex scanning, whereas DVT was evident in only 5% of patients in the absence of leg swelling. This group further confirmed that most patients with high-probability $\dot{V}/\dot{Q}$ scans had no DVT visualized by duplex sonography.

Finally, in a study by Matteson and colleagues,[35] 664 patients who underwent venous duplex examination for the diagnosis of "rule out PE" were reviewed. For all lower extremity duplex examinations, 13% of studies were positive. Although no attempt was made to stratify patients by leg symptoms or risk factors, this study reaffirmed the overall low yield of venous duplex examination in the evaluation of PE and the finding that the majority of patients with confirmed PE do not demonstrate DVT.

In summary, it appears that the lower extremity venous duplex examination is an appropriate primary diagnostic study in the patient who is suspected of having suffered PE and has unilateral lower extremity swelling. In the absence of leg swelling, CT angiography or $\dot{V}/\dot{Q}$ scanning is the first test of choice. Furthermore, if the venous duplex study is negative after a nondiagnostic $\dot{V}/\dot{Q}$ scan, CT or pulmonary angiography must be pursued if clinical suspicion warrants further investigation, because no DVT is demonstrated in more than one half of the patients who have suffered PE.

SUPERFICIAL VENOUS THROMBOSIS

Superficial venous thrombosis has traditionally been considered a relatively benign disease. It is important, however, as a marker of coexistent DVT and hypercoagulability. The diagnosis of superficial venous thrombosis is typically made clinically. Physical findings include a painful superficial cord with surrounding erythema in the course of the vein. Treatment of patients with nonsuppurative superficial venous thrombosis is symptomatic and includes ambulation, heat application, compression, and nonsteroidal anti-inflammatory drug therapy.

Duplex evaluation of superficial venous thrombosis, especially occurring in the greater saphenous vein, is important for two reasons. First, although the clinical examination is useful in establishing the diagnosis, it is not reliable in identifying the extent of the thrombus. Particularly in the proximal thigh, thrombus often extends beyond the apparent area of involvement.[36,37] Duplex sonography documents the proximal extent and can be used to monitor progression. Although data are limited, it appears that a small proportion (approximately 10%) of patients with isolated superficial venous thrombosis of the greater saphenous vein progress to DVT if untreated. Of that group, those with superficial venous thrombosis in the thigh are at highest risk, with 70% of untreated patients progressing to thrombosis of the femoral vein. Most clinicians either disconnect the saphenofemoral junction surgically or institute systemic anticoagulation if proximal saphenous thrombosis progresses to the saphenofemoral junction.

Duplex sonography of extremities with superficial venous thrombosis is also useful to identify concomitant but clinically silent DVT. Some series have demonstrated the presence of unapparent DVT in 20% to 40% of patients with superficial venous thrombosis.[38-40] Treatment is directed at DVT and superficial thrombophlebitis. Many of these patients are hypercoagulable, and the appropriate evaluation should be performed.

Occasionally, an apparent superficial phlebitis is, in fact, a soft tissue infection or hematoma. These conditions can easily be distinguished from superficial venous thrombosis with duplex scanning but may be more difficult to differentiate clinically.

AXILLOSUBCLAVIAN VENOUS THROMBOSIS

Deep venous thrombosis of the upper extremities can be broadly divided into two categories: those caused by central venous catheters and those associated with other causes. Overall, axillosubclavian DVT is increasingly common, resulting from the increased use of central venous catheters.[41] In the absence of central catheters, axillo-subclavian DVT may be seen among patients affected by certain cancers (especially mediastinal lymphomas), trauma, surgery, and radiation therapy. However, spontaneous effort thrombosis, also known as the *Paget-Schroetter syndrome*, is the most common presentation of axillosubclavian DVT in the ambulatory population. This condition may be associated with demonstrable anatomic abnormalities of the thoracic inlet (e.g., cervical rib). Men are affected more often than women, and the incidence is higher in the veins of the dominant arm. Presentation of upper extremity DVT can be dramatic. Marked arm swelling and prominent superficial veins leave little doubt of the diagnosis, and the role of duplex sonography is primarily confirmatory. Sometimes the presentation is more subtle. The patient may complain of vague discomfort, with minimal swelling; in these cases, duplex sonography is an effective screening test to document the status of the deep venous system. Unlike the lower extremities, the proximal upper extremities are drained by a rich collateral venous network around the neck and shoulder, making the indirect evaluation of venous flow by plethysmography even less reliable than in the lower extremities and further emphasizing the value of duplex sonography for upper extremity DVT. Duplex ultrasound is, however, limited by the bony structures in the neck and shoulder, impeding imaging of the proximal subclavian vein. Flow characteristics of the proximal subclavian and innominate veins may offer indirect evidence of vein patency, but at this level, direct visualization and manual compression of the veins is not possible. As in the pelvis, if proximal subclavian DVT is suspected, venography should be performed.

Initial treatment of axillosubclavian thrombosis follows standard guidelines for VTE. If there is no obvious underlying cause, a thrombophilia work-up, including antithrombin III, Factor V Leiden, antiphospholipid antibodies, and protein C and S levels, should be performed. Prompt heparin anticoagulation is undertaken to protect from pulmonary emboli, reported to occur in up to 36% of patients.[42] For thromboses caused by catheters, anticoagulation, along with removal of the catheter, if possible, appears to be sufficient. However, anticoagulation alone among young, healthy patients may lead to an unacceptably high rate of post-thrombotic disability, caused by incomplete recannalization of the axillosubclavian system. Increased arterial flow with use of the arm can lead to venous hypertension from outflow obstruction. In the most severe cases, venous claudication, a bursting sensation in the arm, may develop, leading to significant disability. For this reason, many surgeons advocate local thrombolysis. Follow-up venography demonstrates residual extrinsic or intrinsic lesions that may be present, predisposing to thrombosis. The most common extrinsic cause of axilosubclavian thrombosis is compression of the vein between the clavicle and the first rib. Additional causes of extrinsic compression include hypertrophic scalene or subclavius muscles, the costoclavicular ligament, or the head of the clavicle. Congenital or acquired intrinsic venous lesions also may cause venous stenosis, leading to thrombosis. Extrinsic causes are usually treated by thoracic inlet decompression, typically including first rib resection and resection of the anterior scalene muscle. After thoracic inlet decompression, intrinsic venous lesions can be treated, either concurrently, with open surgical reconstruction, or through endovascular techniques performed 1 to 2 days postoperatively. The timing of decompression after thrombolysis varies with the surgeon's preference. Some prefer to wait 1 to 3 months after lysis while anticoagulating the patient to reduce thrombogenesis of the local venous endothelium. Others advocate decompression 1 to 2 days after lysis to minimize the probability of rethrombosis. Conclusive data are absent; therefore, no firm conclusion can be drawn. Nevertheless, utilizing this general approach, Machleder[43] reported reduced upper extremity disability from 60% to 12%, compared with anticoagulation alone.

SEQUELLAE OF DEEP VENOUS THROMBOSIS

The sequellae of DVT result from proximal chronic venous obstruction, acquired incompetence of the valves of the deep venous system following recannalization, or both. In most patients who have suffered from DVT, the thrombosed vein recannalizes over a period of months, allowing adequate restoration of flow to the central circulation. Despite recannalization, the vein wall and valves are permanently damaged in at least 60% of cases,[44] leaving the valve leaflets immobile and fixed to the vein wall. Incompetence of the system results, and reflux occurs when the standing position is assumed. In some individuals, the thrombosed veins do not recannalize, resulting in chronic obstruction to venous return. Regardless of whether the cause is proximal obstruction, reflux, or both, venous hypertension occurs. The venous hypertension presents clinically as chronic leg swelling, ankle pigmentation, and, ultimately, ankle ulceration in the "gaiter zone," just above the ankle. Collectively, this is known as the *post-thrombotic syndrome* (Fig. 21–1).

The pathophysiology underlying the swelling and discoloration is straightforward. Increased hydrostatic pressure in the deep venous system causes extravasation of protein-rich tissue fluid, presenting clinically as interstitial edema. If venous hypertension persists, acquired incompetence of the valves of the perforating veins results in secondary varicose veins (Fig. 21–2). Red blood cells extravasate and are deposited in the subcutaneous tissue surrounding the perforators. Metabolic breakdown of the hemoglobin is responsible for the characteristic brawny pigmentation of the postphlebitic syndrome. Eventually, ulceration can develop, either spontaneously or as the result of minor trauma. Although the pathophysiology of the ulceration is not clear, it appears to be related to an inflammatory reaction in the tissue, fibrin cuffing, and eventual lipodermatosclerosis. Whatever the cause, ulceration is undoubtedly related to persistent venous hypertension.

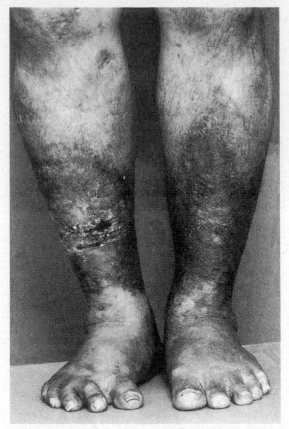

FIGURE 21–1. The *gaiter zone* is located in the lower calf and ankle. In this region, the ambulatory superficial venous pressures are the highest, leading to edema, pigmentation, and ultimately, ulceration. The skin, after years of edema, is difficult to examine for incompetent perforators (both clinically and with duplex sonography) because of extensive fibrosis.

Duplex ultrasound of the postthrombotic extremity is useful for both diagnosis and therapy. First, indirect confirmation of the diagnosis of venous hypertension can be made with duplex ultrasound by direct observation of deep vein valve incompetence or documentation of chronic deep vein obstruction. The perforating veins and the superficial venous system can be similarly assessed. This information assists in planning therapy; for example, if the deep venous system is widely incompetent, valve repair or transplantation may be required. However, if the deep venous system is competent, perforator interruption or stripping of the superficial venous system may suffice.

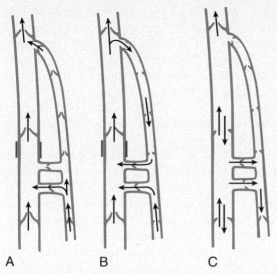

FIGURE 21-2. With incompetent deep veins and perforating veins, venous hypertension below the fascia of the leg is transmitted to the superficial system. *A*, Normal. *B*, Greater saphenous incompetence. *C*, Deep and perforator vein incompetence.

VARICOSE VEINS

Primary varicose veins are abnormally dilated and tortuous components of the superficial venous system, *in the absence of coexisting deep venous disease.* Varicose veins are classified as *secondary* when they are associated with obstruction or incompetence of the deep venous system and *recurrent* if they reappear after ablation. For most patients, the medical history and physical examination provide sufficient information to distinguish between primary and secondary varicose veins. In the patient with primary varicose veins, a history of DVT is rare. Physical signs of the post-thrombotic syndrome, such as brawny edema in the gaiter zone and venous stasis ulcers, are uncommon. However, in the occasional patient, it can be difficult to rule out involvement of the deep venous system by the medical history and physical examination. In this instance, duplex sonography can be especially helpful. Exclusion of pathology of the deep venous system confirms the diagnosis of primary varicose veins and predicts a high likelihood of cure with complete excision of the varicosities.

When ablative treatment of varicose veins is planned, careful assessment of the greater saphenous vein is critical. If the saphenous vein is competent, treatment can be confined to the clinically evident varicosities. Conversely, if greater saphenous incompetence is found, the vein should be ablated to reduce the probability of recurrence, even if it is not clinically apparent that it is varicose. Specific attention must be paid to the saphenofemoral junction. Valvular incompetence at the saphenofemoral junction occurs in most cases of primary varicose veins. Nevertheless, the varicosities may be clinically apparent in only the calf or distal thigh (Fig. 21-3). If the saphenofemoral valve is incompetent, the saphenous vein must be ligated flush at the saphenofemoral junction, and the proximal vein must be

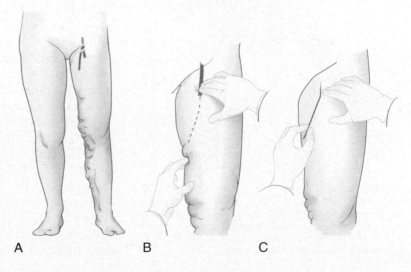

FIGURE 21-3. Varicose veins in the calf may be isolated to the superficial calf veins, or they may be associated with incompetence of the entire saphenous vein (*A*). Physical examination (*B* and *C*) and duplex sonography can determine the extent of superficial venous involvement.

ablated. Failure to do so increases the likelihood of recurrence.

Perforator incompetence may also cause or accompany varicose veins in the absence of deep venous incompetence. Occasionally, an incompetent perforator causes primary varicose veins, even though the deep venous system is intact. Ligation of the incompetent perforator and ablation of the varicosities are the key to successful management of the problem. Incompetent perforator veins are easily localized with duplex sonography.

Recurrence of primary varicose veins is caused either by inadequate initial treatment or by development of new primary varicose veins. Initial treatment unwittingly directed at secondary varicose veins uniformly results in recurrence. The most easily identified and managed cause of recurrent primary varicose veins is inadequate high ligation of the greater saphenous vein at the saphenofemoral junction when an incompetent valve is present at that level (Fig. 21–4). Failure to ligate the greater saphenous vein flush with the common femoral vein preserves the incompetent valve, allowing reflux into the subcutaneous branches at the saphenous bulb. This condition may be identified, either by physical examination or by duplex scanning, as a cluster of veins in the inguinal region. When incompetence and reflux are identified in these veins, flush ligation is curative.

A variety of other causes of recurrent primary varicosities are known, including incomplete ligation of incompetent perforators, a duplicated saphenous system, and failure to differentiate greater from lesser saphenous vein incompetence. As usual, careful physical examination, complemented with duplex sonography, determines the cause of recurrent varicosities. The importance of evaluation of the deep venous system cannot be overstated, because secondary varicose veins, resulting from deep venous incompetence, are a common cause of recurrence.

MAPPING FOR BYPASS SURGERY

Evaluation of the presence, location, and adequacy of a proposed bypass conduit prior to harvest for bypass surgery is often helpful. This is accurately done with duplex sonography. In the obese patient, for example, the course of the vein may be hidden by subcutaneous tissue. Duplex scanning can confirm the patency and location of the veins, avoiding the undesirable consequence of raising large skin flaps. Similarly, in the patient who has suffered previous saphenous vein thrombosis, duplex scanning can identify chronic occlusion or valvular insufficiency, conditions that obviate vein use as a bypass graft. In those patients who have undergone venous surgery or prior vein harvesting, the greater saphenous vein may be absent. A diligent search using the duplex scanner can facilitate identification of alternative bypass conduits for the planned procedure. In our experience, the greater and lesser saphenous, superficial femoral, cephalic, and basilic veins are all potentially useful as bypass conduits and are easily evaluated and mapped with duplex sonography.

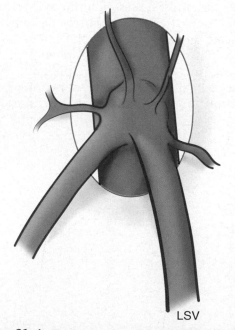

LSV

FIGURE 21–4. The greater (long) saphenous vein (LSV) enters the femoral vein through the fossa ovalis. There are several large superficial branches that enter the saphenous vein at the saphenous bulb. These veins, as well as the greater saphenous vein, must be ligated to prevent recurrence of varicose veins.

References

1. White RH: The epidemiology of venous thromboembolism. Circulation 107:I-4–I-8, 2003.
2. Kroegel C, Reissig A: Principle mechanisms underlying venous thromboembolism: Epidemiology, risk factors, pathophysiology and pathogenesis. Respiration. 70:7–30, 2003.
3. Egeberg O: Inherited antithrombin deficiency causing thrombophilia. Thromb Diath Haemorrh 13:516–530, 1965.
4. Miletich J, Sherman L, Broze G Jr: Absence of thrombosis in subjects with heterozygous protein C deficiency. N Engl J Med 317:991–996, 1987.
5. Svensson PJ, Dahlback B: Resistance to activated protein C as a basis for venous thrombosis. N Engl J Med 330:517–522, 1995.
6. Anderson FA Jr, Spencer FA: Risk factors for venous thromboembolism. Circulation 107: I-9–I-16, 2003.
7. van Hylckama Vlieg A, van der Linden IK, Bertina RM, et al: High levels of factor IX increase the risk of venous thrombosis. Blood 95:3678–3682, 2000.
8. PIOPED Investigators: Value of the ventilation/perfusion scan in acute pulmonary embolism: Results of the prospective investigation of pulmonary embolism (PIOPED). JAMA 263:2753–2759, 1990.
9. Aaro LA, Juergens JL: Thrombophlebitis associated with pregnancy. Am J Obstet Gynecol 109:1128–1136, 1971.
10. Hogberg U. Maternal deaths in Sweden, 1971–1980. Acta Obstet Gynecol Scand 65: 161–167, 1986.
11. Lidegaard O, Edstrom B, Kreiner S: Oral contraceptives and venous thromboembolism: A five-year national case-control study. Contraception 65:187–196, 2002.
12. Ginsburg KS, Liang MH, Newcomer L, et al: Anticardiolipin antibodies and the risk for ischemic stroke and venous thrombosis. Ann Intern Med 117:997–1002, 1992.
13. Ginsberg JS: Management of venous thromboembolism. N Engl J Med 335:1816–1829, 1996.
14. Nicolaides A, Kakkar V, Renney J: The soleal sinuses: Origin of deep vein thrombosis. Br J Surg 58:307–309, 1971.
15. Rollins D, Semrow C, Friedell M, et al: Origin of deep vein thrombi in ambulatory population. Am J Surg 156:122–125, 1988.
16. Sevitt S, Gallagher N: Venous thrombosis and pulmonary embolism. A clinico-pathological study in injured and burned patients. Br J Surg 48:475–489, 1961.
17. Philbrick J, Becker D: Calf vein thrombosis: A wolf in sheep's clothing. Arch Intern Med 148:2131–2138, 1988.
18. Atri M, Herba MJ, Reinhold C, et al: Accuracy of sonography in the evaluation of calf deep vein thrombosis in both postoperative surveillance and symptomatic patients. Am J Roentgenol 166:1361–1367, 1996.
19. Thomas ML, McAllister V: The radiological progression of deep venous thrombus. Radiology 99:37–40, 1971.
20. Doous T: The clinical significance of deep venous thrombosis of the calf. Br J Surg 63:377–378, 1976.
21. Kakkar V, Howe C, Flanc C, Clarke M: Natural history of postoperative deep-vein thrombosis. Lancet 230:230–232, 1969.
22. Kakkar VV, Corrigan TP: Efficacy of low-dose heparin in preventing postoperative fatal pulmonary embolism: Results of an international multicentre trial. In Kakker VV, Thomas DP (eds): Heparin: Chemistry and Clinical Usage. London, Academic Press, 1976, pp 229–245.
23. Lohr J, Kerr T, Lutter K, et al: Lower extremity calf thrombosis: To treat or not to treat? J Vasc Surg 14:618–623, 1991.
24. Moser KM, LeMoine JR: Is embolic risk conditioned by location of deep venous thrombosis? Ann Intern Med 94:439–444, 1981.
25. Dorfman GS, Cronan JJ, Tupper TB, et al: Occult pulmonary embolism: A common occurrence in deep venous thrombosis. Am J Roentgenol 148:263–266, 1987.
26. Solis MM, Ranval TJ, Nix ML, et al: Is anticoagulation indicated for asymptomatic postoperative calf vein thrombosis? J Vasc Surg 16: 414–418, 1992.
27. Haas SB, Tribus CB, Insall JN, et al: The significance of calf thrombi after total knee arthroplasty. J Bone Joint Surg Br 74: 799–802, 1992.
28. Hull RD, Hirsh J, Carter CJ, et al: Pulmonary angiography, ventilation lung scanning, and venography for clinically suspected pulmonary embolism with abnormal perfusion lung scan. Ann Intern Med 98:891–899, 1983.
29. Giachino A: Relationship between deep vein thrombosis in the calf and fatal pulmonary embolism. Can J Surg 31:129–130, 1988.
30. Barnes R: Is anticoagulation indicated for postoperative or spontaneous calf vein thrombosis? In Veith F (ed): Current Clinical Problems in Vascular Surgery. St. Louis, Quality Medical Publishing, 1993, pp 151–155.
31. Beecham R, Dorfman G, Cronan J, et al: Is bilateral lower extremity compression sonography useful and cost-effective in the evaluation of suspected pulmonary embolism? Am J Roentgenol 161:1289–1292, 1993.
32. Glover J, Bendick P: Appropriate indications for venous duplex ultrasonic examinations. Surgery 120:725–731, 1996.

33. Killewich L, Nunless J, Auer A: Value of lower extremity venous duplex examination in the diagnosis of pulmonary embolism. J Vasc Surg 17:934–939, 1993.

34. Eze A, Comerota A, Kerr R, et al: Is venous duplex imaging an appropriate initial screening test for patients with suspected pulmonary embolism. Ann Vasc Surg 10:220–223, 1996.

35. Matteson B, Langsfeld M, Schermer C, et al: Role of venous duplex scanning in patients with suspected pulmonary embolism. J Vasc Surg 24:768–773, 1996.

36. Pulliam C, Barr S, Ewing A: Venous duplex scanning in the diagnosis and treatment of progressive superficial thrombophlebitis. Ann Vasc Surg 5:190–195, 1991.

37. Lohr JM, McDevitt DT, Lutter KS, et al: Operative management of greater saphenous thrombophlebitis involving the saphenofemoral junction. Am J Surg 164:269–275, 1992.

38. Lutter K, Kerr T, Roedersheimer L, et al: Superficial thrombophlebitis diagnosed by duplex scanning. Surgery 110:42–46, 1991.

39. Jorgenson J, Hanel K, Morgan A, Hunt J: The incidence of deep venous thrombosis in patients with superficial thrombophlebitis of the lower limbs. J Vasc Surg 18:70–73, 1993.

40. Ascer E, Lorensen E, Pollina R, Gennaro M: Preliminary results of nonoperative approach to saphenofemoral junction thrombophlebitis. J Vasc Surg 22:616–621, 1995.

41. Martin EC, Koser M, Gordon DH: Venography in axillary-subclavian vein thrombosis. Cardiovasc Radiol 2:261–266, 1979.

42. Prandoni P, Polistena P, Bernardi E, et al: Upper-extremity deep vein thrombosis: Risk factors, diagnosis, and complications. Arch Intern Med 157:57–62, 1997.

43. Machleder HI: Evaluation of a new treatment strategy for Paget-Schroetter syndrome: Spontaneous thrombosis of the axilliary-subclavian vein. J Vasc Surg 17:305–317, 1993.

44. Meissner MH, Manzo RA, Bergelin RO, et al: Deep venous insufficiency: The relationship between lysis and subsequent reflux. J Vasc Surg 18:596–605, 1993.

Chapter 22

Extremity Venous Anatomy, Terminology, and Ultrasound Features of Normal Veins

WILLIAM J. ZWIEBEL, MD

This chapter presents venous anatomy, terminology used in venous diagnosis, and ultrasound features of normal veins. One cannot reasonably examine any part of the body without knowledge of anatomy[1-4]; hence, that is where this chapter begins.

EXTREMITY VENOUS ANATOMY

In this text, the terms *proximal* and *distal* are defined in relation to the heart, in conformance with standard anatomic practice. Structures that are closer to the heart are described as proximal, and those that are farther away are described as distal.

In both the upper and lower extremities, the deep veins are accompanied by arteries and in many areas are paired. In contrast, arteries do not accompany the superficial veins. Both the superficial and deep veins are often of clinical importance in the upper extremities; therefore, the examination of both systems is necessary. In contrast, the deep system is the major area of clinical concern in the lower extremity, and examination of the superficial system frequently is unnecessary, except for the proximal greater saphenous vein at its junction with the deep system.

Deep Upper Extremity Veins

The radial, ulnar, brachial axillary, and subclavian veins comprise the *deep* venous system of the upper extremity. It is custom-

ary in describing venous anatomy to begin distally and proceed proximally, following the course of the flowing blood, so we begin at the wrist and move proximally to the superior vena cava.

The deep veins of the forearm are the radial and ulnar veins, which are paired and accompany the arteries of the same name (Fig. 22–1). Although these veins are small, they are readily detected sonographically because their companion arteries are easily identified.

Just below the elbow, the paired radial veins merge, forming a radial trunk, and the ulnar veins merge in a like manner. These trunks may extend directly into the arm, forming the paired brachial veins, or the trunks may unite, forming a common vein

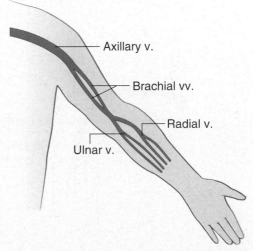

FIGURE 22–1. The deep veins of the upper extremity.

that almost immediately splits again into the paired brachial veins, as shown in Figure 22–1. In any event, the brachial portion almost always consists of a pair of veins, one lying on each side of the brachial artery. These unite proximally, forming a common trunk that continues into the axilla as the axillary vein. The point of transition from brachial to axillary vein is at the lower border of the teres major muscle, but this landmark is not readily detectable sonographically. The axillary vein continues proximally, becoming the subclavian vein at the upper border of the first rib (Fig. 22–2). Again, this point of transition is difficult to identify sonographically. The axillary and subclavian veins usually are single structures but, uncommonly, are paired. When single, these veins normally are slightly larger than the adjacent arteries, but the veins may be substantially larger than the arteries if distended by venous congestion or breath-holding.

Proximally, the subclavian vein joins the internal jugular vein to form the brachiocephalic vein (see Fig. 22–2). The right and left brachiocephalic veins subsequently join in the upper portion of the mediastinum, forming the superior vena cava. The brachiocephalic veins usually cannot be imaged sonographically because they are obscured by the sternum. Likewise, the superior vena cava usually is obscured by the sternum, the ribs, and the air-filled lungs. Because the patency of these veins cannot be confirmed by direct examination, indirect verification of patency is necessary with Doppler sonography through the detection of pulsatility and respiration-induced flow variation in the subclavian vein.

Superficial Upper Extremity Veins

The cephalic and basilic veins (Fig. 22–3) and their tributaries constitute the major superficial veins of the upper extremity. The cephalic vein arises from the lateral portion of the dorsal venous arch of the hand and extends in a subcutaneous location more or less along the lateral aspect of the forearm. At the elbow, it connects with an important branch, called the median cubital vein, which crosses the antecubital fossa obliquely. The cephalic vein continues along the lateral aspect of the arm in a subcutaneous location and then courses over the lateral aspect of the deltoid muscle at the shoulder. Finally, it dives between the upper end of the deltoid and the clavicular portion of the pectoralis muscles to join the subclavian vein.

The basilic vein begins at the dorsal venous arch of the hand and then courses in a subcutaneous location along the medial

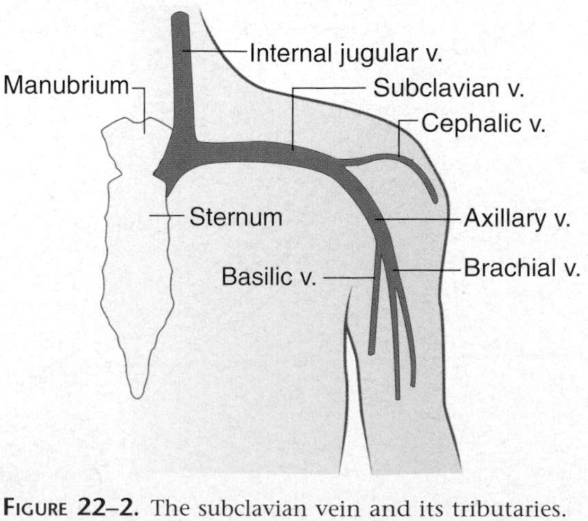

FIGURE 22–2. The subclavian vein and its tributaries.

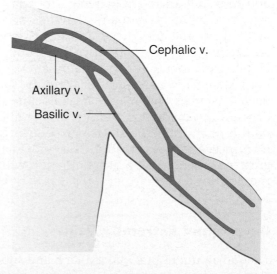

FIGURE 22–3. The superficial veins of the upper extremity.

aspect of the forearm to the elbow, where it crosses the medial side of the anticubital fossa. In the arm, it continues cephalad along the medial border of the biceps muscle and then joins the axillary vein at the lower border of the teres major muscle.

Deep Lower Extremity Veins

As noted previously, most of the venous return from the lower extremities is channeled through the deep system. This system communicates with the superficial veins by means of perforating veins, so named because they perforate the musculature that separates the deep and superficial venous system. In normally functioning perforating veins, valves maintain flow in one direction, *from superficial to deep.* Flow in the opposite direction is always abnormal. Perforating veins are most numerous below the knee and are of clinical importance if incompetent, permitting blood to flow from the deep to the superficial system. Perforator incompetence may be associated with superficial varicosities, as well as discoloration, thickening, and ulceration of the skin.

The deep veins of the lower extremity are the anterior tibial, posterior tibial, and peroneal veins in the calf; the superficial femoral, deep femoral, and common femoral veins in the thigh; and the external and common iliac veins in the pelvis. Please note that the *superficial* femoral vein is, in fact, part of the deep venous system. This nomenclature is occasionally a point of confusion.

Calf and Popliteal Veins

The anterior tibial, posterior tibial, and peroneal veins (Fig. 22–4) drain the calf. In each case, these are paired veins that accompany an artery of the same name. Proximally, the two posterior tibial veins unite, forming a short posterior tibial trunk, and the peroneal pair likewise forms a short trunk. The trunks subsequently unite in the popliteal fossa to form the popliteal vein. There are many variations in the union of

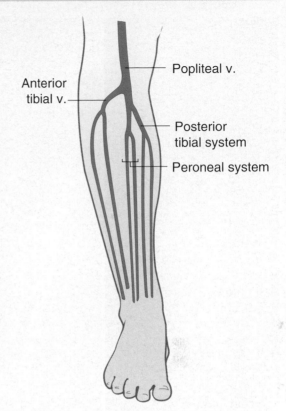

FIGURE 22–4. The popliteal vein and the calf veins.

the posterior tibial and peroneal veins, as discussed later.

The paired anterior tibial veins often join the popliteal vein independently. Alternately, they also may form a short trunk, as shown in Figure 22–4, before joining the popliteal vein. In either case, the anterior tibial veins have a unique anatomic configuration, in that they extend from lateral to medial, behind the proximal tibia, to join the popliteal vein.

Muscular veins often are visible in the calf. As the name implies, these veins drain the calf musculature and may be quite large. The most noteworthy are the gastrocnemius and soleal veins, which are illustrated in Figure 22–5. The gastrocnemius veins are seen in the medial head of the gastrocnemius muscle and drain into either the popliteal vein or the posterior tibial system. The gastrocnemius veins are sites for isolated, symptomatic venous thrombosis.[5,6] The soleal veins (or sinuses) are embedded in the soleus muscle, which is centrally located, posterior to the tibia. These veins, which may be a

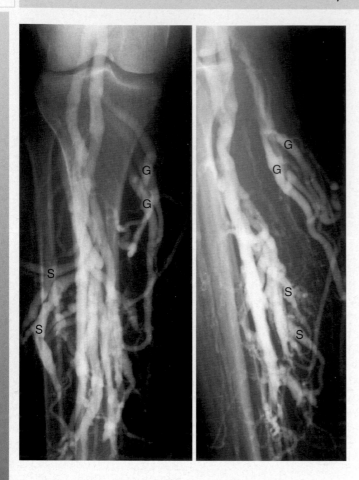

FIGURE 22–5. The gastrocnemius (G) and soleal (S) veins are shown on anteroposterior (*left*) and lateral (*right*) contrast venography images.

centimeter or more in diameter, drain into the posterior tibial or peroneal system. The soleal veins are quite important, as they are thought to be common sites for origin of venous thrombosis in the calf and may be a site of isolated venous thrombosis.[5,6]

The popliteal vein (see Fig. 22–4) is formed by the junction of the posterior tibial and peroneal veins, either in the proximal calf or the inferior aspect of the popliteal fossa. This vein extends longitudinally through the popliteal fossa and then deviates medially through a tunnel in the adductor musculature called the adductor canal. The popliteal vein lies immediately posterior to the popliteal artery; hence, as viewed from the popliteal fossa, it is *superficial* to the artery. Approximately 25% of popliteal veins are duplicated (or bifid).[2] Usually, this results from continuation of the posterior tibial and peroneal trunks high into the popliteal fossa before they unite.

Femoral Venous System

At the proximal end of the adductor canal, the popliteal vein becomes the superficial femoral vein, which continues through the thigh as the primary route of venous drainage. The "superficial" name derives from its location. As it is not covered by muscle tissue, it is quite superficial, except in obese individuals. The superficial femoral vein is bifid in approximately 25% of individuals.[2] As seen sonographically, from the anteromedial thigh, the superficial femoral vein lies deep to the adjacent superficial femoral artery.

In the upper thigh, the superficial femoral vein is joined by the deep femoral vein (also called the profunda femoris vein), forming the common femoral vein (Fig. 22–6). The greater saphenous vein, which is part of the superficial venous system, joins the anteromedial aspect of the

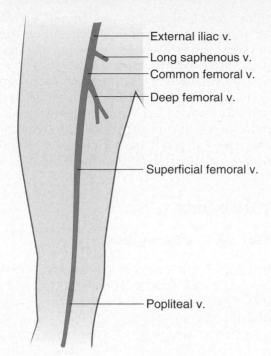

External iliac v.

Long saphenous v.

Common femoral v.

Deep femoral v.

Superficial femoral v.

Popliteal v.

FIGURE 22–6. The femoral venous system.

common femoral vein. Care should be taken not to mistake this vein for the deep femoral vein.

Iliac Veins

After crossing the inguinal ligament, the common femoral vein becomes the external iliac vein, which dives posteriorly into the "bowl" of the pelvis. At the approximate level of the sacroiliac joints, the external iliac vein, draining the leg, is joined by the internal iliac vein, draining the pelvis and gluteal area, forming the common femoral vein. The latter climbs cephalad out of the pelvis for about 5 cm, where it joins the ipsilateral common iliac vein (at the L5 level) to form the inferior vena cava. The major tributaries of the inferior vena cava are shown in Figure 22–7.

Superficial Lower Extremity Veins

The lower extremity is drained by an important superficial venous system, the primary

components of which are the greater and lesser saphenous veins. The greater saphenous vein (Fig. 22–8) is the longest vein in the body; hence, it also is also called the long saphenous vein. It begins in the foot, passes anterior to the medial malleolus, and extends from the ankle to the groin along the medial aspect of the leg and thigh. About 4 cm below the inguinal ligament, it dives through the muscular fascia and joins the common femoral vein. The greater saphenous vein is used commonly as a conduit for coronary and peripheral arterial reconstruction; therefore, it is frequently the subject of ultrasound examination. In spite of its length, it can be "harvested" for bypass surgery without adverse consequences, since it drains only superficial structures and its function is readily replaced by collaterals. Isolated thrombosis of the greater saphenous vein is relatively common. Although painful, greater saphenous thrombosis is usually of little clinical importance. The exceptions are cases in which thrombus extends to the saphenofemoral junction or into the common femoral vein, posing the risk of clinically dangerous embolization of thrombus to the pulmonary circulation.

The lesser saphenous vein (Fig. 22–9) lies between the two heads of the gastrocnemius muscle along the posterior aspect of the calf: It is in the same position as the seam on a stocking. It extends from just above

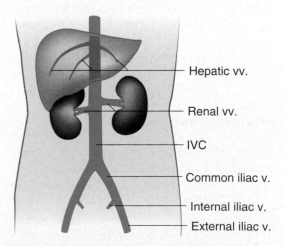

Hepatic vv.

Renal vv.

IVC

Common iliac v.

Internal iliac v.

External iliac v.

FIGURE 22–7. The inferior vena cava (IVC) and the iliac veins.

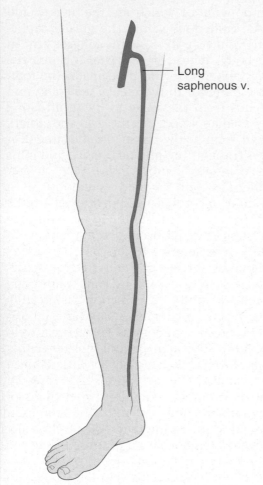

FIGURE 22–8. The greater (long) saphenous vein.

veins are duplicated in approximately 25% of individuals.[2] Venous duplications are important, because the unwary sonographer might overlook thrombus isolated to one of the paired veins. Many variations can occur at the union of the posterior tibial and peroneal veins,[3] and the frequent occurrence of variations at this location requires that care be taken in the course of ultrasound examination of the calf veins.

TERMINOLOGY

Clot versus Thrombus

In essence, the terms *blood clot* and *thrombus* are synonymous and are often used interchangeably, but *clot* refers to any coagulated mass of blood, whereas *thrombus* refers more precisely to a clot that forms within a blood vessel or the heart. Hence, the term *thrombus* is preferred with respect to the venous system.[7]

the ankle to the popliteal fossa, where it empties into the popliteal vein. Like the greater saphenous vein, the lesser saphenous may be used as a conduit for bypass surgery. It also may be a site of thrombus formation, with possible extention of thrombus into the popliteal vein, posing a risk of pulmonary artery embolization.

Anatomic Variants

There are many variations of venous anatomy. For practical reasons, only the more common variations are mentioned here, but the sonographer will undoubtedly encounter other variations. Figure 22–10 illustrates common variations of lower extremity venous anatomy. As noted previously, the superficial femoral and popliteal

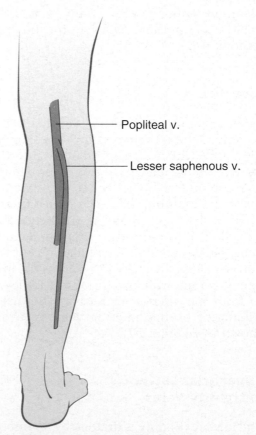

FIGURE 22–9. The lesser saphenous vein.

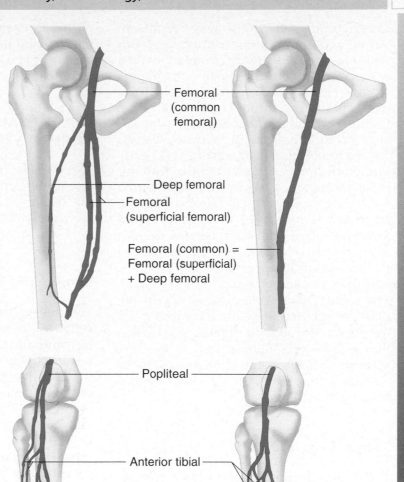

FIGURE 22–10. Common variants of lower extremity venous anatomy. (From DeWeese JA, Rogoff SM, Tobin CE: Radiographic Anatomy of Major Veins of the Lower Limb. Rochester, NY, Eastman Kodak. Reprinted courtesy of Eastman Kodak Company.)

Femoral (common femoral)

Deep femoral
Femoral (superficial femoral)

Femoral (common) = Femoral (superficial) + Deep femoral

Popliteal

Anterior tibial

Peroneal (fibular)

Posterior tibial

Thrombophlebitis

The term *thrombophlebitis* refers to the acute phase of venous thrombosis during which thrombus formation is associated with vein wall inflammation. Thrombophlebitis is thrombosis plus phlebitis or vein wall inflammation.

Acute and Chronic Venous Thrombosis

In terms of risk for pulmonary embolization, *acute* generally refers to a period of about 14 days,[8] during which the vein wall is inflamed and thrombus is loosely attached. Within this period, thrombus may

embolize to the pulmonary circulation, causing clinically significant, or even life-threatening, pulmonary artery occlusion. After about 14 days, thrombus that has not lysed generally adheres to the vein wall as a consequence of inflammation, and the risk of embolization is lessened, unless new thrombus forms. Thus, *acute* refers to approximately the first 14 days following the development of thrombus.

The terms *subacute* and *chronic* do not have a clear pathologic or clinical definition. *Subacute* generally infers weeks to perhaps 6 months, and *chronic*, thereafter. Moreover, there is no identifiable dividing line between the acute, subacute, and chronic phases from a sonographic perspective. The lack of precise clinical and sonographic definitions may result in serious communication errors, and for that reason, these terms should be used with considerable caution in sonographic reports. Perhaps the best way to avoid misrepresentation of thrombus age is to relate, whenever possible, the sonographic appearance of thrombus to the clinical history. For example, I might report, "Recently formed thrombus is present in the posterior tibial and peroneal veins, consistent with a 4-day history of calf pain." I often use the term *recent thrombosis*, or *recently formed thrombus*, rather than *acute*, because *recent* is relatively vague when used in relation to the sonographic appearance of thrombus and does not imply a specific time frame. The term *chronic venous thrombosis*, in my opinion, should not be used, because it is a misnomer. Chronic thrombus is not thrombus at all—it is fibrous scar. It is more accurate to refer to the chronic *sequelae* of venous thrombosis, or chronic venous scarring.

Thigh, Leg, and Calf

The *thigh* is the portion of the lower extremity between the hip and the knee. The *leg* is the segment between the knee and the ankle. The *calf* is the posterior, muscular portion of the leg.[7] The terms *upper leg* and *lower leg*, although used by some authors, are not common anatomic parlance.

Arm and Forearm

The *arm* is the portion of the upper extremity between the shoulder and the elbow, and the *forearm* is the portion from the elbow to the wrist.[7] The terms *upper arm* and *lower arm* are used by some authors, including some contributors to this text.

Proximal and Distal

The terms *proximal* and *distal*,[7] as they apply to the venous system, are somewhat confusing. In the vascular system, *proximal* means nearer to the heart, and *distal* means

farther from the heart. These terms do not reflect blood flow direction, which is a little confusing because venous flow is from distal to proximal.

IMAGE CHARACTERISTICS OF NORMAL VEINS

The B-mode and color flow image are the essence of ultrasound venous examination. The diagnostically important imaging characteristics of normal veins are listed in Table 22–1 and summarized below.

Lumen and Wall

The lumen of a normal vein[9,10] usually is echo free, as seen with gray-scale sonography, and the interior surface of the vein wall is smooth (Fig. 22–11*A*). The wall itself is so thin that it cannot be seen, and thickening of the wall suggests pathology. With many high-resolution instruments, blood flow may be visible on the B-mode image, and in such cases, the vein lumen is faintly echogenic[5] (Fig. 22–12). This normal echogenicity may be differentiated from thrombus, because movement of the blood is readily seen, whereas thrombus is stationary. Blood flow should extend all the way to the vessel margin (Fig. 22–12*B*). This is important, as a "filling defect" in the color flow image suggests thrombus or scarring. Please note that the proper method for examining veins with color flow is to *first visualize the vein wall clearly and then to demonstrate that*

Table 22–1. Sonographic Features of Normal Veins

B-Mode
  Thin (invisible) wall
  Smooth wall
  Anechoic lumen (except with venous stasis)
  Compressible
Spectral and Color Doppler
  Spontaneous flow
  Phasic flow (large veins)
  Flow ceases with the Valsalva maneuver
  Flow augmentation with distal compression
  Unidirectional flow (toward the heart)

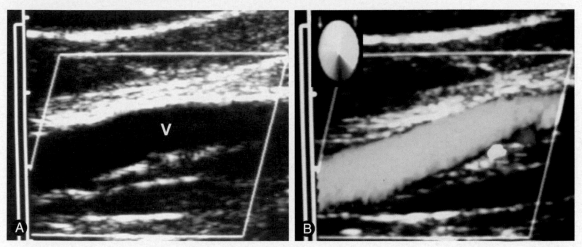

FIGURE 22–11. Color flow features of a normal extremity vein. *A,* The wall of the vein (V) is clearly defined and smooth, but the wall is not visible per se. The lumen is echo free. *B,* Blood flow fills the vein lumen completely (i.e., no flow voids are present within the lumen).

flow is present to the wall. Relying solely on the color flow image can possibly result in diagnostic error, although it is recognized that in the calf it may be possible to see the veins only with color flow.

Valves

Valves, which permit only cephalad flow, are numerous within extremity veins. The number of valves increases from proximal to distal. In the calf, a valve is present approximately every 2 cm along the length of the tibial and peroneal veins, and the valve sinuses in these areas may produce a beaded appearance on ultrasound images. Valves may be seen with ultrasound when image quality is excellent. Valve sinuses are widened areas of the lumen that accommodate the valve cusps. The two cusps that constitute most valves (occasionally there are three) are thin and appear delicate[11] (Fig. 22–13). The free edges of the cusps move symmetrically and freely within the flow stream, coapting in the center of the vessel when closed and folding back parallel to the vein wall when open. If only the base of a cusp, near its attachment, is seen on an ultrasound image, movement of the cusp may appear restricted, even if the valve is normal. Hence, a valve that is thought to be dysfunctional should be viewed from different perspectives, if possible, to determine whether it moves freely. Dysfunctional valves generally permit reflux of blood, which may be visible on the color flow image or the spectrum display. Small, faintly echogenic aggregates of red blood cells may accumulate behind the valve cusps in slow-flow states. These aggregates are easily displaced with vein compression, whereas thrombus in the same location is stationary.

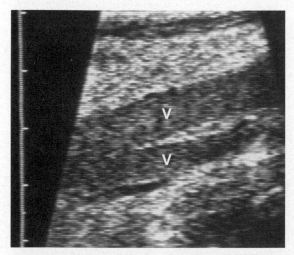

FIGURE 22–12. Echogenic blood. The blood in these veins (V) is echogenic because flow is sluggish and red blood cells have aggregated into larger units that reflect ultrasound effectively. Movement of the blood is visible in real time, differentiating between sluggish flow and thrombus.

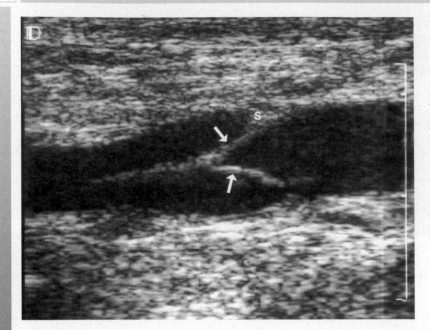

FIGURE 22–13. Venous valve. The two cusps of a valve (*arrows*) are clearly seen in this example. They are curvilinear and coapt in the center of the vessel. (It is uncommon to see venous valves with this level of clarity.) Stasis of blood (S) is evident behind one of the valve cusps. The blood is more echogenic here because of aggregation of red blood cells, as also shown in Figure 22–12.

Compressibility

Veins, as opposed to arteries, have thin walls, and the vein is held open primarily by the pressure of blood within the lumen. Thus, the vein lumen can be obliterated with a small amount of extrinsic pressure (Fig. 22–14). This simple observation is of great diagnostic importance, because the walls do not coapt when the lumen contains thrombus, even when the pressure applied is sufficient to distort the shape of an adjacent artery.[10] Vein compressibility is best tested with short-axis (transverse) images. A false impression of compressibility may occur with long-axis (longitudinal)

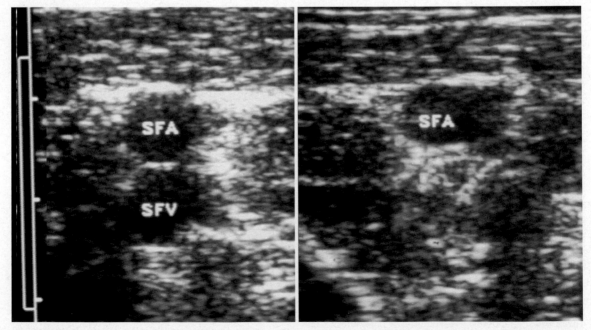

FIGURE 22–14. Vein compression. With pressure from the transducer, the superficial femoral vein (SFV) disappears from view (*right panel*), indicating that it is patent. SFA, superficial femoral artery.

views, because the vein may slip out of the image plane during attempted compression and disappear from view, falsely implying compressibility.

Vein Size

The major veins of the arm and thigh are somewhat larger in diameter than corresponding arteries. If the vein is substantially larger than the artery (i.e., more than twice the arterial diameter) and if the size does not vary with respiration, thrombosis should be suspected, because thrombus distends the vein lumen. Vein size may also be increased by back-pressure from congestive heart failure, proximal venous obstruction, or venous reflux. Furthermore, certain veins, such as the peroneal, soleal, and gastrocnemius veins, may normally be fairly large. Enlargement, therefore, should not be the sole criterion for the diagnosis of venous thrombosis.

Small vein size may be a manifestation of a remote episode of venous thrombosis, but small vein size should not be the only criterion by which abnormality is diagnosed. If the patient is dehydrated or severely vasoconstricted, the veins may be smaller than normal. Furthermore, the paired veins of the calf and forearm may be small for no apparent reason.

Respiratory Changes

The diameter of large veins (e.g., the femoral vein) increases with deep inspiration or with the Valsalva maneuver.[9] Visible respiration-related changes in vein caliber are not used diagnostically, but flow changes detected with Doppler ultrasound have great diagnostic importance, as indicated later.

DOPPLER CHARACTERISTICS OF NORMAL VEINS

Blood flow in normal veins has five important features, as summarized in Table 22–1: It is spontaneous and phasic, ceases with

the Valsalva maneuver, is augmented by distal compression, and is unidirectional (toward the heart).[11–13]

Spontaneous Flow

Blood flow occurs spontaneously in medium and large veins with the patient at rest, even if the extremity is dependent. That is, flow occurs without extrinsic compression of the soft tissues of the limb or muscular activity. The absence of spontaneous flow may result from thrombosis at the site of examination or from obstruction, either proximal or distal to that point. Flow is often *not* spontaneous in small veins, such as the paired tibial branches in the calf or the veins of the foot or hand. This is because the velocity of flow in these vessels, in the absence of muscular activity, is too slow for Doppler ultrasound detection.

Phasic Flow

Normal venous flow is *respirophasic*, meaning that the velocity of flow changes in response to respiration. The abbreviated term *phasic* is usually used, rather than *respirophasic*. Phasic changes in flow velocity are evident in the color flow image, the Doppler spectrum display (Fig. 22–15), and the audible Doppler signal. The Doppler spectrum and audible signal are the best media for assessing the phasic flow pattern, because subtle abnormalities are more apparent with these media than with color flow imaging. When the phasic pattern is absent, flow is described as *continuous* (Fig. 22–16). This flow pattern is significant, for it indicates the presence of substantial obstruction proximal, or sometimes distal, to the site of Doppler examination. With obstruction, blood trickles through diminutive collaterals or recanalization channels, and the phasic changes are lost. *The phasic pattern may persist when thrombus does not substantially obstruct the vein lumen;* therefore, the identification of a phasic flow pattern does not entirely exclude thrombosis, but it does exclude occlusive thrombosis.

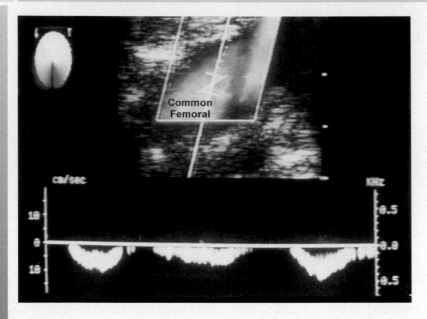

FIGURE 22–15. Spontaneous, phasic flow. The flow velocity fluctuates in response to respiration and right atrial contraction, indicating that the venous system is substantially patent between the point of Doppler examination and the chest.

The Valsalva Response

Deep inspiration followed by bearing down (the Valsalva maneuver) results in the abrupt cessation of blood flow in large- and medium-sized veins (Fig. 22–17). This important response documents the patency of the venous system from the point of Doppler examination to the thorax. Although cessation of flow is visible on color flow images, the Valsalva response is best evaluated with the Doppler spectrum display or from the audible Doppler signal. The Valsalva maneuver is particularly useful for confirming the patency of those segments of the venous system that cannot be examined directly. It should be noted, however, that an abnormal response to the Valsalva maneuver occurs only with *substantial* venous obstruction. A normal response may be observed if the vein lumen is only partially blocked.

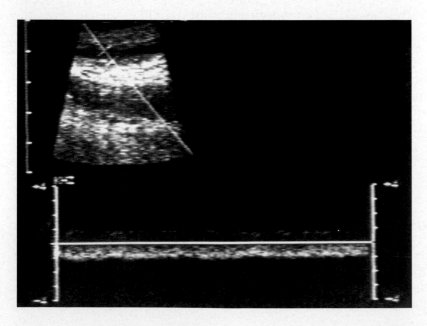

FIGURE 22–16. Continuous flow. The undulating flow pattern seen in Figure 22–15 is absent, indicating venous obstruction. The flow velocity is also low.

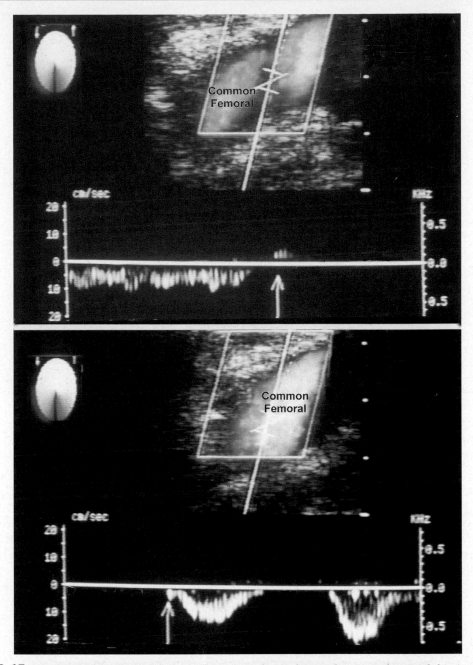

FIGURE 22–17. The Valsalva response. *Top*, As the patient bears down, elevation of intra-abdominal pressure abruptly terminates extremity venous flow (*arrow*). Reversed flow does not occur, indicating that the extremity valves are competent. *Bottom*, Flow resumes promptly with exhalation (*arrow*).

Augmentation

Manual compression of the extremity distal to the site of ultrasound examination increases, or *augments*, venous flow. The resulting gush of blood is recorded as an abrupt increase in the Doppler frequency shift (Fig. 22–18). This response confirms substantial patency of the veins between the site of Doppler examination and the site of venous compression. The absence of this response indicates substantial obstruction *distal* to the site of Doppler examination. Delayed or weak augmentation indicates distal obstruction that is incomplete or is circumvented by collaterals. The

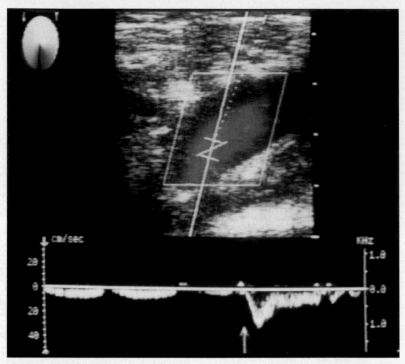

FIGURE 22–18. Flow augmentation. Calf compression results in a dramatic increase in flow velocity (*arrow*) in the common femoral vein. This finding confirms substantial patency of the veins between the calf and the common femoral area.

effects of augmentation are visible on color flow images, but the adequacy of augmentation is best evaluated with the Doppler spectrum or audible Doppler signals. Although augmentation was one of the earliest-described Doppler features of venous flow, it has not proven reliable for excluding thrombosis. This is because augmentation may be normal when a vein is only partially obstructed or when obstruction is circumvented by collateral flow.

Unidirectional Flow

In the normal venous system, blood flows only toward the heart, because the valves prevent flow in the opposite direction (retrograde flow). Normally functioning valves are described as competent, and valves that permit retrograde flow are described as incompetent. Valvular incompetence is diagnosed when retrograde flow occurs in response to the Valsalva maneuver (Fig. 22–19) or manual compres-

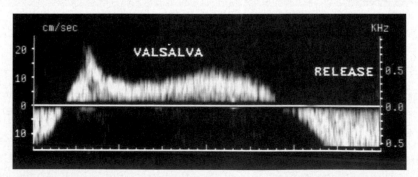

FIGURE 22–19. Venous reflux. Venous flow reverses with the onset of the Valsalva maneuver and remains reversed until the Valsalva maneuver is released, indicating severe, sustained reflux caused by valvular incompetence. Compare with Figure 22–17.

sion *proximal* to the site of ultrasound examination. Reflux is most conveniently assessed with the color flow image and may be documented with Doppler spectrum analysis.

References

1. Hollinshead WH: Textbook of Anatomy, 3rd ed. New York, Harper & Row, 1974, p 75.
2. Kadir S: Diagnostic Angiography. Philadelphia, WB Saunders, 1986, p 541.
3. DeWeese JA, Rogoff SM, Tobin CE: Radiographic Anatomy of Major Veins of the Lower Limb. Rochester, NY, Eastman Kodak.
4. Blackburn DR: Venous anatomy. J Vasc Technol 12:78–82, 1988.
5. Cotton LT, Clark C: Anatomical localisation of venous thrombosis. Ann R Coll Surg 36:214–224, 1965.
6. Nicolaides AN, Kakkar VV, Field ES, et al: The origin of venous thrombosis: A venographic study. Br J Radiol 44:653–663, 1971.
7. Stedman's Medical Dictionary, 20th ed. Baltimore, Williams & Wilkins, 1961, pp 141, 249, 330, 470, 604, 837, 1233, 1527, 1533.
8. Horowitz O, Casey MP, Maslak MM: Venous thrombosis: Pulmonary embolus complex. In Horowitz O, McComb P, Roberts B (eds): Diseases of Blood Vessels. Philadelphia, Lea & Febiger, 1985, pp 263–289.
9. Talbot SR: B-mode evaluation of peripheral veins. Semin Ultrasound CT MR 9:295–319, 1988.
10. Effeney DJ, Friedman MB, Gooding GAW: Iliofemoral venous thrombosis: Real-time ultrasound diagnosis, normal criteria, and clinical application. Radiology 150:787–792, 1984.
11. Zwiebel WJ: Duplex examination of the carotid arteries. Semin Ultrasound CT MR 11:97–135, 1990.
12. Zwiebel WJ: Duplex sonography of the venous system. Semin Ultrasound CT MR 9:269–326, 1988.
13. Barnes RW: Doppler techniques for lower-extremity venous disease. In Zwiebel WJ (ed): Introduction to Vascular Ultrasonography. Orlando, FL, Grune & Stratton, 1986, pp 333–350.

Chapter 23

Technique for Extremity Venous Ultrasound Examination

WILLIAM J. ZWIEBEL, MD

This chapter describes protocols for ultrasound examination of both the upper and lower extremity veins.[1-15] No two ultrasound laboratories perform a given examination in exactly the same way, and it is likely that the protocols described herein will be modified to suit the needs of particular laboratories or patients. A consistent method of examination must be established within each laboratory, however, to ensure that examinations are comprehensive and accurate. The examination protocol should conform to established standards, such as those specified by the organizations listed in Table 23–1.

INSTRUMENTATION

The ultrasound instrument chosen for extremity venous diagnosis should have the following features: (1) excellent spatial resolution, which implies incident ultrasound frequencies in the 5- to 15-MHz range; (2) excellent gray-scale resolution (dynamic range); (3) a Doppler device that is sensitive enough to detect low-velocity venous flow; and (4) color flow/power Doppler. Extremity venous examinations can be performed, in large part, with gray-scale imaging; however, color flow imaging is essential, as it facilitates both the identification of smaller veins and the confirmation of blood flow.

IMAGE ORIENTATION

Terms used in venous ultrasound imaging to describe the orientation of the scan plane are as follows. Images oriented along the length of the vein are described as *long axis* or *longitudinal*. Images perpendicular to the vein axis are described as *short axis* or *transverse*. I generally use the terms *long axis* and *short axis*. *Longitudinal* and *transverse* actually refer to the axis of the body as a whole, but these terms often are acceptable for venous imaging, because many veins run in longitudinal planes. Thus, long-axis images often are truly longitudinal in orientation, and short-axis images often are transverse in orientation.

INTERMITTENT COMPRESSION

A basic method for extremity vein examination with ultrasound is *intermittent compression*, which is conducted as follows. Using a *short-axis view*, pressure is applied with the transducer, causing the vein to collapse. Pressure is then released, the transducer is moved 2 to 3 cm along the course of the vein, and compression is again applied. This process is repeated along the entire course of the vein. Because the vein wall is thin and venous pressure is low, relatively little force is needed to collapse the vein and confirm its patency. If thrombus is present, the vein will not collapse, no matter how much pressure is applied. In practice, intermittent compression is conducted very rapidly, and a lengthy segment of vein can be examined in a short period. Intermittent compression should not be conducted with long-axis views, as the vein may slip out of the image plane, mimicking compressibility.

Table 23–1. Organizations That Set Standards for Vascular Ultrasound Departments

The American Institute of Ultrasound in Medicine: 14750 Sweitzer Lane, Suite 100, Laurel, MD 20707; http://www.aium.org

The Intersocietal Commission for Accreditation of Vascular Laboratories: 8840 Stanford Boulevard, Suite 4900, Columbia, MD 21045; http://www.icavl.org

The American College of Radiology: 1891 Preston White Drive, Reston VA 20191; http://www.acr.org

UPPER EXTREMITY VENOUS PROTOCOL

Patient Position

The patient should be recumbent on a bed or a stretcher that is sufficiently wide to comfortably support the patient's upper extremity and trunk. This is important, because muscular contraction from an uncomfortable patient position can compress and occlude the veins and can limit transducer access. As with all venous examinations, the room and patient should be sufficiently warm as to avoid peripheral vasoconstriction, which reduces the size of extremity veins and makes venous sonography more difficult.

Step 1. The Subclavian Vein

We begin the upper extremity examination with the subclavian vein, which may be approached from above or below the clavicle (Fig. 23–1). The above-clavicle approach may be more effective in one patient and the below-clavicle approach in another. With the below-clavicle view, the vein is visualized through the pectoralis muscles. The subclavian examination is conducted almost exclusively in long-axis views, and color flow is always used. The normal vein is uniform in caliber and is slightly larger than the adjacent artery. Doppler assessment of the vein (Fig. 23–2) is essential. Flow should be spontaneous and somewhat pulsatile (as a result of transmission of right atrial pulsation). Furthermore, flow should

be respirophasic and should respond appropriately to the Valsalva maneuver. (See Chapter 22 for definitions of these terms.) *Verification of normal subclavian flow features is very important*, as it confirms the patency of the innominate vein and the superior vena cava, which generally cannot be examined directly.

After completing the Doppler examination, look for the junction of the subclavian and internal jugular veins and confirm the patency of the latter. We do not examine the internal jugular vein in detail unless there are clinical indications to do so. Note that the size of the internal jugular vein changes substantially with respiration.

Finally, follow the subclavian vein as far distally as possible. Be careful not to slip unknowingly into an enlarged collateral vein. Remember, arteries accompany the major deep veins of the upper extremity. If you do not see an artery near the vein, you may be looking at a collateral vein.

Step 2. The Axillary and Brachial Veins

With the patient's arm abducted and rotated externally, place the transducer high in the axilla and identify the axillary vein in a short- or long-axis view (Fig. 23–3). Use the Doppler flow signals, if needed, to confirm the identity of the vein and the adjacent artery. Then, using short-axis views and intermittent compression, follow the course of the axillary vein into the brachial vein.

No discrete landmark indicates the junction of the axillary and brachial veins. Proceeding distally, it will be noted that the brachial vein splits into two branches, lying on either side of the brachial artery. The brachial vein is almost always duplicated, and both branches must be examined. Continue to examine the brachial veins with intermittent compression to the level of the elbow. Although the axillary and brachial veins may be examined with long-axis, color flow images, it is expedient, and possibly more accurate, to examine them with short-axis intermittent compression. Of course, the short-axis views may be supplemented with long-axis color flow images as needed.

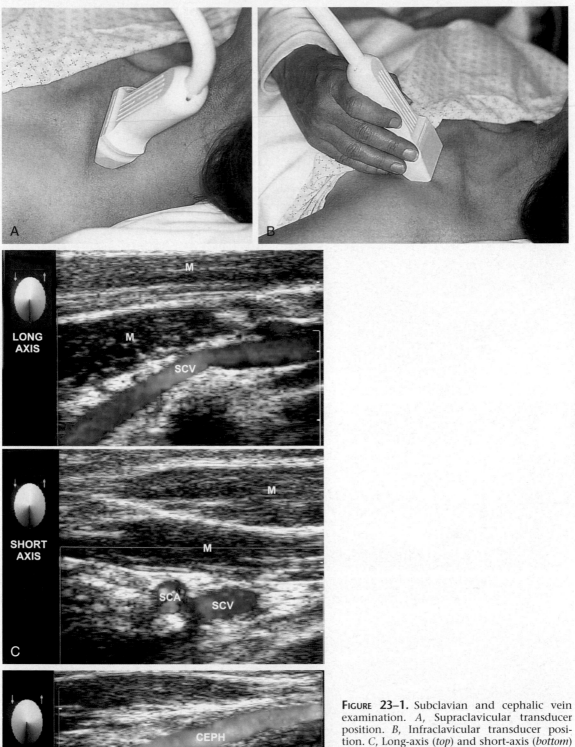

FIGURE 23–1. Subclavian and cephalic vein examination. *A*, Supraclavicular transducer position. *B*, Infraclavicular transducer position. *C*, Long-axis (*top*) and short-axis (*bottom*) views of a normal subclavian vein (SCV). Note that the vein is slightly inferior to the subclavian artery (SCA) and is deep to the pectoralis muscles (M). *D*, Supraclavicular view showing the junction of the cephalic vein (CEPH) with the subclavian vein.

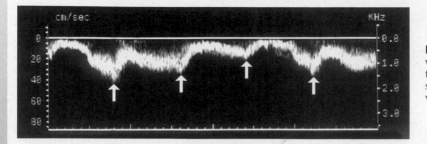

FIGURE 23–2. Normal subclavian vein Doppler signal. Note the cardiac pulsations (*arrows*) superimposed on respiratory variation.

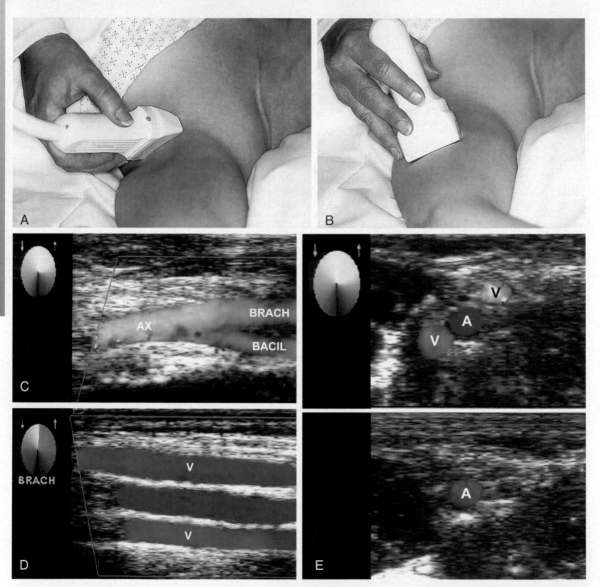

FIGURE 23–3. Axillary, basilic, and brachial vein examinations. *A*, Transducer position for viewing the axillary vein. *B*, Transducer position for viewing the brachial vein. *C*, Junction of the brachial (BRACH) and the basilic (BACIL) veins, forming the axillary vein (AX). *D*, Paired brachial veins (V) lying on each side of the brachial artery (A). *E*, The *upper image* shows the brachial veins adjacent to the brachial artery. The *lower image* was obtained with compression, and only the artery is visible.

Step 3. The Basilic Vein

Next, return to the axillary area and identify the junction of the basilic vein (medial) with the axillary vein, using short- or long-axis images. Then, follow the basilic vein to the elbow, using short-axis intermittent compression. Because the basilic vein is a component of the superficial venous system, it is not accompanied by an artery and lies just under the skin. A light touch with the transducer is important; otherwise the vein will collapse and cannot be identified.

Step 4. The Cephalic Vein

Now, move to the lateral aspect of the arm, a little above the elbow, and locate the cephalic vein, which lies approximately in the groove between the biceps and triceps muscles. If you do not find the vein here, look for it further cephalad, adjacent to the deltoid muscle. As with the basilic vein, the cephalic vein lies just under the skin and is not accompanied by an artery. Minimum transducer pressure is required to avoid compression of the vein, which renders it invisible. Once located, use short-axis views and intermittent compression to confirm vein patency from the elbow to the shoulder. Near its proximal end, the cephalic vein crosses the deltoid muscle and then dives deeply to join the subclavian vein. This proximal portion is best examined with long-axis color flow views, as seen in Figure 23–1D.

Step 5. The Forearm Veins

In most cases, the subclavian vein and arm veins are of primary clinical concern, and the venous ultrasound examination is terminated at the elbow. If there is clinical suspicion of forearm venous thrombosis, the examination is extended to the wrist. The forearm venous examination is simply a continuation of the arm examination, using short-axis views and intermittent compression. At the end of the brachial vein examination, follow the radial and ulnar veins (Fig. 23–4) from the elbow to the wrist, using the corresponding arteries as anatomic guides. If you get lost at the elbow, go to the wrist and follow the radial and ulnar veins proximally. The basilic and cephalic veins in the forearm are examined similarly, by beginning in the arm and continuing into the forearm as far as possible. These veins may become quite small in the forearm and may branch; therefore, it may not be possible to follow the basilic and cephalic veins to the wrist.

Protocol Summary

The protocol for upper extremity venous examination is summarized in Table 23–2.

LOWER EXTREMITY VENOUS PROTOCOL

Patient Position

Clear visualization of the lower extremity veins requires adequate distention of the venous system. To this end, the lower extremity must be dependent, which may be accomplished by steeply elevating the head of the examination table or by examining the patient in the sitting position (Fig. 23–5). The patient and the examining room should be sufficiently warm to prevent vasoconstriction, which results in poor venous distention.

Step 1. The Iliac Veins

The iliac veins are not routinely examined. Instead, it is customary practice to rely on Doppler signals obtained at the groin to exclude more proximal venous obstruction. When Doppler signals are abnormal or there are other suggestions of obstruction, the iliac veins can be examined directly. A 3- to 5-MHz transducer is generally required for iliac vein examination. First, identify the external iliac vein at the groin, and then, using long-axis views, follow it cephalad as it dives deeply into the pelvis. You should trace the external and common iliac veins cephalad as far as possible, with a goal of following the iliac system all the

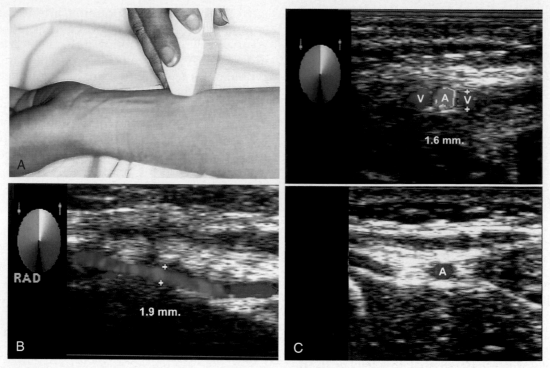

FIGURE 23–4. Forearm vein examination. *A,* Transducer position for viewing the ulnar veins. *B,* Long-axis view of ulnar veins (V). Note the small size (1.9 mm). *C,* The upper image is a short-axis view of the paired ulnar veins adjacent to the ulnar artery (A). Note the small size of the veins (1.6 mm). In the lower image, obtained with compression, only the artery is visible.

way to the inferior vena cava. The junction of the external and common iliac veins often cannot be identified, but this junction approximates the point where the iliac vessels lie most deeply within the pelvis.

In most cases, the iliac system is best visualized from an anterolateral approach, with the transducer lateral to the rectus muscle, as shown in Figure 23–6. Examination of the iliac veins seems impossible to neophyte

---

Table 23–2. Protocol for Upper Extremity Venous Examination

Step 1.   The Subclavian Vein
            Visualize with long-axis images from the manubrium as far distally as possible. Check
               subclavian Doppler signals. Examine the internal jugular vein.

Step 2.   The Axillary and Brachial Veins
            Examine the axillary and brachial veins principally with short-axis views and intermittent
               compression, supplemented by long-axis color flow views. Be sure to examine both
               branches of the brachial vein.

Step 3.   The Basilic Vein
            Identify the junction of the basilic and brachial veins and follow the basilic vein to the
               elbow, using transverse compression. Supplement with long-axis views as needed.

Step 4.   The Cephalic Vein
            Identify the cephalic vein in the forearm and examine it with short-axis views and
               transverse compression. Use long-axis, color flow views to visualize its junction with the
               subclavian vein.

Step 5.   The Forearm Veins
            Follow the radial, ulnar, basilic, and cephalic veins to the wrist if symptoms suggest
               abnormality in these segments. Short-axis views with intermittent compression is the
               primary mode of examination.

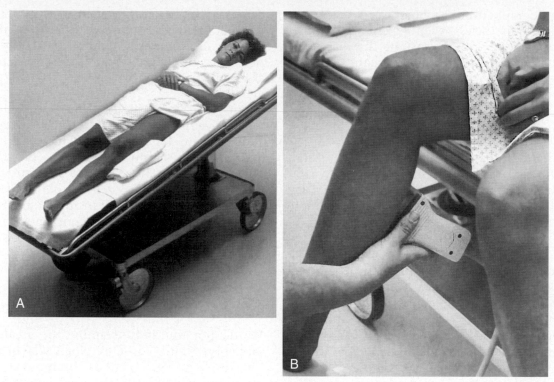

FIGURE 23–5. Patient positions for lower extremity venous examination. *A*, Supine, reverse Trendelenburg's position. *B*, Upright position. (*A*, *B*, Modified from Zwiebel WJ, Priest DL: Color duplex sonography of extremity veins. Semin Ultrasound CT MR 11:136–167, 1990.)

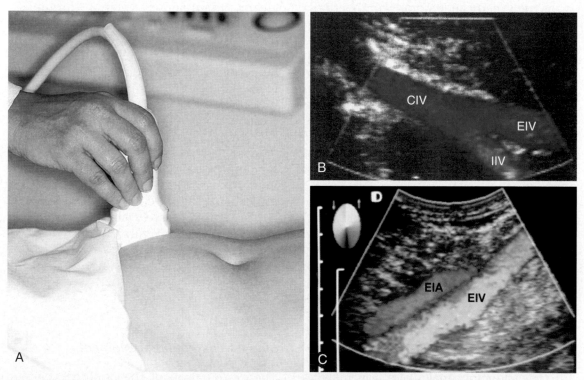

FIGURE 23–6. Iliac vein examination. *A*, The transducer is positioned lateral to the rectus muscle for visualization of the iliac veins. *B*, Junction of the external (EIV) and internal (IIV) iliac veins, forming the common iliac vein (CIV). *C*, The external iliac vein, as seen just caphalad to the inguinal ligament. EIA, external iliac artery.

sonographers but becomes easier with practice; nonetheless, even experienced sonographers cannot demonstrate the iliac veins in all patients, and image quality may be suboptimal.

Step 2. The Femoral Segment

The examination of the venous system from the femoral level distally is usually conducted with a 5- to 10-MHz linear array transducer. Begin the examination at the groin with long-axis views of the distal external iliac vein. Move caudad into the common femoral vein (Fig. 23–7) and look for two important landmarks: (1) the junction of the superficial and deep femoral veins, forming the common femoral vein, and (2) the entry of the greater saphenous vein into the common femoral vein. These are the first of several landmarks that should be identified during each venous examination, in order to avoid misdiagnoses. (For instance, I have seen a sonographer proceed from the common femoral vein into a dilated greater saphenous vein and mistake it for the superficial femoral vein, overlooking thrombus in the latter.)

Next, confirm the patency of the greater saphenous and deep femoral veins with color flow imaging and then evaluate flow in the common femoral vein with Doppler (see Fig. 23–7C). Check for spontaneous and phasic flow and, if needed, a normal Valsalva response. These measures are used to exclude occlusion of the iliac veins or the inferior vena cava, as mentioned previously.

After the Doppler examination is complete, switch to short-axis views and begin the intermittent compression examination of the common and superficial femoral veins. This is the primary method used for lower extremity venous examination. Starting as high as possible in the common femoral vein and continuing into the superficial femoral vein, sequentially test vein compressibility (Fig. 23–8) to the point at which the superficial femoral vein dives into the adductor canal. Color flow imaging often is used for the transverse compression

examination, but gray-scale imaging is quite adequate and in some cases may provide greater information than color flow. Abnormal (noncompressible) areas may be assessed further with long-axis color flow views.

Just above the knee, the superficial femoral vein dives through a tunnel in the adductor muscles called the adductor canal and emerges behind the knee in the popliteal space. The adductor segment of the superficial femoral vein is too deep to be compressed effectively in most patients (Fig. 23–9), and this segment must be examined only with long-axis color flow images.

Step 3. The Greater Saphenous Vein

We do not routinely examine the greater saphenous vein[15] in detail when searching for lower extremity venous thrombus, but we *always* examine the proximal 5 cm or so below its junction with the common femoral vein. When symptoms (painful, palpable subcutaneous "cord") suggest greater saphenous vein thrombosis, however, this vessel should be examined in detail. Short-axis intermittent compression is generally the most efficient means of saphenous vein examination. A superficially focused, high-frequency (7- to 10-MHz) transducer and a very light touch are required for this examination. Too much pressure obliterates the vein lumen and renders it invisible. Note that the greater saphenous vein is located just outside of the muscular fascia (i.e., at the junction of the muscle and the subcutaneous fat) and that two fascial planes are visible adjacent to the vein, as shown in Figure 23–10. If the vein lies just below the skin and is not invested by fascia, it probably is not the greater saphenous vein but, rather, is a subcutaneous branch or collateral.

Step 4. The Popliteal Segment

The examination of the popliteal segment necessitates repositioning of the patient as

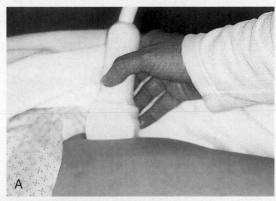

FIGURE 23–7. Long-axis femoral vein examination. *A*, Transducer position, upper thigh. *B*, The junction of the greater (long) saphenous vein (LSV) with the common femoral vein (CFV) is an important landmark. *C*, Doppler signals are obtained routinely in the common femoral vein. (Phasic, spontaneous flow, with augmentation at the *arrow*.) *D*, The junction of the superficial femoral vein (SFV) and the deep femoral veins (DFV), forming the common femoral vein, is another important landmark.

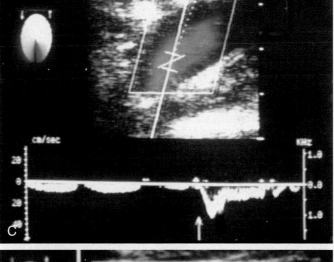

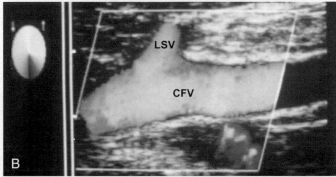

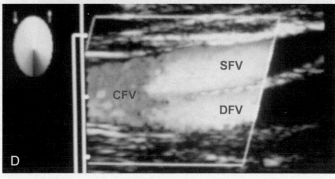

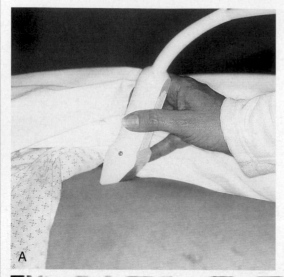

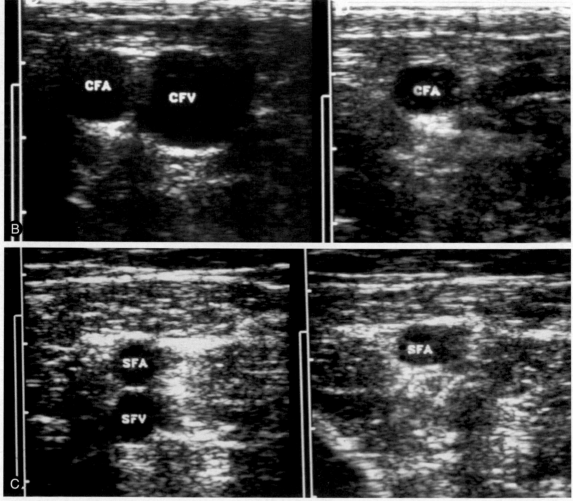

FIGURE 23-8. Short-axis femoral vein examination. *A*, Transducer position, upper thigh. *B*, Short-axis views of the common femoral vein (CFV), without (*left*) and with (*right*) compression. Note that the vein is *medial* to the common femoral artery (CFA). *C*, Short-axis view of the superficial femoral vein (SFV), without (*left*) and with (*right*) compression. Note that the vein is *deep* to the superficial femoral artery (SFA).

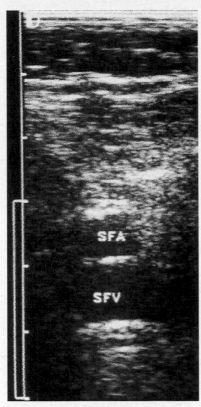

FIGURE 23–9. The adductor segment. The superficial femoral vein (SFV) is generally too deep for effective transverse compression. SFA, superficial femoral artery.

shown in Figures 23–11A and 23–12. Begin the examination with long-axis views of the popliteal vein (Fig. 23–11B) and move upward into the adductor canal to examine the distal part of the superficial femoral vein. It is important to go as high in the adductor canal as possible to ensure that a segment of this vessel is not missed. The junction of the superficial femoral and popliteal veins is arbitrarily designated as the distal end of the adductor canal, but no convenient sonographic landmarks identify this junction. Return to the popliteal segment, noting that the popliteal vein lies *superficial* to the popliteal artery from this perspective. This is the *reverse* of the relationship seen during the superficial femoral examination. Next, test the patency of the popliteal vein with short-axis intermittent compression (see Fig. 23–11C). Begin as high as possible in the popliteal fossa and continue distally into the posterior tibial and peroneal trunks.

Step 5. The Paired Calf Veins

The transducer positions for calf vein examination are shown in Figure 23–12. There are two basic approaches to the calf veins: beginning at the knee or beginning at the ankle. It is efficient to begin at the knee, as the transducer is already located there at the

FIGURE 23–10. Short-axis view of the greater (long) saphenous vein (LSV). Note the fascial planes (*arrows*) adjacent to the vein.

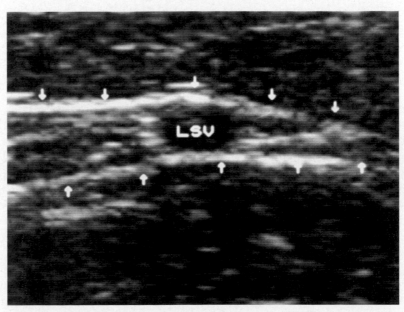

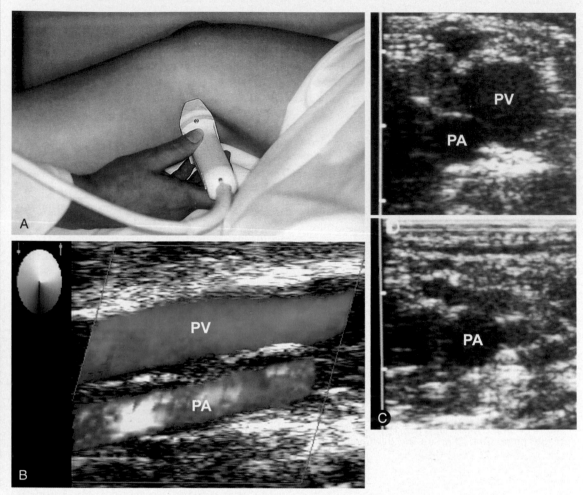

FIGURE 23–11. Popliteal vein examination. *A,* Transducer position. *B,* Long-axis view of the popliteal vein (PV). Note that the vein is *superficial* to the popliteal artery (PA). *C,* Short-axis view of the popliteal vein and artery, without (*top*) and with (*bottom*) compression.

end of the popliteal examination. We frequently experience difficulty following the calf veins from the knee down, however, in which case, we go to the ankle and proceed back up to the knee.

In most instances, calf vein examination combines transverse compression and long-axis color flow imaging. Because calf vein examination requires technologic creativity, it is not possible to describe a consistent examination protocol for the calf veins. The goal, however, is to ensure that all three calf vein pairs (anterior tibial, posterior tibial, and peroneal) are adequately visualized.

We usually start the calf vein examination with transverse compression, which works particularly well for the paired posterior tibial and peroneal veins. The corresponding arteries are important orienting landmarks,

and when the arteries are occluded by atherosclerosis, the calf vein examination is often compromised. In many cases, the transverse compression examination must be supplemented with long-axis color flow imaging, especially in the upper calf area, where the paired branches unite to form common trunks. Note that blood flow is generally *not* spontaneous in the calf veins, and flow must be augmented by periodic manual compression of the foot or the lower portion of the calf, below the site of examination.

Approach to the Posterior Tibial and Peroneal Veins

The posterior tibial veins actually lie posteromedial to the tibia and are best approached from the posteromedial aspect

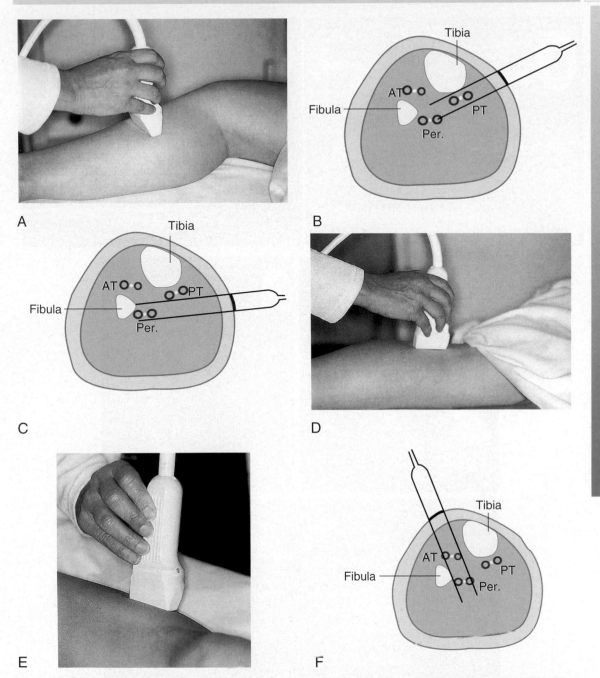

FIGURE 23–12. Calf vein transducer positions. *A*, Posteromedial position for viewing the posterior tibial and peroneal veins. *B* and *C*, Posterior tibial (PT) and peroneal (Per.) vein image planes. *D*, "Stocking seam" transducer approach to the peroneal veins. *E*, Anterolateral transducer position for viewing the anterior tibial veins. *F*, Anterior tibial (AT) vein image plane.

of the leg, as shown in Figures 23–12 and 23–13. The peroneal veins are imaged from the same transducer position but are seen deep to the posterior tibial veins. In spite of their deep location, they are well seen if the calf is not too large or edematous.

If the posterior tibial or peroneal veins are not well seen from a posteromedial approach, try a straight posterior approach with the patient prone, as shown in Figure 23–12D. In addition, the peroneal trunk sometimes can be seen from the

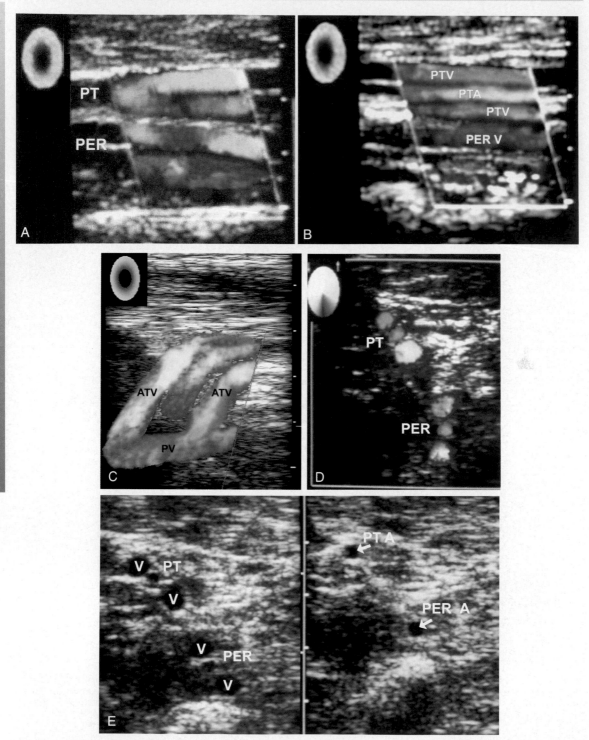

FIGURE 23–13. Representative images of normal calf veins. *A*, Power Doppler view of the junction of the paired posterior tibial and peroneal veins, forming the common posterior tibial (PT) and peroneal (PER) trunks. *B*, Power Doppler view of the paired posterior tibial veins (PTV) adjacent to the posterior tibial artery (PTA). One of the peroneal veins (PER V) is also visible. *C*, Power Doppler view showing the junction of the anterior tibial veins (ATV) with the popliteal vein (PV). The anterior tibial artery lies between the anterior tibial veins. *D*, Short-axis color flow view of the posterior tibial and peroneal veins. *E*, On the *left* is a short-axis view of the paired posterior tibial and peroneal veins (V) without compression. With compression (*right*), only the posterior tibial and peroneal arteries are visible (PT A and PER A, respectively).

anterolateral approach that is used routinely to visualize the anterior tibial system (Figs. 23–12E and 23–12F).

Approach to the Anterior Tibial Veins

The anterior tibial veins are best visualized from an anterolateral transducer approach, with the transducer positioned between the tibia and the fibula (Figs. 23–12 and 23–13). In many cases, the paired anterior tibial veins drain separately into the popliteal vein. Alternatively, the paired veins unite and enter the popliteal vein as a common trunk. In either case, they veer off from the popliteal vein at an acute angle and then turn inferiorly after penetrating the interosseous ligament between the tibia and the fibula. The anterior tibial branches are small, and isolated thrombosis of this system is relatively uncommon, leading to the suggestion by some that their examination is unnecessary.[13,15,16] Nevertheless, routine examination of the anterior tibial vein is generally recommended and usually requires little time.

Step 6. The Gastrocnemius and Soleal Veins

In our department, we do not attempt to visualize the gastrocnemius and soleal veins routinely, but sonographers should be aware of the general location of these veins, as shown in Figure 22–5 (see Chapter 22), in order to identify thrombus within these muscular branches. The gastrocnemius and soleal veins (Fig. 23–14) are fairly common sites of isolated thrombus formation. It is especially important to look for thrombus in these veins when the patient has focal calf pain and/or tenderness and the remainder of the deep venous system is normal.

Protocol Summary

The examination protocol for the lower extremity venous system is summarized in Table 23–3.

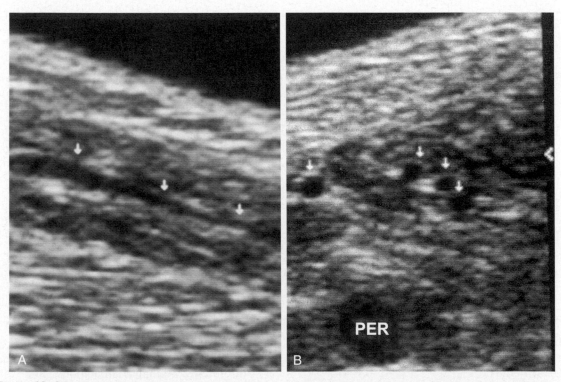

FIGURE 23–14. Soleal veins (*arrows*), as seen in long-axis (A) and short-axis (B) images. PER, peroneal vein.

Table 23–3 Protocol for Lower Extremity Venous Examination

Step 1.   The Iliac Segment
Identify the external iliac vein at the groin and follow it cephalad with long-axis images. Locate the iliac bifurcation or its approximate position. Follow the common iliac vein cephalad to the inferior vena cava. If you lose track of the vein, start at the inferior vena cava and follow the iliac vein inferiorly.

Step 2.   The Femoral Segment
Use long-axis images to identify the external iliac vein at the groin and follow it distally into the common femoral vein. Note the entrance of the greater saphenous vein. Check Doppler characteristics at the common femoral level. Identify the deep femoral vein and confirm its patency. Return to the groin and check vein compressibility with short-axis images and intermittent compression from the femoral level to the adductor canal. Watch for superficial femoral vein duplication.

Step 3.   The Greater Saphenous Vein
Confirm that the proximal portion of the greater saphenous vein is patent with long-axis color flow views. Examine as much of the vein as is clinically indicated, using short-axis intermittent compression.

Step 4.   The Popliteal Segment
Using long-axis views, locate the distal portion of the superficial femoral vein as high as possible in the adductor canal. Follow the superficial femoral vein distal into the popliteal segment to the junction of the tibial trunks. Confirm the compressibility of the popliteal vein and the tibial trunks with short-axis views and intermittent compression. Watch for popliteal vein duplication.

Step 5.   The Calf Veins
Examine the posterior tibial veins and trunk in their entirety, starting either at the popliteal space or at the ankle. Use short-axis intermittent compression as the primary mode and supplement with long-axis color flow images parallel to veins. Examine the peroneal veins similarly. Examine the anterior tibial veins with long-axis color flow images. Examine the gastrocnemius and soleal veins as clinically indicated, using long- or short-axis views.

References

1. Talbot SR: B-mode evaluation of peripheral veins. Semin Ultrasound CT MR 9:295–319, 1988.
2. Lensing AWA, Prandoni P, Brandjes D, et al: Detection of deep-vein thrombosis by real-time B-mode ultrasonography. N Engl J Med 320: 341–345, 1989.
3. Effeney DJ, Friedman MB, Gooding GAW: Iliofemoral venous thrombosis: Real-time ultrasound diagnosis, normal criteria, and clinical application. Radiology 150:787–792, 1984.
4. Barnes RW: Doppler techniques for lower-extremity venous disease. In Zwiebel WJ (ed): Introduction to Vascular Ultrasonography. Philadelphia, Grune & Stratton, 1986, pp 333–350.
5. Sullivan ED, Peters BS, Cranley JJ: Real-time B-mode venous ultrasound. J Vasc Surg 1:465–471, 1984.
6. Oliver MA: Duplex scanning in venous disease. Bruit 9:206–209, 1985.
7. Raghavendra BN, Horii SC, Hilton S, et al: Deep venous thrombosis: Detection by probe compression of veins. J Ultrasound Med 5:89–95, 1986.
8. Dauzat MM, Laroche JP, Charras C, et al: Real-time B-mode ultrasonography for better specialty in the noninvasive diagnosis of deep venous thrombosis. J Ultrasound Med 5:625–631, 1986.
9. Cronan JJ, Dorfman GS, Scola FH, et al: Deep venous thrombosis: US assessment using vein compression. Radiology 162:191–194, 1987.
10. Vogel P, Laing FRC, Jeffrey RB, et al: Deep venous thrombosis of the lower extremity: US evaluation. Radiology 163:747–751, 1987.
11. Appelman PT, De Jong TE, Lampmann LE: Deep venous thrombosis of the leg: US findings. Radiology 163:743–746, 1987.
12. Rose SC, Zwiebel WJ, Nelson BD, et al: Symptomatic lower extremity deep venous thrombosis: Accuracy, limitations, and role of color-duplex flow imaging in diagnosis. Radiology 175:639–644, 1990.

13. Rose SC, Zwiebel WJ, Miller FJ: Distribution of acute lower extremity deep venous thrombosis in symptomatic and asymptomatic patients: Imaging implications. J Ultrasound Med 13:243–250, 1994.
14. Zwiebel WJ, Priest DL: Color duplex sonography of extremity veins. Semin Ultrasound CT MR 11:136–167, 1990.
15. Hatch W, Hatch-Wunderle V (eds): Phlebography and Sonography of the Veins. Berlin, Springer-Verlag, 1997, pp 6–16.
16. Kazmers A, Groehn BA, Meeker-Ferguson C: Is interrogation of the anterior tibial veins necessary during venous duplex? J Vasc Tech 25:7–9, 2001.

Chapter 24

Ultrasound Diagnosis of Venous Thrombosis

William J. Zwiebel, MD

The primary focus of this chapter is ultrasound detection and assessment of venous thrombosis, which is the principal pathology that affects the venous system. Also included is a discussion of arteriovenous fistula, which is a less common but important condition.

THROMBOSIS AND THROMBOLYSIS

Thrombus originates focally within the venous system, perhaps in an area of stagnation, such as the region at the base of a valve cusp. Once formed, thrombus induces additional thrombosis, and, as a result, thrombus propagates along the vein lumen. In some cases, the lumen is only partially filled, while in others, the lumen is occluded. During the acute phase, the presence of thrombus induces an inflammatory response in the adjacent vein wall. Thus, the term *thrombophlebitis* is applicable, *phlebitis* referring to inflammation of the vein wall. The inflammatory component is the cause of cramping, focal pain, and tenderness associated with acute thrombophlebitis. Many factors may initiate venous thrombosis, but in most cases, vein wall inflammation follows the formation of thrombus. In some cases, however, and especially with respect to indwelling venous catheters, injury of the vein wall initiates an inflammatory response that causes thrombus to form within the vein lumen secondarily.

In response to the presence of thrombus, an enzyme called plasminogen is released from the blood and chemically lyses thrombus. In some cases, plasminogen may com-pletely lyse the thrombus over a period of days to weeks, leaving no trace and no adverse sequelae. Clinical experience with venous sonography suggests, however, that this is a relatively uncommon course, and in many cases, lysis is incomplete.

Within about 7 to 14 days, the inflammatory reaction resolves, and a process begins through which residual thrombus that does not lyse subsequently is transformed into fibrous tissue. The thrombus is invaded by fibroblasts, and these cells slowly convert the remaining thrombus to fibrous tissue that persists indefinitely. If only a small amount of thrombus remains unlysed, the resulting fibrous scar may take the form of small plaquelike areas or thickening of the vein wall. With more extensive scarring, the caliber of the vein is reduced, or the vein may be become an occluded fibrous cord.

ULTRASOUND FINDINGS

Thrombus within the venous system is hypoechoic during the first few days after its formation but becomes more echogenic with time. This and additional changes permit the age of the thrombus to be approximated in many patients. The detection of thrombus and the assessment of its age require familiarity with the ultrasound findings described later.

Acute Thrombosis

As noted in Chapter 22, the term *acute* refers to approximately the first 14 days after thrombus forms,[8] during which the vein wall is inflamed and thrombus is loosely attached. Within this period, thrombus may embolize to the pulmonary circulation, causing clinically significant, or even life-threatening, pulmonary artery occlusion. By the end of the acute period and into the subacute stage, thrombus is adherent to the vein wall, and the risk of embolization is lessened. The term *acute thrombosis* must be used with great caution, because sonographic findings provide only a general time frame and do not clearly separate the acute and subacute phases. During the acute period, thrombus has the following ultrasound appearance.[1–9]

Low Echogenicity

Recently formed thrombus generates only low-level echoes and may be virtually anechoic (Fig. 24–1A). Because of its low echogenicity, small thrombi may be difficult to visualize. The presence of such thrombi is indicated, however, by a flow void on color flow images and a lack of vein compressibility (discussed later). As thrombus ages during the course of the acute period, echogenicity increases slightly, but the intensity of the echoes remains low and is less than that of the surrounding muscle. Blood flow persists in veins that are incompletely filled with acute thrombus. Even when the vein lumen is filled, blood flow may be demonstrated in tiny residual channels adjacent to the vein wall (Fig. 24–1B and C), producing a "train track" appearance. Flow may also be seen within the thrombus with recanalization (Fig. 24–1C).

Venous Distention

Recently thrombosed veins are generally distended to an abnormally large size and are substantially larger than the adjacent artery (Fig. 24–1D). The exception to this rule occurs if the thrombus is small and nonocclusive or if the vein is scarred and incapable of dilation. Venous distention is a significant finding because it helps to differentiate between recently formed thrombus and older thrombus. In the latter case, the vein and artery either are similar in size or the vein is smaller than the artery. Distention of the vein persists throughout the acute period and into the subacute period.

Loss of Compressibility

When thrombus of any age is present, the vein lumen cannot be obliterated with compression. Lack of compressibility of the vein (Fig. 24–2) is perhaps the single most reliable finding for differentiating between thrombosed and normal veins. Excellent results for diagnosing venous thrombosis have been reported on the basis of this diagnostic criterion alone.[5–7] It should be noted that thrombus can be *excluded* only when compression causes the vein to disappear *completely.* If the vein does not collapse completely, the lumen may be partially filled with thrombus. Resistance from surrounding musculoskeletal structures may prevent adequate compression of the vein and may result in a false-positive diagnosis of thrombosis. To judge if compression is adequate, look at the adjacent artery. If pressure is sufficient to deform the artery substantially, the vein should collapse. To confirm your impression, attempt compression from another transducer position and check for a flow void within the vein using color flow imaging.

Free-Floating Thrombus

The proximal end of an acute thrombus, representing the most recently formed coagulum, may not adhere to the vein wall, and in such cases, the thrombus is said to float freely within the lumen. The visualization of free-floating thrombus provides unequivocal evidence of acuity. The ultrasound image of free-floating thrombus (Fig. 24–3) is dramatic and frightening, for it vividly depicts the potential for embolization to the pulmonary circulation. Whenever acute thrombus is identified sonographically, and particularly when the thrombus is free floating, care must be taken

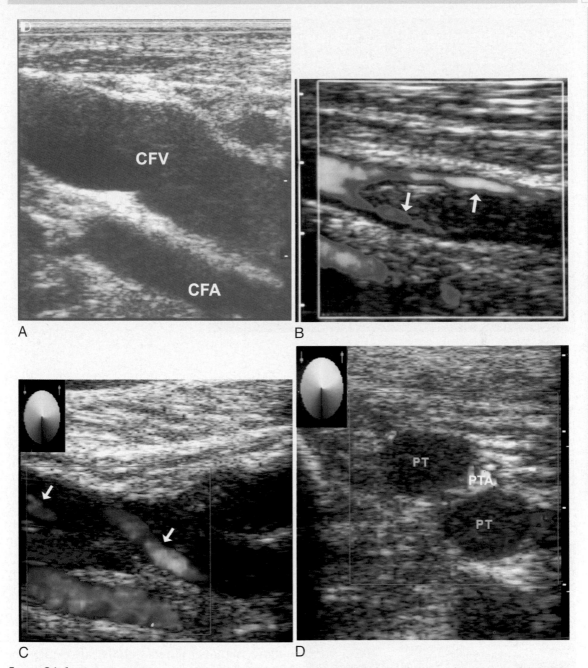

FIGURE 24–1. *A*, Acute thrombus in the common femoral vein (CFV) is less echogenic than surrounding tissues. (In this reproduction, the thrombus is barely visible.) CFA, common femoral artery. *B*, With color flow imaging, blood flow (*arrows*) is seen around the thrombus. *C*, Restoration of flow (*arrows*) is apparent in this 1-week-old thrombus. *D*, Marked dilation of acutely thrombosed posterior tibial (PT) veins is apparent. Compare with the posterior tibial artery (PTA).

not to dislodge the thrombus by unnecessary manipulation. The extent of thrombosis should be evaluated with as little manipulation as possible. Thereafter, the patient should remain recumbent and quiet. Do not allow the patient to walk or to move from the examining table to a wheelchair! Dislodgement of thrombus during ultrasound examination has been reported,[10] resulting in pulmonary embolization, but this appears to occur rarely, as discussed in Chapter 25.

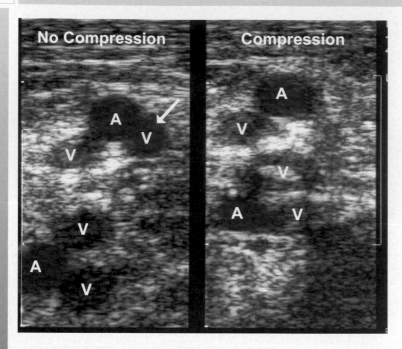

No Compression

Compression

FIGURE 24–2. Lack of compressibility. Four veins (V) are visible in this illustration, but only one collateral vein (*arrow*) responds to compression. The others are filled with thrombus approximately 1 week of age. A, artery.

Doppler Signal Abnormality

When thrombus of any age substantially occludes the vein lumen, Doppler flow abnormalities may be detected. Proximal to the thrombosed segment (i.e., downstream), flow augmentation is diminished or absent. Distal to a thrombosed segment, flow is continuous (see Chapter 22) rather than phasic, and the Valsalva response is diminished or absent.[11] This lack of respiratory variation is a particularly important finding when seen in the common femoral vein or the subclavian vein, as it implies obstruction of more proximal venous segments that cannot be examined directly. The importance of continuous flow cannot be overemphasized. It may provide the only sonographic evidence of venous obstruction that is of great clinical significance.

Venous flow abnormalities occur only when the vein lumen is substantially blocked by thrombus or other causes, such as extrinsic compression. Localized, partially occlusive thrombus may not affect flow signals. Flow signals also may be normal, or nearly so, if large collateral veins circumvent the region of obstruction.

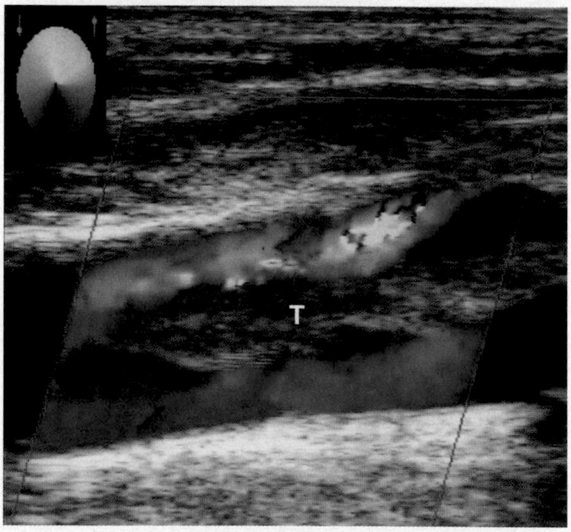

Collateralization

Collateral venous channels enlarge rapidly during the acute phase of venous thrombosis, and these channels are often visible during ultrasound examination. The collaterals may be located either adjacent to the thrombosed vein or more distantly. Collaterals typically are much smaller than the

FIGURE 24–3. Free-floating thrombus. Flowing blood surrounds free-floating thrombus (T) within the common femoral vein. This thrombus originated in the greater saphenous vein and extended into the common femoral vein.

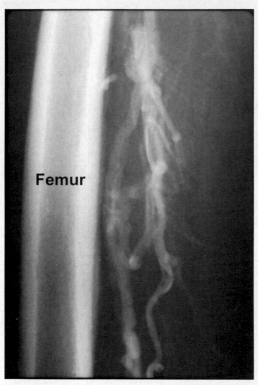

FIGURE 24-4. Collateralization. An extensive network of venous collaterals is shown on this contrast venogram. The superficial femoral vein is occluded.

normal vein and often are tortuous or braided (Fig. 24–4). It is important not to mistake a collateral for the original vein and thereby overlook venous thrombosis.

Subacute Thrombosis

The length of the subacute phase is not clearly defined. By *subacute,* I mean that thrombus is older than 2 weeks and is potentially as old as six months. The transition from recently formed (acute) to subacute thrombosis occurs gradually, and the sonographic abnormalities referable to acute thrombosis persist to varying degrees into the subacute phase. As unlysed thrombus ages, the following changes may be seen.[1–8]

Increased Echogenicity

The thrombus gradually becomes more echogenic throughout the subacute period (Fig. 24–5A and B). Unfortunately, this change is variable, and it is not possible to determine the age of thrombus precisely by means of echogenicity. In my experience, thrombus that is several days old may sometimes be similar in echogenicity to thrombus that is weeks or even months old. The echogenicity of thrombus is helpful in only two circumstances. Anechoic or very poorly echogenic thrombus can reliably be diagnosed as acute and usually is only days old. Highly echogenic material, on the other hand, represents scar that develops in unlysed thrombus. Everything in between is undefined with respect to age.

Decreased Thrombus and Vein Size

Retraction and lysis may noticeably reduce the size of thrombus during the subacute period, and this is especially noticeable on serial examinations (Fig. 24–5A and B). Decreased thrombus size may be evident both on short-axis views that show a decrease in vein diameter and on long-axis views that show a decrease in the linear extent of thrombus. With retraction and lysis of thrombus, the vein becomes less distended and returns to a normal caliber.

Adherence of Thrombus

Free-floating acute thrombus becomes attached to the vein wall during the acute period, and thrombus is not free-floating in the subacute period.

Resumption of Flow

When thrombus retracts and lyses, the lumen may be restored to patency and the resumption of blood flow is seen with color flow imaging (Fig. 24–5C and D). This does not necessarily mean that the vein will return to normal, however. Thickened walls and reduced vein caliber are common following venous thrombosis, and such changes may be permanent. In other cases, the vein may remain occluded.

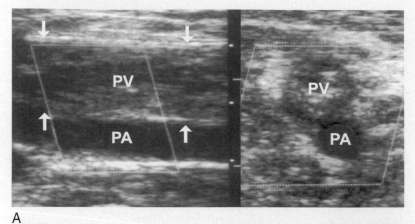

A

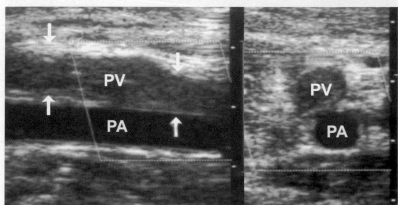

B

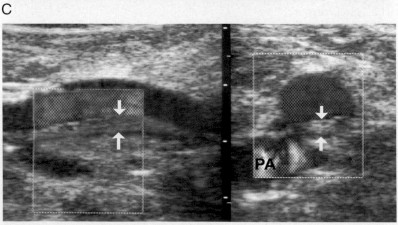

C

D

FIGURE 24–5. Changes in thrombus with time (long- and short-axis views). *A*, One-month-old thrombus within the popliteal vein (PV, *arrows*) is moderately echogenic, and the vein is substantially larger than the popliteal artery (PA). *B*, At 4 months, thrombus echogenicity is unchanged, but the size of the popliteal vein (*arrows*) has decreased and is about equal to the popliteal artery. *C*, At 11 months, substantial recanalization of the vein lumen (L) is evident in the popliteal vein (*arrows*). *D*, At 18 months, an echogenic area of scar (*arrows*) is all that remains at the site of popliteal vein thrombosis.

Collateralization

Collateral venous channels (see Fig. 24–4) continue to enlarge during the subacute phase and may become increasingly obvious sonographically.

The Chronic Phase

As noted in Chapter 22, the term *chronic thrombosis* is a misnomer: The proper term is *chronic post-thrombotic scarring*. Whereas *chronic* is not defined with respect to venous thrombosis, you could consider it to mean longer than 6 months after the acute episode. By this time, thrombus that has not lysed has been invaded by fibroblasts and is in the process of becoming organized as fibrous tissue that will persist indefinitely. Complete lysis of venous thrombus occurs in only about 20% of cases.[12] It is not surprising, therefore, that persistent abnormality is observed sonographically in many patients who have suffered venous thrombosis.[13] The following abnormalities may be seen in the chronic phase.[1,4,8,13–15]

Wall Thickening

Diffuse thickening of the vein wall (Fig. 24–5D and Fig. 24–6A) is a common chronic finding following venous thrombosis. The thick-walled, scarred vein also is reduced in caliber, and flow may be obstructed if the vein is small. The echogenicity of the thickened vein wall is variable but typically is less than that of muscle.

Echogenic Intraluminal Material

In many cases, post-thrombotic fibrous scars produce focal plaquelike areas along the vein wall that project into the vein lumen, as shown in Figure 24–6B. These areas may be quite echogenic (i.e., more echogenic than the adjacent muscle). In some cases, calcification may be present that produces focal strong reflections and acoustic shadows.

Another manifestation of chronic venous scarring is the formation of weblike synechiae that project into the vein lumen (Fig. 24–6C and D). Synechiae are formed from unlysed thrombus that is attached only along one side of the vein. The thrombus is gradually transformed into a fibrous band attached in the same location as the thrombus from which it arose.

Fibrous Cord

If the vein lumen does not recanalize but instead remains substantially narrowed or occluded, the vein may be reduced during the chronic period to an echogenic cord of much smaller diameter than a normal vein. A tiny residual lumen, or no lumen at all, may be present. In some cases, the scarred vein may disappear from view sonographically. It seems that one determinant of whether a vein recanalizes is the degree of adhesion of the thrombus to the vein wall. If the thrombus is adherent around its entire circumference, recanalization must occur in the center of the vessel. Unlysed residual thrombus subsequently is converted to a thickened fibrous vein wall, and the vein size is permanently reduced, as seen in Figure 24–6A. If recanalization does not occur in cases of diffusely adherent thrombus, the vein becomes a fibrotic cord. Alternatively, if the thrombus is attached only along one side of the vein, the lumen is more readily reestablished as the unlysed thrombus is converted to fibrous tissue only along the side where the thrombus adheres, as shown in Figure 24–6C and D.

Valve Abnormality

Thrombus is thought to commonly originate in the vicinity of valves. Considering this location and the fact that incomplete lysis and subsequent fibrosis are the rule, it is not surprising that valve damage is a frequent sequela of venous thrombosis. Valve damage is manifested by thickening of the cusps, adherence of the cusps to the vein wall, restricted cusp motion (Fig. 24–7), and failure of apposition of the cusps in the center of the vessel. The physiologic consequences of valve damage are reflux and persistent venous stasis that results from reflux-induced back-pressure. Valvular re-

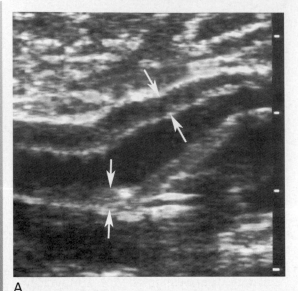

A

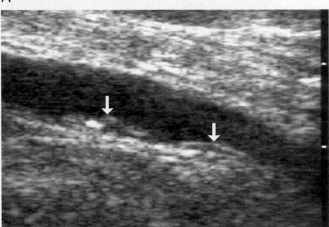

B

FIGURE 24–6. Chronic sequelae of venous thrombosis. *A*, Diffuse wall thickening (*arrows*) of up to 4 mm is seen in this popliteal vein. The appearance was stable over a 3-year period. *B*, Plaquelike scars (*arrows*) are present 2 years after an episode of thrombophlebitis. *C* and *D*, Weblike scars called synechiae (*arrows*) are shown in long- and short-axis views. (Images are from different patients, each about 1 year post-thrombophlebitis.)

flux is evident on the color flow image, in the audible Doppler signal, and on the Doppler spectrum display. Reflux may result in varicosities, which are abnormally large and tortuous veins; chronic edema; skin thickening and discoloration; and skin ulceration. Ultrasound assessment of these and other aspects of venous insufficiency is covered in detail in Chapter 26.

Doppler Flow Abnormalities

In addition to venous reflux, other Doppler flow abnormalities may be encountered with chronic venous thrombosis because of venous obstruction. These are lack of spontaneous flow, lack of phasicity, absence of

the Valsalva response, and subnormal or absent augmentation.[11]

SUPERFICIAL VERSUS DEEP VENOUS THROMBOSIS

It is important to differentiate between superficial and deep venous thrombosis (DVT). With superficial thrombosis, a palpable cord may be readily apparent in the subcutaneous tissues. On ultrasound examination, this cord reveals typical findings of venous thrombosis (Fig. 24–8). In the upper extremities, it is important to examine both the superficial and deep venous systems sonographically. In the lower extremity, however, the deep system is the primary

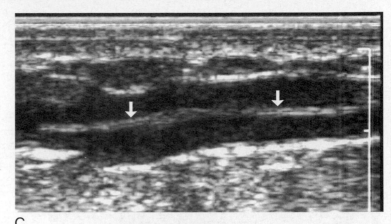

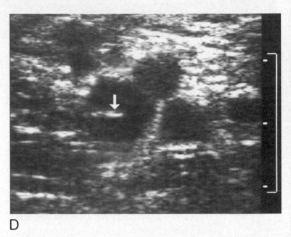

FIGURE 24–6—cont'd. See legend opposite.   C

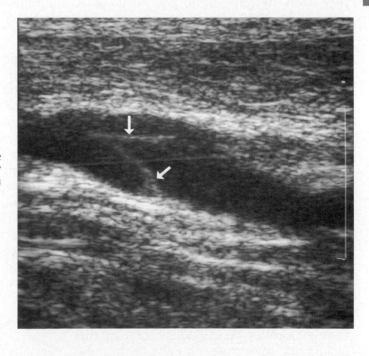

D

FIGURE 24–7. Immobile, or stuck, valve cusps (*arrows*) are embedded in recently formed thrombus, which is barely visible on this reproduction.

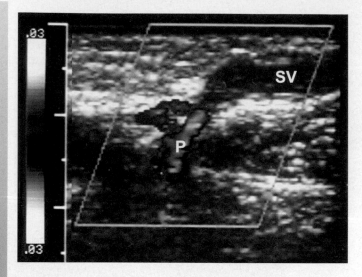

FIGURE 24–8. An acutely thrombosed superficial vein (SV) is visible just below the skin. This vein communicates with a patent perforator vein (P).

subject of ultrasound examination, and the superficial system is examined in detail only when symptoms or signs suggest thrombosis of this system.

Only supportive therapy is generally necessary when thrombus is confined to the superficial veins of the lower extremity. This is because there is risk of pulmonary embolization only when thrombus is present near the attachment of the greater or lesser saphenous veins to the deep system or when thrombus actually extends into the deep system from the saphenous veins. Superficial venous thrombosis can, however, be of clinical importance as a source of stasis problems and varicocities that can result from chronic superficial vein occlusion or valve damage.

DIAGNOSTIC PITFALLS

This section represents a catalog of mistakes or near-mistakes that we have made in the course of ultrasound venography. Fortunately, we have learned to avoid most of these errors through years of experience.

Suboptimal Image Quality

When the quality of the color flow image is suboptimal, it may be possible to confirm venous patency grossly, but nonocclusive thrombi cannot be excluded. Some of the factors that affect image quality are beyond the sonographer's control, such as obesity and soft-tissue edema, but many factors can be controlled by the sonographer, including the use of transducers with proper frequency, attention to instrument settings, and efforts to attain image planes that clearly delineate the veins. It is noteworthy that one of the reporting requirements of the vascular laboratory accrediting organizations listed in Chapter 23 concerns the quality of the examination. Venous ultrasound reports should clearly indicate the areas adequately visualized and should state whether technical problems, such as poor visualization, limit the diagnostic potential of the examination.

Compression Difficulties

The iliac veins cannot be examined with intermittent compression due to interference from abdominal contents. The adductor segment of the superficial femoral vein usually cannot be compressed due to resistance from the surrounding muscles. In addition, the proximal calf veins are difficult to compress in many patients because of muscular resistance. Compression difficulties can lead the unwary to a false-positive diagnosis of venous thrombosis, but this can be avoided with color flow demonstration of venous patency.

Mistaken Identity

Serious errors may occur if veins are misidentified. I have seen the long saphenous vein mistaken for the superficial femoral vein, the cephalic vein mistaken for the axillary vein, and the basilic vein mistaken for the brachial vein, as well as cases of mistaken vein identity in the calf. Misidentification of veins usually occurs when the technologist is inexperienced, when the technologist does not pay proper attention to venous anatomy, or when a large collateral is visualized and the occluded vein is overlooked. To prevent errors of identity, *always locate and document major anatomic landmarks* that confirm the identity of veins. (These landmarks have been described in preceding chapters.) In the deep system, be mindful that arteries should always be seen adjacent to the veins.

Duplication

Unrecognized venous duplication may be a source of diagnostic error when the patent member of the duplicated pair is identified and the occluded member is not. Venous duplication (Fig. 24–9) should be suspected in areas where duplication is common (brachial, superfical femoral, popliteal), when the visualized vein is smaller than normal (it is smaller because it is half of a pair), and whenever the location of a vein is atypical.

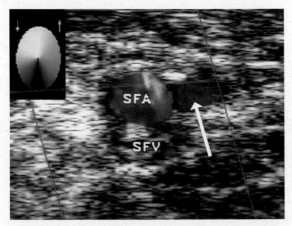

FIGURE 24–9. Duplicated superficial femoral vein (SFV). The main portion of the SFV is occluded by 2-month-old thrombus, but the vein is duplicated and the other branch (*arrow*) is patent. SFA, superficial femoral artery.

Assessment of Thrombus Age

Thrombus that is extremely fresh (a few days old) is easily recognized as acute on ultrasound examination because it is anechoic or poorly echogenic. Chronic, postthrombotic scar that is years old also is readily identified by its strong echogenicity. Between these extremes, the age of thrombus can be only broadly approximated. A practical approach to this problem is to always ask, "Does the appearance of thrombus correlate with the duration of the patient's symptoms?" The sonographic findings should be reported along similar lines; e.g., "moderately echogenic thrombus is present, consistent with a 2-week history of leg swelling." Even though the age of thrombus cannot be determined precisely with ultrasound, it is often possible to correlate its appearance with the duration of symptoms.

Recurrent Deep Venous Thrombosis

The residua of preceding episodes of DVT pose a significant limitation for ultrasound examination, because subacute or chronic vein wall thickening may mimic acute thrombosis. In a follow-up study of patients with DVT, Cronan and Leen[13] found persistent thrombus or wall thickening in 53% of extremities examined 6 to 31 months after the acute thrombotic episode. Furthermore, in many of these cases, it would not have been possible to differentiate between chronic abnormalities and those associated with more recent thrombosis.

In patients with prior venous thrombosis, an important indication that thrombosis is new is its detection in previously unaffected portions of the venous system. Unfortunately, one can recognize new thrombus in this way only if a good "road map" exists of the preceding episode of thrombosis, as illustrated in Figure 24–10. It is important for the technologist to accurately depict the location of thrombus on this road map. Of particular value is a *post-treatment road map*

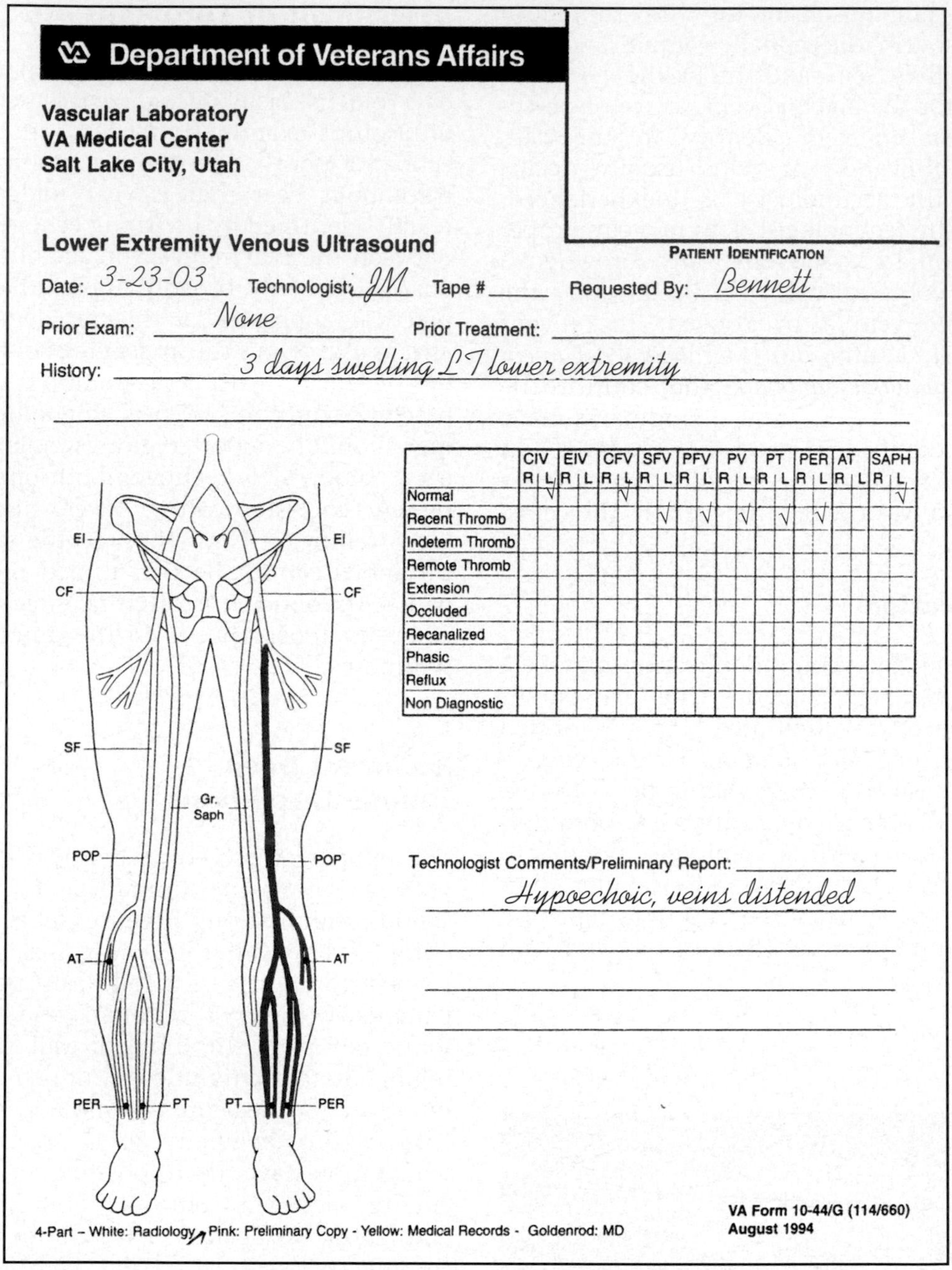

Department of Veterans Affairs

Vascular Laboratory
VA Medical Center
Salt Lake City, Utah

Lower Extremity Venous Ultrasound

PATIENT IDENTIFICATION

Date: 3-23-03   Technologist: JM   Tape # _____   Requested By: Bennett

Prior Exam: None   Prior Treatment: _____

History: 3 days swelling LT lower extremity

	CIV		EIV		CFV		SFV		PFV		PV		PT		PER		AT		SAPH	
	R	L	R	L	R	L	R	L	R	L	R	L	R	L	R	L	R	L	R	L
Normal		✓				✓														✓
Recent Thromb								✓		✓		✓		✓		✓				
Indeterm Thromb																				
Remote Thromb																				
Extension																				
Occluded																				
Recanalized																				
Phasic																				
Reflux																				
Non Diagnostic																				

EI — EI
CF — CF
SF — SF
Gr. Saph
POP — POP
AT — AT
PER — PT   PT — PER

Technologist Comments/Preliminary Report: _____
Hypoechoic, veins distended

4-Part – White: Radiology, Pink: Preliminary Copy - Yellow: Medical Records - Goldenrod: MD

VA Form 10-44/G (114/660)
August 1994

A

FIGURE 24–10. Thrombosis "road maps." Diagrams showing the extent of thrombus are made routinely in our department. In this hypothetical example, *A* shows the initial extent of thrombus, and *B* shows the extent of organizing thrombus at the end of anticoagulant therapy.

obtained 3 to 6 months after an episode of DVT, showing areas that are or are not patent and the locations of unlysed thrombus.

We do not have the benefit of a post-therapy baseline in many patients who present with recurrent DVT, because they were treated previously in other institutions. And even when we have a baseline, we sometimes cannot differentiate between old and new thrombus. In such cases, we are forced to resort to contrast venog-

FIGURE 24–10—cont'd. See legend opposite.

raphy, which also may be of limited diagnostic value in patients with recurrent DVT. Magnetic resonance venography has yet to be proven of value in differentiating between recent and remote thrombus.

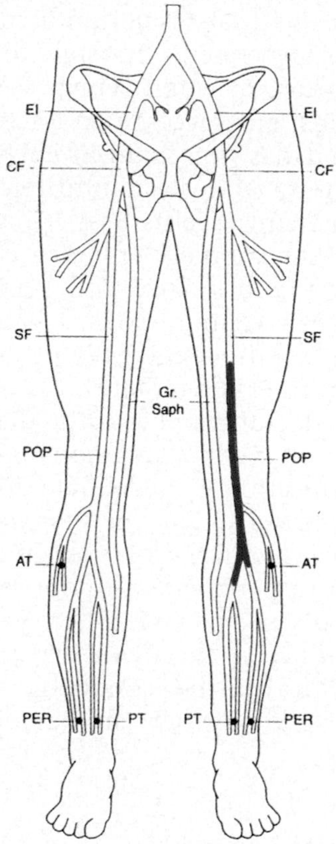

Improper Use of the Color Flow Image

Color flow scanning is a valuable asset in venous imaging, but it may be a source of misdiagnosis if used improperly. If the sensitivity or gain levels of the Doppler image are set too high, color "blooming" occurs, causing the flow information to bleed into the B-mode image. Small or even moderately sized thrombi may be obscured by blooming. Conversely, false-positive diagnosis of thrombus may occur if spurious flow voids are generated by an improper gain setting, an inadequate Doppler angle, or the use of the wrong velocity range.

Poor Venous Distention and Reduced Flow

The final pitfall to be considered is suboptimal venous distention. We have occasionally encountered patients without prior venous disease who were ideal candidates for ultrasound venography, yet visualization of the calf veins was extremely limited because of small vein caliber. This problem may be caused by vasoconstriction, which may result from an excessively cool examining room or a lack of dependency of the limb. In other instances, the lack of venous distention may be a result of hypovolemia. In still other instances, we have no explanation for the lack of venous distention.

The sonographer should do everything possible to distend the leg veins. Examination in a sitting position can be especially helpful for distending the calf veins.

REPORTED ACCURACY

Iliofemoral and Popliteal Regions

A large volume of data is available that attests to the accuracy of ultrasound for diagnosis of DVT in the iliofemoral and popliteal areas.[3–8,14,16–22] These data leave little or no doubt that sonography of the femoral and popliteal veins is highly reliable in symptomatic patients. Sensitivity and specificity for acute symptomatic DVT exceed 90% in most studies and approach 100% in some series.

Calf Veins

Sonography is also highly accurate for the diagnosis of acute calf venous thrombosis in *symptomatic* patients, *when the calf veins can be seen adequately.* In this circumstance, sensitivity and specificity are reported to exceed 90%.[4,8,21–23] The term *adequate visualization* is of great importance, however. In our patient population, all three pairs of calf veins can be seen adequately in only about 60% of patients, which is similar to success rates reported by others in the medical literature (range, 60%–90%).[8,23–26] Furthermore, it seems that visualization rates are population dependent. In spite of ultrasound instrument improvement over the past 15 years, our success rate for calf vein visualization has not changed appreciably. The use of intravenously administered ultrasound-enhancing agents (see Chapter 4) appears to substantially enhance calf vein visualization and reduce the number of indeterminate examinations,[26] but these agents are expensive and presently are not available in the United States.

It is well documented that the diagnostic results of calf vein sonography are poor when visualization is inadequate. However, the good news is that the *specificity* and *positive predictive value* of sonography are high, even in patients with poor visualization.[27–35] This means that when veins will not compress, or when you see thrombus directly, you can be confident of your diagnosis, and further studies are not needed.

Results in Asymptomatic Patients

It must be emphasized that the excellent published results for venous sonography refer principally to symptomatic patients. Subsequent to the glowing initial reports, it was noted that sonography was generally less accurate in asymptomatic patients than in symptomatic individuals.[24,27–35] Sonographic accuracy seems to be particularly poor in postoperative joint replacement patients, in whom sensitivity ranges from 25% to 77% overall and from 11% to 54%

for calf vein thrombi.[21,22,27–35],* Furthermore, the results of recently published articles are no better than those published in the late 1980s and early 1990s.

There are three main reasons that ultrasound results are relatively poor in asymptomatic patients.[36–38] First, small, localized, nonocclusive thrombi are more prevalent in asymptomatic patients, as compared with symptomatic individuals, who tend to have large, segmental thrombi (e.g., the entire superficial femoral vein). Second, in some asymptomatic patient populations, the prevalence of isolated calf vein thrombosis, which is inherently difficult to detect, is substantially greater than in symptomatic patients. (This has not been observed universally.[39,40]) Because the examination success rate in the calf is relatively poor, the sensitivity for isolated calf vein thrombus is reduced accordingly. Finally, the clarity of vein visualization may be poor in certain asymptomatic cohorts, such as postoperative orthopedic patients who have considerable leg edema.

The bright side of ultrasound examination in asymptomatic patients is a high level of specificity. I have yet to read a published study with an ultrasound specificity of less than 90%. As noted previously, this means that when you see acute thrombus, you can be confident in your diagnosis. It also means that the use of ultrasound as an initial examination tool for asymptomatic patients has merit. If thrombus is seen, then treatment may be initiated. If not, it may be advisable to proceed to other studies, such as contrast venography.

Upper Extremity Veins

The use of ultrasound venography in the upper extremities has increased substantially during the past decade, largely due to more frequent uses of indwelling upper exteremity catheters for intravenous therapy. Such catheters are a significant risk factor for thrombophlebitis. In hospitalized children, thrombosis occurs more commonly in upper extremity veins than in lower extremity veins.[41,42]

Although the overall incidence of upper extremity venous thrombosis remains low in hospital patients (< 1/1000 patients), the incidence is high in patients with upper extremity symptoms, such as pain and swelling.[41,43,44] In these patients, thrombophlebitis is found to be the cause in about 40% of cases.[43]

Fortunately, ultrasound is a very effective means of diagnosis of *symptomatic* upper extremity venous thrombosis, with reported sensitivity and specificity in the range of 82% to 100%.[45,46] Furthermore, the great majority of upper extremity venous examinations are technically successful in our experience and in that of others.[47]

The bad news about upper extremity venous sonography potentially concerns *asymptomatic* patients, in whom there appears to be a large problem with false-negative examinations. An article by Male and colleagues[42] reports only 35% sensitivity for ultrasound detection of asymptomatic thrombi in pediatric patients as compared with contrast venography. Almost all of the undetected thrombi were nonocclusive and located in the central veins or superior vena cava, where sonographic visualization was not possible. Although this is only one report based on a specific patient population, caution is advised in the use of sonography to search for asymptomatic upper extremity thrombosis.

VENOUS ULTRASOUND CONTROVERSIES

Over the years that venous sonography has been used clinically, a number of controversial issues have arisen regarding the clinical applications of this diagnostic technique. These important controversies are addressed in Chapter 25.

References

1. Talbot SR: B-mode evaluation of peripheral veins. Semin Ultrasound CT MR 9:295–319, 1988.

---

*The exception is a report of 92% sensitivity for asymptomatic calf vein thrombi.[24]

2. Effeney DJ, Friedman MB, Gooding GAW: Iliofemoral venous thrombosis: Real-time ultrasound diagnosis, normal criteria, and clinical application. Radiology 150:787–792, 1984.

3. Sullivan ED, Peters BS, Cranley JJ: Real-time B-mode venous ultrasound. J Vasc Surg 1:465–471, 1984.

4. Oliver MA: Duplex scanning in venous disease. Bruit IX:206–209, 1985.

5. Raghavendra BN, Horii SC, Hilton S, et al: Deep venous thrombosis: Detection by probe compression of veins. J Ultrasound Med 5:89–95, 1986.

6. Dauzat MM, Laroche JP, Charras C, et al: Real-time B-mode ultrasonography for better specialty in the noninvasive diagnosis of deep venous thrombosis. J Ultrasound Med 5:625–631, 1986.

7. Cronan JJ, Dorfman GS, Scola FH, et al: Deep venous thrombosis: US assessment using vein compression. Radiology 162:191–194, 1987.

8. Vogel P, Laing FRC, Jeffrey RB, et al: Deep venous thrombosis of the lower extremity: US evaluation. Radiology 163:747–751, 1987.

9. Zwiebel WJ, Priest DL: Color-duplex sonography of extremity veins. Semin Ultrasound CT MR 11:136–167, 1990.

10. Schroder WB, Bealer JF: Venous duplex ultrasonography causing acute pulmonary embolism: A brief report. J Vasc Surg 15:1082–1083, 1992.

11. Barnes RW: Doppler techniques for lower-extremity venous disease. In Zwiebel WJ (ed): Introduction to Vascular Ultrasonography. Philadelphia, Grune & Stratton, 1986, pp 333–350.

12. Hirsh J, Genton E, Hall R: Venous thromboembolism. New York, Grune & Stratton, 1981, pp 1–4.

13. Cronan JJ, Leen V: Recurrent deep venous thrombosis: Limitations of US. Radiology 170:739–742, 1989.

14. Appelman PT, De Jong TE, Lampmann LE: Deep venous thrombosis of the leg: US findings. Radiology 163:743–746, 1987.

15. Zwiebel WJ: Sources of error in duplex venography and an algorithmic approach to the diagnosis of deep venous thrombosis. Semin Ultrasound CT MR 9:286–294, 1988.

16. O'Leary DO, Kane R, Pinel D, et al: A prospective study of the efficacy of B-scan sonography in the detection of deep venous thrombosis in the lower extremity. Presented at the American Institute of Ultrasound in Medicine Annual Convention, Las Vegas, NV, September 16–19, 1986.

17. Nix ML, Nelson CL, Harmon BH, et al: Duplex venous scanning: Image vs. Doppler accuracy. Presented at the Eleventh Annual Meeting of the Society of Vascular Technology, Chicago, IL, June 8–12, 1988.

18. Lensing AWA, Prandoni P, Brandjes D, et al: Detection of deep-vein thrombosis by real-time B-mode ultrasonography. N Engl J Med 320:341–345, 1989.

19. Foley WD, Middleton WD, Lawson TL, et al: Color Doppler ultrasound imaging of lower-extremity venous disease. Am J Roentgenol 152:371–376, 1989.

20. Rose SC, Zwiebel WJ, Murdock LE, et al: Insensitivity of color Doppler flow imaging for detection of acute calf deep venous thrombosis in asymptomatic postoperative patients. J Vasc Interv Rad 4:111–117, 1993.

21. Polak JF, Culter SS, O'Leary DH: Deep vein of the calf: Assessment with color Doppler flow imaging. Radiology 171:481–485, 1989.

22. Comeroto AJ, Katz ML, Hasheim MA: Venous duplex imaging for the diagnosis of acute deep venous thrombosis. Hemostasis 23(suppl 1): 61–71, 1993.

23. Semrow CM, Friedell ML, Buchbinder D, et al: The efficacy of ultrasonic venography in the detection of calf vein thrombosis. Presented at the Tenth Annual Meeting of the Society of Non-Invasive Vascular Technology, Toronto, Canada, June 4–6, 1987.

24. Atri M, Herba MK, Reinhold C, et al: Accuracy of sonography in the evaluation of calf deep vein thrombosis in both postoperative surveillance and symptomatic patients. Am J Roentgenol 166:1361–1367, 1996.

25. Rose SC, Zwiebel WJ, Nelson BD, et al: Symptomatic lower extremity deep venous thrombosis: Accuracy, limitations, and role of color Doppler flow imaging in diagnosis. Radiology 175:639–644, 1990.

26. Bucek RA, Kos T, Schober E, et al: Ultrasound with Levovist in the diagnosis of suspected calf vein thrombosis. Ultrasound Med Biol 27:455–460, 2001

27. Dauzat MM, Laroche JP, Charras C, et al: Real-time B-mode ultrasonography for better specificity in the noninvasive diagnosis of deep venous thrombosis. J Ultrasound Med 5:625–631, 1986.

28. Borris LC, Christiansen JM, Lassen MR, et al: Comparison of real-time B-mode ultrasonography and bilateral ascending phlebography for detection of postoperative deep vein thrombosis following elective hip surgery. Thromb Haemost 61:363–365, 1989.

29. Manninen R, Manninen H, Soimakallio S, et al: Asymptomatic deep venous thrombosis in the calf: Accuracy and limitations of ultrasonography as a screening test after total knee arthroplasty. Br J Radiol 66:199–202, 1993.

30. Yucel EK, Fisher JS, Egglin TK, et al: Isolated calf venous thrombosis: Diagnosis with compression US. Radiology 179:443–446, 1991.

31. Midgette AS, Stuikel TA, Littenberg F: A meta-analytic method for summarizing diagnostic test performance: Receiver-operating-characteristic-summary point estimates. Med Decis Making 13:253–257, 1993.

32. Agnelli G, Volpato R, Radicchia S, et al: Detection of asymptomatic deep vein thrombosis by real-time B-mode ultrasonography in hip surgery patient. Thromb Haemost 68:257–260, 1992.

33. Lensing AW, Doris CI, McGrath FP, et al: A comparison of compression ultrasound with color Doppler ultrasound for the diagnosis of symptomless postoperative deep vein thrombosis. Arch Intern Med 157:765–768, 1997.

34. Lausen I, Jensen R, Wille-Jorgensen P: Colour Doppler flow imaging ultrasonography versus venography as screening method for asymptomatic postoperative deep venous thrombosis. Eur J Radiol 20:200–204, 1995.

35. Westrich GH, Allen ML, Tarantino SJ, et al: Ultrasound screening for deep venous thrombosis after total knee arthroplasty: 2-year reassessment. Clin Orthop 356:125–133, 1998.

36. Cogo A, Lensing AW, Prandoni B, Hirsh J: Distribution of thrombosis in patients with symptomatic deep vein thrombosis. Arch Intern Med 153:2777–2780, 1993.

37. Markel A, Manzo RA, Bergelin RO, Strandness DE: Pattern and distribution of thrombi in acute venous thrombosis. Arch Surg 127:305–309, 1992.

38. Rose SC, Zwiebel WJ, Miller FJ: Distribution of acute lower extremity deep venous thrombosis in symptomatic and asymptomatic patients: Imaging implications. J Ultrasound Med 13:243–250, 1994.

39. Hill SL, Holtzman GI, Martin D, et al: The origin of lower extremity deep vein thrombi in acute venous thrombosis. Am J Surg 173:485–490, 1997.

40. Flinn WR, Sandager GP, Silva MB Jr, et al: Prospective surveillance for perioperative venous thrombosis. Experience in 2643 patients. Arch Surg 131:472–480, 1996.

41. Chan AK, Deveber G, Monagle P, et al: Venous thrombosis in children. J Thromb Haemost 1:1443–1455, 2003.

42. Male C, Chait P, Ginsberg JS, et al: Comparison of venography and ultrasound for the diagnosis of asymptomatic deep vein thrombosis in the upper body in children: Results of the PARKAA study. Prophylactic Antithrombin Replacement in Kids with ALL treated with Asparaginase. Thromb Haemost 87:593–598, 2002.

43. Kroger K, Schelo C, Gocke C, Rudofsky G: Colour Doppler sonographic diagnosis of upper limb venous thromboses. Clin Sci (Lond) 94:657–661, 1998.

44. Mustafa S, Stein PD, Patel KC, et al: Upper extremity deep venous thrombosis. Chest 123:1953–1956, 2003.

45. Baxter GM, Kincaid W, Jeffrey RF, et al: Comparison of colour Doppler ultrasound with venography in the diagnosis of axillary and subclavian vein thrombosis. Br J Radiol 64:777–781, 1991.

46. Koksoy C, Kuzu A, Kutlay J: The diagnostic value of colour Doppler ultrasound in central venous catheter related thrombosis. Clin Radiol 50:687–689, 1995.

47. Baarslag HJ, van Beek EJ, Koopman MM, Reekers JA: Prospective study of color duplex ultrasonography compared with contrast venography in patients suspected of having deep venous thrombosis of the upper extremities. Ann Intern Med 136:865–872, 2002.

Chapter 25

Controversies in Venous Ultrasound

John J. Cronan, MD

Practice patterns in the past decade have defined venous ultrasound as the initial diagnostic modality to assess for deep venous thrombosis (DVT). There are many unexplored ideas and also very novel concepts that have developed as venous ultrasound has become universally utilized. This chapter reviews new, and sometimes controversial, principles that are integral to understanding and utilizing venous ultrasound in clinical practice.

THE ROLE OF THE UNILATERAL VENOUS ULTRASOUND EXAMINATION IN THE PATIENT WITH UNILATERAL SYMPTOMS

In the era of venography, when the radiologist was requested to evaluate a patient for acute DVT, only the leg in question was studied.[1] Because of the risk of reactions to intravenous contrast material and the invasiveness of venography, the asymptomatic leg was not studied. Historically, noninvasive vascular laboratories employing plethymsography routinely evaluated both the symptomatic and the asymptomatic leg. These laboratories, which are usually directed by surgeons, not radiologists, utilized the information obtained from the asymptomatic leg as a frame of reference to help diagnose any thrombus that might be present in the symptomatic leg. Following the introduction of venous ultrasound, radiologists continued to evaluate only the symptomatic leg. Alternatively, many vascular laboratories, which had developed a pattern of noninvasively evaluating both the symptomatic and the asymptomatic leg, continued this practice as the transition occurred from plethysmography to venous ultrasound.

Contemporary reports in the literature regarding the need to evaluate the asymptomatic leg are conflicting. Of interest, until 1995, a Correct Procedural Terminology (CPT) code existed only to evaluate bilateral lower extremities. In 1995, a code for a unilateral or limited examination of the leg was provided (CPT 93971). Also in 1995, the Intersocietal Commission for Accreditation of Vascular Laboratories (ICAVL) acknowledged the need for limited unilateral studies with the publication of revised guidelines. Up until that modification, the Intersocietal Commission for Accreditation of Vascular Labor had indicated that an examination of a symptomatic extremity also required a study of the asymptomatic leg.

Controversy exists regarding the importance and frequency of finding thrombus in the asymptomatic leg.[2,3] Historically, the literature has indicated that the asymptomatic leg does not harbor thrombus. More recently, articles have been published suggesting that thrombus can be found in the asymptomatic leg, but the frequency of this finding in a patient with a negative evaluation of the symptomatic leg occurred in less than 1% of cases.[1,4–6] Certainly, finding thrombus in the asymptomatic leg of a patient with thrombus in the symptomatic leg will not alter treatment. The likelihood of finding thrombus solely in the asymptomatic leg is between 0% and 1%. I suggest that this low frequency of thrombus does not justify a routine evaluation of the asymptomatic leg in a patient presenting with a symptomatic extremity.

BILATERAL SYMPTOMS: THE ROLE OF THE BILATERAL VENOUS EXAMINATION

As discussed previously, the situation of a patient presenting with bilateral lower leg swelling or bilateral leg pain would have been handled in the era of venography with reevaluation of the patient or, more likely, with a contrast venogram of only one extremity. It has been suggested that most of these patients have cardiac disease or peripheral vascular disease as the dominant cause of their swelling.[6] However, a recent article presents an alternative opinion, suggesting that a significant percentage of these patients harbor lower extremity venous thrombus.[5]

Certainly, the important factor to consider is the subgroup of patients with bilateral swelling who would be risk factors.[1] If a patient has a significant underlying risk for DVT, such as malignancy, then the bilateral examination should be performed. If there are no risk factors for DVT, the first assumption should be that the patient has heart disease or underlying peripheral vascular disease as the cause of the bilateral leg swelling. The probability of finding thrombus in the leg is related to the presence of risk factors for DVT. In the absence of any risk factors for DVT, it is unusual to find extremity thrombus. It has been stated that the majority of patients with DVT have one or more recognized risk factors.[7]

THE EXTENT OF THE ULTRASOUND EXAMINATION: HOW MUCH NEEDS TO BE STUDIED?

Proper technique for ultrasound evaluation of the vein, as stated both in the American College of Radiology standards in 1993 (revised in 2001) and by the Intersocietal Commission for Accreditation of Vascular Laboratories, indicates that a patient with a symptomatic extremity should be evaluated from the level of the inguinal ligament to the popliteal fossa in as continuous a manner as possible (Fig. 25–1).[8]

Recently, it has been demonstrated that *symptomatic* patients have lengthy thrombi involving one or more venous segments.[9,10] Symptomatic thrombus involves multiple venous segments and is different from that which develops in the asymptomatic high-risk patients, in whom thrombus often develops focally on valve cusps in the calf.[11] This observation was demonstrated on retrospective review of venograms and has been confirmed in our ultrasound laboratory. We demonstrated that in approximately 99% of symptomatic cases, evaluation of the femoral or popliteal vein, employing the "two-point" compression

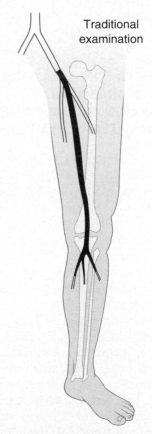

FIGURE 25–1. Topographic delineation of the lower extremity venous system as examined in routine evaluation.

technique, would detect thrombus that extends above the knee. This two-point evaluation requires only examination of the common femoral and popliteal venous areas (Fig. 25–2).[12]

This very abbreviated study detects a high percentage of cases with DVT. The overall decrease in the examination time is slightly in excess of 50%. The potential of the two-point technique has been confirmed by others who have demonstrated that approximately 95.4% of thrombus would be detected using a two-point compression technique.[13] Obviously, there is some degree of compromise with the two-point technique, balancing simplicity versus accuracy. This limited-compression technique is not the accepted standard but would have utility in the emergency department or when evaluating the patient with extremely restricted mobility. When unable to evaluate the entire leg, this "two-point" technique provides a high degree of certainty.

SIGNIFICANCE OF A NEGATIVE ULTRASOUND EXAMINATION

Evidence exists that a negative compression ultrasound study of a symptomatic lower extremity, employing complete evaluation of both the femoral and popliteal veins, provides sufficient validation to withhold anticoagulation.[4,14] The need for any follow-up studies in these cases is somewhat less well defined, but the evidence suggests that if the patient remains symptomatic, a repeat study of the lower extremity should be performed 3 to 5 days after the initial examination. In rare cases, small focal calf thrombi might propagate upward in this time frame and cause symptoms. As will be mentioned in the next section, the potential for direct evaluation of the calf veins needs to be considered as a more direct approach to immediate diagnosis.

CALF VEIN THROMBOSIS

The clinical acceptance of venous ultrasound as a diagnostic technique in the evaluation of the symptomatic patient occurred based on clinical series that did not attempt direct evaluation of calf veins. The initial reports and literature were based only on evaluation of the femoral and popliteal veins. It was with this examination format that the compression ultrasound examination was acknowledged as clinically useful.[15] Although calf thrombi are common, they rarely cause clinical problems and usually do not produce extensive clinical symptoms.

Eighty-eight percent of calf thrombus occurs in the asymptomatic patient, and this accounts for 50% of thrombi in the asymptomatic population. Similarly, the presence of calf thrombus is unlikely to lead to clinically significant pulmonary embolus (PE).[16] As pointed out by Moser and LeMoine,[17] patients with calf thrombus are

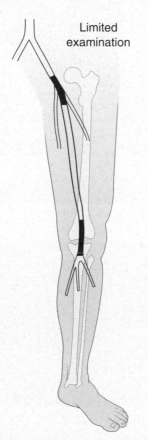

FIGURE 25–2. Proposed "two-point" lower extremity venous evaluation.

Limited examination

unlikely to have signs or symptoms of PE. Pulmonary embolism that originates from the calf is usually asymptomatic. Alternatively, patients with above-knee thrombus have PE in more than 50% of cases, despite the fact that they may not have any signs or symptoms of this phenomenon and evidence of PE is detected only on ventilation/perfusion scans or pulmonary arteriograms.[18–20]

If thrombus is isolated to the calf veins, it is perceived that upward propagation into the popliteal veins eventually occurs in approximately 20% of cases.[21–23] The poten-

tial exists to detect this propagating thrombus when it enters the popliteal veins if serial studies are performed at 3- to 5-day intervals (Fig. 25–3).[16] However, based on technical success in evaluating the calf veins, there has been an impetus to employ direct evaluation of the calf veins, which is now technically possible. This permits the diagnosis or exclusion of calf thrombus on the day of clinical presentation. Clinical series have suggested that ultrasound evaluation of the calf veins in both the symptomatic and the asymptomatic patient is as accurate as evaluating above-knee veins.[24]

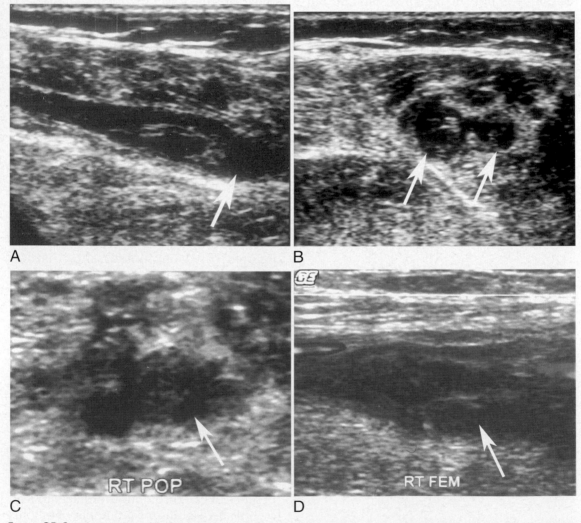

FIGURE 25–3. Propagation of calf vein thrombus. Long-axis (*A*) and short-axis (*B*) views of a distended, thrombus-filled gastrocnemius vein (*arrows*). The popliteal and femoral veins were normal. *C*, Compression of the popliteal (POP) vein (*arrow*) 12 days later demonstrates the presence of acute thrombus. *D*, The femoral (FEM) vein (*arrow*) now is also filled with thrombus, which has propagated upward from the calf.

Therapeutic management of patients with documented calf thrombus is debatable. Some suggest that observation of the thrombus with serial ultrasound studies is all that is necessary. A second examination, performed at 3 to 5 days from the baseline study, detects upward propagation of thrombus into the popliteal system, and if this occurs, treatment begins. However, there is now convincing evidence that calf thrombus does contribute to subclinical pulmonary embolism.[17-20]

Another issue that may strongly endorse the importance of evaluating the calf veins and treating calf thrombus relates to the development of chronic venous insufficiency. Most venous valves are located below the knee. If thrombus develops in the calf area, this could lead to destruction of the valves and initiate chronic venous insufficiency. Therefore, logic strongly endorses direct evaluation of the calf veins to search for thrombus. Detection of thrombus permits treatment to be initiated so that the extent of valve destruction in the calf veins is minimized.

This belief that calf thrombus does embolize and produces valve destruction is a forceful argument to support early diagnosis and treatment of thrombus isolated to calf veins.[21-24] If a patient has signs or symp-toms of calf thrombus, venous ultrasound of the calf should be performed.[25] Detection of thrombosis in the deep calf veins should prompt initiation of treatment.

COMPRESSION ULTRASOUND CAUSING PULMONARY EMBOLUS

Compression ultrasound has always had the potential to break off thrombus in the femoral vein and lead to pulmonary embolization. While this has been a theoretical consideration, only recently have several reports surfaced noting that patients who had diagnostic compression ultrasound were subsequently found to have developed PE.[26,27] The temporal relationship of the ultrasound examination to the actual occurrence of PE is somewhat uncertain. This is particularly noteworthy given the fact that patients with above-knee DVT have clinically unsuspected PE in greater than 50% of cases.[14] It should be noted that the risks of compression ultrasound are quite small if one takes care to avoid excessive venous compression and manipulation of the vein beyond that which is necessary for diagnosis. When concerns are raised about the risk for causing PE, the

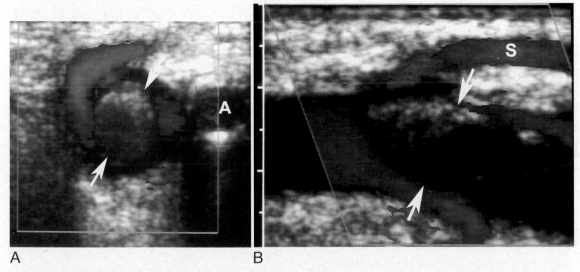

A   B

FIGURE 25-4. Short-axis (A) and long-axis (B) views showing free-floating thrombus (*arrows*) in the femoral vein at the level of the saphenous vein inflow (S). Caution should be exercised when applying compression to the veins. A, femoral artery.

scenario typically involves free-floating thrombus in the upper femoral vein (Fig. 25–4), which is at particularly great risk of embolization.

DVT IN OCCULT MALIGNANCY

Trousseau's sign concerns hypercoagulability associated with cancer and is based on the finding of spontaneous venous thrombosis in patients with underlying malignancy. When patients present with DVT and have no known risk factors, there is an underlying concern that they may indeed have an occult malignancy. Several published series have looked at this issue and observed a 10% to 34% incidence of cancer developing in patients who lack any apparent cause for thrombosis.[28–31] The controversy regarding the actual percentage of patients with underlying malignancy is less important. The real issue is that all sources support a causal relationship. DVT associated with malignancy tends to be much more extensive and aggressive than DVT in the nonmalignant setting.[32] The clinical examination demonstrates an extremity that is very swollen and painful (Fig. 25–5).

Controversy also exists regarding whether a diagnostic workup should be initiated following documentation of DVT in a patient without risk factors (Fig. 25–6). There is evidence to indicate that a workup searching for occult malignancy is not cost effective and that the cancers are already metastatic.[33] Alternatively, there is an opinion that an aggressive workup is warranted in these situations.[34,35] Patients with DVT related to Trousseau's syndrome usually clinically manifest the cancer within 1 to 2 years. Malignancies associated with venous thrombosis typically arise in the breast, the gastrointestinal or genitourinary tracts, the lung, and the brain. Of note, if a patient presents with recurrent episodes of DVT and has no known risk factors, the risk of an underlying malignancy is markedly increased.[34]

ULTRASOUND FOR THE ASSESSMENT OF PULMONARY EMBOLUS

Clinicians have developed a reluctance to perform pulmonary angiography to confirm or exclude the presence of PE. The workup of PE, therefore, often terminates following an indeterminate ventilation/perfusion (V/Q) lung scan result. After a ventilation/perfusion scan, 75% of patients fail to fit into a normal- or high-probability category for PE, and thus, the potential for PE remains uncertain.[36,37] Because the majority of PEs are felt to originate from the lower extremity, a teleological assessment employing noninvasive venous imaging to clarify an indeterminate lung scan or to confirm that a clinical impression of PE has then been utilized.[38] By establishing the presence of thrombus in the lower extremity, adequate therapy could be initiated, as the treatment for DVT and PE is essentially the same (i.e., anticoagulation). However, it has been observed for several decades that even when bilateral venography is employed, nearly a third of patients who have documented PE will not demonstrate any thrombus in the lower extremities.[14] Hence, *a negative lower extremity venous ultrasound study cannot exclude PE.* This is an important concept to convey to the clinician, as he or she should not terminate consideration of PE based on a negative noninvasive

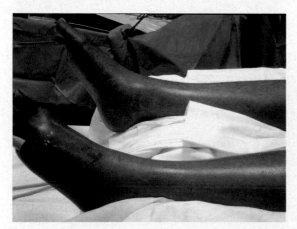

Figure 25–5. Malignancy-induced venous thrombosis is often associated with extreme leg swelling and a tense appearance.

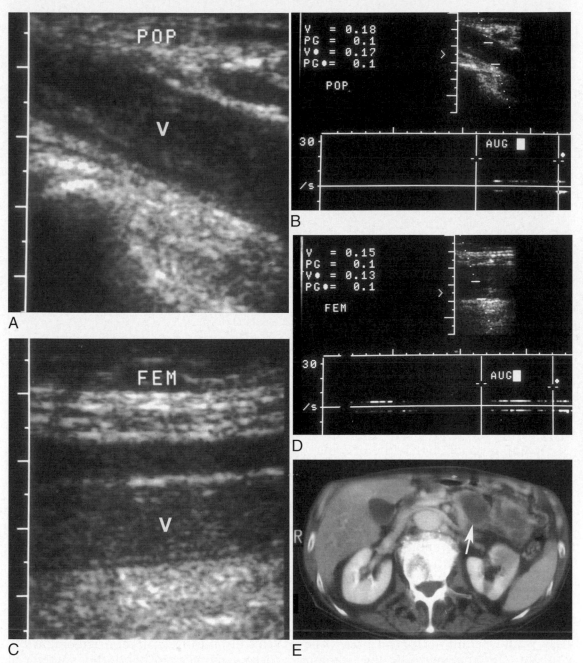

FIGURE 25–6. A patient without a known history of malignancy presents with a tensely swollen extremity, which demonstrates occlusion of all the veins. *A*, The popliteal (POP) vein (V) is markedly distended with occlusive thrombus. *B*, Pulsed Doppler indicates absence of flow in the popliteal vein. *C* and *D*, Likewise, the entire femoral (FEM) vein (V) is occluded by thrombus. *E*, CT image obtained several days after the venous examination demonstrates a 5-cm pancreatic tail mass (*arrow*). This was biopsied and yielded adenocarcinoma of the pancreas.

study if there is a strong clinical suspicion for PE. Similarly, the value of employing lower extremity venous ultrasound in the absence of leg symptoms, to diagnose PE, is questionable.[39–41]

The venous ultrasound examination of the lower extremity in a setting of possible PE should be focused. In the absence of any symptoms or signs in the lower extremities, only the femoral-popliteal system needs

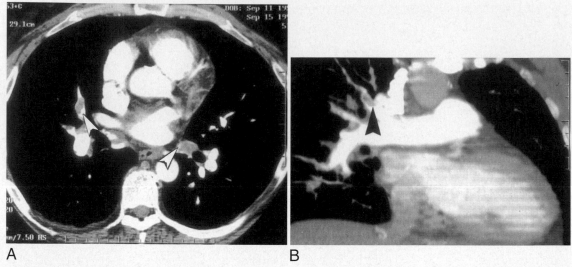

FIGURE 25–7. Pulmonary thromboembolus. A middle-age man presented with leg pain and swelling. Ultrasound (not shown) demonstrated acute thrombus in the right femoral vein. *A,* The onset of chest pain the same day led to CT pulmonary angiography, which confirmed pulmonary embolization (*arrowheads*). *B,* This reformatted coronal CT image shows acute thrombus in the right pulmonary artery (*arrowhead*).

to be evaluated. As discussed in the calf section, symptomatic PE from calf thrombus is very rare. Also, asymptomatic legs rarely harbor thrombus.

A recent proposal has been to employ spiral computed tomography (CT) in the workup of PE and to complement pulmonary contrast spiral CT with compression ultrasound (Fig. 25–7).[42,43] The suggestion has been made that if a patient presents with symptoms of DVT and PE, ultrasound of the lower extremities should be obtained first. If the test is positive for thrombus, treatment for venous thromboembolic disease should be initiated. A negative venous ultrasound study would permit anticoagulation to be withheld. Alternatively, if the patient presented with symptoms of PE, a multidetector CT scan would be done initially; if that test's results were negative, ultrasound could then be done to determine whether there was thrombus in the lower extremities. Either a multidetector CT scan demonstrating pulmonary artery thrombus or compression ultrasound demonstrating lower extremity DVT would permit treatment to be started. Negative studies would permit anticoagulation to be withheld.[44]

There is clearly a move to reassess the diagnostic methods of evaluating for PE. This new approach, using multidetector CT and compression ultrasound, indicates that clinicians are searching for an alternative to pulmonary angiography and to the ventilation/perfusion scan.

CONFUSING TERMINOLOGY

Proper anatomic terminology in the venous system is important because many primary care physicians misconstrue examination reports generated by radiologists. Radiologists have often identified the veins distal to the common femoral as the "deep femoral vein" and the "superficial femoral vein." This can create confusion, as *the superficial femoral vein* is actually a *component of the deep venous system.* A thrombus in this location requires treatment. When this venous segment is labeled as "superficial," a clinician unfamiliar with the terminology might assume that it is not an important vein (because it is a superficial vein) and decide not to initiate treatment.

The suggestion has been made that the femoral vein be called the femoral vein

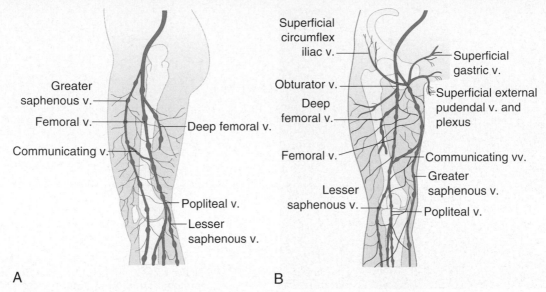

FIGURE 25–8. Correct terminology. Avoid reference to the femoral vein as "superficial." Lateral (A) and anterior (B) lower extremity views illustrating preferred terminology.

throughout its length (Fig. 25–8).[45] A permissible alternative is to refer to that portion of the femoral vein below the inguinal ligament and prior to the bifurcation as the common femoral vein. This is certainly worth pondering, as it would be unfortunate for a casual definition of venous anatomy to prevent a patient from being appropriately treated.

RISK FACTORS FOR DEEP VENOUS THROMBOSIS

Our knowledge regarding the causation of DVT is expanding, revealing our initial ignorance regarding the etiology of venous thrombosis. A recognizable cause for DVT is evident in nearly 70% of cases.[46] Our knowledge gap is manifested in the 30% of patients in whom no known risk factor is apparent.

Most imagers are familiar with the established causes of DVT: immobilization, trauma, pregnancy, and childbirth, as well as malignancy (Fig. 25–9).[47,48] The relationship between estrogen and DVT has been established for 25 years.[49] In the past decade, mutations and conditions associated with thrombophilia have been defined—antithrombin, protein C or protein S deficiency, Factor V Leiden, pro-

thrombin G20210A mutation, hyperhomocysteinuria, and lupus anticoagulants.[50,51]

Within the past year, a link between DVT and atherosclerosis has been established.[46] The actual etiological relationship is uncertain, but a diffuse underlying inflammation involving both the arterial and venous systems is possible. There is confirmation of a relationship between asymptomatic atherosclerotic lesions and spontaneous venous thrombosis of the legs.

Eventually, all cases of DVT will have a definable etiology. Presently, it is important that the clinician be aware of the many causes and realize that unless they are corrected, repeat episodes of DVT will occur. In fact, a risk factor for DVT is a prior episode of DVT.

CONCLUSIONS

I have presented several issues that are in evolution and remain somewhat controversial. However, it is important to realize that this is by no means an all-inclusive list of controversial topics, and many other issues could be discussed. However, in spite of these controversies, ultrasound for evaluation of the venous system, particularly in the acute situation, remains the dominant diagnostic technique.

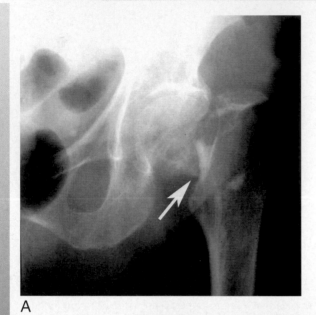

A

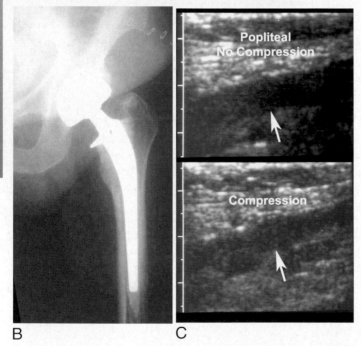

B   C

FIGURE 25–9. Acute hip fracture and immobilization as risk factors for DVT. This 69-year-old woman developed acute DVT 1 week after falling (risk = trauma) and surgery (risk = immobilization + trauma). *A,* Hip film demonstrating acute left hip fracture (*arrow*). *B,* Hemiarthroplasty was performed. *C,* One week later, the popliteal vein (*arrows*) is occluded by acute thrombus.

References

1. Cronan JJ: Deep venous thrombosis: One leg or both legs? Radiology 200:323–324, 1996.
2. Sheiman RG, McArdle CR: Bilateral lower extremity US in the patient with unilateral symptoms of deep venous thrombosis: Assessment of need. Radiology 194:171–173, 1995.
3. Strotham G, Blebea J, Fowl RJ, Rosenthal GR: Contralateral duplex scanning for deep venous thrombosis is unnecessary in patients with symptoms. J Vasc Surg 22:543–547, 1995.
4. Cronan JJ: Controversies in venous ultrasound. Semin Ultrasound CT MR 18:33–38, 1997.
5. Naidich JB, Torre JR, Pellerito JS, et al: Suspected deep venous thrombosis: Is US of both legs necessary? Radiology 200:429–431, 1996.
6. Sheiman RG, Weintrub JL, McArdle CR: Bilateral lower extremity US in the patient with bilateral symptoms of deep venous thrombosis: Assessment of need. Radiology 196:379–381, 1995.
7. Anderson FA, Wheeler HB: Physician priorities in the management of venous thromboem-

bolism: A community wide survey. J Vasc Surg 15:707–714, 1992.

8. ACR Standards for the performance of peripheral venous ultrasound examination (revised 2001). ACR Standards 2002–2003; 579–581.

9. Cogo A, Lensing AW, Prandoni P, Hirsh J: Distribution of thrombosis in patients with symptomatic deep vein thrombosis. Arch Intern Med 153:2777–2780, 1993.

10. Markel A, Manzo RA, Bergelin RO, Strandness DE: Patterns and distribution of thrombi in acute venous thrombosis. Arch Surg 127:305–309, 1992.

11. Rose SC, Zwiebel WJ, Miller FJ: Distribution of acute lower extremity deep venous thrombosis in symptomatic and asymptomatic patients: Imaging implications. J Ultra Med 13:243–250, 1994.

12. Pezzullo JA, Perkins AB, Cronan JJ: Symptomatic deep vein thrombosis: Diagnosis with limited compression US. Radiology 198:67–70, 1996.

13. Frederick MG, Hertzberg BS, Kliewer MA, et al: Can the US examination for lower extremity deep venous thrombosis be abbreviated? A prospective study of 755 examinations. Radiology 199:45–47, 1996.

14. Cronan JJ: Venous thromboembolic disease: The role of US. Radiology 186:619–630, 1993.

15. Vaccaro JP, Cronan JJ, Dorfman GS: Outcome analysis of patients with normal compression US examinations. Radiology 175:645–649, 1990.

16. Huisman MV, Büller HR, Ten Cate JW, Vreeken J: Serial impedance plethysmography for suspected deep venous thrombosis in outpatients. N Engl J Med 314:823–828, 1986.

17. Moser KM, LeMoine JR: Is embolic risk conditioned by location of deep venous thrombosis? Ann Intern Med 94:439–444, 1981.

18. Huisman MV, Büller HR, Ten Cate JW, et al: Unexpected high prevalence of silent pulmonary embolism in patients with deep venous thrombosis. Chest 95:498–502, 1989.

19. Philbrick JT, Becker DM: Calf deep vein thrombosis: A wolf in sheep's clothing? Arch Intern Med 148:2131–2138, 1988.

20. Lohr JM, Kerr TM, Lutter KS, et al: Lower extremity calf thrombosis: To treat or not to treat? J Vasc Surg 14:618–623, 1991.

21. Kakkar VV, Howe CT, Flanc C, et al: Natural history of postoperative deep venous thrombosis. Lancet 2:230–232, 1969.

22. Langerstedt CL, Olsson CG, Fagher BO, et al: Need for long-term anticoagulant treatment in symptomatic calf vein thrombosis. Lancet 2:515–518, 1985.

23. Cornuz J, Pearson SD, Polak JF: Deep venous thrombosis: Complete lower extremity venous US examination in patients without known risk factors—outcome study. Radiology 211:637–641, 1999.

24. Atri M, Herva MJ, Reinhold C, et al: Accuracy of sonography in the evaluation of calf deep vein thrombosis in both postoperative surveillance and symptomatic patients. AJR 166:1361–1367, 1996.

25. Gottlieb RH, Voci S, Syed L, et al: Randomized prospective study comparing routine versus selective use of sonography of the complete calf in patients with suspected deep venous thrombosis. AJR 180:241–245, 2003.

26. Perlin SJ: Pulmonary embolism during compression US of the lower extremity. Radiology 184:165–166, 1992.

27. Schroder WB, Bealer JF: Venous duplex ultrasonography causing acute pulmonary embolism: A brief report. J Vasc Surg 15:1082–1083, 1992.

28. Silverstein RL, Nachman RL: Cancer and clotting—Trousseau's warning. N Engl J Med 327:1163–1164, 1992.

29. Goldberg RJ, Seneff M, Gore JM, et al: Occult malignant neoplasm in patients with deep venous thrombosis. Arch Intern Med 147:251–253, 1987.

30. Aderka D, Brown A, Zelikovski A, Pinkhas J: Idiopathic deep vein thrombosis in an apparently healthy patient as a premonitory sign of occult cancer. Cancer 57:1846–1849, 1986.

31. Monreal M, Lafoz E, Casals AN, et al: Occult cancer in patients with deep venous thrombosis. Cancer 67:541–545, 1991.

32. Schulman S, Lindmarker P: Incidence of cancer after prophylaxis with warfarin against recurrent venous thromboembolism. N Engl J Med 342:1953–1958, 2000.

33. Sorenson HT, Mellemkjaer L, Olsen J, Baron JA: Prognosis of cancers associated with venous thromboembolism. N Engl J Med 343:1846–1850, 2000.

34. Prandoni P, Lensing AWA, Büller HR, et al: Deep-vein thrombosis and the incidence of subsequent symptomatic cancer. N Engl J Med 327:1128–1133, 1992.

35. Prins MH, Lensing AWA, Hirsh J: Idiopathic deep vein thrombosis. Is a search for malignant disease justified? Arch Intern Med 154:1310–1312, 1994.

36. Stein PD, Hull RD, Saltzman HA, Pineo G: Strategy for diagnosis of patients with suspected acute pulmonary embolism. Chest 103:1553–1559, 1993.

37. Killewich LA, Nunnelee JD, Auer AI: Value of lower extremity venous duplex examination in the diagnosis of pulmonary embolism. J Vasc Surg 17:934–939, 1993.

38. Smith LL, Iber C, Sirr S: Pulmonary embolism: Confirmation with venous duplex US as

adjunct to lung scanning. Radiology 191: 143–147, 1994.

39. Turkstra F, Kuijer PMM, van Beek EJR, et al: Diagnostic utility of ultrasonography of leg veins in patients suspected of having pulmonary embolism. Ann Intern Med 126:775–781, 1997.

40. Sheiman RG, McArdle CR: Clinically suspected pulmonary embolism: Use of bilateral lower extremity US as the initial examination—a prospective study. Radiology 212:75–78, 1999.

41. MacGilavry MR, Sanson B, Büller HR, Brandjes DPM: Compression ultrasonography of the leg veins in patients with clinically suspected pulmonary embolism. Is a more extensive assessment of compressibility useful? Thromb Haemost 84:973–976, 2000.

42. Rosen MP, Sheiman RG, Weintraub J, McArdle C: Compression sonography in patients with indeterminate or low-probability lung scans: Lack of usefulness in the absence of both symptoms of deep vein thrombosis and thromboembolic risk factors. AJR 166:285–289, 1996.

43. Hull RD, Hirsh J, Carter CJ, et al: Pulmonary angiography, ventilation lung scanning, and venography for clinically suspected pulmonary embolism with abnormal perfusion lung scan. Ann Intern Med 98:891–899, 1983.

44. Goodman LR, Lipchik RJ: Diagnosis of acute pulmonary embolism: Time for a new approach. Radiology 199:25–27, 1996.

45. Bundens WP, Bergan JJ, Halasz NA, et al: The superficial femoral vein: A potentially lethal misnomer. JAMA 274:1296–1298, 1995.

46. Prandoni P, Bilora F, Marchiori A, et al: An association between atherosclerosis and venous thrombosis. N Engl J Med 348:1435–1441, 2003.

47. Geerts WH, Code KI, Jay RM, et al: A prospective study of venous thromboembolism after major trauma. N Engl J Med 331:1601–1606, 1994.

48. Toglia MR, Weg JG: Venous thromboembolism during pregnancy. N Engl J Med 335:108–114, 1996.

49. Vandenbroucke JP, Rosing J, Bloemenkamp KWM, et al: Oral contraceptives and the risk of venous thrombosis. N Engl J Med 344: 1527–1535, 2001.

50. Seligsohn U, Lubetsky A: Genetic susceptibility to venous thrombosis. N Engl J Med 344:1222–1231, 2001.

51. Den Heijer M, Koster T, Blom HJ, et al: Hyperhomocysteinemia as a risk factor for deep-vein thrombosis. N Engl J Med 334:759–762, 1996.

Chapter 26

Ultrasound Diagnosis of Venous Insufficiency

MARSHA M. NEUMYER, BS, RVT

The term *chronic venous insufficiency* is associated with a form of venous dysfunction that has been widely researched and yet is poorly understood. Most often, the term refers to venous valvular incompetence in the superficial, deep, and/or perforating veins. Incompetence of the vein valves permits reversal of flow and promotes venous hypertension in distal segments. This form of venous dysfunction may be the result of recanalization of thrombosed venous segments, pathologic dilation of the vein, or the congenital absence of competent valves. It is important to understand that venous valvular incompetence may occur alone or in association with venous obstruction. Venous insufficiency is associated with physical findings that are characteristic, yet these findings are nonspecific with respect to cause. They do not differentiate between obstruction and valvular incompetence, nor do they define the location or extent of valvular dysfunction.

Historically, chronic venous insufficiency was evaluated using methods that were inaccurate, nonspecific for incompetence or obstruction, or were invasive and associated with patient discomfort and poor acceptance. For these reasons, investigators have pursued a variety of noninvasive vascular procedures that have defined lower extremity venous flow dynamics globally or segmentally. As a pathway to understanding these laboratory procedures, it is important to review the mechanism of venous valvular incompetence.

PATHOPHYSIOLOGY OF VENOUS INSUFFICIENCY

Normal venous anatomy and physiology were described in Chapter 22. It is necessary to appreciate that venous valves are present throughout the lower extremity venous system in the deep, superficial, and perforating veins. The concentration of valves is higher in the calf veins than in the deep veins of the thigh.

Ambulation results in activation of the calf muscle pump. With calf muscle contraction, venous blood is propelled, or augmented toward the heart. The valves distal to the contracting muscles, and those in the perforating veins, close to prevent reflux. This reduces venous pressure in the foot from approximately 90 mm Hg during standing at rest to 20 to 30 mm Hg during walking. During muscular relaxation, there is slow filling of the venous system from arterial inflow, but venous pressure remains low. In the limb with chronic venous insufficiency, incompetent valves allow blood to move from the deep to the superficial system during muscle contraction. During relaxation, incompetent valves in the deep, superficial, and perforating veins allow blood to flow in a retrograde direction. This results in an uninterrupted column of blood under the influence of gravity and hydrostatic pressure, causing persistently elevated venous pressure, both at rest and during exercise. Venous hypertension may lead to leakage of protein-rich fluid and blood cells through the capillary walls into the intercellular space. The immediate result is soft tissue edema, but the long-term result is skin thickening and hyperpigmentation, and, ultimately, skin ulceration. The pathogenesis of stasis-related ulceration is not well understood, but the chronic debilitating effects of ulceration are easily appreciated.

Chronic venous insufficiency may affect only the superficial veins or it may be a sequel to deep venous thrombosis. The valves below the knee are most often implicated in the clinical sequelae of venous thrombosis. Patients who develop ulceration following an episode of deep vein thrombosis quite often exhibit both deep venous incompetence and incompetence of the greater and lesser saphenous veins. It is of interest to note that patients with significant incompetence of the deep veins below the knee may not suffer from ulceration if there is normal valvular function in the superficial veins.

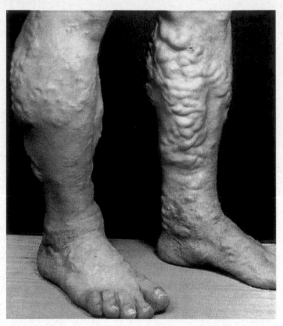

FIGURE 26–1. Lower limb demonstrating dilated superficial veins and varicosities on the medial aspect of the calf and around the ankle.

CLINICAL SIGNS AND SYMPTOMS

Most commonly, patients with chronic venous insufficiency present with symptoms that may include edema, dilated veins, leg pain, and changes in the skin in the region of the ankle. Patients with incompetence involving the superficial, perforating, and deep venous systems may demonstrate the full spectrum of symptoms, while those with only segmental incompetence of the superficial veins may experience lesser degrees of disability.

Mild swelling in the region of the ankle is usually the first sign noted by patients with valvular dysfunction. The edema usually resolves with bed rest or with elevation of the limb. In patients with severe venous insufficiency, the swelling may involve the lower limb to the midcalf level and may or may not be associated with pitting in response to moderate pressure applied to the skin.

The increased venous pressure that results from incompetence of the superficial vein valves causes dilation of the superficial veins in the distal extremity (Fig. 26–1). This is generally noted first on the medial aspect

of the lower calf and around the ankle. With progressively worsening dysfunction, the veins become enlarged and tortuous.

Patients with valvular dysfunction frequently complain of a feeling of heaviness and aching in the legs after prolonged standing or after sitting with the legs dependent. In patients with valvular incompetence in the absence of venous obstruction, the feeling may subside with walking or with elevation of the limb, actions that relieve venous congestion. In contrast, if the deep veins are obstructed, exercise results in venous claudication, consising of severe cramping, burning pain that persists as long as the veins remain congested. Several investigators have shown that venous claudication is caused by a rapid increase in pressure in both the superficial and deep venous systems.[1,2] This is most often the result of obstruction of the iliofemoral venous segment with inadequate collateral flow.

The goals of the noninvasive vascular laboratory in evaluating patients with venous insufficiency symptoms are to define which venous systems are involved (superficial and/or deep), the anatomic level of dysfunction, and whether the pathologic process includes both incompetence and obstruction.

VASCULAR LABORATORY TEST PROCEDURES

Historically, investigators relied on the invasive procedures (namely, ascending and descending venography and ambulatory venous pressure measurements) to evaluate chronic venous insufficiency. Venography was considered to be the gold standard for visualization of anatomy, confirmation of the presence of venous obstruction and collateralization, and definition of the location and extent of valvular reflux. Ambulatory venous pressure measurements were used as a hemodynamic complement to the anatomic information obtained from venography.[3] Pressures could be measured with the patient at rest in a supine position, while standing, and during exercise. This procedure had value as a means for recording venous pressure recovery time, which has been used as the basis for more recent plethysmographic studies.

The modern vascular laboratory evaluation of venous insufficiency has evolved steadily from continuous-wave Doppler velocimetry to indirect, plethysmographic procedures and finally, to the quantification of venous reflux using duplex ultrasound imaging. Although duplex sonography is currently the most accurate method for assessing venous incompetence, continuous-wave Doppler remains in use as a convenient, "low-tech" method for diagnosing venous reflux. Therefore, its inclusion in this chapter is worthwhile. Plethysmographic methods also remain in clinical use as a means of assessing venous hemodynamics, and for that reason, they too are discussed.

Bi-directional Continuous Wave Doppler

Equipment

Bi-directional, continuous-wave Doppler uses separate transmitting and receiving crystals that operate continuously to detect

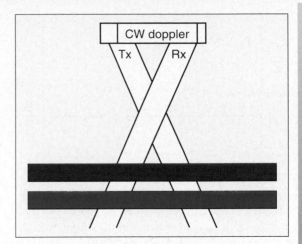

FIGURE 26–2. Diagram of a continuous wave Doppler demonstrating transmitting and receiving crystals with the ultrasound beam intersecting both an artery (red) and a vein (blue). Rx, receiving crystal; Tx, transmitting crystal.

flow at all depths along the emitted sound beam (Fig. 26–2). Because of this, the signal that is received may contain echoes from more than one vessel lying within the beam path. The depth of penetration of a sound beam is inversely proportional to the carrier Doppler frequency. For this reason, lower-frequency transducers (3–5 MHz) are required for studying the deeper veins of the thigh, while higher frequencies (8–10 MHz) may be used for the superficial and calf veins in patients with normal body habitus.

Quadrature phase separation is used to detect the direction of flow. The analog waveform of the Doppler signal is displayed using a frequency-to-voltage converter and a zero-crossing detector. The voltage output is proportional to the number of zero crossings (Fig. 26–3). This display method is highly dependent on the signal-to-noise ratio and on the amplitude of the return signal.[4,5]

Patient Positioning

Patients are examined in a warm room while lying supine in a reversed Trendelenburg (10–15 degrees) position, or standing to promote venous filling. In the supine position, the patient's head is slightly elevated and the legs are externally rotated at the hip with the knees comfortably flexed.

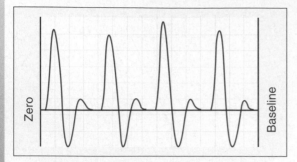

FIGURE 26–3. Analog waveform from a continuous-wave Doppler, using a zero-crossing detector and quadrature phase separation to show direction of flow. (Modified from Scissons R: Physiological Testing Techniques and Interpretation. North Kingstown, RI, Unetixs Educational Publishing, 2003.)

In the upright position, the patient should initially face the examiner with the body supported mainly on the contralateral leg. The limb must remain immobile throughout the examination to prevent muscle contraction and inadvertent augmentation of venous flow. The examination is facilitated if the patient stands on a platform that is approximately 2 feet high with a support railing on three sides.

Examination Technique and Diagnostic Criteria

The examination is initiated with the continuous-wave Doppler probe placed in a cephalad direction over the femoral vein at an angle approximating 45 degrees to the skin. The identification of the vein is confirmed by first insonating the common femoral artery (noting the pulsatile, multiphasic, caudad flow signal) and then moving the probe in a medial direction to locate the common femoral vein. Care must be taken to avoid pressure on the probe, because the veins are quite easily compressed.

Normal venous flow is spontaneous and phasic with respiration, yielding a "wind-like" audible Doppler signal. Manual compression of the limb below the probe should augment forward flow, with resultant increased amplitude of the audible Doppler signal. When the limb is compressed above the probe, the Doppler signal will normally cease, because competent valves restrict retrograde venous flow. When compression above the probe is released, an augmented, forward flow signal should be noted. The same effects will normally occur if the patient coughs or performs a Valsalva maneuver. Both actions cause an increase in intra-abdominal pressure, which restricts escape of blood from the lower limb. The same compression and/or respiration procedure is repeated over the superficial femoral, popliteal, and posterior tibial veins and in the regions of the saphenofemoral and saphenopopliteal junctions. Spontaneous signals are most often present in the larger-diameter thigh and popliteal veins. If the patient is examined in a cool room, however, vasoconstriction may reduce extremity blood flow and augmentation of flow may be required to confirm patency of the small-diameter tibial veins.

If the valve immediately *distal* to the site of probe placement is incompetent, retrograde flow will be noted with compression of the limb *above* the probe. Given this, a retrograde flow signal over the common femoral vein following an appropriately performed Valsalva maneuver would suggest an incompetent valve immediately *proximal* to that site. Moreover, the presence of a single competent valve at any site proximal to the probe will prevent reflux and may lead to a falsely negative result.

The anatomic location of valvular incompetence can be inferred by simple compression maneuvers that exclude the superficial venous system during the examination. The continuous-wave Doppler probe is placed over the region of the saphenofemoral junction, and the presence of retrograde flow is confirmed with release of compression of the limb *below* the level of the probe. A tourniquet is placed around the limb approximately 10 cm distal to the expected location of the saphenofemoral junction and tightened sufficiently to compress the greater saphenous vein (Fig. 26–4). Compression of the limb below the level of the probe is repeated. The continued presence of retrograde flow suggests incompetence of the common femoral and/or proximal superficial femoral vein(s). If retrograde flow is abolished by tourniquet application, incompetence of the greater saphenous vein

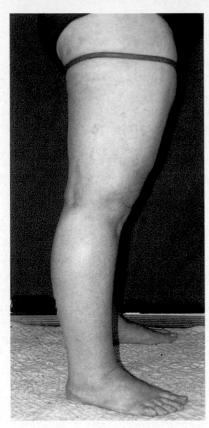

FIGURE 26–4. Lower extremity showing placement of the upper thigh tourniquet for compression of the greater saphenous vein.

is suggested. The saphenopopliteal junction should be examined in a similar manner to distinguish popliteal/gastrocnemius reflux from incompetency of the lesser saphenous vein.

Absence of a flow signal along the anatomic course of a vein suggests occlusion of the vessel. Remembering that the major arteries and deep veins course together through the lower extremity, a venous signal found at a distance of more than 1 cm from the corresponding artery suggests a large collateral and occlusion of the primary vein. Low-amplitude Doppler signals may imply partial thrombosis, a collateralized venous occlusion, or a recanalized vein.

Advantages

In the hands of experienced examiners, bi-directional, continuous-wave Doppler velocimetry has been shown to have excellent sensitivity (92%) with acceptable specificity (73%) for the assessment of venous incompetence.[6] While some applaud this method as a valuable, portable tool for detection of valvular incompetence or obstruction of the deep and superficial veins,[7-9] others note that the continuous-wave Doppler test is extremely operator dependent and subjective.[10]

Limitations

It is important to be aware of the considerable limitations associated with continuous-wave Doppler examination of the extremity veins. Because this is a nonimaging modality, there is no way to be certain which veins are being insonated. Duplication of the deep and superficial veins is common, and a signal may be elicited from a patent vein that lies adjacent to a thrombosed venous segment or from a large collateral vein. It is often quite difficult to differentiate reflux in the deep venous system from reflux in a superficial vein or a major tributary at the saphenofemoral or saphenopopliteal junctions. Similarly, incompetency in large perforating veins may be confused with reflux in the saphenous or deep veins. Finally, standardization of the testing protocol is not possible because of the variability associated with tourniquet application. There is no assurance that the superficial veins are adequately compressed or that the compression does not obliterate flow in the deep venous system or perforating veins.

Photoplethysmography

Equipment

Photoplethysmography is a relatively simple tool used to screen for valvular incompetence. This technique employs an infrared light–emitting diode, with a second diode used to sense light reflected from subdermal venous flow. The photoplethysmographic probe is most commonly affixed to the skin in the supramalleolar region, using double-stick tape (Fig. 26–5). The plethysmograph is coupled to a direct current

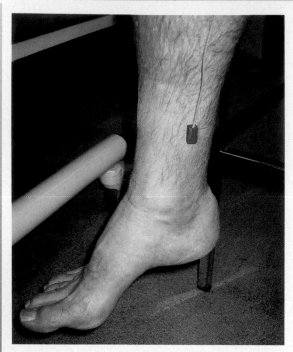

FIGURE 26–5. Lower extremity demonstrating correct placement of a photoplethysmographic sensor for evaluation of venous refill time.

recorder (DC mode) to track the average changes in reflected light that occur over time in association with alterations in blood flow volume. In the normal limb, the volume of blood in the skin decreases in response to manual compression of the calf or dorsiflexion of the foot and ankle. In the absence of obstruction to arterial inflow, the venous microcirculation refills slowly. If venous valves are incompetent, however, reflux occurs and the microcirculation refills rapidly. The quality of venous emptying with calf muscle compression can be assessed subjectively, and the length of time required for venous refill can be calculated from the calibrations on the strip chart recording.

Patient Positioning

The patient is seated forward on a bed or examination table with the legs unsupported. The photoplethysmographic sensors are affixed to the medial aspect of the leg above the malleolus. Care is taken to avoid positioning the sensor over regions of inflammation or ulceration.

Examination Technique and Diagnostic Criteria

The patient is initially requested to relax the limb while a baseline tracing is recorded on the plethysmographic strip chart recorder. The stylus for the recorder is positioned near the top of the tracing.

The patient is then requested to dorsiflex the foot four or five times. This causes the calf muscles to contract, simulating ambulation, and empties the calf veins in normal individuals. Manual calf compression can be used for patients who are unable to achieve adequate emptying of the venous pool with dorsiflexion. When the leg is relaxed and immobile, the calf veins refill. The venous refilling time is defined as the number of seconds required for the photoplethysmographic tracing to reach a stable endpoint for at least 5 sec. The refill time is measured from the time exercise ceases to the stable endpoint (Fig. 26–6A). As noted previously, normally there is a rapid reduction of venous volume (and venous pressure) with limb exercise. Capillary refilling is primarily a function of arterial inflow when vein valves are competent and venous refilling is relatively slow. In patients with competent deep and superficial veins, the venous refill time is lengthened and usually exceeds 20 seconds.

A venous refill time less than 20 sec suggests venous insufficiency (Fig. 26–6B). Superficial venous reflux can be differentiated from deep venous reflux by application of tourniquets to compress the greater and lesser saphenous veins. A tourniquet (latex tubing or blood pressure cuff inflated to 45 mm Hg) is initially placed above the knee. The test is repeated as described previously. If the venous refill time normalizes to longer than 20 sec, the superficial venous system is implicated as the source of incompetence. If the refill time improves but does not normalize, the data imply that both the deep and superficial systems are incompetent. The tourniquet is then moved below the knee. If the refill time normalizes, this is diagnostic of superficial venous incompetence alone. If the refill time remains less than 20 sec with tourniquet compression of

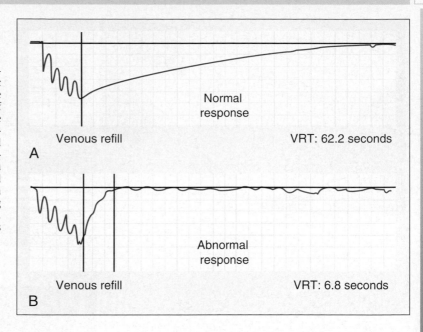

FIGURE 26–6. Strip chart recordings of photoplethysmographic measurement venous refill time (VRT). Note the placement of calipers at completion of the exercise and at a stable endpoint. *A,* Normal venous refill time, exceeding 20 sec. *B,* Abnormal response consistent with venous reflux. Venous refill time is only 6.8 sec. (From Scissons R: Physiological Testing Techniques and Interpretation, North Kingstown, RI, Unetixs Educational Publishing, 2003.)

the superficial veins, this suggests deep venous insufficiency.

Advantages

Photoplethysmographic determination of venous refill time correlates with ambulatory venous pressure measurements.[11] The application is technically simple and the equipment is inexpensive and portable. This modality serves as a useful screening tool for evaluation of patients in whom venous insufficiency is suspected on the basis of history or physical findings.

Limitations

While attractive as a screening tool because of its technical simplicity, photoplethysmographic assessment of venous refill time has significant limitations. Most notable is the fact that it is a subjective, nonquantitative modality. It also is not capable of anatomically localizing the site of incompetence. As with bi-directional continuous-wave Doppler, the technique cannot be standardized because of variability in sensor placement and tourniquet pressure. The sensor may be placed over

incompetent perforators or a region of localized inflammation or ischemia. There is no assurance that the superficial veins are compressed or that the deep veins remain patent with tourniquet application. Additionally, it must be recognized that the results of photoplethysmographic studies may be influenced by body temperature, with alterations of blood flow and filling time occurring in response to vasodilation and/or vasoconstriction.

Air Plethysmography

Air plethysmography (APG) was first introduced in the 1960s to study lower extremity volume changes that occur in response to alterations in posture and muscular exercise. Once it became possible to calibrate the system, interest was hightened in this noninvasive modality that could replace the older diagnostic devices such as strain gauge segmental volume and water plethysmographs. Christopoulos and colleagues[12] introduced APG as a diagnostic tool in 1987 to detect global limb volume changes that occur with exercise and gravity.

With respect to venous competence, APG measures the following: (1) calf venous volume, (2) the rate at which calf venous

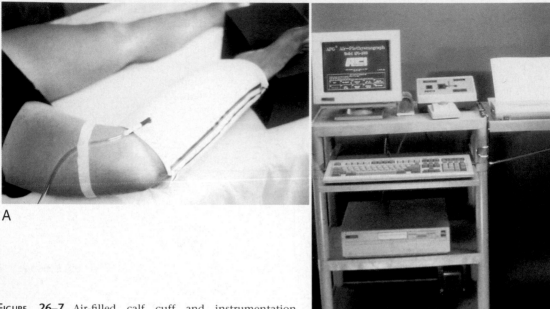

FIGURE 26–7. Air-filled calf cuff and instrumentation required for air plethysmographic evaluation. *A,* Correct placement of the air-filled cuff on the patient's calf. *B,* Air-calibrated pressure transducer, amplifier, recorder, and display system.

volume is restored normally or as a result of reflux, (3) the effectiveness of the calf muscle pump, and (4) ambulatory venous pressure (indirectly).

Equipment

Air plethysmography uses an air-filled, polyvinyl cuff, which surrounds the calf and functions as a sensing device to detect calf volume changes. The cuff is connected to an air-calibrated pressure transducer, amplifier, and recorder (Fig. 26–7).

Patient Positioning

The patient initially reclines in the supine position with the heel slightly elevated on a support and with the limb externally rotated and flexed to allow application of the cuff. Volume changes in the limb are recorded during limb elevation (which empties the veins), venous refilling, and a series of maneuvers with the patient upright, as shown in Figure 26–8 and described in the following section.

TECHNIQUE AND DIAGNOSTIC CRITERIA

With the patient's heel supported and the limb properly positioned, the air-filled cuff is adjusted over the calf so that it encloses

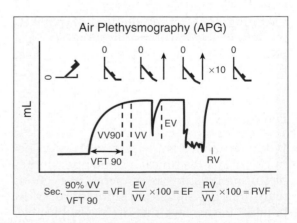

FIGURE 26–8. The protocol for air plethysmographic study and tracings for measurement of the venous filling index (VFI), ejection fraction (EF), and residual volume fraction (RVF). EV, ejection volume; RV, residual volume; VFT, venous filling time; VV, venous volume. (From Christopoulos DG, Nicolaides AN, Szendro G, et al: Air plethysmography and the effects of elastic compression on venous hemodynamics of the leg. J Vasc Surg 5:148–150, 1987.)

the calf from the knee to the ankle. The patient's limb is elevated 45 degrees to empty the calf veins (Fig. 26–8). Maximal venous emptying is indicated when the baseline recording stabilizes. The patient is then quickly brought to a standing position with the body weight supported on the opposite limb. Filling of the calf veins is recorded continuously until a steady baseline is again obtained. This indicates that functional *venous volume* (VV) has been reached. Venous filling should result in an increase in leg venous volume of 100 to 150 mL in limbs with competent vein valves and 100 to 350 mL in limbs with venous insufficiency.

The *venous filling index* (VFI) is the ratio of 90% of the VV divided by the time required to achieve 90% venous filling (*venous filling time*, or VFT90%). The venous function index, which evaluates overall valvular competence, is calculated from the equation 90% VV/VFT90%. This measurement of average filling rate is expressed in milliliters per second. A VFI of 2 mL/sec or less indicates normal valvular function, while a VFI greater than 7 mL/sec is consistent with deep and/or superficial incompetence and is associated clinically with symptoms of chronic venous insufficiency. Application of a narrow, below-knee tourniquet to occlude the lesser and greater saphenous veins may reduce the VFI to less than 5 mL/sec in limbs with incompetent common femoral vein valves but competent popliteal valves.[13] Christopoulos and associates[12] found that a VFI between 2 and 30 mL/sec was associated with superficial venous incompetence, while patients with a VFI between 7 and 28 mL/sec had evidence of deep venous insufficiency.

After the measurements cited previously are obtained, the patient is asked to rise up once on the toes and return to normal position. This maneuver activates the calf muscle pump, which decreases venous volume. The *ejection volume* (EV) measures the decrease in venous volume achieved with one heel raise exercise and represents the volume of blood expelled by the calf with a single calf muscle contraction. The *ejection fraction* (EF) represents the emptying power of a single calf contraction and

normally exceeds 60% of the baseline venous volume. The ejected volume and ejection fraction can be calculated from the equation EF = (EV/VV) × 100.

The patient then performs 10 heel raises to completely empty the calf veins and returns to the resting position. The *residual venous volume* (RV) is recorded at the end of the exercise. The *residual venous volume fraction* (RVF) is calculated as RV/VV × 100 to determine the percentage of total calf blood volume that remains following this level of exercise. Normally, this value is less than 35% and represents overall calf muscle pump function. While some investigators believe that this value correlates with ambulatory venous pressure,[12] others have challenged this opinion.[14,15]

Advantages

Air plethysmography has value as a tool for studying the calf muscle pump function and global lower limb venous hemodynamics. As such, it can be used to select patients who will benefit from surgical intervention to correct venous valvular dysfunction, and to evaluate the effect of noninvasive therapeutic measures, such as limb compression.

Limitations

While APG has shown value as a noninvasive means for assessing global venous hemodynamics in the lower extremity, specific incompetent valve sites cannot be identified. While the technique has merit for quantification of venous reflux and outflow obstruction, it is difficult for many patients to move from the supine to upright position rapidly and to perform the heel raise maneuvers. A small number of patients cannot undergo testing because of extensive limb swelling and discomfort or their inability to perform the exercise routine.

Duplex Ultrasonography

Duplex ultrasound, the combination of B-mode (gray-scale) imaging and pulsed Doppler velocity spectral analysis, has become the primary diagnostic procedure for identification of deep vein thrombosis and superficial thrombophlebitis. This technique, complemented with color flow imaging, provides an excellent tool for demonstrating venous obstruction and reflux. The B-mode image allows definition of the vein lumen, vein valve leaflets, and vein wall morphology, as well as compressibility of the vein and assessment of the acoustic properties of thrombus. Pulsed Doppler velocity spectral analysis is used to ensure accurate differentiation of venous and arterial flow, to document venous flow patterns and flow direction, and for timing the duration of venous reflux through incompetent valves. Color flow imaging is used to differentiate venous occlusion from partial thrombosis of the vein, to distinguish reflux in the deep veins from reflux in the superficial system at the saphenofemoral and saphenopopliteal junctions, to identify incompetent perforating veins, and to demonstrate recanalization and collateralization of chronically thrombosed venous segments.

Equipment

Accurate assessment of lower extremity venous morphology and hemodynamics requires a high-resolution ultrasound system equipped with pulsed Doppler transducers ranging in frequency from 3 to 10 MHz. This frequency range allows interrogation of the inferior vena cava, deep pelvic veins, and veins of the thigh and calf. Excellent spatial resolution is necessary to ensure identification of acute, acoustically homogeneous thrombus. Additionally, Doppler spectral and color wall filters must be independently controlled to ensure detection of low-amplitude, low-velocity flow associated with partially occlusive thrombus, recanalized venous segments, and venous collaterals.

Patient Positioning

The patient is placed in the supine position with the head slightly elevated and the examination table in the reverse Trendelenburg position (feet 10–15 degrees below the level of the heart) to maximize venous pooling in the lower limbs. The patient's hips are externally rotated, and the knees are slightly flexed. This position permits easy access to the common femoral, superficial femoral, deep femoral, posterior tibial, peroneal, and greater saphenous veins. Moving the patient to the lateral decubitus position facilitates examination of the common iliac, external iliac, popliteal, and lesser saphenous veins. The popliteal and lesser saphenous veins may also be interrogated with the patient lying prone with the feet elevated slightly on a rolled towel or pillow. Elevation in this manner prevents hyperextension of the knee and resulting extrinsic compression of the popliteal vein and the sapheno-popliteal junction. The inferior vena cava may be evaluated with the patient lying in the supine position, or a coronal image plane can be used with the patient in a left lateral decubitus position.

Technique and Diagnostic Criteria

The examination is initiated with a longitudinal, B-mode image of the common femoral vein. Confirmation of venous flow is ensured by placing the Doppler sample volume within the vein lumen. Normal venous flow signals are spontaneous and phasic with respiration (Fig. 26–9). As described in the discussion of bi-directional, continuous-wave Doppler, forward (cephalad) flow occurs when the limb is compressed *distal* to the probe. There should be no evidence of retrograde flow with release of distal compression, with a Valsalva maneuver, or with limb compression *proximal* to the probe.

The venous competency examination may be complemented with color flow imaging to facilitate the recognition of flow direction, the identification of anatomic landmarks and flow patterns, and the detection of morphologic and hemodynamic abnormalities (Fig. 26–10). Color flow imaging parameters must be optimized for detection of low-velocity flow by decreasing the color velocity scale and wall filters and

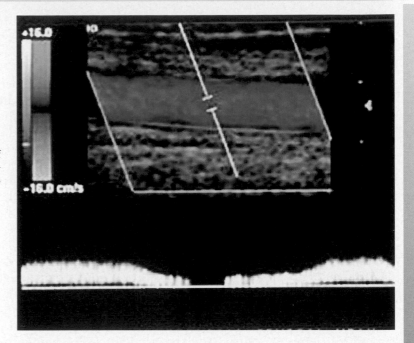

FIGURE 26–9. Color flow image of the common femoral vein demonstrating appropriate flow direction and spontaneous respirophasicity.

taking care to use an appropriately angled, narrow color box. Doppler spectral waveforms should confirm normal flow direction at rest and the absence of retrograde flow with application of distal limb compression or release of proximal compression. Abnormal flow direction can also be confirmed with color flow imaging.

The B-mode examination of the femoral area is continued by moving the transducer slightly distally or proximally to identify the saphenofemoral junction. The common femoral vein and the saphenofemoral junction are interrogated carefully for evidence of intraluminal echoes that suggest the presence of thrombus. Care should be taken to identify valve sinuses in the common femoral and proximal greater saphenous veins. The sinuses most commonly have an elliptical configuration. By imaging perpendicular to the anterior wall of the vein, the thin, mobile valve leaflets can be visualized (Fig. 26–11). Compression of the limb proximal to the probe, a Valsalva maneuver, or

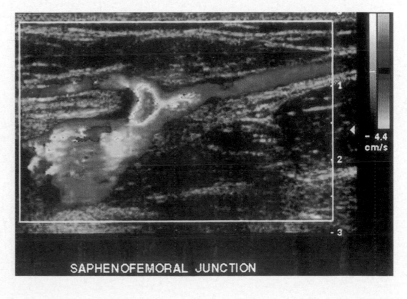

FIGURE 26–10. Color flow image of the saphenofemoral junction demonstrating slight elevation of velocities and minimal reflux in a proximal branch of the greater saphenous vein.

SAPHENOFEMORAL JUNCTION

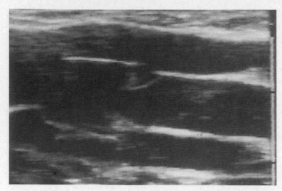

FIGURE 26–11. B-mode image of a valve sinus demonstrating the thin, echogenic valve leaflets.

release of distal compression will normally elicit no evidence of retrograde venous flow (Fig. 26–12). The scan is continued throughout the common femoral vein to its bifurcation into the profunda femoris and superficial femoral veins. The profunda femoris vein is examined as far along its course as possible, with careful attention to the absence of thrombus and reflux. The superficial femoral vein is examined throughout its length in a similar manner to evaluate the valve sinuses, to confirm the absence of intraluminal echoes, and to ensure valvular competency. B-mode image resolution may be compromised in the distal thigh because of the depth of the vein. To overcome this obstacle, the transducer is placed in the popliteal fossa to image the popliteal vein longitudinally.

Counterpressure is applied to the patient's knee while the scan is continued in a cephalad direction into the distal superficial femoral vein.

The transducer is returned to the popliteal fossa to insonate the popliteal vein throughout its length, ensuring the absence of thrombus and confirming the competence of this important valve site. The scan is continued distally to identify the anterior tibial and tibioperoneal trunks. In a manner identical to that used for examination of the proximal veins, posterior tibial and peroneal veins are interrogated throughout their length. The anterior tibial veins may be interrogated only proximally or throughout their length, as clinically indicated. Color flow imaging may facilitate identification of the tibial veins, duplicated venous segments, and the absence of reflux.

Following the longitudinal examination of the deep veins, the transducer is returned to the level of the common femoral vein and a transverse image of the vein is obtained at the saphenofemoral junction. Compressibility of the vein is then tested with by applying pressure with the ultrasound transducer, both proximal and distal to the junction. The walls of a vein coapt with pressure in the absence of thrombosis or abnormal venous pressure resulting from extrinsic compression of the vein proximal to the image site. Compressibility is then assessed sequentially throughout all venous

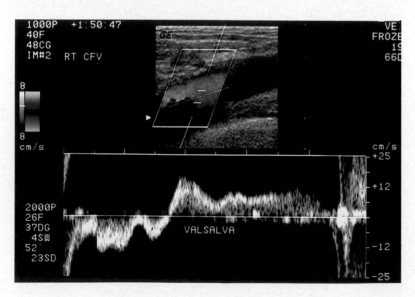

FIGURE 26–12. Color flow image and Doppler spectral waveform demonstrating significant reflux through an incompetent valve in the common femoral vein. (Courtesy of Providence Surgical Care Group, Providence, RI.)

segments, from the common femoral vein distally to the tibial veins at ankle level.

When assessment of the deep system is complete, the greater and lesser saphenous veins are insonated in an identical manner. Longitudinal and transverse B-mode imaging is used to ensure the absence of thrombus, evaluate valve sites, and assess venous compressibility.

Intraluminal echogenicity suggests venous thrombosis, and affected venous segments are noncompressible or partially compressible (Fig. 26–13). As described in Chapter 24, acute thrombus most often appears lightly echogenic with a spongy texture and may be poorly attached to the vein wall. As the thrombus organizes in the subacute and chronic phases, it becomes more echogenic, because of the increased collagen content, and it becomes more rigid. It then is well attached to the vein wall, and as it continues to organize, it contracts, pulling the walls of the vein inward. The vein may appear to be small in diameter with thickened, irregular walls. Over time, recanalization may occur or collateral veins may develop (Fig. 26–14).

Doppler spectral waveforms become continuous and nonphasic when venous outflow is obstructed by thrombus or extrinsic compression. Augmentation of flow with

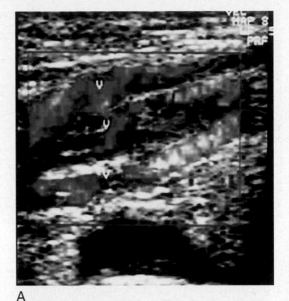

A

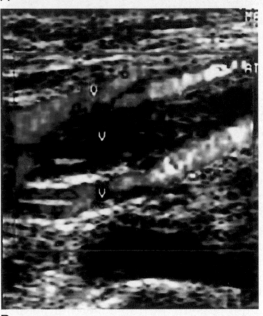

B

FIGURE 26–14. Color flow images of a thrombosed venous segment. *A*, Recanalized venous segment. Note small channels of flow within the thrombus. *B*, Collateralized venous segment. Note the small channels that parallel the thrombosed segment. V, venous channels.

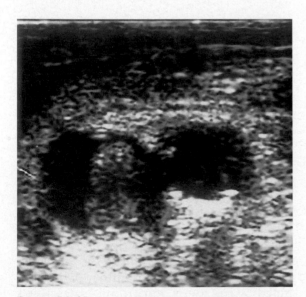

FIGURE 26–13. Cross-sectional image of the femoral vein demonstrating partially occlusive, organized thrombus.

distal limb compression also is diminished, as compared with flow at the same level in a normal contralateral limb. Color flow imaging is useful in differentiating a totally thrombosed vein from one that is partially obstructed (Fig. 26–15). Careful imaging is necessary to ensure that flow characteristics

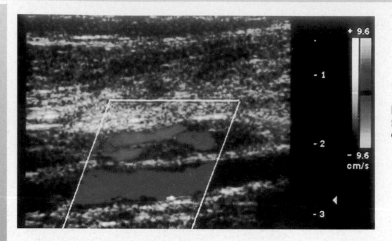

FIGURE 26–15. Color flow image of a femoral vein demonstrating partially occluding thrombus.

are recorded from the original superficial and deep veins, rather than from large venous collaterals.

Quite often, deep vein thrombosis damages the vein valves, causing them to thicken and scar. As a result, the valve leaflets cannot function properly, leading to reflux of blood through incompetent sites. Improperly functioning valve leaflets can be identified with B-mode imaging, and retrograde flow at such valves is demonstrated with spectral and color Doppler (Fig. 26–16).

Incompetent perforating veins can be identified with duplex sonography complemented by color flow imaging (Fig. 26–17). Perforating veins connect the superficial and deep systems and have one-way valves that normally allow blood flow *only* from the superficial to the deep veins. Large perforating veins are commonly found in the distal calf and in the proximal and mid-thigh. In the thigh, identification of the medially located perforating veins is best accomplished with transverse B-mode imaging beginning at the level of the common femoral vein. The perforating veins penetrate the deep fascia and connect the greater saphenous vein to the deep veins of the thigh.[16-18] When a perforating vein is identified, manual compression of the limb above and below the transducer can be used to detect retrograde flow.[17,19] Color flow imaging can identify retrograde blood flow toward the transducer, consistent with valvular incompetence. Incompetent perforating veins are usually larger than competent ones. Phillips and associates[20] noted

that all perforating veins larger than 4 mm in diameter were incompetent, while those smaller than 3 mm were competent.

In the calf, there are major groups of medially located perforating veins that are rather constant in their anatomic location. They are typically located 6, 12, 18, 24, and 28 to 32 centimeters above the heel. The first three groups are referred to as the Cockett's perforators, and the highest (antero-medial) perforating vein is called the Boyd perforator.[21] Identification of these medial perforating veins should be included in the scanning protocol for venous insufficiency, because they account for approximately 40% of incompetent perforating veins.[18]

Lateral calf perforating veins vary in location. Imaging in the transverse plane with color Doppler, beginning at the level of the proximal lesser saphenous and peroneal veins, facilitates localization of the major lateral perforators. In the proximal calf, two perforating veins connect the lesser saphenous vein to the gastrocnemius veins.[18] In the distal calf, there are usually two lateral perforating veins located approximately 5 and 12 cm above the ankle.

When venous insufficiency is suggested during the recumbent ultrasound examination, confirmation is obtained by moving the patient to the standing position to impose the usual circumstances of valve function. The standing examination is facilitated by the use of a platform, as described previously in the discussion of continuous wave Doppler. Color flow imaging is

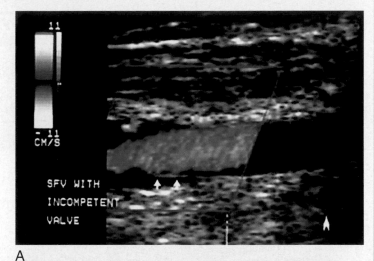

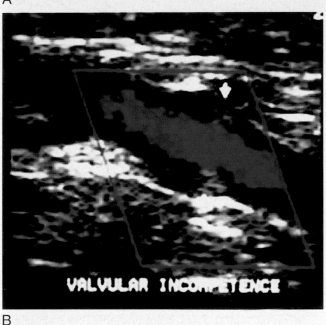

A

B

FIGURE 26–16. Color flow images demonstrating valvular incompetence. *A*, Venous flow is antegrade through an incompetent valve when manual compression is applied distal to the valve. *B*, Flow direction is retrograde (reflux) through the incompetent valve when manual compression is released. (Color assignment is *red* for flow toward the transducer and *blue* for flow away from the transducer.)

repeated in the longitudinal plane over the saphenofemoral and saphenopopliteal junctions and along the deep and superficial venous segments where valvular incompetence was previously suggested. If the patient is able to perform an adequate Valsalva maneuver, this method may be used to produce reflux. Otherwise, manual limb compression proximal and distal to the suspect valve sites is employed.

With the Doppler sample volume placed centerstream in the vein distal to a valve site that appears to be incompetent on color flow examination, Doppler spectral waveforms are recorded during normal respira-

tion and with manual limb compression or the Valsalva maneuver. The duration of retrograde venous flow is determined. Welch and colleagues [22] have termed this the valve closure time. The University of Washington vascular laboratory team [23,24] has shown that the normal valve closure time is less than 0.5 sec (Fig. 26–18).

Venous valves close when reversal of the normal transvalvular pressure gradient results in sufficient retrograde flow velocity to force the valve leaflets to coapt. Van Bemmelem and associates [23] noted that valve closure was achieved when the reverse velocities exceeded 30 cm/sec. During ultra-

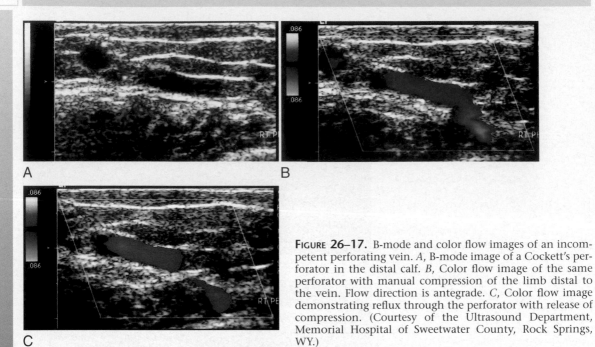

A

B

C

FIGURE 26–17. B-mode and color flow images of an incompetent perforating vein. *A*, B-mode image of a Cockett's perforator in the distal calf. *B*, Color flow image of the same perforator with manual compression of the limb distal to the vein. Flow direction is antegrade. *C*, Color flow image demonstrating reflux through the perforator with release of compression. (Courtesy of the Ultrasound Department, Memorial Hospital of Sweetwater County, Rock Springs, WY.)

sound examination, the velocity of retrograde flow is related to the external pressure on the vein. Reflux can be demonstrated only when a significant transvalvular pressure gradient is present. It must be noted that sufficient pressure is not uniformly achieved with either the Valsalva maneuver or manual compression, particularly in the more distal veins. This can result in failure to detect venous incompetence.

Advantages

Duplex ultrasound, complemented with color flow imaging, has been validated as a sensitive and specific modality for the identification of superficial and deep vein thrombosis.[26–28] Valvular incompetence can be confirmed with spectral and color Doppler, and, unlike photoplethysmography and APG, venous insufficiency can be

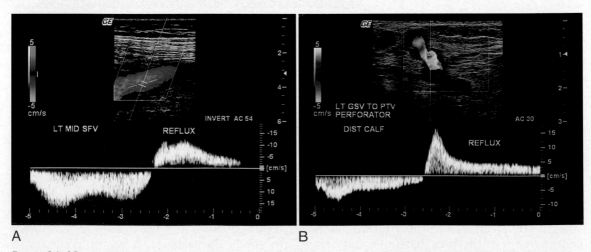

A

B

FIGURE 26–18. Color flow images and velocity spectral waveforms demonstrating clinically significant reflux (duration longer than 0.5 sec) (*A*) in a femoral vein and (*B*) in a calf perforating vein. The duration of reflux is determined using the timing monitor on the bottom of the image display. (Courtesy of the Hershey Vascular Laboratory, The Penn State Vascular Institute, Hershey, PA.)

localized to specific valve sites in the deep and superficial veins. Incompetent perforators can similarly be identified and mapped prior to intervention.

Limitations

The accuracy of the technique is entirely dependent on the experience of the sonographer and physician interpreter. In parallel with continuous-wave Doppler and photoplethysmography, the intensity of the Valsalva maneuver or manual compression cannot be standardized and may be insufficient to produce reflux. This was shown by van Bemmelen and colleagues[25] to be a significant problem, particularly in the distal veins. Because of the inability to ensure adequate venous pressure to produce reflux with Valsalva or manual compression, the severity of venous insufficiency cannot be quantitated.

Quantitative Measurement of Venous Incompetence

Given the inability to standardize duplex ultrasound identification of reflux using the Valsalva maneuver or manual compression, investigators sought a method that would remove the variability of the procedure and permit quantification of valvular incompetence. In 1989, the vascular laboratory teams in Seattle at the University of Washington and at St. Mary's Hospital in London published reports using cuff-deflation techniques.[23,29] The method proposed by van Bemmelen and colleagues[23] has been adopted by many laboratories as a reliable, reproducible procedure for the identification and quantification of segmental venous reflux.

Equipment

Quantitative measurement of venous insufficiency requires a high-resolution ultrasound system and a range of pulsed Doppler transducers identical to those used for duplex scanning. Although not required for accurate testing, color flow imaging facili-

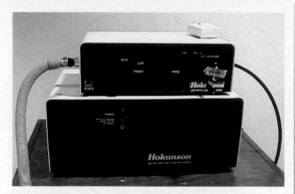

FIGURE 26–19. A rapid cuff inflator and air source are required to rapidly fill the large thigh and calf cuffs.

tates venous identification and recognition of retrograde flow.

A rapid cuff inflator and air source are required to insure inflation of large (24-cm) thigh cuffs within 0.3 sec (Fig. 26–19). In addition, a 12-cm cuff is applied to the patient's calf, and a 7-cm cuff is wrapped around the foot.

Patient Positioning

The patient stands on a platform, facing the examiner, with the body weight shifted to the leg opposite that being investigated for duplex ultrasound examination of the common femoral and proximal superficial femoral veins and the saphenofemoral junction. For evaluation of the popliteal vein and the proximal lesser saphenous vein, the patient faces away from the examiner, again standing in a non–weight bearing position. The knee is flexed slightly to prevent extrinsic compression of the popliteal vein. This position also may be used for examination of the mid-segment of the greater saphenous vein, the anterolateral and accessory posterior branches of the greater saphenous vein, and the posterior tibial and peroneal veins.

Technique

A large (24-cm) blood pressure cuff is placed around the patient's thigh. This is connected to the air source with the automatic cuff inflator and is intermittantly inflated to

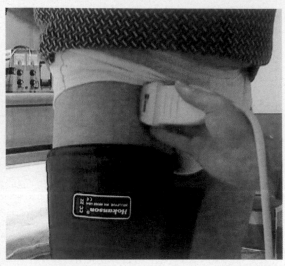

FIGURE 26–20. Appropriate positioning of the patient, thigh cuff, and transducer for obtaining Doppler spectral recordings from the common femoral, superficial femoral, and proximal greater saphenous veins.

80 mm Hg pressure during the course of the examination.

Step 1. The examination begins with identification of the common femoral vein in the longitudinal plane with B-mode imaging (Fig. 26–20). Color flow imaging may be used to facilitate identification of the vein and the recognition of flow direction. The Doppler sample volume is placed centerstream in the common femoral vein, and spectral waveforms are obtained during normal respiration. The thigh cuff is then inflated for 3 sec and then rapidly deflated while Doppler spectral waveforms are continuously recorded. Careful attention should be given to the direction of flow during cuff deflation and, if present, the length of time during which retrograde venous flow persists. Calipers associated with the ultrasound calculation software can be used to determine the duration of reflux. Reflux that persists for longer than 0.5 sec is considered to be clinically significant.[25]

Step 2. The saphenofemoral junction is identified, and the inflation and deflation procedure is repeated in a manner identical to that used for evaluation of the common femoral vein. Doppler spectral waveforms are recorded continuously throughout inflation and deflation of the cuff. This procedure is next repeated with Doppler spectral waveform recordings from the proximal superficial femoral vein (Fig. 26–21).

Step 3. The patient is now turned to face away from the examiner, and the 12-cm blood pressure cuff is placed around the calf (Fig. 26–22). The popliteal vein is imaged in the longitudinal plane, and Doppler spectral waveforms are obtained during normal respiration. The cuff is then inflated to 100 mm Hg pressure for 3 sec and then rapidly deflated. Spectral waveforms are recorded continuously during inflation and deflation (Fig. 26–23).

Step 4. Following completion of the popliteal recording, the mid- and distal segments of the superficial femoral vein

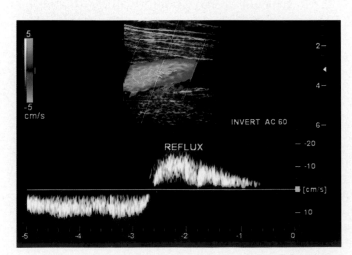

FIGURE 26–21. Color flow image and Doppler spectral waveforms demonstrating significant reflux in the proximal superficial femoral vein. (Courtesy of The Hershey Vascular Laboratory, the Penn State Vascular Institute, Hershey, PA.)

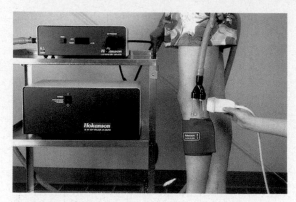

FIGURE 26–22. Appropriate positioning of the patient, calf cuff, and transducer for recording Doppler spectral tracings from the popliteal, distal superficial femoral, and perforating veins. (Courtesy of D. E. Hokanson, Incorporated, Bellevue, WA.)

and the major perforating veins along the medial side of the thigh are tested in an identical manner.

Step 5. The confluence of the lesser saphenous vein with the popliteal vein is identified and imaged in the longitudinal plane. Doppler spectral waveforms are recorded during normal respiration and during cuff inflation to 100 mm Hg pressure and rapid deflation. Careful attention is given to flow direction and, if present, to the duration of retrograde venous flow.

Step 6. The mid-segment of the greater saphenous vein is identified on the medial aspect of the knee and imaged in its longitudinal plane. Using a cuff

inflation pressure of 100 mm Hg, the presence of reflux is confirmed in a manner similar to that used for the deep veins of the thigh. Next, the anterolateral branch of the greater saphenous vein is located on the lateral aspect of the knee and evaluated in the longitudinal plane in an identical fashion.

Step 7. The blood pressure cuff is moved to the level of the ankle. The posterior tibial and peroneal veins are identified using B-mode and/or color flow imaging. Doppler spectral waveforms are recorded from the posterior tibial veins during normal respiration and with the cuff inflated to 100 mm Hg. Waveforms are continuously recorded during rapid cuff deflation. The test is repeated in an identical manner for evaluation of the peroneal veins.

Step 8. The posterior arch vein and the mid-segment of the lesser saphenous vein should be examined using a cuff inflation pressure of 100 mm Hg, with the cuff at ankle level.

Step 9. A 7-cm-wide blood pressure cuff is wrapped around the foot. Color flow imaging is used to locate the posterior tibial veins in long axis just anterior to the medial malleolus. The blood pressure cuff is inflated to 120 mm Hg pressure. Doppler spectral waveforms are recorded during cuff inflation and deflation. The peroneal veins and the distal segment of the greater saphenous vein

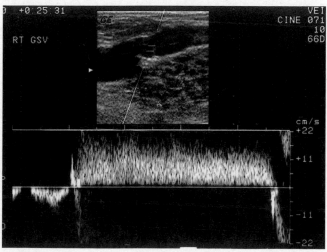

FIGURE 26–23. Color flow image and Doppler spectral waveforms demonstrating significant reflux in the superficial femoral vein. (Courtesy of Providence Surgical Care Group, Providence, RI.)

are interrogated for reflux in an identical fashion.

Step 10. Large perforating veins associated with the posterior arch vein that were identified in the distal calf during the initial duplex evaluation of the limb may be tested using the 7-cm metatarsal cuff and an inflation pressure of 120 mm Hg.

Diagnostic Criteria

As noted previously, reflux that persists for longer than 0.5 sec at any level is considered to be clinically significant. In addition, O'Donnell and associates[18] have shown that a sum of the venous closure times from the superficial femoral and popliteal veins exceeding 4 sec is accurate in predicting severe venous reflux.

Advantages

The standing cuff inflation-deflation technique, combined with duplex ultrasonography, provides a quantitative estimate of valve closure time in specific segments of the deep and superficial venous systems. All venous segments, including major perforating veins, can be studied using this method, which mimics venous valvular physiology. The deficiencies of the Valsalva maneuver and manual compression techniques, cited previously, are overcome by use of distal limb cuff compression to ensure adequate extrinsic venous pressure and transvalvular pressure gradients. The accuracy of the cuff inflation-deflation technique does not depend on the presence of incompetent valves proximal to the venous segment being studied, as does the Valsalva's maneuver.

Limitations

While they are relatively inexpensive items, an automatic cuff inflator and an air source capable of rapid cuff inflation are not common to all noninvasive vascular laboratories. Some laboratories find it helpful to have one sonographer perform the imaging component of the study while a second member of the staff assists with the cuff inflation and deflation procedures. Additionally, patient and sonographer comfort is best achieved if the patient is examined while standing on a platform that is 18 to 24 inches in height surrounded on three sides by a support railing. This places the patient's lower limb at a level approximating the ultrasound system controls and allows the sonographer to assume an ergonomically correct position throughout the procedure. Such platforms are not universally available and may need to be specially constructed to meet individual laboratory designs.

Care must be taken to observe the patient throughout the examination, as a small percentage of patients with impaired venous function and venous dilation may experience dizziness, as noted by Ballard and associates.[30] This is most likely the result of deceased venous return during the cuff inflation procedure.

SEGMENTAL VENOUS INCOMPETENCE

It is not uncommon to find segmental valvular dysfunction in both the deep and superficial veins. Patients with venous ulceration most often have three or four incompetent segments, involving either the deep or superficial systems.[31] Incompetence of the superficial veins is present in at least 92% of cases with ulceration, while incompetence of the deep veins at the ankle level is least common.[12]

van Bemmelen and Bergan[31] have described the distribution of incompetent segments of the greater saphenous vein in patients with superficial venous insufficiency. The greater saphenous vein was incompetent at knee level in 61% of limbs, at calf level in 49%, and in the proximal thigh in 32% of limbs. This finding emphasizes the prevalence of distal superficial incompetence while the more proximal valves of the greater saphenous vein remain functional. In patients with incompetence of the greater saphenous vein at knee level, van Bemmelen and Bergan noted that less than 50% had multisegmental incompetence from the saphenofemoral confluence to the level of the knee. A total of 34% of patients with greater saphenous incompetence at knee level and functional proximal superficial venous segments demonstrated deep venous reflux in the superficial femoral and popliteal veins. In these cases, an incompetent perforating vein was identified at the upper end of the incompetent segment of the greater saphenous vein.

Lesser saphenous venous reflux is often found to occur segmentally. Incompetency of the proximal segment of the lesser saphenous vein has been reported in 36% of lower limbs, while 31% of limbs demonstrated reflux in the calf segments.[31] If the valves in the distal segments remain competent, flow from incompetent proximal valves is diverted to superficial branches.

CONCLUSIONS

The vascular laboratory approach to the diagnosis of venous insufficiency is dependent on the clinical questions that are to be answered. The question of whether the patient has venous insufficiency can be answered with a thorough medical history, physical examination, and photoplethysmographic refill time. Air plethysmography is reserved for patients whose global limb venous hemodynamics and the effectiveness of the calf muscle pump must be determined to define therapeutic options. To accurately assess the deep, superficial, and perforating venous systems for valvular incompetence and to exclude residual venous obstruction, a complete venous duplex ultrasound examination should be performed, complemented by color flow imaging. To ensure the most accurate, site-specific definition of clinically significant valvular incompetence, segmental quantitative measurement of reflux using the standing cuff inflation-deflation technique should be employed.

References

1. Negus D, Cockett FB: Femoral vein pressures in post-phlebitic iliac vein obstruction. Br J Surg 54:522, 1967.

2. Killewich LA, Martin R, Cramer M: Pathophysiology of venous claudication. J Vasc Surg 1:502, 1984.

3. Nicolaides AN, Zukowski AJ: The value of dynamic venous pressure measurements. World J Surg 10:919–924, 1986.

4. Johnston KW, Maruzzo BC, Cobbold RSC: Inaccuracies of a zero-crossing detector for recording Doppler signals. Surg Forum 28:201–203, 1977.

5. Strandness DE Jr.: Doppler ultrasonic techniques in vascular disease. In EF Bernstein (ed): Noninvasive Diagnostic Techniques in Vascular Disease, 3rd ed. St. Louis, CV Mosby, 1985, pp 13–18.

6. Raju S, Fredericks R: Evaluation of methods for detecting venous reflux. Perspectives in venous insufficiency. Arch Surg 125:1463–1467, 1990.

7. Barnes RW: Noninvasive tests for chronic venous insufficiency. In Bergan JJ, Yao JST (eds): Surgery of the Veins. Orlando, FL, Grune & Stratton, 1985, pp 99–109.

8. Sigel B, Popky GL, Wagner DK, et al: Doppler ultrasound method for diagnosing lower extremity venous disease. Surg Gynecol Obstet 127:339–350, 1968.

9. Miller SS, Foote AV: The ultrasonic detection of incompetent perforating veins. Br J Surg 61:653–656, 1974.

10. O'Donnell TF, Burnand KG, Clemenson G, et al: Doppler examination versus clinical and phlebographic detection of the location of incompetent perforating veins. Arch Surg 112:31–35, 1977.

11. Abramowitz HB, Queral LA, Flinn WR, et al: The use of photoplethysmography in the assessment of venous insufficiency: A comparison to venous pressure measurements. Surgery 86:434–441, 1979.

12. Christopoulos DG, Nicolaides AN, Szendro G, et al: Air plethysmography and the effects of elastic compression on venous hemodynamics of the leg. J Vasc Surg 5:148–159, 1987.

13. Herman RJ, Neiman HL, Yao JST, et al: Descending venography: A method of evaluating lower extremity valvular function. Radiology 137:63–69, 1980.

14. Payne S, Thrush A, London N, et al: Venous assessment using air plethysmography: A comparison with clinical examination, ambulatory venous pressure measurement, and duplex scanning. Br J Surg 80:967–970, 1993.

15. Lees TA, Lambert D: A comparative study of air plethysmography and Doppler colour flow imaging with ambulatory venous pressure measurements in the diagnosis of venous reflux in the lower limb. In Raymond-Martinbeau R, Prescott RM, Zummo M (eds): Phlebologie 92. Paris, John Libbey Eurotext, 1992, pp 594–596.

16. Oliver MA: Anatomy and physiology. In Talbot SR, Oliver MA (eds): Techniques of Venous Imaging. Pasadena, CA, Appleton Davies, 1992, pp 11–20.

17. Masuda EM, Kistner RL, Eklof B: Prospective study of duplex scanning for venous reflux: Comparison of Valsalva and pneumatic cuff techniques in the reverse Trendelenburg and standing position. J Vasc Surg 20:711–719, 1994.

18. O'Donnell TF: Surgical treatment of incompetent communicating veins, In Bergan JJ, Kistner RL (eds): Atlas of Venous Surgery. Philadelphia, Saunders, 1992, pp 111–124.

19. Lees TA, Lambert D: Patterns of venous reflux in limbs with skin changes associated with chronic venous insufficiency. Br J Surg 6:725–728, 1993.

20. Phillips GWL, Paige J, Molan MP: A comparison of colour duplex ultrasound with venography and varicography in the assessment of varicose veins. Clin Radiol 50:20–25, 1995.

21. Mozes G, Gloviczki P, Menawat S, et al: Surgical anatomy for endoscopic subfascial division of perforating veins. J Vasc Surg 23:800–808, 1996.

22. Welch HJ, Faliakoa EC, McLaughlin RL, et al: Comparison of descending phlebography with quantitative photoplethysmography, air plethysmography, and duplex quantitative valve closure time in assessing deep venous reflux. J Vasc Surg 16:913–919, 1993.

23. van Bemmelen PS, Bedford G, Beach K, Strandness DE: Quantitative segmental evaluation of venous valvular reflux with duplex ultrasound scanning. J Vasc Surg 10:425–431, 1989.

24. Markel A, Meissner MH, Manzo RA, et al.: A comparison of the cuff deflation method with Valsalva's maneuver and limb compression in detecting venous valvular reflux. Arch Surg 129:701–705, 1994.

25. van Bemmelen PS, Beach K, Bedford G, Strandness DE Jr.: The mechanism of venous valve closure. Arch Surg 125:617–619, 1990.

26. Talbot SR: Use of real time imaging in identifying deep venous obstruction: A preliminary report. Bruit 6:41–44, 1984.

27. Mattos MA, Londrey GL, Leutz DW, et al: Color flow duplex scanning for the surveillance and diagnosis of acute deep venous thrombosis. J Vasc Surg 15:366–376, 1992.

28. Kerr TM, Cranley JJ, Johnson JR, et al: Analysis of 1084 consecutive lower extremities involved with acute venous thrombosis diagnosed by duplex scanning. Surgery 108:520–527, 1990.

29. Vasdekis SN, Clarke GH, Nicolaides AN: Quantification of venous reflux by means of duplex scanning. J Vasc Surg 10:670–677, 1989.

30. Ballard JL, Bergan JJ, DeLange M: Venous imaging for reflux using duplex ultrasonography. In AbuRahma AF, Bergan JJ (eds): Noninvasive Vascular Diagnosis. London, Springer-Verlag, 2000, pp 329–334.

31. van Bemmelen PS, Bergan JJ: Segmental duplex reflux examination and color flow imaging. In Medical Intelligence Unit: Quantitative Measurement of Venous Incompetence. Austin, TX, R.G. Landes Company, 1992, pp 51–66.

Chapter 27

Nonvascular Pathology Encountered During Venous Sonography

WILLIAM J. ZWIEBEL, MD

There are many things that may cause pain or swelling of the leg besides venous thrombosis, and a number of these conditions may be detected sonographically. Additionally, a variety of asymptomatic conditions may be discovered in the course of venous ultrasound imaging. It is important, therefore, that ultrasound practitioners recognize nonvascular pathology that is encountered in the course of venous ultrasound examinations.[1-12] In this chapter, we cover the more commonly encountered conditions; namely, venous congestion, abscess, hematoma, adenopathy, soft tissue tumor, popliteal cyst, joint effusion, and lymphedema.

VENOUS CONGESTION

Bilateral lower extremity edema may result from elevated hydrostatic pressure within the venous system induced by congestive heart failure. The inability of the heart to pump blood adequately leads to backpressure in the venous system, subsequently resulting in tissue edema and leg swelling. A second cause for venous congestion is fluid overload, which may result from renal failure or iatrogenic overhydration. Heart failure and fluid overload cannot be differentiated sonographically, as the end results in the extremities are the same—venous congestion and soft tissue edema.

In the presence of venous congestion, the Doppler signals in large veins (e.g., iliac and common femoral) are pulsatile[4] (Fig. 27–1).

In some cases, pulsatility may be so striking that it is difficult, at first glance, to know whether Doppler signals are venous or arterial. However, vessel identification is easily accomplished by comparing the Doppler signals in the vein and the adjacent artery and by noting the direction of blood flow (cephalad in the venous system).

Soft tissue edema associated with venous congestion produces a reticulated pattern in the subcutaneous fat, as seen in Figure 27–2, caused by the accumulation of fluid among subcutaneous fat globules. Although less obvious, fluid also accumulates among the muscle bundles. Edema has devastating effects on sonographic resolution. The interfaces between tissue and fluid reflect and refract the sound beam in myriad directions, attenuating both the incident and reflected waves and introducing noise. The result is a "snowy," low-resolution image that is especially problematic for imaging calf veins.

Ultrasound venography is requested frequently in patients with bilateral leg swelling and dyspnea, in whom pulmonary thromboembolism is a consideration. Although it is logical, for reasons of simplicity and noninvasiveness, to begin the search for pulmonary thromboembolism with venous ultrasound, the likelihood of finding thrombus in patients with bilateral leg swelling is very low (5% or less).[5] Therefore, the potential for overutilization of venous ultrasound in dyspneic patients with leg swelling is considerable. It has been shown that most such patients have con-

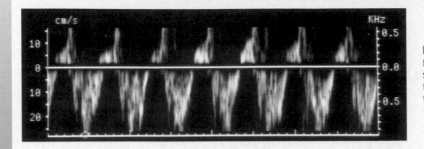

FIGURE 27–1. Pulsatile venous flow. Common femoral vein flow signals are markedly pulsatile in this patient with leg swelling due to right heart failure.

gestive heart failure. Proper clinical screening is the only means for avoiding unnecessary venous ultrasound examinations, and a number of protocols have been developed that test the likelihood that a patient may have deep vein thrombosis/pulmonary embolus, but achieving a consistent level of screening is difficult to accomplish.[6,7]

This is a good opportunity to emphasize an important fact about pulmonary thromboembolism: *A negative venous ultrasound examination does not exclude pulmonary embolus.* About 25% to 30% of patients with documented pulmonary embolism do not have lower extremity venous thrombosis.[6,7] In such cases, the thrombus may already have embolized from the leg veins to the lungs, or the thrombus may have originated from other venous sources, including the pelvic and upper extremity veins.

LYMPHEDEMA

Lymphedema is another condition that may mimic the manifestations of venous thrombosis.[5] Neoplastic or postsurgical obstruction of the lymphatic system may cause extremity swelling and pain that are difficult to differentiate from the effects of venous thrombosis. The sonographic manifestations of lymphedema are no different from edema caused by venous congestion, as described previously. In the absence of detectable lymph node enlargement, no specific ultrasound findings point to lym-

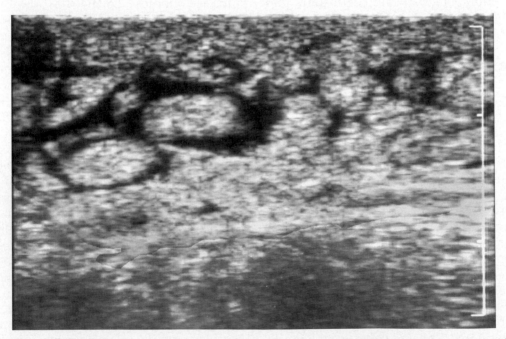

FIGURE 27–2. Massive soft tissue edema gives the subcutaneous fat a marbled appearance in this patient with renal failure and fluid overload.

phatic obstruction as the etiology. Sonography generally serves well, however, to confirm that the venous system is patent and is not the cause of the problem.

ABSCESS AND CELLULITIS

Abscess and cellulitis are both manifestations of bacterial infection. The term *abscess* implies the formation of an enclosed collection of pus, whereas *cellulitis* refers to diffuse soft tissue infection without a focal purulent collection. Abscess and cellulitis cause swelling, skin erythema, pain, and tenderness. These signs and symptoms may closely mimic the manifestations of acute venous thrombosis, and for that reason, ultrasound is commonly used to sort out the two possibilities by ensuring that the venous system is patent.

The soft tissue edema that accompanies cellulitis cannot be differentiated from edema generated by other conditions, such as congestive heart failure or fluid overload. If an abscess is present (Fig. 27–3A),

FIGURE 27–3. Various appearances of soft tissue abscesses. *A*, This is an incisional abscess that developed after arterial bypass graft. Note the thick, irregular walls and low-level internal echoes. Enhanced through-transmission of ultrasound is present, as the contents are watery and produce little attenuation. *B*, Composite image of an extensive, poorly defined medial arm abscess in a diabetic patient. This abscess is much different than that shown in *A*. The borders of the abscess are not visualized at all. The presence of infection is indicated only by heterogeneous material (*arrows*) containing myriad tiny air bubbles that produce tiny bright reflections. Enhanced through-transmission is absent due to the echogenic, attenuating nature of the abscess contents. Magnetic resonance imaging was needed to demonstrate the full extent of the abscess, which was not encapsulated.

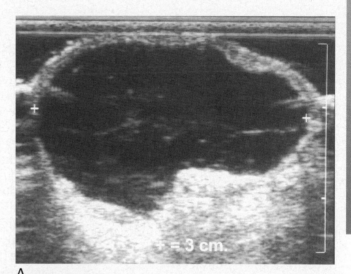

A

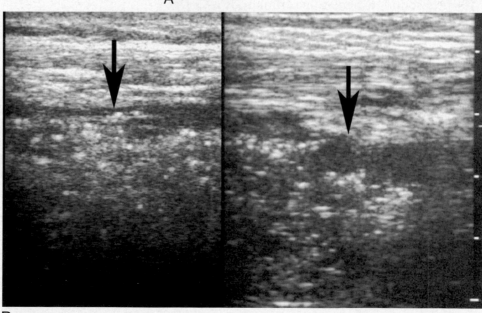

B

however, it can usually be identified with ultrasound as a circumscribed fluid collection. Typically, the fluid contains low-level echoes or a layer of echogenic debris. Tiny gas bubbles within an abscess may produce myriad tiny bright reflections (Fig. 27–3B), and larger gas bubbles may occasionally generate focal bright reflections accompanied by acoustic shadowing. The margins of an abscess may be smooth and well defined or shaggy and poorly defined. Extremity abscesses tend to spread out longitudinally, along the confines of the fascial planes. Therefore, they may have an elongated, fusiform shape.

HEMATOMA

Extremity soft tissue hematomas usually occur in association with trauma (violent or iatrogenic), anticoagulation, or vigorous exercise (usually in athletes). Hematomas may cause pain and extremity swelling that are difficult to distinguish clinically from the effects of venous thrombosis. Once again, sonography plays an important diagnostic role in documenting the patency of the venous system. In addition, an acute hematoma may be directly visualized with ultrasound (Fig. 27–4), assuming that the blood collects locally and does not spread out within the tissues (ecchymosis). As seen with ultrasound, a hematoma initially is a hypoechoic mass that usually has ill-defined borders and is slightly heterogeneous. With time, the hematoma retracts and serum is exuded; at that point, the hematoma is a heterogeneous collection in which the echogenic thrombus is surrounded by anechoic fluid. With lysis of the thrombus, a hematoma may become an entirely anechoic fluid collection. Large hematomas may compress the venous system, causing venous distention and sluggish flow. In some cases, stagnation may lead to secondary venous thrombosis.

MUSCLE INJURY

Muscle injury may result from a blow (contusion), from a penetrating injury, or from a "muscle pull," which is a tearing of a muscle bundle in response to vigorous exercise or abrupt straining. Tearing of the muscle is accompanied initially by varying degrees of bleeding and, subsequently, by inflammation. Kim and colleagues[8] report that injured muscle initially is hyperechoic and either homogeneous or heterogeneous. By about 7 days after injury, the affected muscle is intermediate to low in echogenicity and heterogeneous. These findings persist for at least 3 weeks after injury (Fig. 27–5). Long-term follow-up information is not available. With a muscle pull, the area of injury may be quite focal and possibly fusiform in shape. Larger areas of abnormality may be seen with contusion.

ADENOPATHY

The term *adenopathy* refers to pathological enlargement of lymph nodes, whether from inflammatory or neoplastic causes. Adenopathy may cause extremity swelling, either by associated obstruction of lymphatic drainage or by compression of the venous system. In some cases, the enlarged lymph nodes are tender.

Massive adenopathy generates hypoechoic confluent nodal masses that are readily identified sonographically (Fig. 27–6A). These masses can generally be differentiated from abscesses or hematomas because blood flow can be demonstrated within the mass with color flow ultrasound. In addition, adenopathy tends to occur at specific sites, particularly in the axilla, in the groin, along the iliac vessels, or adjacent to the inferior vena cava and the aorta. In patients with extremity swelling, the sonographers should be mindful that lymphadenopathy may be the cause, through venous compression and restriction of venous flow. It is important to examine Doppler signals carefully for a continuous flow pattern indicative of proximal obstruction (see Chapter 22). If venous compression is suspected, the sonographer may also search directly for adenopathy in the axilla, groin, or abdomen.

Not all lymphadenopathy is seen in the form of a coalescent mass of nodes. Individual enlarged nodes may also be detected

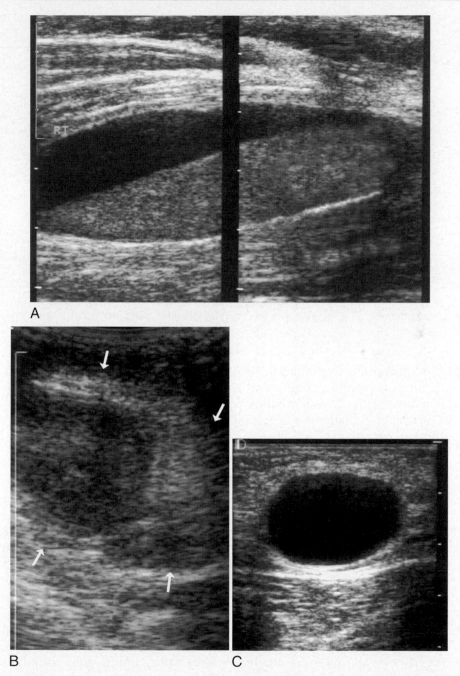

FIGURE 27–4. Various appearances of soft tissue hematomas. *A,* Composite image of an acute (hours-old) arm hematoma related to poorly controlled Coumadin therapy. Note the fluid/fluid level resulting from settling of non-clotted blood cells. *B,* An acute (12-hours-old) hematoma (*arrows*) in the popliteal fossa. This hematoma is fairly echogenic, consistent with its acute state and coagulation of the blood. *C,* Two-month-old asymptomatic hematoma at a saphenous vein harvest site. The well-defined collection is anechoic because the clot has lysed and the collection has become a hygroma containing blood breakdown products.

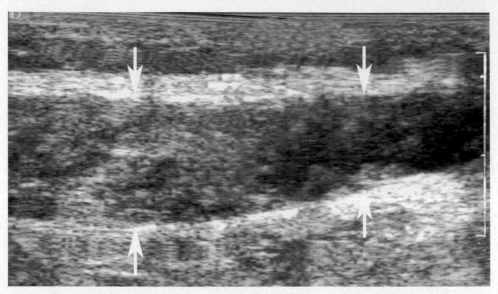

FIGURE 27–5. Muscle injury. A fusiform, heterogeneous region (*arrows*) is seen within the calf musculature at a site of pain and tenderness. The symptoms began one day previous, after the patient helped push a stalled automobile.

during venous ultrasound examination. In such cases, it often is possible to differentiate between a neoplastic or inflammatory etiology by noting the shape of the node and the pattern of vascularity[9–11] (Fig. 27–6 B and C). With benign lymph node enlargement, the normal ovoid nodal shape is maintained, with the short-axis diameter not exceeding half of the length of the node. In addition, fat is present in the hilum of the node, producing bright echoes that are surrounded by the low-level echoes of the nodal tissue. Finally, as seen with color flow imaging, blood vessels enter the node only through the hilum. With neoplastic enlargement, tumor cells infiltrate the node and the normal architecture is replaced. The node becomes abnormally rounded, with the short-axis diameter exceeding half of the length. The fat within the hilum may be replaced by tumor, and in such cases, the bright fat echoes are no longer seen. In substantially enlarged malignant nodes, central anechoic or low-echogenicity zones may be seen due to necrosis. Finally, malignant nodes show substantial alteration of vascularity. The orderly branching of vessels from the hilum to the periphery is lost. Instead, irregular vessels follow a disorderly pattern, accompanied by nonperfused areas of necrosis.

In addition, blood vessels enter through the periphery of the node as well as the hilum.

SOFT TISSUE TUMORS

Benign or malignant soft tissue tumors[1,12–14] may be encountered in the course of ultrasound venous examination, either as subjects of the examination or as incidental findings. The latter situation is particularly true of popliteal fossa or groin masses that are thought clinically to be cysts or aneurysms but instead are found to be tumors. Primary soft tissue tumors include leiomyomas, a variety of sarcomas, squamous cell carcinomas, and melanomas. Metastatic tumors may originate from a wide variety of sources, but those that metastasize to the extremity soft tissues are usually highly malignant. The ultrasound appearance of soft tissue tumors is variable. Some are solid, but others may contain large areas of liquefactive necrosis or hemorrhage. The latter may resemble hematomas, abscesses, or cysts, but differentiation is commonly possible through the demonstration of blood flow in solid portions of the mass (Fig. 27–7). Some tumors are well defined, while others appear to infiltrate the

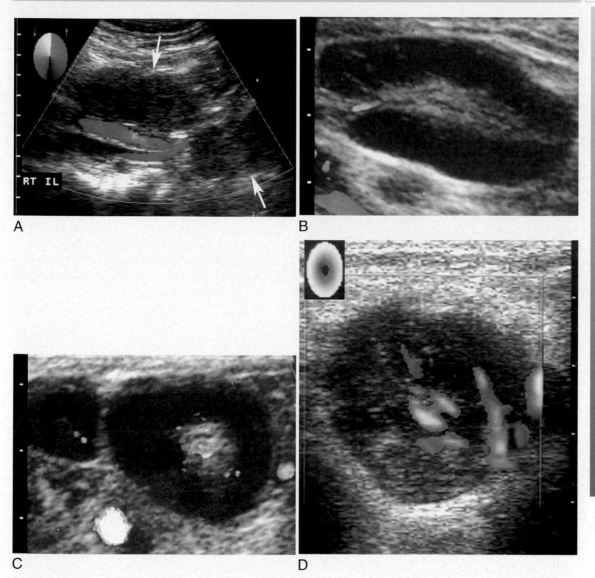

FIGURE 27–6. Adenopathy. *A*, Markedly enlarged lymph node masses (*arrows*) are seen adjacent to the iliac (IL) vessels in a patient with lymphoma. *B* and *C*, Hilar and short-axis color flow views of an enlarged inguinal lymph node with normal architecture found during venous sonography. Note that the echogenic hilar fat is surrounded by hypoechoic nodal parenchyma and that vascularity is both central and orderly appearing. *D*, Power Doppler view of a lymphomatous inguinal node discovered incidentally during venous sonography. No hilum is visible, and the vasculature is disorganized. On orthogonal views (not shown) the node was spherical rather that ovoid, and several other abnormal nodes were seen in the same area.

surrounding tissues. Color and spectral Doppler ultrasound have been used to assess the vascularity of soft tissue masses. Although Doppler features do not accurately differentiate between benign and malignant masses, malignant lesions tend to have irregularly distributed vessels that are oddly angulated and tortuous and change caliber abruptly. In addition, malignant lesions may contain prominent avascular areas due to necrosis.[13] Finally, high flow velocity (exceeding 50 cm/sec) in afferent tumor arteries suggests malignancy, as does a low-resistance spectral waveform pattern.

POPLITEAL CYSTS

With chronic knee joint dysfunction, certain bursae that communicate with the knee may dilate, forming cysts in the

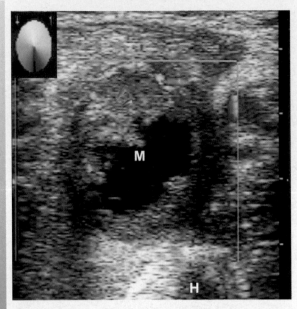

FIGURE 27–7. Soft tissue tumor. A partially necrotic mass (M) is seen adjacent to the humerus (H). Disorderly blood flow is evident in the lesion. This is a squamous cell carcinoma metastasis from an ipsilateral digital primary.

vicinity of the popliteal fossa.[15,16] Popliteal cysts are particularly common in patients with severe degenerative joint disease and those with rheumatoid arthritis, but they are by no means exclusive to these conditions. The gastrocnemius-semimembranosus bursa most commonly becomes cystic, and when this occurs, the dilated bursa is called a Baker's cyst. This bursa lies *posterior and medial* to the knee joint, between the muscles of the same names. Cysts at other locations in the popliteal fossa should not be called Baker's cysts. Instead, they should simply be referred to as popliteal cysts. As popliteal cysts enlarge, they dissect between the fascial planes and may extend down into the calf musculature. Large cysts are prone to spontaneous rupture, which causes pain, tenderness, and swelling in the calf. These signs and symptoms are indistinguishable from the manifestations of acute deep venous thrombosis.

Ultrasound is the primary modality for differentiation between popliteal cysts and acute deep venous thrombosis. Popliteal cysts (Fig. 27–8) are usually well defined, rounded, and anechoic, but some chronic cysts may contain echogenic debris or may be diffusely echogenic. In the latter case, soft tissue neoplasms are a differential consideration. It is helpful in such cases to look for blood flow within the mass, which is not present in a cyst but may be seen in a tumor.

Because it is the most common popliteal cyst, it is worthwhile to describe the specific features of a Baker's cyst: (1) The cyst is medially located and closely associated with the medial head of the gastrocnemius muscle; (2) the cyst is crescentic, as seen in transverse images; and (3) the upper end of the cyst is at the level of the knee joint. Unfortunately, not all popliteal cysts have this typical location, but they usually have a typical cystic appearance.

Popliteal cyst rupture probably cannot be confirmed absolutely with ultrasound, but certain features suggest cyst rupture; namely, irregular or ill-defined cyst borders (due to loss of turgor) and a pointed inferior end of the cyst. Normally, popliteal cysts have rounded borders. With rupture, the cyst fluid dissects inferiorly into the calf among the muscle bundles, giving the inferior end of the fluid collection a pointed configuration. It should be remembered that the principal role of sonography is to determine whether the venous system is the cause of calf pain. If the venous system is patent, rupture of a Baker cyst becomes one of several diagnostic possibilities.

Popliteal artery aneurysms may be mistaken clinically for Baker's cysts, but differentiation is simple because blood flow is detected in the aneurysm (with the assumption that the vessel is patent), and continuity with the popliteal artery is easily demonstrated.

JOINT EFFUSION

A final condition that may mimic extremity venous thrombosis is acute knee arthropathy or trauma. Although the primary joint abnormality cannot generally be diagnosed with ultrasound, a joint effusion accompanying the knee problem can easily be recognized. Fluid may be seen to distend the

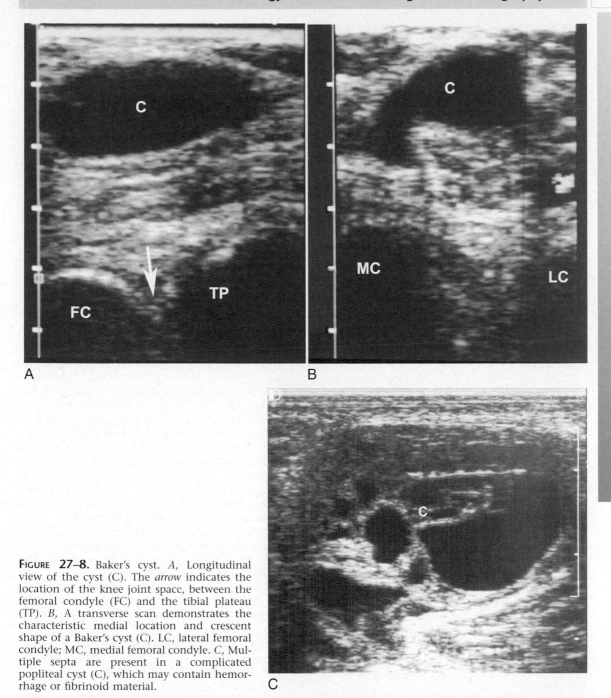

FIGURE 27–8. Baker's cyst. *A*, Longitudinal view of the cyst (C). The *arrow* indicates the location of the knee joint space, between the femoral condyle (FC) and the tibial plateau (TP). *B*, A transverse scan demonstrates the characteristic medial location and crescent shape of a Baker's cyst (C). LC, lateral femoral condyle; MC, medial femoral condyle. *C*, Multiple septa are present in a complicated popliteal cyst (C), which may contain hemorrhage or fibrinoid material.

joint capsule laterally, medially, or above the patella in the quadriceps bursa (Fig. 27–9). With a little diligence, fluid also may be recognized in other joints, including the elbow and ankle.[17] At the knee, differentiation between joint effusion and a popliteal cyst is not difficult, as the fluid is confined adjacent to the borders of the patella laterally, medially, or superiorly. Sonographic identification of joint effusion is important, as this finding may direct clinical investigation toward the knee joint and away from the deep venous system, which is assumed to be normal.

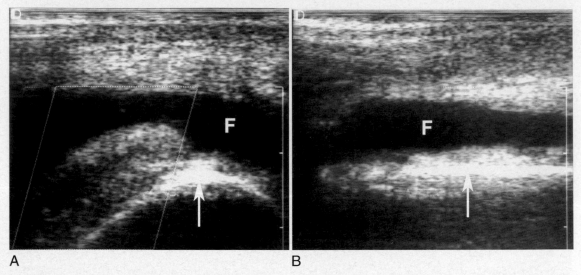

FIGURE 27–9 Knee joint effusion. Images obtained along the medial (*A*) and lateral (*B*) borders of the patella show joint fluid (F), which would not be visible in a normal knee. Note that the bony structure of the knee (*arrows*) is quite close to the fluid.

REFERENCES

1. Borgstede JP, Clagett BS: Types, frequency and significance of alternative diagnoses found during duplex Doppler venous examination of the lower extremities. J Ultrasound Med 11: 85–89, 1992.
2. Borgstede JP, Clagett BS: Types, frequency and significance of alternative diagnoses found during duplex Doppler venous examination of the lower extremities. J Ultrasound Med 11: 85–89, 1992.
3. Drinman KJ, Wolfson PM, Steinitz D, et al: Duplex imaging in lymphedema. J Vasc Technol 17:23–26, 1993.
4. Abu-Yousef MM, Kakish ME, Mufid M: Pulsatile venous Doppler flow in lower limbs: Highly indicative of elevated right atrium pressure. Am J Roentgenol 167:977–980, 1996.
5. Sheiman RG, Weintraub JL, McArdle CR: Bilateral lower extremity US in the patient with bilateral symptoms of deep venous thrombosis: Assessment of need. Radiology 196:379–381, 1995.
6. Goldhaber SZ: Pulmonary embolism. N Engl J Med 339:93–104, 1998.
7. Weinman EE, Salzman EW: Deep-vein thrombosis. N Engl J Med 331:1630–1641, 1994.
8. Kim HG, Ryu KN, Sung DW, Park YK: Correlation between sonographic and pathologic findings in muscle injury; experimental study in rabbits. J Ultrasound Med 21:1113–1119, 2002.
9. Ott G, Schang T, Seelbach-Goebel B, et al: Lymphadenopathy: Differentiation of benign from malignant disease—color Doppler US assessment of intranodal angioarchitecture. Radiology 208:117–123, 1998.
10. Ying M, Phil M, Ahuja A, et al: Power Doppler sonography of normal cervical lymph nodes. J Ultrasound Med 19:511–517, 2000.
11. Tschammler A, Heuser B, Ott G, et al: Pathological angioarchitecture in lymph nodes: Underlying histopathologic findings. Ultrasound Med Biol 26:1089–1097, 2000.
12. Belli P, Costantini M, Mirk P, et al: Role of color Doppler sonography in the assessment of musculoskeletal soft tissue masses. J Ultrasound Med 19:823–830, 2000.
13. Needleman L, Nack TL: Vascular and nonvascular masses. J Vasc Technol 18:299–306, 1994.
14. Mitchell DG, Merton DA, Liu JB, Goldberg BB: Superficial masses with color flow Doppler imaging. J Clin Ultrasound 19:555–560, 1991.
15. Ward EE, Jacobson JA, Fessell DP, et al: Sonographic detection of Baker's cysts: Comparison with MR imaging. Am J Roentgenol 176: 373–380, 2001.
16. Langsfeld M, Matteson B, Johnson W, et al: Baker's cysts mimicking the symptoms of deep vein thrombosis: Diagnosis with venous duplex scanning. J Vasc Surg 25:658–662, 1997.
17. Fessell DP, Jacobson JA, Craig J, et al: Using sonography to reveal and aspirate joint effusions. Am J Roentgenol 174:1353–1362, 2000.

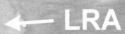

SECTION V
ABDOMEN AND PELVIS

Chapter 28

Anatomy and Normal Doppler Signatures of Abdominal Vessels

WILLIAM J. ZWIEBEL, MD

The correct identification of abdominal vessels and the accurate assessment of blood flow in the abdomen require knowledge of vascular anatomy and of the Doppler characteristics of specific vessels. This fundamental information is presented in this chapter. The reader should be familiar with concepts of arterial pulsatility and Doppler spectrum analysis, as presented in Section I, "Basics."

CELIAC ARTERY

The celiac artery, also called the *celiac trunk* or *celiac axis*, is the most cephalad visceral branch of the abdominal aorta. It arises from the anterior aortic surface, between the diaphragmatic crura (Fig. 28–1). It then bifurcates about 1 to 3 cm from its origin into the common hepatic and splenic arteries, which are readily visualized with ultrasound. The celiac artery also gives rise to the left gastric artery, which is generally not visible sonographically. The branching pattern of the celiac artery is quite constant, occurring in approximately 93% of individuals. In the most common variations, one or more of the celiac branches arise separately from the aorta or from the superior mesenteric artery (SMA). In less than 1% of individuals, the celiac artery and the SMA arise from the aorta as a common trunk. In such cases, the common trunk splits into the celiac artery and the SMA within 1 or 2 cm from the aorta.[1,2]

Ultrasound visualization of the celiac artery is best in the transverse plane (Fig. 28–2), in which the T-shaped bifurcation of

the vessel is characteristic. In older individuals with tortuous vessels, the "T" configuration may droop to the patient's left and be less apparent. The celiac artery origin is also seen readily in longitudinal images, but the branches are not well seen in this plane. Celiac artery Doppler signals have a characteristic low-resistance flow pattern, with a large amount of continuous forward flow throughout diastole, but a slightly higher resistance pattern is seen near the origin of the vessel. The splenic and hepatic branches also exhibit a low-resistance flow pattern, caused by the low flow resistance within the microcirculation of the liver and spleen.[3]

If the celiac artery is occluded, collateralization occurs through the pancreaticoduodenal arterial arcade, which is a network of small vessels surrounding the pancreas and

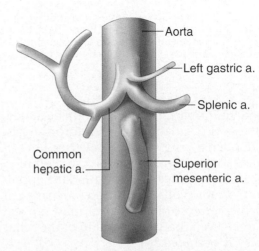

FIGURE 28–1. The celiac artery and its branches.

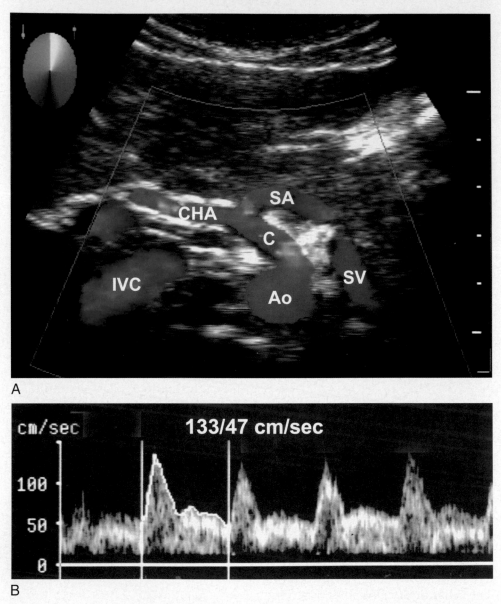

A

B

FIGURE 28–2. Celiac artery ultrasound. *A*, Transverse sonogram of the celiac axis (C) as it divides into the common hepatic artery (CHA) and splenic artery (SA). Ao, aorta; IVC, inferior vena cava; SV, a segment of the splenic vein. *B*, Normal, low-pulsatility Doppler signal in the distal portion of the celiac artery. Peak systolic velocity is 133 cm/sec, and end diastolic velocity is 47 cm/sec.

duodenum. With the celiac trunk occluded, these vessels enlarge and feed into the gastroduodenal artery, which reverses flow in order to supply blood to the common hepatic artery. Because of abundant opportunities for collateralization, hepatic or splenic artery blood flow may appear normal, even though the origin of the celiac artery is occluded.[4]

SPLENIC ARTERY

The splenic artery (limb of the celiac T toward patient's left) follows a tortuous course along the posterosuperior margin of the pancreatic body and tail (Fig. 28–3A) and terminates by splitting into a number of branches in the hilum of the spleen. Along the way, the splenic artery gives

FIGURE 28–3. *A*, Splenic artery anatomy. *B*, Normal, low-pulsatility Doppler signal from the splenic artery. Peak systolic velocity is 110 cm/sec, and end-diastolic velocity is 45 cm/sec.

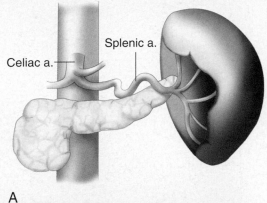

A

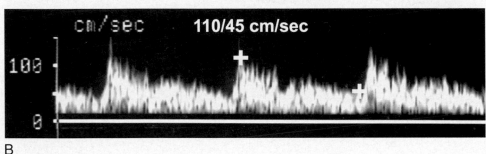

B

rise to several pancreatic branches, short gastric branches, and the left gastroepiploic artery. None of these vessels can be seen with ultrasound. Transverse scans from a midline approach usually reveal the proximal portion of the splenic artery (see Fig. 28–2A). The course of the distal portion of the splenic artery is difficult to image because of tortuosity. The distal-most portion of the splenic artery may be visualized through the spleen from a left lateral approach. Because of the tortuous course of the splenic artery, flow in this vessel is typically turbulent,[5] as seen in Figure 28–3B.

HEPATIC ARTERY

The common hepatic artery (Fig. 28–4) is the limb of the celiac T that heads toward the patient's right. After running a short distance along the superior border of the pancreatic head, the common hepatic artery gives rise to the gastroduodenal artery, which can often be seen with ultrasound at the anterosuperior border of the pancreatic head. Beyond the gastroduodenal artery origin, the *common* hepatic artery becomes the *proper* hepatic artery, which follows the portal vein to the porta hepatis (entrance to the liver). At this point, it divides into the left and right hepatic arteries, which penetrate into the hepatic substance. The anatomic relationships among the hepatic artery, the portal vein, and the extrahepatic bile ducts are shown in Figure 28–4B.

The classic hepatic artery configuration just described is seen in 72% of individuals.[5] A number of alternative patterns may occur, the most noteworthy of which are the following: (1) the common (4%) or right (11%) hepatic artery may arise from the SMA, and (2) the left hepatic artery may arise from the left gastric artery (10%).[2]

The hepatic arteries are usually well visualized sonographically from an anterior abdominal approach. The common hepatic artery is most easily identified at its origin from the celiac artery (see Fig. 28–2A). The proper hepatic artery is seen on ultrasound

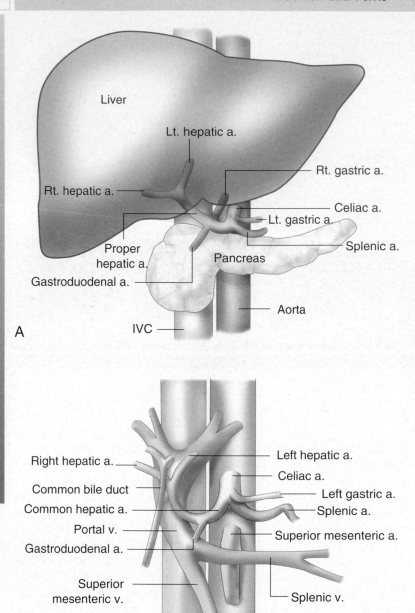

Liver

Lt. hepatic a.

Rt. gastric a.

Rt. hepatic a.

Celiac a.

Lt. gastric a.

Proper hepatic a.

Pancreas

Splenic a.

Gastroduodenal a.

Aorta

A

IVC

Figure 28–4. *A,* The hepatic artery and its branches. *B,* Anatomic relationships among the hepatic artery, the portal vein, and the extrahepatic bile ducts. IVC, inferior vena cava.

Right hepatic a.

Left hepatic a.

Common bile duct

Celiac a.

Common hepatic a.

Left gastric a.

Portal v.

Splenic a.

Gastroduodenal a.

Superior mesenteric a.

Superior mesenteric v.

Splenic v.

IVC

Aorta

B

images near the porta hepatis that show the portal vein in short or long axes, as can be seen in Figure 28–5*A.* The right and left hepatic artery branches can be followed into the substance of the liver to a variable distance from the porta hepatis. As noted previously, the hepatic arterial system has low-resistance flow characteristics, with a large amount of continuous forward flow throughout diastole (Fig. 28–5*B*).

SUPERIOR MESENTERIC ARTERY

The SMA arises from the anterior surface of the aorta, immediately distal to the origin of the celiac artery (Fig. 28–6). The SMA generally consists of a short, anteriorly directed segment and a much longer inferiorly directed segment that ends in the vicinity of the ileocecal valve. SMA branches supply the jejunum, ileum, cecum, and ascending

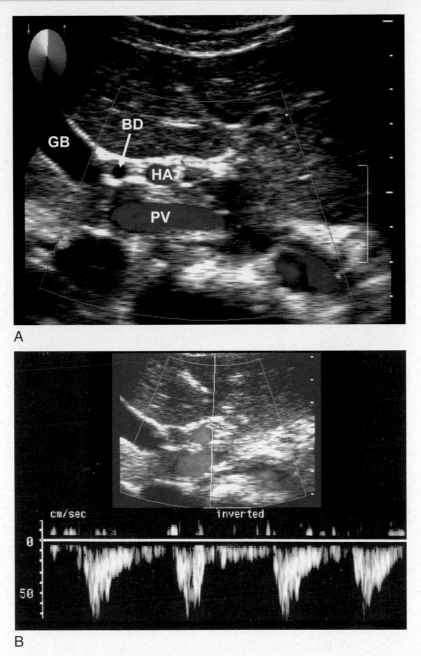

FIGURE 28–5. Ultrasonography of the hepatic artery. *A,* At the porta hepatis, the hepatic artery (HA) can be differentiated from the bile duct (BD), because blood flow is present in the former and not in the latter. Blood flow is also seen in the portal vein (PV). GB, gallbladder. *B,* Doppler examination confirms the identity of the (proper) hepatic artery, which has low-resistance arterial signals.

colon, as well as the proximal two thirds of the transverse colon and portions of the duodenum and pancreatic head. As noted previously, the SMA may also give rise to an aberrant right hepatic artery (11%) or common hepatic artery (4%).[1]

The SMA is easily identified on longitudinal or transverse ultrasound images (Fig. 28–7). The SMA serves as an important orienting landmark for scanning upper abdominal vessels because it has characteristic anatomic relationships with several epigastric structures that are well seen on transverse ultrasound images. Please review Figure 28–7*A* and note the following. First, observe that the SMA is surrounded by a

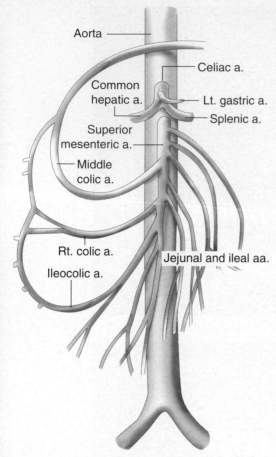

FIGURE 28–6. Superior mesenteric artery anatomy.

Labels on figure: Aorta; Celiac a.; Common hepatic a.; Lt. gastric a.; Splenic a.; Superior mesenteric a.; Middle colic a.; Rt. colic a.; Jejunal and ileal aa.; Ileocolic a.

distinctive, triangular mantle of fat that is very useful for identifying this vessel. Second, the SMA lies to the right of the superior mesenteric vein. Third, the pancreas and the splenic vein lie anterior to the SMA. In contrast, the left renal vein (discussed later) lies posterior to the SMA (between the SMA and the aorta). These anatomic features are very distinctive, making the SMA an excellent point of orientation for abdominal scanning.

SMA blood flow is best evaluated with longitudinal ultrasound images, because a lengthy segment of the vessel is visualized from a single perspective. The SMA Doppler spectrum shows turbulent flow near the arterial origin; however, as one moves distally, flow becomes more uniform. In a fasting patient, a high-resistance flow pattern is seen in the SMA (see Fig. 28–7C), with sharp systolic peaks and absent late diastolic flow. Within 30 to 90 minutes after eating, however, the SMA flow assumes a low-resistance pattern (see Fig. 28–7D), with broad systolic peaks and continuous diastolic flow.[3] These fasting/postprandial flow features have important diagnostic implications, as discussed in Chapter 31.

PORTAL VENOUS SYSTEM

The portal venous system transports blood from the bowel and spleen to the liver. The portal vein (Fig. 28–8) begins at the junction of the splenic and superior mesenteric veins, which converge immediately posterior to the pancreatic neck. The portal vein courses obliquely toward the right to terminate at the porta hepatis, where it divides into right and left portal branches. Each branch enters the corresponding lobe of the liver.

The splenic vein lies immediately posterior to the pancreas and follows a straight course (unlike the tortuous splenic artery) to the hilum of the spleen. The body and tail of the pancreas "follow" the course of the splenic vein; hence, the pancreas is a good landmark for finding the splenic vein.

The superior mesenteric vein extends almost straight caudad from the portal vein junction and parallels the course of the SMA, which lies to its left. The superior mesenteric vein is best seen with ultrasound in longitudinal veiws.

Other tributaries of the portal venous system include the coronary vein and the inferior mesenteric vein, which are illustrated in Figure 28–8. The inferior mesenteric vein empties into the splenic vein in 38% of individuals. Alternatively, it may terminate at the splenic–superior mesenteric vein junction (32%) or into the superior mesenteric vein itself (25%).[2] The coronary vein runs along the posterior aspect of the stomach toward the gastroesophageal junction. This vein usually enters the superior aspect of the portal vein near the portosplenic junction,[2] where it can be seen with ultrasound. The coronary vein may shunt blood from the portal to the systemic circulation in cases of portal hypertension (see Chapter 32).

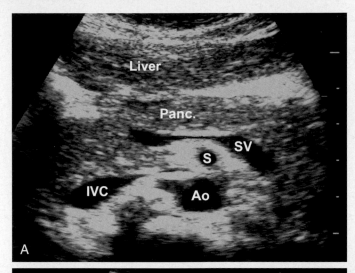

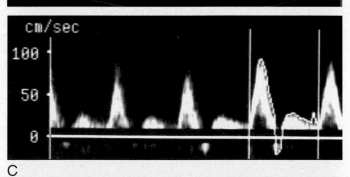

FIGURE 28–7. Ultrasound of the superior mesenteric artery. *A,* Anatomic relationships of the SMA (superior mesenteric artery; S). Note that the SMA is surrounded by a distinctive layer of echogenic fat. The pancreas (Panc.) is anterior to the SMA. The aorta (Ao) is posterior to the SMA. IVC, inferior vena cava; SV, splenic vein. *B,* A long-axis view shows the origin of the celiac artery and the SMA from the aorta (Ao). *C,* Normal, high-resistance Doppler signal in the SMA of a fasting patient. *D,* Normal low-resistance postprandial SMA Doppler signals.

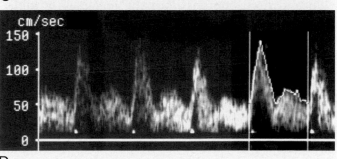

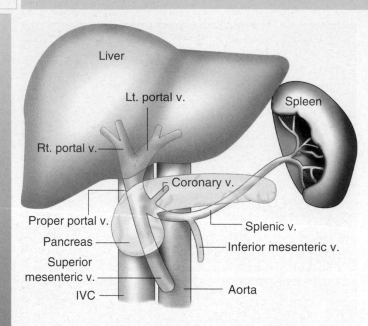

Liver

Lt. portal v.

Spleen

Rt. portal v.

Coronary v.

FIGURE   28–8. Portal venous system
anatomy. IVC, inferior vena cava.

Proper portal v.

Splenic v.

Pancreas

Inferior mesenteric v.

Superior
mesenteric v.

IVC

Aorta

Doppler assessment of portal vein flow is clinically important. This assessment is usually conducted with ultrasound views along the axis of the portal vein, as shown in Figure 28–9. Flow in the portal vein and its tributaries is normally *toward* the liver. Portal vein Doppler waveforms exhibit subtle phasic variation caused principally by respiration-related changes in thoracic pressure. The phasic pattern generates a "windstorm" sound in the audible Doppler signal, which is quite distinct from the pulsatile sound of the hepatic artery and other epigastric arterial branches. With right heart failure and fluid overload, right atrial pulsations may be transmitted through the liver to the portal vein, which then exhibits pulsatile Doppler waveforms.

The normal portal vein measures up to 13 mm in diameter during quiet respiration in a supine patient.[6] The caliber of the portal vein and its tributaries normally increases substantially during sustained deep inspiration. This is best seen in the splenic and superior mesenteric veins, which normally increase 50% to 100% in diameter from quiet respiration to deep inspiration.[7,8] With portal hypertension, the portal vein may dilate and respiratory variation in the splenic/superior mesenteric veins may be obliterated.

HEPATIC VEINS

Typically, there are three major hepatic veins (Fig. 28–10), which converge on the inferior vena cava (IVC) at the diaphragm. The right hepatic vein runs in a coronal plane between the anterior and posterior segments of the right hepatic lobe. The middle hepatic vein lies between the right and left hepatic lobes and may be seen prominently on sagittal or parasagittal images of the liver. The left hepatic vein runs between the medial and lateral segments of the left hepatic lobe. In 96% of individuals, the middle and left hepatic veins join to form a common trunk before entering the IVC.[9] The caudate lobe has its own venous drainage, directly into the IVC. The hepatic veins and other anatomical structures are important landmarks that define hepatic lobar anatomy, as listed in Table 28–1 and illustrated in Figure 28–11.

The left hepatic vein frequently is duplicated, and a number of other variations of hepatic vein anatomy may occur.[9] Accessory hepatic veins, which enter the IVC in locations other than at the diaphragm (Fig. 28–10), occur commonly, although they are rarely identified sonographically.[10] Occasionally, one of the three major hepatic veins is absent, typically, the right hepatic

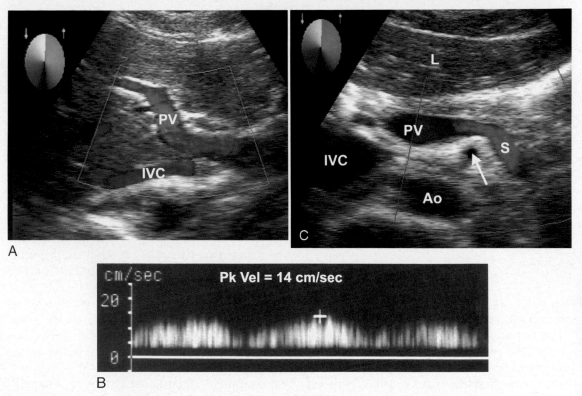

FIGURE 28–9. Ultrasound of the portal vein and its tributaries. *A*, Long-axis view of the portal vein (PV). IVC, inferior vena cava. *B*, Normal phasic Doppler spectrum in the portal vein. Peak velocity (Pk Vel) is 14 cm/sec. *C*, The splenic vein (S) is seen at its junction with the portal vein (PV). *Arrow* represents the superior mesenteric artery. Ao, aorta; IVC, inferior vena cava; L, liver.

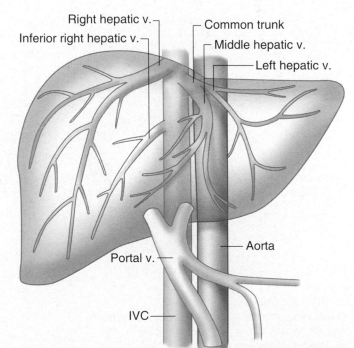

FIGURE 28–10. Hepatic vein anatomy. IVC, inferior vena cava.

Table 28–1. Structures Defining Hepatic Lobar Anatomy

Structure	Location
Right hepatic vein	Separates anterior and posterior segments, right lobe
Middle hepatic vein	Separates right and left lobes
Gallbladder fossa	Separates right and left lobes
Ascending branch, left portal vein	Separates lateral and medial segments, left lobe
Falciform ligament	Separates lateral and medial segments, left lobe

vein (6%), or less commonly, the middle or left hepatic veins.

The hepatic veins are best visualized with ultrasound using a transverse subxiphoid approach, which yields an image of the three main hepatic trunks converging on the IVC, such as is seen in Figure 28–12. From this perspective, however, blood flow often cannot be visualized in the right hepatic vein, because the axis of this vein is perpendicular to the ultrasound beam. The

right hepatic vein is seen to greatest advantage using a coronal scan plane and an intercostal transducer position (Fig. 28–12C). The right hepatic vein is the only major venous trunk that can be seen from this perspective.

The normal hepatic veins are sonolucent structures embedded within the liver parenchyma. Hepatic veins may be differentiated from portal veins by the following sonographic features:

1. Course: Hepatic veins are more or less longitudinally oriented, whereas portal veins run in transverse planes.
2. Convergence: The hepatic veins converge on the IVC at the diaphragm, whereas the portal veins converge on the porta hepatis.
3. Changes in size: The hepatic veins enlarge progressively toward the diaphragm, whereas the portal veins become larger as they approach the porta hepatis.
4. Margins: Hepatic veins have "naked" margins, whereas the portal veins are surrounded by a heavy sheath of echogenic fibrous tissue (see Fig. 28–12B).

Hepatic vein Doppler signals are quite different from those typically seen in the

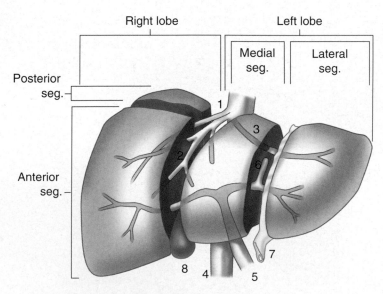

FIGURE 28–11. Anatomical landmarks that define the major hepatic lobes and segments (seg). V, vein.

1. Right hepatic v.
2. Middle hepatic v.
3. Left hepatic v.
4. Inferior vena cava
5. Portal v.
6. Ascending left portal v.
7. Falciform lig.
8. Gallbladder

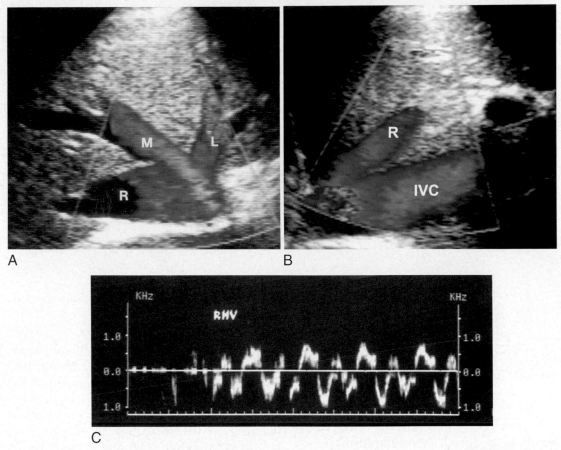

FIGURE 28–12. Hepatic vein sonography. *A,* Transverse view of the three main hepatic vein trunks as they enter the inferior vena cava. L, left hepatic vein; M, middle hepatic vein; R, right hepatic vein. *B,* Coronal view showing the right hepatic vein (R) at its junction with the inferior vena cava (IVC).

portal vein. Blood flow in the hepatic veins has a somewhat chaotic, pulsatile pattern that results from transmission of right atrial pulsations into the veins. The Doppler spectrum (see Fig. 28–13) reflects a combination of phasic variation and transmitted pulsations.

INFERIOR VENA CAVA

The normal IVC is situated anterior to the spine and to the right of the aorta. The IVC begins at the junction of the common iliac veins and terminates in the right atrium (Fig. 28–14).

FIGURE 28–13. Normal hepatic vein Doppler signals. Note that these pulsatile signals are quite different from normal portal vein Doppler signals.

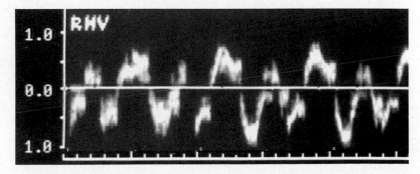

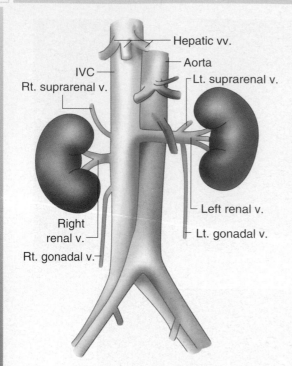

Figure 28–14. The inferior vena cava (IVC) and its tributaries.

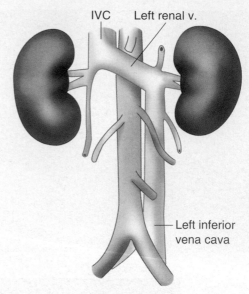

Figure 28–15. Anomalous, left-sided inferior vena cava.

The upper abdominal portion of the IVC is easily visualized sonographically,[11–13] using the liver as an acoustic window (see Chapter 29). The inferior portion of the IVC may be difficult to visualize, depending on the body habitus of the patient and the amount of overlying bowel gas. The size of the IVC varies markedly with respiration and throughout the cardiac cycle, but the IVC seldom exceeds 2.5 cm in diameter.[13] Deep inspiration limits venous return to the chest, markedly dilating the IVC. Expiration has the opposite effect. The IVC diameter is also dependent on patient size and right atrial pressure (diameter is increased with fluid overload or heart failure).

Doppler flow signals in the IVC are somewhat pulsatile near the heart because of reflected right atrial pulsations. Farther distally, the flow pattern is phasic and is similar to the pattern seen in extremity veins.

Most anomalies of the IVC occur at and below the level of the renal veins.[10] Of these, the most common are duplication (0.2%–3.0%) and transposition (0.2%–0.5%). In both of these anomalies, the left-sided IVC usually crosses over to join the normal right-sided IVC at the level of the left renal vein (Fig. 28–15). Interruption of the IVC with azygos or hemiazygos continuation (0.6%) results from failure of the intrahepatic segment of the IVC to form. Flow is diverted to the heart via the azygos and hemiazygos veins, and the hepatic veins drain directly into the right atrium.

RENAL ARTERIES

The renal arteries (Fig. 28–16) arise from the aorta, slightly below the origin of the SMA. The origin of the right renal artery is usually

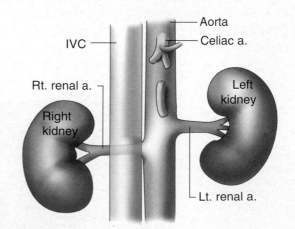

Figure 28–16. Renal artery anatomy. IVC, inferior vena cava.

slightly superior to the left, but this relationship is not constant. The right renal artery arises from the anterolateral aspect of the aorta and then passes *posterior* to the IVC as it courses toward the right renal hilum. The left renal artery arises from the lateral or posterolateral aspect of the aorta and follows a posterolateral course to the left renal hilum.

Almost one third of kidneys are supplied by two or more arteries arising from the aorta.[14] In some of these cases, the main renal artery is duplicated. In other instances, accessory renal arteries arise from the aorta superior or inferior to the main renal artery and may enter the kidneys either at the renal hilum or at the poles of the kidney. Extrahilar accessory arteries also may arise from the ipsilateral renal artery, the ipsilateral iliac artery, the aorta, or, occasionally, from other arteries in the retroperitoneum.

The branching pattern of the renal arteries is illustrated in Figure 28–17. The renal arteries typically divide into anterior and posterior divisions that lie, respectively, anterior and posterior to the renal pelvis. The anterior division branches into four segmental arteries, whereas the posterior division supplies only a single renal segment. The segmental arteries branch farther within the renal sinus, forming interlobar arteries that penetrate the renal parenchyma. These terminate in arcuate arteries that curve around the corticomedullary junction, giving rise to cortical branches.[14]

With ultrasound, the renal artery origins (Fig. 28–18A and B) are usually best visualized by scanning transversely from a midline anterior approach. The right renal artery can usually be followed to the kidney with this approach, but visualization of the left renal artery may not be possible from this transducer position. In such cases, coronal scans from a posterolateral transducer position is a useful alternative. This approach works best in lean individuals and is especially useful in infants and small children (see Fig. 28–18C). In large adults, the distal renal artery may be seen using the posterolateral transducer position, but it may not be possible to follow the renal artery back to the aorta.

Renal artery Doppler signals have a low-resistance flow pattern, as seen in Figure 28–18D. Continuous forward flow is present in diastole because of low resistance in the renal vascular bed. This flow pattern is evident at all locations in the renal arteries, including the intrarenal branches.[5]

RENAL VEINS

Each renal vein is formed from tributaries that coalesce in the renal hilum. As illustrated in Figure 28–14, the left renal vein usually receives the left suprarenal (adrenal) vein from above and the left gonadal (ovarian or testicular) vein from below. The left renal vein then passes anterior to the aorta and posterior to the SMA, to enter the left side of the IVC. The right renal vein, which is shorter than the left renal vein, extends directly to the IVC from the right renal hilum and usually receives no tributaries.

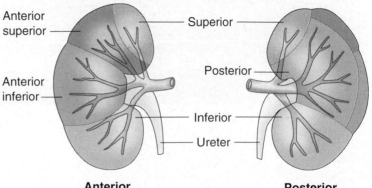

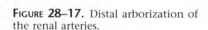

FIGURE 28–17. Distal arborization of the renal arteries.

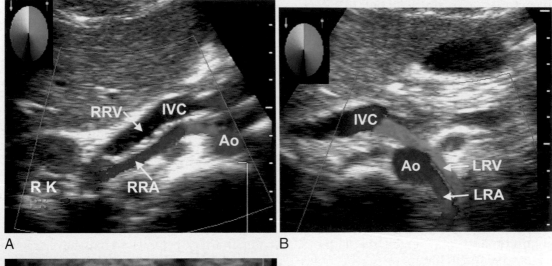

A

B

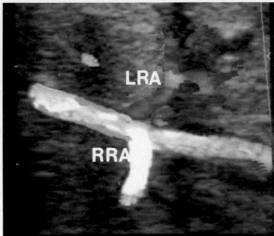

C

FIGURE 28–18. Sonographic appearance of the renal arteries and veins. A, Transverse image of the right renal artery (RRA) and right renal vein (RRV). Note that the artery lies posterior to the inferior vena cava (IVC) and the renal vein. Ao, aorta; RK, right kidney. B, Transverse image of the left renal artery (LRA) and the left renal vein (LRV). Once again, the renal artery is posterior to the renal vein. It is important not to mistake the vein for the artery. Ao, aorta; IVC, inferior vena cava. C, Coronal view of the left (LRA) and right (RRA) renal arteries in a premature infant (head to left). D, Normal, low-pulsatility renal artery Doppler spectrum. Peak systolic velocity (PSV) is 82 cm/sec. E, Normal phasic renal vein Doppler spectrum. Peak velocity (Pk Vel) is 22 cm/sec.

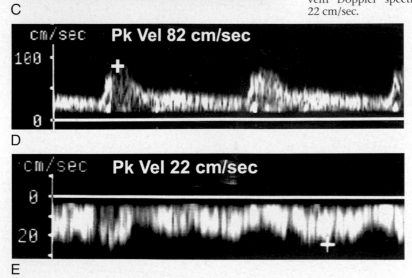

D

E

The left renal vein may be circumaortic (1.5%–8.7%), with separate veins passing anterior and posterior to the aorta. The left renal vein may also be retroaortic in location (1.8%–2.4%), with a single branch passing posterior to the aorta, rather than anterior. Accessory renal veins are commonly present on the right side, draining directly into the IVC.[11,14]

The renal veins can best be visualized with ultrasound (see Fig. 28–18A, B) on transverse scans from an anterior approach. In small children and lean adults, the renal veins also may be seen coronally from a posterolateral approach. Sonographers should be mindful that the left renal vein crosses the midline *between* the aorta and the SMA. This differentiates the left renal vein and the nearby splenic vein, which lies anterior to the SMA.

Doppler signals in the renal veins (see Fig. 28–18E) show the same phasic flow variation as the IVC. Transmitted cardiac pulsations may be evident in the renal veins near the IVC.

References

1. Ruzika FF Jr, Rossi P: Normal vascular anatomy of the abdominal viscera. Radiol Clin North Am 8:3–29, 1970.
2. Michels NA: Blood Supply and Anatomy of the Upper Abdominal Organs. Philadelphia, JB Lippincott, 1955.
3. Lewis BD, James EM: Current applications of duplex and color Doppler ultrasound imaging: Abdomen. Mayo Clin Proc 64:1158–1169, 1989.
4. Geelkerken RH, Delahunt TA, Schulte-Kool LJ, et al: Pitfalls in the diagnosis of origin stenosis of the coeliac and superior mesenteric arteries with transabdominal color duplex instrumentation. Ultrasound Med Biol 22:695–700, 1996.
5. Taylor KJW, Burns PN, Woodcock JP, Wells PNT: Blood flow in deep abdominal and pelvic vessels: Ultrasonic pulsed Doppler analysis. Radiology 154:487–493, 1985.
6. Weinreb J, Kumari S, Phillips G, Pochaczevsky R: Portal vein measurements by real-time sonography. Am J Roentgenol 139:497–499, 1982.
7. Bolondi L, Gandolfi L, Arienti F, et al: Ultrasonography in the diagnosis of portal hypertension: Diminished response of the portal vessels to respiration. Radiology 142:167–172, 1982.
8. Bellamy EA, Bossi MC, Cosgrove DO: Ultrasound demonstration of changes in the normal portal venous system following a meal. Br J Radiol 57:147–149, 1984.
9. Cosgrove DO, Arger PH, Coleman BG: Ultrasonic anatomy of hepatic veins. J Clin Ultrasound 15:231–235, 1987.
10. Makuuchi M, Hasegawa H, Yamazaki S, et al: The inferior right hepatic vein: Ultrasonic demonstration. Radiology 148:213–217, 1983.
11. Kellman GH, Alpern MB, Sandler MA, Craig BM: Computed tomography of vena caval anomalies with embryologic correlation. Radiographics 8:533–556, 1988.
12. Needleman L, Rifkin MD: Vascular ultrasonography: Abdominal applications. Radiol Clin North Am 24: 461–484, 1986.
13. Mintz GS, Kotler MN, Parry WR, et al: Real-time inferior vena caval ultrasonography: Normal and abnormal findings and its use in assessing right-heart function. Circulation 64:1018–1024, 1981.
14. Hollinshead WH: Textbook of Anatomy, 3rd ed. Hagerstown, MD, Harper & Row, 1974, pp 521–523.

Chapter 29

Ultrasound Assessment of the Aorta, Iliac Arteries, and Inferior Vena Cava

WILLIAM J. ZWIEBEL, MD

THE AORTA AND ILIAC ARTERIES

The focus of this chapter is on the aorta, and especially aortic aneurysm. In the early days of sonography, the aorta represented a success story, for it could be successfully examined with ultrasound, even in the bistable ultrasound days prior to the development of gray-scale instrumentation. The ability to reliably visualize the iliac arteries with ultrasound came much later, with the development of real-time ultrasound instruments, and especially with the emergence of color flow sonography.

Normal Anatomy

Aortic and iliac artery anatomy is illustrated in Chapter 28, but there are a few details that require emphasis. The normal abdominal aorta[1–5] (Fig. 29–1) has a clearly defined wall and smooth margins and tapers very slightly below the level of the renal arteries. The maximum infrarenal aortic diameter averages 2 cm in adults and varies little with respect to age, gender, race, and body size.[4,5] The abdominal aorta lies adjacent to the spine throughout its course, slightly to the left of midline. In contrast, the inferior vena cava (IVC) lies to the right of the midline and gradually moves away from the spine as it passes through the liver and diaphragm. In the upper abdomen, therefore, it is possible to differentiate between the aorta and the IVC at a glance, by simply noting the

position of the vessels relative to the spine. The normal iliac arteries (Fig. 29–2) are smoothly marginated and uniform in caliber. The maximum diameter of the common iliac artery (outer to outer) is 15 mm in men and 13 mm in women. The external iliac and common femoral arteries are slightly smaller, measuring up to 12 mm in men and 11 mm in women.[6] In older individuals, the iliac arteries may be quite tortuous.

Terminology

An artery is considered aneurysmal when its diameter equals or exceeds 1.5 times the normal diameter. Considering that the normal aorta does not exceed 2 cm in diameter distally, it is considered aneurysmal at 3 cm.[1–7] Aneurysmal dilatation is often localized, but some aneurysms may extend over long segments of an artery. Certain terms, including *saccular* and *fusiform*, are used to describe the shape of aneurysms. Other terms, including *true aneurysm*, *false aneurysm*, and *mycotic aneurysm*, describe the pathologic type or causes of aneurysms. It is useful to review some of these terms, as their meaning is not self-evident.

True Aneurysm

The composite layers of the vessel wall are intact but stretched in true aneurysms

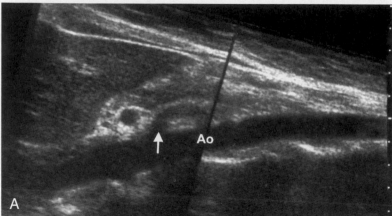

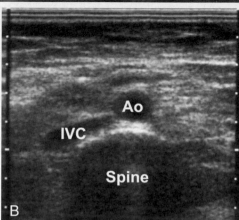

FIGURE 29-1. The normal aorta. *A*, A composite, longitudinal view demonstrates the entire aorta (Ao) from the diaphragm, on the left, to its termination, on the right. Note that the aorta tapers slightly below the level of the superior mesenteric artery (*arrow*), and that the aorta follows the course of the spine. *B*, Transverse view of the aorta (Ao), the inferior vena cava (IVC), and the spine. The aorta measures only about 1.5 cm in this individual.

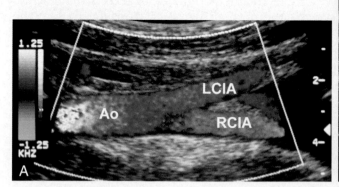

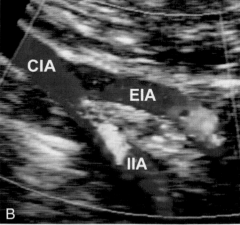

FIGURE 29-2. Normal iliac arteries. *A*, This coronal view shows the bifurcation of the aorta (Ao) into the right (RCIA) and left (LCIA) common iliac arteries. *B*, The common iliac artery (CIA) is seen to divide into the external (EIA) and internal (IIA) iliac arteries.

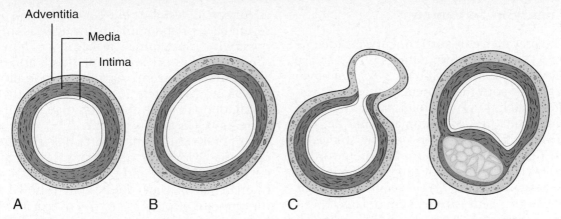

FIGURE 29–3. Aneurysms and dissection. *A,* Normal arterial wall components are shown. *B,* In a true aneurysm, the components of the arterial wall are "stretched." *C,* In a false aneurysm, a hole is present in the arterial wall, with an adjacent confined collection of blood. *D,* In arterial dissection, a hematoma forms between components of the wall.

(Fig. 29–3). The great majority of aortic and iliac aneurysms are true aneurysms. Aneurysms represent focal weakening and stretching of the arterial wall. The precise pathogenic cause of aortic and iliac aneurysms is unknown. They frequently occur in association with atherosclerosis, but they are not caused by atherosclerosis per se.[8,9]

False Aneurysm

A false aneurysm occurs when a hole in the arterial wall permits the escape of blood, which is subsequently confined by surrounding tissues (see Fig. 29–3C). The extravasated blood forms a hematoma into the center of which blood continues to circulate. The aneurysm is "false" because it is not confined by an arterial wall. Most false aneurysms result from iatrogenic arterial puncture followed by inadequate hemostasis, but false aneurysms may also result from violent trauma or localized destruction of the arterial wall by an infectious agent. The term *mycotic aneurysm* is used for infection-related lesions. False aneurysms also may occur at graft anastomoses.

Arterial Dissection

The term *dissecting aneurysm* is a misnomer, for the artery affected by dissection is not always aneurysmal (dilated). The preferred term, therefore, is *arterial dissection.*[10] This condition occurs when blood enters the media of the vessel through a rent in the intima and then dissects along the length of the artery (see Fig. 29–3D). The intima, and in some cases part of the media, are stripped away, and a new lumen, called the false lumen, is formed. Blood may flow freely through both the false lumen and the original (true) lumen to supply branch vessels. Arterial dissection requires two processes: the weakening of the media of the vessel and the development of a rent in the intima through which blood gains access to the media. Certain uncommon conditions, such as Marfan's syndrome, weaken the arterial media and predispose individuals to arterial dissection, but the most important predisposing condition is age and its associated weakening of the arterial media. Although arterial dissection occurs commonly in atherosclerotic vessels, atherosclerosis is not a causative factor.

Aortic dissection begins almost invariably in the chest and extends into the abdomen. If the dissection begins in the ascending aorta, it may extend into the brachiocephalic vessels. The most common site at which aortic dissection begins, however, is just below the left subclavian artery. The second most common site is the ascending aorta.

Aneurysm Screening

The prevalence of aortic aneurysms (diameter >3 cm) in Western nations is 4.5% at age 65 yr and 10.8% at 80 yr.[11,12] For unknown reasons, aortoiliac aneurysms occur predominately (76%) in men.[13] Up to 60% of aneurysms are asymptomatic and are discovered incidentally on imaging studies or on physical examination. It is noteworthy, however, that physical examination is only 58% sensitive and 75% specific for detecting aortic aneurysms of 3 cm or larger. Even for aneurysms 5 cm or larger, physical examination is only 82% sensitive.[7,13-15] It is good practice, therefore, to check for "silent" aortic aneurysms in all elderly patients (especially men) who present for abdominal or retroperitoneal ultrasound examination. Recent interest in screening for aortic aneurysms has shown that most aortic aneurysms evolve between ages 60 and 70 yr, and that if the abdominal aorta measures no more than 2.5 cm by age 70 yr, the likelihood of developing a clinically significant aneurysm is very low.[11,16-18] Therefore, a single screening ultrasound examination between ages 65 and 70 showing an aortic diameter of 2.5 cm or less virtually excludes aortic aneurysm for the rest of an individual's life.

Aortic aneurysms are usually localized to the infrarenal portion of the aorta and the common iliac arteries. They can, of course, occur elsewhere in the aorta and extremity arteries. The tendency for aortic aneurysms to occur infrarenally (below the renal arteries) is of great clinical importance, because the surgeon may conveniently maintain perfusion of the kidneys during surgical repair by cross-clamping the aorta below the renal arteries. Surgical repair is complex for aneurysms that extend cephalad to the renal arteries and may involve reimplantation of the renal arteries or mesenteric vessels.

Aneurysm Presentation

Symptomatic aneurysms present with abdominal, back, or leg pain. The presence of pain does not necessarily mean that the aneurysm is leaking, but sudden onset of severe back or abdominal pain suggests this possibility. Substantial leakage, or frank rupture, causes prostration or shock and is a catastrophic event carrying a mortality rate of approximately 50%.[19-21] The risk that an abdominal aortic aneurysm may rupture increases with aneurysm size.[7,10,12,19-24] In a large 1998 study, the potential rupture rate was 2%/yr for aneurysms less than 4.5 cm in diameter and growth rates of less than 1 cm/yr.[21] Older studies have shown a rupture rate of only 3% to 5% over a 10-yr period for aneurysms that remain less than 5 cm in diameter. In contrast, the rupture rate is increased substantially for aneurysms measuring 4.5 to 6 cm, with a rupture rate of 10%/yr reported for aneurysms of this size.[20] This figure is higher than previously reported estimates of 5%/yr for aneurysms of 5 cm or larger.[7] Surgical repair is generally recommended for abdominal aortic aneurysms measuring 5 cm or greater in diameter and becomes more imperative at 6 cm in diameter because the risk of rupture increases substantially for aneurysms of this size.[24,25]

On average, the diameter of an abdominal aortic aneurysm grows 2 to 5 mm per year.[7,22,26-30] Average expansion rates are not very meaningful, however, because considerable individual variation exists. When an aneurysm is discovered, therefore, serial ultrasound measurements are usually made at 6-mo intervals to determine the rate of expansion. The usual interval for follow-up is 6 mo, but the follow-up may be yearly for aneurysms that are small and stable in size.

Most iliac artery aneurysms occur in association with distal aortic aneurysms, and in such cases, the aortic aneurysm is generally the source of clinical concern. Isolated iliac artery aneurysms* are uncommon but may be deadly for two reasons. First, they often cannot be palpated, even when they are large, and therefore are not detected on physical examination. Second, rupture of an iliac artery aneurysm generates nonspecific symptoms of abdominal or pelvic pain, the cause of which may not be

*Not associated with aortic aneurysm.

recognized until the patient becomes hypotensive or dies. Iliac artery aneurysms 3 cm or larger are generally believed to pose significant risk of rupture, and surgical repair or percutaneous stenting is recommended for iliac aneurysms of this size. Iliac artery aneurysms are usually located in the proximal or distal portion of the common iliac arteries. It is important, therefore, to visualize both areas in the course of aneurysm evaluation.

Aneurysm Diagnosis

The primary criterion for the sonographic diagnosis of an arterial aneurysm[27,29,31–34] is a focal increase in the caliber of the artery, with the diameter of the dilated segment measuring at least 1.5 times greater than adjacent unaffected segments. For aortic aneurysms, an additional feature is the absence of tapering of the aorta below the mesenteric and renal vessels.

Aortic aneurysms have various gross configurations. Some are bulbous, with a sharp junction, or neck, between the normal and aneurysmal portions. Others are fusiform, with a gradual transition between the normal and aneurysmal portions. Many aneurysmal aortas are tortuous, for the aorta typically elongates as it dilates. Tortuous aortas usually deviate to the left of the spine, as shown in Figure 29–4, but some may deviate anteriorly, creating a prominent kink at the aneurysm neck.

Concentric layers of thrombus usually line the interior of large aortic or iliac aneurysms (Fig. 29–5), and this thrombus may generate emboli that occlude distal arteries. Because of the presence of thrombus, the outer dimensions of an aneurysm are often much greater than the dimensions of the lumen. Therefore, catheter arteriography usually underestimates the size of an aortic aneurysm because this technique visualizes only the arterial lumen.[31,32] Ultrasound, computed tomography, and magnetic resonance imaging show both the wall and the lumen; therefore, they can accurately evaluate aneurysm size. Aneurysm thrombus contains a sparse cellular matrix,

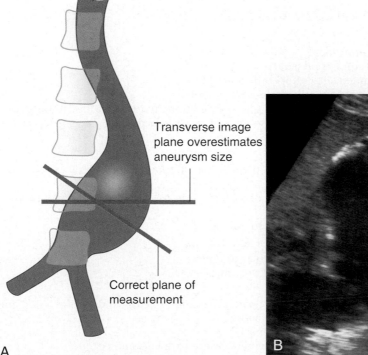

Transverse image plane overestimates aneurysm size

Correct plane of measurement

A

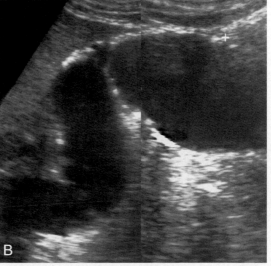

B

FIGURE 29–4. Measurement difficulties caused by aortic tortuosity. *A*, Note that the diameter of this tortuous aorta is exaggerated with a true transverse view and is correctly measured only in an oblique view. Coronal images eliminate this problem. *B*, Composite coronal view of a markedly tortuous, aneurysmal aorta.

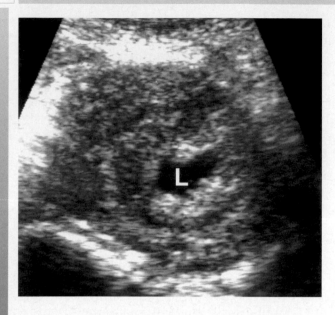

FIGURE 29–5. Thrombus within an aneurysm. Concentric layers of thrombus surround the arterial lumen (L).

but a substantial supporting structure is absent and the material is jelly-like in consistency. Although some evidence indicates thrombus may reduce wall stress,[27] it has no structural support per se, and the presence or absence of thrombus does not affect clinical decision making with respect to aneurysm repair.[19] The laminated structure of the thrombus can create lucent areas that occasionally mimic arterial dissection.[34–36]

Examination Protocols

I recommend the ultrasound examination protocol presented in Table 29–1 for

Table 29–1. Examination Protocol for Aortic and Iliac Aneurysms

1. Longitudinal
Examine aorta, diaphragm to bifurcation.
Use color flow to identify dissection, if present.
Determine location and longitudinal extent of aortic aneurysm.
Measure aortic aneurysm anteroposterior diameter, outer to outer.
Examine iliac arteries to iliac bifurcation. Use color flow, at least briefly to detect flow disturbances associated with iliac artery stenosis. Document severity of stenosis, if present, as per Chapter 18.
Measure iliac artery aneurysm(s), if present, outer to outer.

2. Transverse
Document the maximum diameter of the aorta at the diaphragm, superior mesenteric artery, and distally near the aortic bifurcation.
Measure aneurysm anteroposterior and transverse diameters, outer to outer.
Visualize the iliac arteries.
Measure iliac artery aneurysm(s), if present, outer to outer.

3. Coronal
Measure aortic aneurysm, transverse dimension, outer to outer.
Examine iliac arteries and measure aneurysm(s), if present.

4. Color Doppler examination
If examination time permits, confirm patency of superior mesenteric, celiac, and renal arteries, and examine for flow disturbances associated with stenosis.
Measure distance from renal arteries to aneurysm neck.
Alternatively, measure distance from superior mesenteric artery to aneurysm neck.

5. Kidneys: longitudinal and transverse views
Document kidney length and normal features.
Document hydronephrosis, if present.

assessment of aortic and iliac aneurysms. To attain the best results, the following points should be noted with respect to this protocol.[33,35,37]

1. Always measure an aneurysm the way a surgeon does in the operating room, from the outer surfaces of the vessel (outer to outer) (Fig. 29–6).
2. Sagittal and coronal planes are recommended for aneurysm measurement, as well as the transverse plane (see Fig. 29–6). I do not have scientific proof that this method enhances accuracy, but in my experience, the use of these planes shows the point of maximum dilatation clearly in a way that is reproducible from one examination to the next. It also avoids error resulting from oblique transverse measurements.
3. Coronal views are generally easier to obtain from the left side of the aorta than from the right side.
4. The maximum interobserver variability for aortic measurement is approximately 5 mm (95% confidence limits), and the mean variability is about 2.5 mm.[33] Therefore, an increase in size of less than 5 mm from one examination to another may not be significant. Gradual size increase on serial examination is important.
5. Remember, aneurysms do not decrease in size! To avoid looking foolish, be aware of the measurements reported previously before giving current measurements.
6. Always determine whether an aneurysm extends to, or above, the renal arteries. This is done best by directly visualizing the renal artery origins and measuring the distance from these vessels to the aneurysm. Time constraints often do not permit direct visualization of the renal arteries, but their location may be quickly inferred by measuring the distance from the superior mesenteric artery to the aneurysm (see Fig. 29–6D). The renal arteries arise no more than 2 cm below the superior mesenteric artery; therefore, the renal arteries should be unaffected if the aneurysm begins 2 cm or more below the superior mesenteric artery.[37]
7. The entire abdominal aorta must be examined to ensure that suprarenal aneurysms are not overlooked.
8. An aneurysm at the bifurcation of the iliac arteries (Figs. 29–7 and 29–8) can easily be overlooked, because this area is difficult to visualize. A transducer position lateral to the rectus muscles (Fig. 29–9) aids iliac artery visualization.
9. Color flow imaging should always be used at some point in the aortic examination to exclude aortic dissection and to identify iliac artery stenosis.

Aneurysm Complications

Potential complications of aortic aneurysms are atherosclerotic renal and mesenteric artery obstruction, hydronephrosis (from aneurysm compression of a ureter), retroperitoneal fibrosis, and aneurysm rupture.

Renal artery obstruction is not due to the aneurysm but is caused by coexisting atherosclerosis. If severe, such obstruction may result in shrinkage of the affected kidney. This finding, as well as hydronephrosis, is easily identified with ultrasound, and for this reason, the kidneys are always evaluated in the course of aortic examination.

Retroperitoneal fibrosis[38,39] is a rare complication of unknown etiology. Fibrosis is manifested as a hypoechoic soft-tissue mantle that partially or completely surrounds the aorta and may extend bilaterally into the retroperitoneum. The ureters may be entrapped in the fibrotic mass, leading to hydronephrosis.

The most disastrous complication of aortic or iliac aneurysm is rupture.[5,7,40,41] Sonography is only rarely used when aneurysm rupture is suspected, because immediate surgery is often required to maintain life. In some cases, however, leakage of blood is contained by surrounding tissues, lessening the acuteness of the clinical situation. In such instances, imaging is used to confirm that aneurysm leakage is the cause of the patient's symptoms. Computed tomography is the preferred method for this task,[42] but as an expedient, sonography sometimes is used

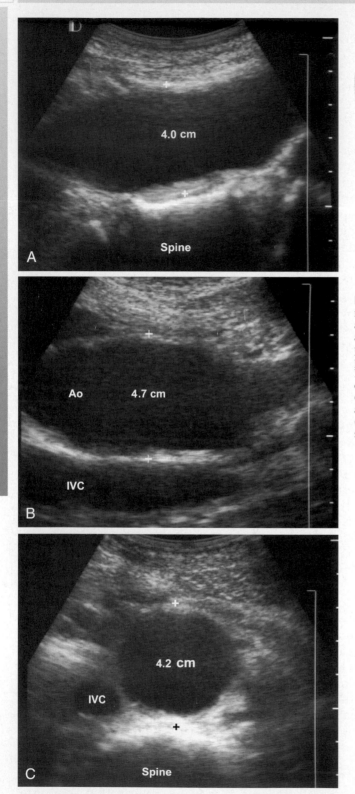

FIGURE 29–6. Aneurysm measurement technique. *A,* Longitudinal view of a distal aortic aneurysm measuring 4 cm in maximum anteroposterior dimension. The spine is visible posteriorly. *B,* As seen in the coronal scan plane, the transverse dimension is 4.7 cm. Note that both the aorta (Ao) and inferior vena cava (IVC) are visible in the coronal plane. *C,* A transverse view demonstrates the anterior and posterior surfaces of the aneurysm clearly (4.2 cm). The lateral surfaces are less clearly seen.

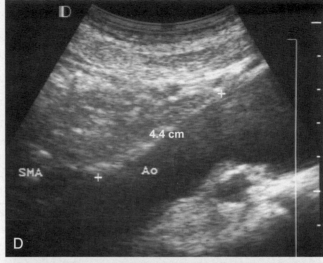

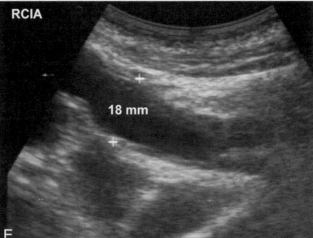

FIGURE 29–6—cont'd. *D,* The distance from the superior mesenteric artery (SMA) to the neck of the aneurysm is 4.4 cm. *E,* Long-axis view of the right common iliac artery (RCIA), with focal dilatation of 18-mm diameter. *F,* Long-axis view of the left common iliac artery (LCIA), with focal dilation of 16-mm diameter.

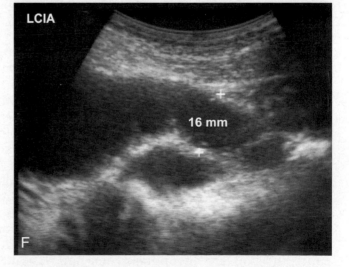

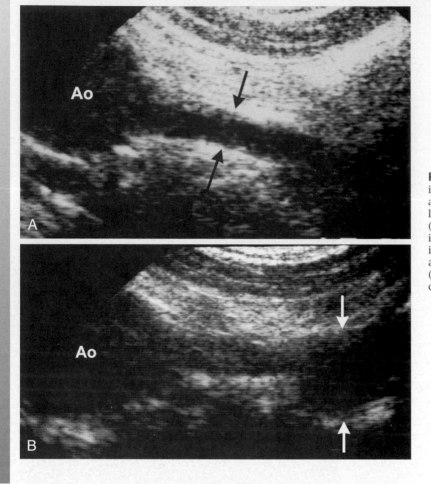

FIGURE 29–7. Aneurysms at the iliac bifurcation. *A*, An aortic aneurysm (Ao) is visible at the left. The common iliac artery (*arrows*) looks normal but the iliac bifurcation is not visualized. *B*, By tracing the iliac artery distally, an aneurysm (arrows) is identified in the distal common iliac artery.

merely to confirm the presence of an aortic aneurysm, implying that rupture is the cause of symptoms. The demonstration of a retroperitoneal hematoma provides direct evidence of aortic rupture (see Fig. 20–1, page 382). The hematoma is hypoechoic and is usually unilateral or asymmetric. It typically displaces the ipsilateral kidney. Peritoneal fluid may also be present if the aneurysm has leaked into the peritoneal space.

Arterial Dissection

Computed tomography and magnetic resonance imaging are the primary imaging methods used for detecting and evaluating arterial dissection, in both the thorax and the abdomen. Arterial dissection may be encountered incidentally, however, during ultrasound examination, and it is important, therefore, for sonographers to recognize this condition. The distinguishing ultrasound finding in arterial dissection is a membrane that divides the arterial lumen into two compartments (Fig. 29–10). This membrane consists of the intima and, in some cases, a portion of the media. The membrane moves freely with arterial pulsations if it is thin and if both the true and false lumens are patent. However, if the membrane is thick, or if one lumen is thrombosed, the membrane may move little or not at all. Duplex examination may demonstrate flow in both lumens, but different flow rates may be present, and in some cases, flow in the false lumen may be too slow to be detected. The dissection membrane may be difficult to appreciate on gray-scale examination; therefore, color flow should be used at least briefly in all

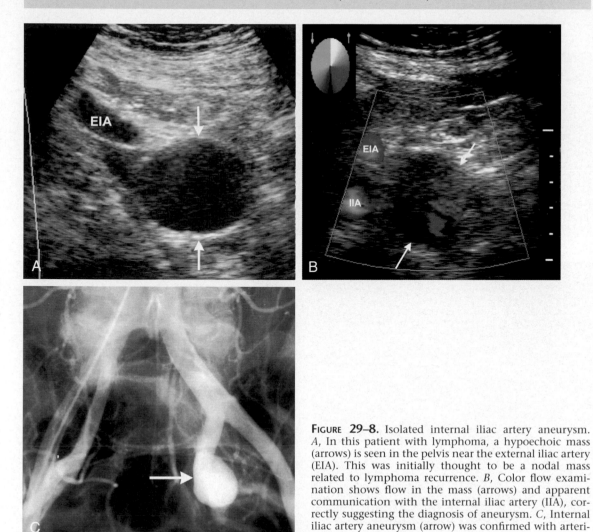

FIGURE 29–8. Isolated internal iliac artery aneurysm. A, In this patient with lymphoma, a hypoechoic mass (arrows) is seen in the pelvis near the external iliac artery (EIA). This was initially thought to be a nodal mass related to lymphoma recurrence. B, Color flow examination shows flow in the mass (arrows) and apparent communication with the internal iliac artery (IIA), correctly suggesting the diagnosis of aneurysm. C, Internal iliac artery aneurysm (arrow) was confirmed with arteriography and treated by embolization.

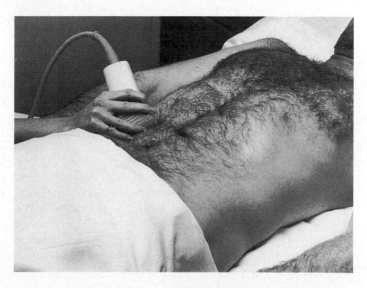

FIGURE 29–9. Transducer position lateral to the rectus muscle, for visualization of the iliac arteries.

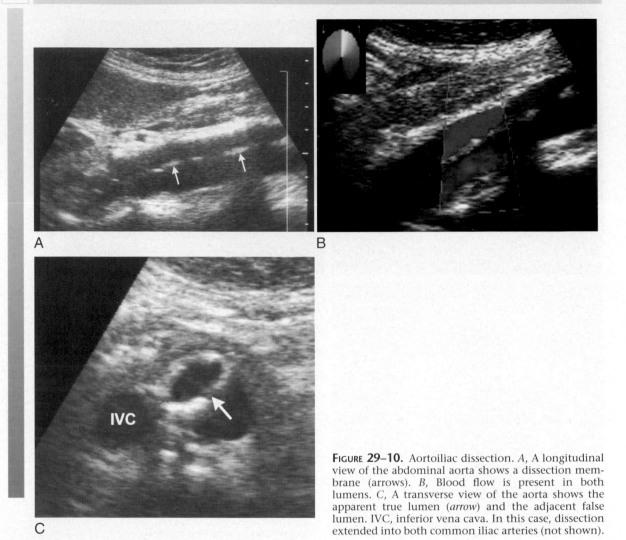

A

B

IVC

C

FIGURE 29–10. Aortoiliac dissection. *A*, A longitudinal view of the abdominal aorta shows a dissection membrane (arrows). *B*, Blood flow is present in both lumens. *C*, A transverse view of the aorta shows the apparent true lumen (*arrow*) and the adjacent false lumen. IVC, inferior vena cava. In this case, dissection extended into both common iliac arteries (not shown).

aortic examinations, as dissection is made readily apparent by color flow.

The diameter of the aorta is generally increased by dissection but not as dramatically as with a true aneurysm. In addition, the proximal and distal ends of the dissection may not be sharply defined, as with true aneurysms. Aortic dissection virtually always originates in the chest and extends into the abdominal aorta. Dissection also commonly extends into the iliac arteries or into the other aortic branches. The sonographer should try to determine the extent of dissection within the abdomen (if this is not already known) and should look for extension into major aortic branches. Stenosis or occlusion of branch vessels commonly accompanies dissection, and duplex

sonography can provide valuable information about these complications.

Aneurysms of Epigastric Aortic Branches

Aneurysms form uncommonly in aortic branch arteries, including the superior mesenteric artery, the splenic artery, the hepatic artery, and the renal arteries.[42,43] Although these aneurysms are uncommon, they are of considerable importance, for they may be mistaken for abdominal masses arising from the pancreas, the liver, or other epigastric structures. This error is particularly apt to occur if the aneurysm does not pulsate because of surrounding fibrosis or

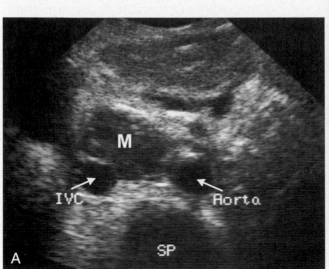

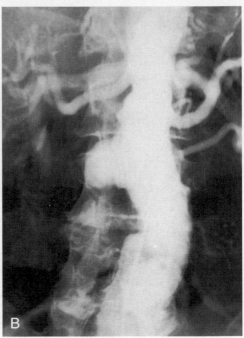

FIGURE 29–11. Masslike epigastric aneurysm at aortic graft anastomosis. This 75-yr-old man, who presented with upper abdominal pain, had undergone aortic aneurysm repair approximately 15 yr prior, but he had not received regular follow-up and could not remember his surgical history at the time of ultrasound examination. *A*, Sonography demonstrated a hypoechoic mass (M) located slightly to the right of the aorta, in the vicinity of the pancreatic head. The mass did not pulsate, and Doppler examination was not done. Initially, the mass was thought to be a pancreatic pseudocyst or a necrotic tumor in or near the pancreatic head. IVC, inferior vena cava; SP, spine. *B*, An arteriogram showed that the mass communicated with the aortic lumen, confirming the diagnosis of pseudoaneurysm arising from the graft/aorta anastomosis.

intraluminal thrombus. The correct diagnosis in such cases can be made only if "aneurysm" comes to the sonographer's mind and Doppler imaging is used to detect flow within the lesion, as shown in Figure 29–11.

Postoperative Assessment

The traditional method of aortic aneurysm repair is surgical bypass grafting, using synthetic graft material. Within the past 5 yr, a second repair method has come into widespread clinical use; namely, endoluminal aortic stent grafting.[23] The new procedure is less invasive and traumatic than abdominal surgery and requires only a brief hospital stay; therefore, it has been widely adopted as a primary aneurysm repair method. It is important, nevertheless, for sonographers to be familiar with the older surgical repair method, as a great number of patients

remain alive who have had surgical repair. Furthermore, aortic aneurysm surgery will continue to be used in the future when stent grafting is not possible. Sonographic assessment of aortic bypass grafts is included here. Ultrasound evaluation before and after stent grafting is the subject of the chapter that follows.

Three types of surgical graft procedures have commonly been used for aortic aneurysm repair (Fig. 29–12): (1) simple tube grafts for aneurysms limited to the aorta; (2) aortoiliac grafts; and (3) aortobifemoral grafts. In some cases, the aneurysmal aorta is opened longitudinally, the graft is placed inside, and the native aorta is wrapped around the graft. This is done to isolate the graft and the duodenum, lessening the chance of graft infection. The wrapping procedure creates a potential space that normally contains fluid during the immediate postoperative periods.[44,45] Most aortic grafts have two components: the

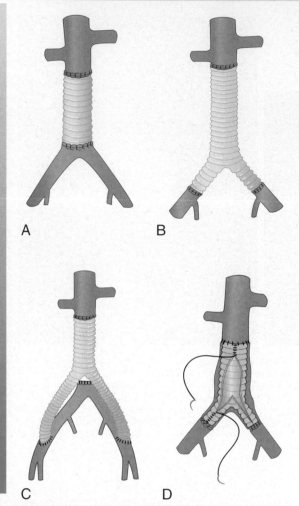

FIGURE 29–12. Types of aortic grafts. *A*, Tube graft with end-to-end proximal and distal anastomoses. *B*, Aortobifemoral graft with end-to-end distal anastomoses. *C*, Aortobifemoral graft with end-to-side distal anastomoses. *D*, The native aorta is wrapped around the graft and sewn closed.

Technique and Normal Appearance of Grafts

The objectives of postoperative ultrasound examination are to examine the full length of the graft, to evaluate blood flow for stenosis, and to detect pathologic fluid collections and aneurysm formation. The ultrasound graft examination generally is fairly quick and easy. The sonographer begins at the proximal end and follows the graft to the distal end (or vice versa) using color flow imaging. As long as there are no flow disturbances indicating stenosis in the graft or the native arteries adjacent to the graft, we simply document the appearance of the proximal and distal anastomoses as well as the diameter of the graft body and limbs, and we document Doppler waveforms and velocities in the runoff vessels, just beyond the distal anastomoses.

The graft material used for aortic bypass generally has a textured, or tram track, appearance, and is fairly echogenic (Fig. 29–13); therefore, the graft can usually be identified easily. The exception to this rule is an old graft (e.g., >8 yr) that is invested with fibrous tissue or atherosclerotic plaque. These grafts can be difficult to identify. Slight puckering of the graft and the native artery is seen normally at the suture lines, causing visible thickening of the artery wall at the anastomosis. A small layer of fluid is normally present around the graft during the postoperative period. This fluid may be focal or diffuse and may persist for more than a week. Large fluid collections may be present postoperatively around the body of an aortic graft if the native aorta is wrapped around it (Fig. 29–14), and this fluid may persist for months. The important thing about postoperative fluid is that it should decrease in volume with time and ultimately disappear. Increasing fluid volume suggests graft infection.

Complications

Complications of aortic graft surgery may be divided into early and late periods. In the early period (weeks/months), surgery-

body, which is attached to the aorta, and the limbs, which are attached to the common or external iliac arteries. Tube grafts, of course, have only one part. The proximal end of the graft is usually attached to the aorta end-to-end, but occasionally an end-to-side anastomosis is used (end of graft to side of aorta). The distal anastomosis is end-to-end for aortoiliac grafts and end-to-side for aortofemoral grafts. Femoral attachment is used when atherosclerosis or aneurysm precludes iliac attachment of the graft limbs. The end-to-side configuration permits retrograde external iliac artery flow needed to supply blood to the internal iliac branches.

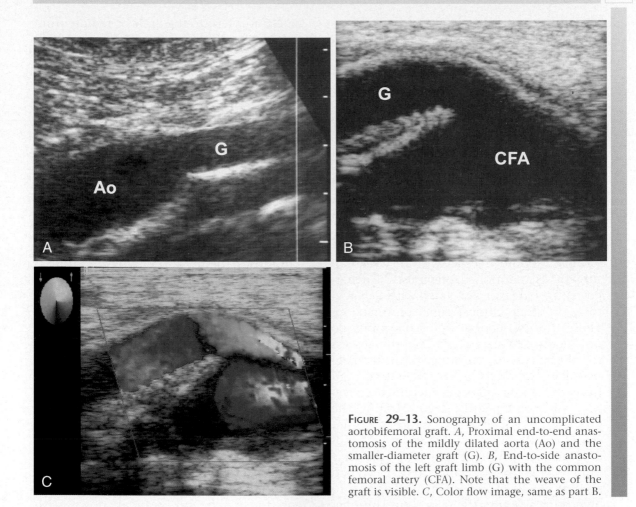

FIGURE 29–13. Sonography of an uncomplicated aortobifemoral graft. *A*, Proximal end-to-end anastomosis of the mildly dilated aorta (Ao) and the smaller-diameter graft (G). *B*, End-to-side anastomosis of the left graft limb (G) with the common femoral artery (CFA). Note that the weave of the graft is visible. *C*, Color flow image, same as part B.

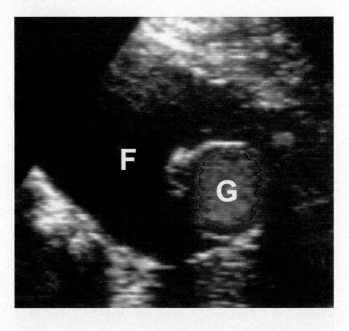

FIGURE 29–14. A large postoperative fluid collection (F) is present between the aneurysm sac and the body of this graft (G).

related hematomas and seromas, as well as infection, are the principal problems. Hematomas are collections of blood, and seromas are collections of tissue fluid or serum. Either type of fluid is normally present adjacent to the graft in the days following surgery, and these fluid collections occasionally may be large focally or may be located somewhat distant from the graft within the retroperitoneum. The sonographic appearance is that of any fluid collection: anechoic or mildly echogenic; homogeneous or heterogeneous. Although they cannot be differentiated from abscesses, postoperative hematomas and seromas should recede within weeks of surgery, as mentioned previously. Furthermore, they are not associated with leukocytosis or other clinical signs of infection. These inconsequential fluid collections do not increase in size, and if they do, abscess should be considered. Abscess can be diagnosed in two ways: (1) by aspirating fluid from the sonographically identified collection and subsequently demonstrating the presence of bacteria via culture or Gram stain, or (2) by a combination of sonographic and clinical findings (e.g., perigraft fluid, leukocytosis, and fever). When abscess is diagnosed, it is important to determine whether the collection is imme-

diately adjacent to the graft or remote from it. A remote abscess (e.g., in a surgical incision) may be drained percutaneouusly without significant clinical consequences, while a perigraft abscess necessitates graft removal (Fig. 29–15). Finally, it should be noted that graft infection may not be accompanied by sonographic abnormalities if the infection is indolent. In such cases, infection may be accompanied only by perigraft inflammation that is not visible sonographically. Chronic infection is generally diagnosed by a combination of laboratory findings, clinical symptomatology, and computed tomography findings.

In most patients, aortic bypass grafting is a durable procedure, and the graft may be expected to function without complications for 10 yr or more. Late graft failure may occur, however, from a variety of causes.[23,46] With time, the graft material may weaken due to fatigue imposed by the repeated stress of arterial pulsation. Fatigue may cause the graft to stretch and dilate, like an old sock, or it may lead to localized failure and the development of a leak accompanied by a pseudoaneurysm. These modes of failure are uncommon, however. The majority of long-term complications occur instead at the distal anastomoses, which tend to stretch and/or break down with

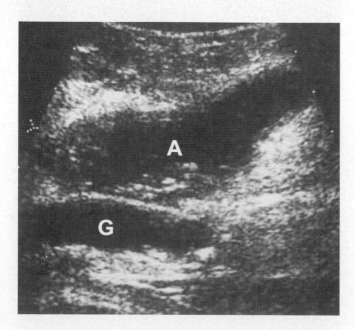

FIGURE 29–15. An abscess (A) is present in a groin incision. Unfortunately, the abscess extends to the graft (G), implying that the graft is infected as well.

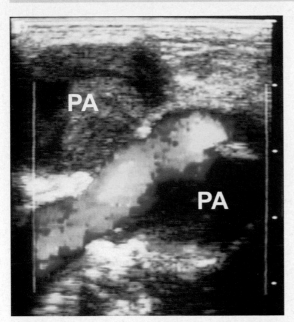

FIGURE 29–16. Graft pseudoaneurysm. A large pseudoaneurysm (PA) extends both superficial and deep to the distal anastomosis of an aortoexternal iliac bypass graft.

time (Figs. 29–16 and 29–17). Stretching causes a true aneurysm to form at the anastomosis, involving both the graft and the native artery. Breakdown of the sutured graft-artery interface leads to pseudoaneurysm formation. While these complications may occur at any ansatomosis, they are usually seen at the distal anastomosis and are particualrly common at aorto-femoral anastomoses. The fact that most graft complications occur at the anastomoses is the reason for emphasizing the identification of the proximal and distal anastomoses in the course of every sonographic graft examination.

Aortic grafts are also subject to the development of stenosis and occlusion. Again, these are usually late problems and almost invariably occur at the distal anastomosis or in the runoff vessel. Stenoses usually occur not in the graft, but in the runoff vessel at or beyond the distal anastomosis. Occasionally, however, stenosis develops in a graft limb. Regardless of location, severe stenosis may cause stagnation of flow and thrombus formation in a graft limb, leading to occlusion. On ultrasound examination, stenosis is indicated by focal high velocity and disturbed flow that is readily detected with color flow sonography. Stenosis severity is judged with Doppler velocity measurements, as discussed in Chapter 18. Occlusion is diagnosed by the absence of flow and the presence of echogenic material in the graft lumen.

THE INFERIOR VENA CAVA

The IVC is evaluated with ultrasound mainly to determine whether this vessel is patent and, if it is not patent, to determine the cause of obstruction. The pathologic condition that most often affects the IVC is thrombosis. Thrombus usually propagates into the IVC from a tributary vessel, but thrombosis can also develop secondary to obstructive processes that reduce IVC flow. In current medical practice, IVC filter placement is a relatively common cause of IVC thrombosis. Neoplasia is probably the second most common pathologic condition affecting the IVC. Primary tumors of the IVC are rare, but extrinsic tumors that compress or invade the IVC are more common. These include renal cell carcinoma, hepatocellular carcinoma, and a host of other neoplasms that metastasize to paracaval lymph nodes. Congenital anomalies of the IVC are rare, but sonographers should be aware of several of the more common anomalies, as described later.

Ultrasound evaluation of the IVC[42,47] is carried out in both longitudinal and transverse planes, but in my experience, longitudinal color flow images (Fig. 29–18) are most convenient and informative. If the IVC is the focus of interest, the vessel should be examined in its entirety, including the suprahepatic, intrahepatic, and infrahepatic portions. If obstruction is found, an attempt should be made to determine its cause. If the IVC is thrombosed, the extent of thrombosis and involvement of tributary vessels should be ascertained. The suprahepatic and intrahepatic portions are readily examined with ultrasound, but the infrahepatic portion may be obscured by bowel contents.

The mean diameter of the IVC in normal individuals[43,48] is 17.2 mm, as measured just below the renal veins during quiet respira-

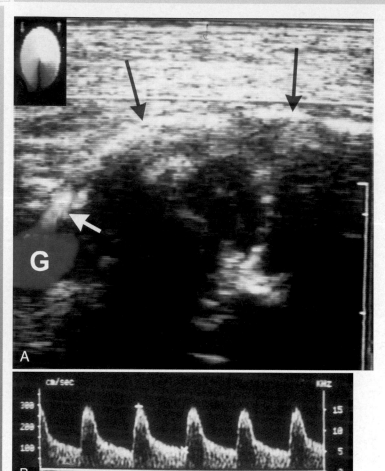

FIGURE 29–17. Graft aneurysm and stenosis (68-yr-old man with claudication, 8 yr after aortobifemoral graft). *A,* A large aneurysm (black arrows) is present at the right femoral anastomosis of an aortofemoral graft (G). Only the near surface of the aneurysm is visible because extensive calcification of the aneurysm obscures deeper structures. A tiny residual lumen is present along the near surface of the aneurysm (white arrow). *B,* Doppler investigation of the stenotic segment shows a peak systolic velocity of 298.4 cm/sec and an end-diastolic velocity of 102.8 cm/sec, consistent with severe narrowing.

tion. The IVC ranges in diameter from 5 to 29 mm during quiet respiration, and the diameter increases about 10% during deep inspiration. The proximal portion of the IVC has a pulsatile Doppler flow pattern contributed by right atrial pressure changes occurring during each cardiac cycle.[42,47] Farther distal, near the confluence of the iliac veins, only respiratory variation may be observed on Doppler examination. Partial obstruction of the IVC may eliminate normal flow variation. In such cases,

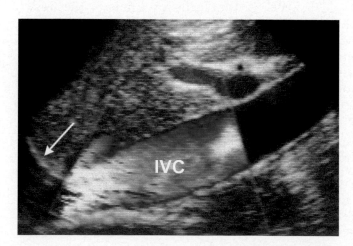

FIGURE 29–18. Normal inferior vena cava (IVC). The proximal end of the IVC is seen deep to the liver in a longitudinal view. The arrow marks the diaphragm.

Doppler flow signals distal to the point of obstruction are described as continuous, because a uniform flow velocity is present, without respiratory or cardiac variation. Continuous flow is a significant finding that should prompt investigation for obstruction of more proximal portions of the IVC.

Acute Thrombosis

The ultrasound findings in acute IVC thrombosis[42-44,47-49] are distention, absence of flow, and the presence of material within the vein lumen. The echogenicity of thrombus varies with its age, as discussed in Chapter 24. In a typical case, the IVC is substantially or completely occluded by thrombus, but thrombus may occasionally propagate from a tributary vessel and float freely within the IVC lumen without blocking flow.[45,50] The pitfalls for sonographic diagnosis are the following: (1) Acute IVC thrombus may be so hypoechoic that it is overlooked in the absence of color flow examination, and (2) false-positive diagnosis of thrombosis may occur in very low-flow states in which Doppler flow detection is difficult.

Inferior Vena Cava Filters

Sonography is commonly used to evaluate devices called filters, which prevent thrombus originating in lower extremity or pelvic veins from embolizing to the pulmonary circulation. These devices are placed in the IVC percutaneously, via the common femoral or jugular veins. When released from the cannula used for its insertion, the filter expands and attaches to the cava wall via small hooks projecting from its periphery. These devices do not significantly obstruct blood flow, but they trap thrombus, preventing it from flowing farther cephalad. Filters are used in patients at risk for pulmonary embolization in whom anticoagulation is contraindicated.

Perhaps the most important function of ultrasound occurs before filter insertion—to ensure that the venous system is thrombus-free from the insertion site to the IVC. The presence of thrombus along the insertion course not only prevents filter placement, but it also imposes a significant risk that attempted insertion will dislodge thrombus and cause dangerous pulmonary embolization. The insertion site (common femoral or internal jugular vein) is examined directly with color flow and compression sonography, and the patency of more proximal venous segments is assessed indirectly with Doppler, as described in Chapter 22.

Inferior vena cava filter insertion may be complicated by thrombosis at the insertion site, inadequate position of the filter, IVC thrombosis, and pericaval hematoma resulting from perforation of the cava.[42,47,49-56] After filter placement, ultrasound is used when complications are suspected. Most often, this is to exclude or detect thrombosis of the introducer vein or the IVC or to assess the location of the filter relative to the renal veins. IVC filters should be positioned below the renal veins, as seen in Figure 29–19, and the IVC should be patent distal to the filter. Although the filters trap thrombus, the visualization of thrombus below the filter is considered abnormal.[53,56] IVC perforation is uncommon, and although the resulting hematoma might be visible with ultrasound, computed tomography is likely to be more useful for diagnosis of this complication.

Neoplastic Obstruction

Neoplastic obstruction of the IVC may result from compression by an extrinsic mass, tumor extension from the hepatic or renal veins, and, rarely, from a tumor arising in the wall of the IVC (most frequently leiomyosarcoma). Ultrasound diagnosis of neoplastic IVC obstruction is made through the visualization of intraluminal tumor or an extrinsic tumor mass that compresses and secondarily obstructs the IVC.[42,44,47-49,57-59] In the case of intraluminal tumor extension (Fig. 29–20), the origin of the tumor from either a renal or hepatic vein is usually readily apparent. Intraluminal tumor is moderately echogenic and has a characteristic color flow finding that dif-

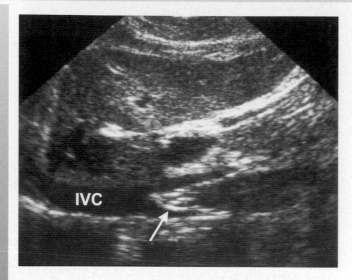

FIGURE 29–19. Inferior vena cava (IVC) filter. A longitudinal view of the IVC shows the proximal end of a filter device (arrow).

ferentiates it from thrombus. Small vessels are visible within the tumor on color flow examination. These, of course, are not present in thrombus, which is avascular. In most instances, it is not difficult to differentiate between intraluminal tumor extension and extrinsic IVC compression by a neoplastic mass (Fig. 29–21).

Intrinsic or extrinsic neoplastic obstruction may cause secondary IVC thrombosis, but this does not always occur. In such cases, IVC flow may be antegrade at a very slow rate, or flow may be reversed as a result of collateralization (Fig. 29–22). Whether patent or occluded, the IVC and tributary veins are likely to be dilated below the level of obstruction. Doppler examination of patent areas below the point of obstruction reveals continuous flow, as described previously.

Anomalies

Several anomalies of the IVC are noteworthy: duplication, left-sided IVC, absence of the intrahepatic portion, and membranous obstruction of the intrahepatic portion. Because these conditions are rare, they are considered only briefly.

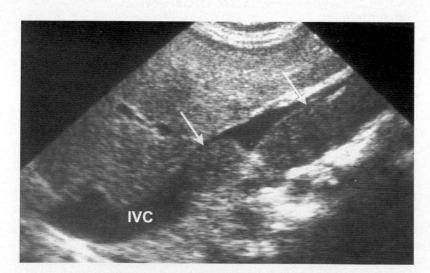

FIGURE 29–20. Extension of renal cell carcinoma (arrows) into the inferior vena cava (IVC).

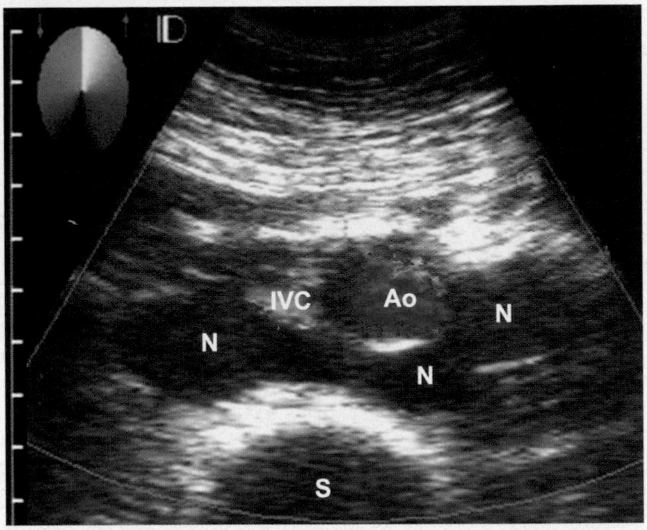

FIGURE 29-21. Extrinsic tumor compressing the inferior vena cava (IVC). Lymph nodes (N), enlarged by lung cancer metastasis, substantially compress the IVC and elevate the aorta (Ao) from the spine (S). The patient presented with bilateral leg swelling.

Duplication occurs in the infrarenal portion of the IVC.[48,60] Two IVCs are seen, one on each side of the aorta. Each vessel continues cephalad as a direct extension of the ipsilateral iliac vein. In most cases, duplication ends at the level of the renal veins, with the left IVC draining into the left renal vein and subsequently into the right IVC, which describes a normal course through the upper abdomen. A variant of this anomaly is a left-sided IVC that extends cephalad into the azygous system. In such cases, the right-sided IVC may continue through the liver, or this portion may be absent, with flow crossing over to the left via the left renal vein.

The intrahepatic portion of the IVC may be absent on a congenital basis.[49,50,61,62] In such cases, flow from the renal veins and the lower extremities may be carried back to the heart by a number of conduits, but the most common are the azygous or hemiazygous veins. With the latter conduits, blood is subsequently discharged into the superior vena cava, from whence it enters the right atrium. Ultrasound diagnosis is based on absence of the intrahepatic portion of the IVC and direct drainage of the hepatic veins into the right atrium, with or without a short common trunk. This anomaly may be isolated and of no consequence, but it may also be a component of more serious conditions that include congenital heart disease, cardiac situs anomalies, and visceral situs disorders.

Membranous obstruction of the IVC is rare in the United States, but worldwide, this peculiar condition is the most common cause of hepatic outflow obstruction.[54,55,63,64] The IVC is present in this condition but is interrupted by an oblique or transverse fibrous septum that is typically located just cephalad to the insertion of the right hepatic vein. The middle and left hepatic veins may insert above or below the membrane and therefore may or may not be obstructed. The right hepatic vein is almost always obstructed. Although membranous IVC obstruction is thought to be a congenital anomaly, it typically does not present until early or middle adulthood, or it may be an asymptomatic, incidental finding. Typical presenting signs and symptoms are bilateral lower extremity swelling and signs of hepatic vein obstruction (see Chapter 32). Ultrasound findings are diagnostic. The obstructing membrane is visible at the diaphragm, and blood flow is reversed in the IVC, which is markedly dilated. The obstructed hepatic veins are dilated and demonstrate sluggish, continuous flow. In addition, intrahepatic venous collateralization may be apparent, as well as findings of portal venous hypertension.

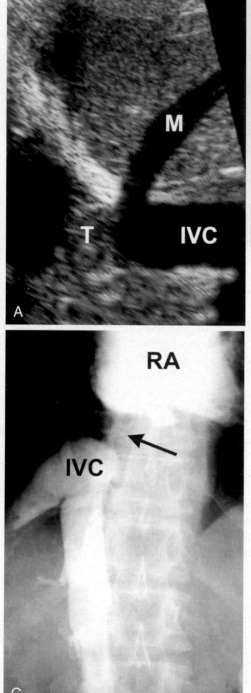

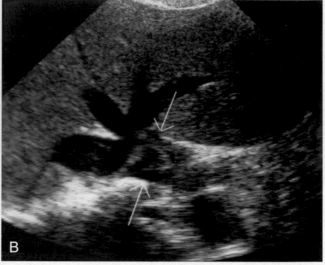

FIGURE 29-22. Inferior vena cava (IVC) occlusion. *A*, Localized growth of a hepatocellular carcinoma (T) obstructs the IVC at the diaphragm. Both the IVC and the middle hepatic vein (M) are markedly dilated. On real-time observation (not shown), blood from the hepatic veins was seen to flow retrograde in the IVC, ultimately to lumbar and iliac collaterals. *B*, A transverse view shows the tumor mass (arrows) and marked distention of the hepatic veins. *C*, A venogram shows the obstructed segment of the IVC (*arrow*) located just below the right atrium (RA).

References

1. Bluth EI: Ultrasound of the abdominal aorta. Arch Intern Med 144:377–380, 1984.
2. Steiner E, Rubens D, Weiss SL, et al: Sonographic examination of the abdominal aorta through the left flank: A prospective study. J Ultrasound Med 5:499–502, 1986.
3. Scott RAP, Ashton HA, Kay DN: Abdominal aortic aneurysm in 4237 screened patients: Prevalence, development and management over 6 years. Br J Surg 78:1122–1124, 1991.

4. Ricci MA, Kleeman M, Case T, Pilcher DB: Normal aortic diameter by ultrasound. J Vasc Technol 19:17–19, 1995.

5. Lederle FA, Johnson GR, Wilson SE, et al: Relationship of age, gender, race and body size to infrarenal aortic diameter. J Vasc Surg 25:595–601, 1997.

6. Paivansalo MJ, Merikanto J, Jerkkola T, et al: Effect of hypertension and risk factors on diameters of abdominal aorta and common iliac and femoral arteries in middle-aged hypertensive and control subjects: A cross-sectional systematic study with duplex ultrasound. Atherosclerosis. 153:99–106, 2000.

7. Hallett JW: Abdominal aortic aneurysm: Natural history and treatment. Heart Dis Stroke 1:303–308, 1992.

8. Blanchard JF, Armenian HK, Friesen PP: Risk factors for abdominal aortic aneurysm: Results of a case-control study. Am J Epidemiol 151:575–583, 2000.

9. Sonesson B, Hansen F, Lanne T: Abdominal aortic aneurysm: A general defect in the vasculature with focal manifestations in the abdominal aorta? J Vasc Surg 26:247–254, 1997.

10. DeSanctis RW, Doroghazi RM, Austen G, et al: Aortic dissection. N Engl J Med 317:1060–1067, 1987.

11. Lawrence-Brown MM, Norman PE, Jamrozik K, et al: Initial results of ultrasound screening for aneurysm of the abdominal aorta in Western Australia: Relevance for endoluminal treatment of aneurysm disease. Cardiovasc Surg 9:234–240, 2001.

12. Scott RAP, Ashton HA, Kay DN: Abdominal aortic aneurysm in 4237 screened patients: Prevalence, development and management over 6 years. Br J Surg 78:1122–1124, 1991.

13. Blau SA, Kerstein MD, Deterling RA: Abdominal aortic aneurysm. In Kerstein MD, Moulder MD, Webb WR (eds): Aneurysms. Baltimore, Williams & Wilkins, 1983, pp 127–196.

14. Fink HA, Lederle FA, Roth CS, et al: The accuracy of physical examination to detect abdominal aortic aneurysm. Arch Intern Med 160:833–836, 2000.

15 Chervu A, Clagett GP, Valentine RJ, et al: Role of physical examination in detection of abdominal aortic aneurysms. Surgery 117:454–457, 1995.

16 Kyriakides C, Byrne J, Green S, Hulton NR: Screening of abdominal aortic aneurysm: A pragmatic approach. Ann R Coll Surg Engl 82:59–63, 2000.

17 Crow P, Shaw E, Earnshaw JJ, et al: A single normal ultrasonographic scan at age 65 years rules out significant aneurysm disease for life in men. Br J Surg 88:941–942, 2001.

18 Wilmink AB, Hubbard CS, Day NE, Quick CR: The incidence of small abdominal aortic aneurysms and the change in normal infrarenal aortic diameter: implications for screening. Eur J Vasc Endovasc Surg 21:165–170, 2001.

19. Garrett HE, Ilabaca PA: The ruptured abdominal aortic aneurysm. In Bergan JJ, Yao JST (eds): Aneurysms, Diagnosis and Treatment. New York, Grune & Stratton, 1982, pp 302–326.

20. Cronenwett JL, Murphy TF, Zelenock GB, et al: Actuarial analysis of variables associated with rupture of small abdominal aortic aneurysms. Surgery 98:462–483, 1985.

21. Scott RAP, Tisi PV, Ashton HA, Allen DR: Abdominal aortic aneurysm rupture rates: A 7-year follow-up study of the entire abdominal aortic aneurysm population detected by screening. J Vasc Surg 28:124–128, 1998.

22. Takamyia M, Hirose Y: Growth curve of ruptured aortic aneurysm. J Cardiovasc Surg 39:9–13, 1998.

23. Rutherford RB (ed): Abdominal aortic aneurysms: New approaches to a continuing problem. Semin Vasc Surg 8:83–167, 1995.

24. Nevitt MP, Ballard DJ, Hallett JW: Prognosis of abdominal aortic aneurysms. N Engl J Med 321:1009–1014, 1989.

25. Bernstein EF, Chan EL: Abdominal aortic aneurysm in high-risk patients: Outcome of selective management based on size and expansion rate. Ann Surg 200:255–263, 1984.

26. Sterpetti AV, Shultz RD, Feldhaus RJ, et al: Abdominal aortic aneurysms in elderly patients: Selective management based on clinical status and aneurysmal expansion rate. Am J Surg 150:772–776, 1985.

27. LaRoy LL, Cormier PJ, Matalon TAS, et al: Imaging of abdominal aortic aneurysms. Am J Roentgenol 152:785–792, 1989.

28. Hirose Y, Hamada S, Takamiya M, et al: Aortic aneurysms: Growth rates measured with CT. Radiology 185:249–252, 1992.

29. Paivansao M, Lahde S, Myllyla V, et al: Ultrasonography in the diagnosis of abdominal aortic aneurysms. Fortschr Röntgenstr 140:683–685, 1984.

30. Mower WR, Quiñones WJ, Gambhir SS: Effect of intraluminal thrombus on abdominal aortic aneurysm wall stress. J Vasc Surg 26:602–608, 1997.

31. Harter LP, Gross BH, Callen PW, et al: Ultrasonic evaluation of abdominal aortic thrombus. J Ultrasound Med 1:315, 1982.

32. King PS, Cooperberg PL, Madigan SM: The anechoic crescent in abdominal aortic aneurysms: Not a sign of dissection. Am J Roentgenol 146:345–348, 1986.

33. Yucel EK, Fillmore DJ, Knox TA, Waltman AC: Sonographic measurement of abdominal aortic diameter: Interobserver variability. J Ultrasound Med 10:681–683, 1991.

34. Cramer MM: Color flow duplex examination of the abdominal aorta: Atherosclerosis, aneurysm, and dissection. J Vasc Tech 19:249–260, 1995.

35. Crotty JM, Timken MJ: Pseudodissection of the abdominal aorta on color Doppler imaging. J Ultrasound Med 14:853–857, 1995.

36. Nguyen BD, Hamper UM: False positive dissection of abdominal aortic aneurysm by color Doppler duplex ultrasonography. J Ultrasound Med 14:467–469, 1995.

37. Hanley M, Ryley NG, Lewis P, Currie I: Can duplex accurately assess the relationship between the renal arteries and an abdominal aortic aneurysm using the superior mesenteric artery as a fixed point? J Vasc Technology 25:97–101, 2000.

38. Bundy AL, Ritchie WGM: Inflammatory aneurysm of the abdominal aorta. J Clin Ultrasound 12:102–104, 1984.

39. Cullenward MJ, Scanlan KA, Pozniak MA, et al: Inflammatory aortic aneurysm (periaortic fibrosis): Radiologic imaging. Radiology 159:75–82, 1986.

40. Clayton MJ, Walsh JW, Brewer WH: Contained rupture of abdominal aortic aneurysms: Sonographic and CT diagnosis. Am J Roentgenol 138:154–156, 1982.

41. Rosen A, Korobkin M, Silverman PM, et al: CT diagnosis of ruptured abdominal aortic aneurysm. Am J Roentgenol 143:265–268, 1984.

42. Falkoff GE, Taylor KJW, Morse S: Hepatic artery pseudoaneurysm: Diagnosis with real-time and pulsed Doppler US. Radiology 158:55–56, 1986.

43. Huey H, Cooperberg PL, Bogoch A: Diagnosis of giant varix of the coronary vein by pulsed-Doppler sonography. Am J Roentgenol 143:77–78, 1984.

44. Mark A, Moss A, Lusby R, et al: CT evaluation of complications of abdominal aortic surgery. Radiology 145:409–414, 1982.

45. Hilton S, Megibow AJ, Naidich DP, et al: Computed tomography of the postoperative abdominal aorta. Radiology 145:403–407, 1982.

46. Marin ML, Hllier LH: Endovascular grafts. Semin Vasc Surg 12:64–73, 1999.

47. Sandager GP, Flinn WR: Technical considerations for evaluation of the inferior vena cava. J Vasc Technol 19:263–268, 1995.

48. Sykes AM, McLoughlin RF, So CBB, et al: Sonographic assessment of infrarenal inferior vena caval dimensions. J Ultrasound Med 14:665–668, 1995.

49. Park JH, Lee JB, Han MC, et al: Sonographic evaluation of inferior vena caval obstruction: Correlative study with vena cavography. Am J Roentgenol 145:757–762, 1985.

50. Sonnenfeld M, Finberg HJ: Ultrasonographic diagnosis of incomplete inferior vena caval thrombosis secondary to periphlebitis: The importance of a complete survey examination. Radiology 137:743–744, 1980.

51. Fox AD, Whiteley MS, Murphy P, et al: Comparison of magnetic resonance imaging measurements of abdominal aortic aneurysms with measurements obtained by other imaging techniques and intraoperative measurements: Possible implications for endovascular grafting. J Vasc Surg 24:632–638, 1996.

52. Blum U, Voshage G, Lammer J, et al: Endoluminal stent-grafts for infrarenal abdominal aortic aneurysms. N Engl J Med 336:12–20, 1997.

53. Golzarian J: Imaging of abdominal aortic aneurysms after endoluminal repair. Semin Ultrasound CT MRI 20:16–24, 1999.

54. Aswad MA, Sandager GP, Pais SO, et al: Early duplex scan evaluation of four vena caval interruption devices. J Vasc Surg 24:809–818, 1996.

55. Mohan CR, Hoballah JJ, Sharp WJ, et al: Comparative efficacy and complications of vena caval filters. J Vasc Surg 21:235–246, 1995.

56. Pasto ME, Kurtz AB, Jarrell BE, et al: The Kimray-Greenfield filter: Evaluation by duplex real-time pulsed Doppler ultrasound. Radiology 148:223–226, 1983.

57. Johnson BL, Harris EJ, Fogarty TJ, et al: Color duplex evaluation of endoluminal aortic stent grafts. J Vasc Technol 22:97–104, 1998.

58. Slovis TL, Philippart AI, Cushing B, et al: Evaluation of the inferior vena cava by sonography and venography in children with renal and hepatic tumors. Radiology 140:767–772, 1982.

59. Pussell SJ, Cosgrove DO: Ultrasound features of tumour thrombus in the IVC in retroperitoneal tumours. Br J Radiol 54:866–869, 1981.

60. Goss CM (ed): Gray's Anatomy, 29th American ed. Philadelphia, Lea & Febiger, 1973.

61. Garris JB, Hooshang K, Sample F: Ultrasonic diagnosis of infrahepatic interruption of the inferior vena cava with azygos (hemiazygos) continuation. Radiology 134:179–183, 1980.

62. Ritter SB, Bierman FZ: Noninvasive diagnosis of interrupted inferior vena cava: Gated pulsed Doppler application. Am J Cardiol 51:1796–1798, 1983.

63. Simson IW: Membranous obstruction of the inferior vena cava and hepatocellular carcinoma in South Africa. Gastroenterology 82:171–178, 1982.

64. Kimura C, Matsuda S, Koie H, Hirooka M: Membranous obstruction of the hepatic portion of the inferior vena cava: Clinical study of nine cases. Surgery 72:551–559, 1972.

Chapter 30

Ultrasound Imaging Assessment Following Endovascular Aortic Aneurysm Repair

GEORGE L. BERDEJO, BA, RVT, AND EVAN C. LIPSITZ, MD

In contrast to open abdominal aortic aneurysm (AAA) repair, objective follow-up and frequent assessment is critical after endovascular aneurysm repair. Because these devices (endografts), sometimes referred to as endovascular grafts, stent-grafts, or transluminally placed endovascular grafts, are relatively new and still evolving, patients undergoing endovascular AAA repair require routine, lifelong follow-up and imaging surveillance.

Color Doppler ultrasound has been used for aortic endovascular graft evaluation and has the advantage of being noninvasive, inexpensive, rapid, safe, nontoxic, and well tolerated by patients. This technique has already become an important tool in both the planning and the postoperative evaluation of endovascular grafts placed for a variety of occlusive, traumatic, and aneurysmal vascular lesions and complications.[1-9] Color Doppler ultrasound combines many of the ideal features of both angiography and spiral computed tomography (CT). It allows the examiner to make both quantitative and qualitative assessments of blood flow through the endovascular graft, and, via a combination of pulsed-wave and color flow Doppler, ultrasound can easily demonstrate normal or abnormal flow patterns that are associated with pathology. Because color Doppler is also relatively inexpensive, easily repeatable, and without known risks, it has become a primary means of surveillance for endovascular interventions.[2,4,5,7,10]

The **primary** objectives of the color Doppler examination following endovascular AAA repair are to:
1. Determine whether there is any persistent perigraft flow in the aneurysm sac (endoleak).
2. Measure maximal residual aneurysm sac diameter.
3. Assess the flow through the endovascular graft and identify any areas of stenosis or occlusion.

If flow is identified within the aneurysm sac, it is important to determine the origin of this flow (endoleak source, Table 30–1), as the source of the flow and the flow characteristics may determine subsequent treatment. Cross-sectional diameter measurements are recorded at each study occasion to determine maximum aneurysm size. When excluded from blood flow, an aneurysm should remain stable or decrease in size over time.[10,11] Any increase in size suggests the presence of flow into the aneurysm sac (endoleak) and therefore a continued risk of rupture,[11,12] although increases in size have been reported without CT, angiographic, or color Doppler evidence of endoleak (endotension).[13-15]

It is also important to determine that the distal arterial circulation has been preserved, by ensuring that there are no graft-threatening abnormalities within the body of the endovascular graft, the graft limb(s), or the inflow or outflow vessels. We have previously described a protocol for evaluation of endovascular grafts placed at the aortoiliac level.[2]

Table 30–1. Endoleak Types

Type 1a, 1b	Endoleak whose origin is at the proximal (1a) or distal (1b) stent attachment site.
Type 2	Endoleak originating from a branch vessel. Possible sources include patent lumbar (posterior to the endovascular graft sonographically), inferior mesenteric (anterolateral to the endovascular graft sonographically), accessory renal or hypogastric arteries, or other patent branches of the abdominal aorta. These are best seen in the transverse orientation.
Type 3	Endoleak that originates at the junctions between components of modular devices or from fabric tears within the graft.
Type 4	Transgraft flow or flow that fills the aneurysm sac due to porosity of the graft.
Endotension	Increase in aneurysm size in the absence of endoleak.

If abnormalities are detected by color Doppler, contrast arteriography and spiral CT can be used to further define the problem in instances in which intervention is considered. This chapter describes a protocol for identifying and characterizing findings associated with endovascular grafts performed for the repair of abdominal aortic and aortoiliac aneurysms.

ENDOVASCULAR GRAFTS: OVERVIEW AND GENERAL CONSIDERATIONS

The endoluminal placement of stent-grafts in sites remote from where the graft is introduced allows for repair of a variety of complex lesions while reducing the relatively high morbidity and mortality associated with traditional open operative repair. In 1991, the first series of transluminally placed endovascular grafts for the repair of abdominal aortic aneurysms in high-risk patients was reported.[16] Since that time, significant advances in the design of endovascular stents and grafts have facilitated their application in aortic and aortoiliac aneurysms, permitting a larger percentage of patients to be treated with these devices.[17–20] The Montefiore Endovascular Graft System (MEGS) is the device we have the most experience with; however, a number of endovascular grafts for the treatment of AAA have been tested and validated in multicenter studies both in the United States and around the world (Fig. 30–1). Currently, three devices (Table 30–2) have been granted U.S. Food and Drug Administration approval for the treatment of aortoiliac aneurysms and are available for widespread use in the United States.[21–23]

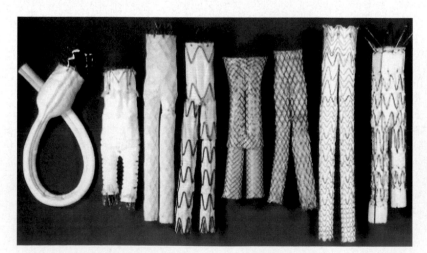

FIGURE 30–1. Endovascular grafts that have undergone trials in the United States. *Left to right*, Montefiore Endovascular Graft System (MEGS), Ancure, Vanguard, Talent, Corvita, AneuRx, Excluder, Zenith. Note the different configurations and designs. Some are fully supported by metal (inside or outside). The MEGS device seen here has a stent only at the proximal attachment site.

Table 30–2. Food and Drug Administration–Approved Grafts for Endovascular Abdominal Aortic Aneurysm Repair

AneuRx (Medtronic, Sunnyvale, CA)
Excluder (WL Gore, Flagstaff, AZ)
Zenith (Cook, Inc., Bloomington, IN)

Endovascular grafts are a combination of intravascular stent and prosthetic graft technologies. The stent itself, in addition to any other adjuncts such as hooks or barbs, functions as the anchoring component of the endovascular graft and provides fixation to the attachment point as well as support for the body of the endovascular graft. The stent can be attached to an assortment of prosthetic grafts. Endovascular grafts use either self-expanding or balloon-expandable modified stents, with Gore-Tex or Dacron as the fabric most commonly used in the finished device. Once the endovascular graft is fixed into position within the vasculature, it permits direct flow through the endovascular graft only, avoiding communication with the native arterial circulation, thus excluding the aneurysm. These endovascular grafts come in many types and configurations (Fig. 30–2). It is not uncommon for endovascular aortic aneurysm repair to be supplemented by other ancillary procedures, such as femorofemoral bypass, intra-arterial coil vessel occlusion, or other vessel occlusion procedures (Fig. 30–3).

Ideally, the endovascular graft is deployed immediately distal to the lowest renal artery proximally and as close to the iliac bifurcation as possible distally. In grafts with hooks or barbs, these penetrate a variable distance

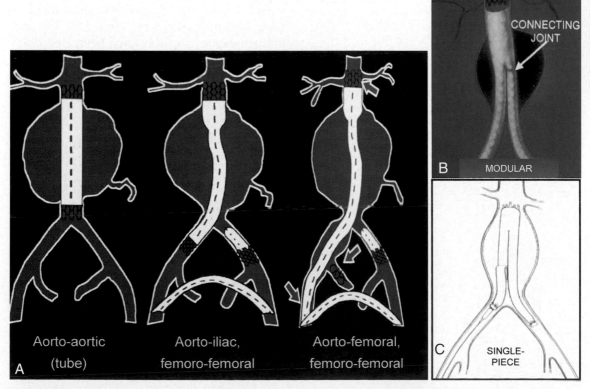

FIGURE 30–2. Examples of the various configurations of endovascular grafts that may be encountered. *A*, On the left is a simple tube graft with stent attachments at the proximal and distal aneurysm necks. In the center is an aortoiliac endovascular graft, and on the right, an aortofemoral endovascular graft is shown (used for complex aortoiliac aneurysm repair). Note the use of occluder devices and coils in the grafts in the center and right. Also note that the proximal stent crosses the renal arteries in the figure on the the right. *B*, A bifurcated modular device with a connecting joint. *C*, A single-piece, aortobiiliac design.

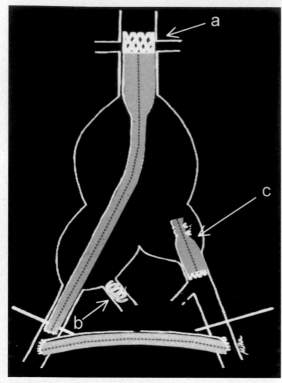

FIGURE 30–3. Example of multiple interventions performed in conjunction with an endovascular graft (aortounifemoral, femorofemoral). The proximal fixation site is located at the level of the renal arteries, and the stent crosses the renal arteries (a). Coils have been deployed in the right internal iliac artery (b), and an occluder device is deployed in the contralateral common iliac artery (c). Both devices prevent backflow into the aneurysm sac. An endoluminal anastomosis is performed at the distal end of the endovascular graft, in the right femoral artery. Outflow to the extremities is via the ipsilateral (right) common femoral artery and the right-to-left femoro-femoral graft. Retrograde flow in the left external iliac artery perfuses the pelvis.

Table 30–3. Advantages of Endovascular Graft Exclusion of Abdominal Aortic Aneurysms

- Procedure is performed from remote site and avoids laparotomy.
- Small incisions (femoral, brachial, or carotid artery cutdown for access).
- No prolonged aortic clamping.
- Decreased or no stay in intensive care unit.
- Decreased length of stay (1–2 d for endovascular vs. 6–8 d for open repair).
- Decreased time to resumption of normal activity level.

into the aortic wall at the proximal and/or distal fixation zones. In patients with no distal aortic neck or coincident iliac artery aneurysms, the endovascular graft is extended to the iliac artery as dictated by the morphology of the aortoiliac aneurysm (Fig. 30–4).

While the endovascular repair of AAAs offers many benefits, (Table 30–3), there are several potential complications associated with this technique. The most significant of these complications are endoleak[24,25] and graft migration, which have been described for all of the endovascular grafts that have been used to date for endovascular AAA repair.

An endoleak is defined as flow outside of the endovascular graft that perfuses and pressurizes the aneurysm sac. This ongoing pressurization of the aneurysm sac carries

Type II

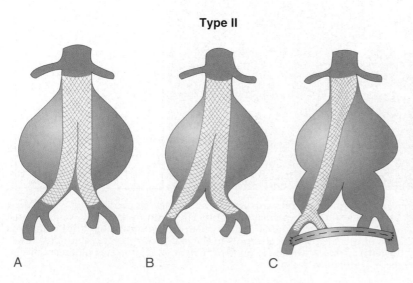

A   B   C

FIGURE 30–4. Various configurations seen in patients with coexisting aortic and iliac artery aneurysms. In type IIA, there is distal aortic involvement, and an aortobiiliac bifurcated endovascular graft extending to the *proximal* common iliac artery is used. In type IIB, there is common iliac artery involvement, and the bifurcated graft is extended to the *distal* common iliac artery bifurcation. In type IIC, there is extensive iliac artery involvement, and the endovascular graft configuration described in Figure 30–3 is used.

Table 30–4. Complications Associated with Endovascular Repair of Abdominal Aortic Aneurysms

Aneurysm growth
Embolization
Fabric tears
Graft infection
Graft migration
Hook fracture
Limb thrombosis
Limb separation
Endoleak*

*Common to all endovascular grafts used to date.

with it the persistent risk of aneurysm enlargement and rupture. The presence of an endoleak, therefore, negates the primary goal of the endovascular procedure and results in an aneurysm that remains inadequately treated.[11,24–30] Although other complications of endovascular AAA repair have been described (Table 30–4), considerable progress in patient selection and surgical technique has reduced the overall rate of these problems. Currently, the optimal method for postendovascular graft screening and the most reliable method for detecting complications are subject to debate. CT is favored in some centers, and color Doppler ultrasound in others.[31,32]

COLOR DOPPLER ULTRASOUND TECHNIQUE

Patient Preparation

As with all abdominal scanning, the quality of the examination may be degraded in the obese or gaseous patient, and preprocedural patient preparation may be necessary. The patient may be required to fast overnight or for at least 8 hr prior to the study to avoid the problems that can be introduced by intestinal gas. Usually, no other patient preparation is necessary.

Technologist Preparation

Prior to ultrasound evaluation, the technologist/sonographer performs a brief history for symptoms of claudication (hip, buttock,

or lower extremity) and impotence (as applicable) and a physical examination that includes palpation of the aortic and femoral pulses. An ankle-brachial index and/or pulse volume recording is obtained bilaterally and compared with the preoperative measurement, where available, to ensure that baseline blood flow to the extremities has been maintained.

To perform a thorough and optimal examination of the endovascular graft, the examiner must have considerable knowledge of the endovascular technique and of the various endovascular graft designs and configurations that are available and must also be familiar with the details of the surgical procedure.

To this end, a review of all previous imaging studies is mandatory. This includes any preoperative or postoperative CT scans, color Doppler scans or angiograms, as well as any intraoperative imaging studies that have been performed. This review is important because the examiner must be familiar with the configuration and specific anatomy of the endovascular graft,[17,33,34] including the level of the proximal and distal attachment sites. This information is used to document endovascular graft migration (if it occurs) and to identify all possible endoleak sources *in advance* of the color Doppler examination (Fig. 30–5). Additionally, review of the operative report or discussion with the operating surgeon is recommended to determine the following: (1) if there has been coil embolization of branch vessels or use of other vessel occlusion devices; (2) if supplemental proximal or distal arterial reconstructive procedures have been performed; and (3) if any other vessels have been treated with stents, either within the endovascular graft to support a portion to the graft or in the native artery to treat occlusive disease. Sonographic examination concerns not only the aortic/iliac stent graft but also all other related arterial occlusion/reconstruction procedures.

Ultrasound Equipment

The examination is performed using a high-resolution, *state-of-the-art* duplex scanner

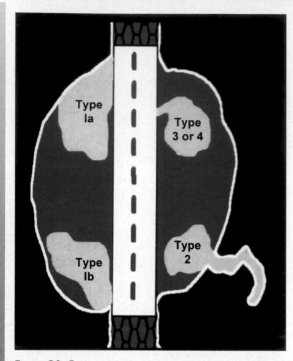

FIGURE 30–5. Potential endoleak sites. Types Ia and Ib: Leakage occurs at the proximal or distal stent attachment sites, as shown in yellow. Type 2: Backflow enters the aneurysm sac from a patent aortic branch or from back-bleeding through the iliac arteries. Type 3 or 4: Flow through the graft body itself.

that provides color flow capability. The equipment selected must allow enough penetration to permit adequate insonation of the deep structures in the abdomen and pelvis with color flow sensitivity that allows the detection of slow flow velocities seen in endoleak, all at reasonable frame rates. A low-frequency (2.5- to 4-MHz) sector or curved array transducer is necessary to visualize these deep structures. Often, however, a variety of differently configured (linear) and higher-frequency transducers are needed to accomplish a complete study.

In our department, all studies are videotaped for review by an interpreting physician, review by the sonographer/technologist prior to follow-up studies, and archiving purposes.

Technical Protocol[4,5]

Patients are generally scanned in the supine position using a midline approach; however, a left lateral decubitus position often facilitates visualization of the entirety of the aneurysm sac. Occasionally, a right lateral decubitus approach may be necessary.

Any examination that does not achieve visualization of the entire aneurysm sac is considered of limited diagnostic value, and the examination is repeated to correct the limitation or as deemed necessary by the interpreting physician.

Ultrasound assessment begins with identification of the intra-aneurysm sac portion of the endovascular graft in a transverse plane (Fig. 30–6). The endovascular graft is then followed proximally to the superior attachment site, where the endovascular graft–artery interface is seen. This site is typ-

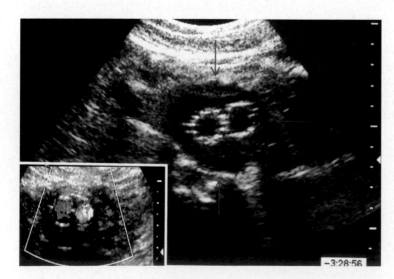

FIGURE 30–6. Transverse image of an abdominal aortic aneurysm treated with a bifurcated endovascular graft. The *red arrows* mark the outer dimensions of the aortic sac. A color flow image is seen in the lower left of the figure.

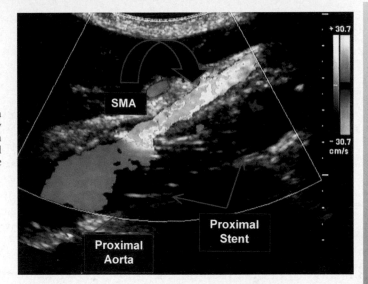

FIGURE 30-7. Long-axis image of the aorta at the level of the superior mesenteric artery (SMA) origin. The proximal stent has been deployed distal to the SMA origin. The renal arteries, crossed by the proximal stent, are not seen in this projection.

ically at, or immediately distal to, the level of the renal arteries, which are visible in the transverse plane. The renal arteries are important landmarks in the evaluation of an endovascular AAA repair.

When the superior end of the endovascular graft is identified, the transducer is turned longitudinally to view the long axis of the aorta. Alternatively, longitudinal assessment of the aorta is begun immediately inferior to the xiphoid process in the midline or slightly to the left.[35] After iden-

tification of the origins of the celiac or superior mesenteric arteries (Fig. 30–7), scanning distally permits visualization of the stent or fixation component of the endovascular graft, which may cross the orifices of both renal arteries or may be deployed immediately below the takeoff of the *lowest* renal artery (Fig. 30–8).

The endovascular graft should be closely apposed to the arterial wall at the proximal end of the prosthesis. The aortic diameter at this site (proximal neck of the aneurysm) is

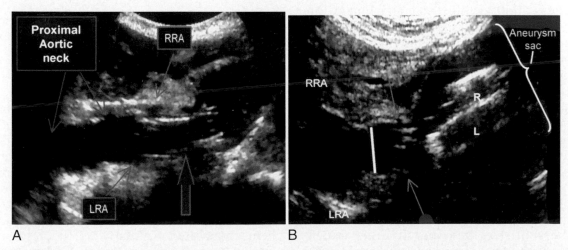

FIGURE 30-8. Proximal stent attachment. *A*, This long-axis image shows the neck of an abdominal aortic aneurysm. The uncovered part of the stent has been deployed across the right and left renal arteries (RRA, LRA) in this patient. The large *open arrow* identifies the proximal stent. *B*, This long-axis image of an endovascular graft was obtained at the level of the proximal fixation site. On the left side of the image is the aortic neck, the diameter of which is measured using electronic calipers (*solid white line*). The *red arrows* connote the stent. The right (R) and left (L) limbs of the endovascular graft are seen to the right of the image.

measured and compared on follow-up examinations to assess for dilation of the aneurysm neck, as this can result in endovascular graft migration and/or endoleak (see Fig. 30–8). Occasionally, the endovascular graft takes a sharp turn immediately distal to the proximal attachment site. This occurs because the endovascular graft follows the tortuous course of the aorta caused by the adjacent aneurysm.

After the proximal fixation site is identified and evaluated, the transducer is moved proximally, and the suprarenal aorta is visualized and examined for defects, such as dissection and intimal flaps, that may have resulted from the introduction and manipulation of devices used during endovascular graft deployment (e.g., catheters, guidewires, sheaths). Blood flow velocity is recorded immediately proximal to the endovascular graft device. The body of the endovascular graft is then scanned along its entire length in the color Doppler mode, and a search is made for flow abnormalities and associated intraluminal defects. The maximal and minimal graft diameters also are measured. Flow velocities and waveforms are recorded in the intra-aneurysm portion of the graft body, with particular attention given to any sites of kinking and/or twisting that may result in stenosis and decreased distal flow.

In straight or tube grafts (i.e., without iliac artery limbs), the distal attachment site, which corresponds to the distal neck of the aneurysm, is identified and the aortic diameter is measured at this point. Dilation can occur at this site, potentially resulting in endoleak or migration of the endovascular graft. For aortoiliac or aortofemoral endovascular grafts, the iliofemoral segment of the endovascular graft (and the femorofemoral crossover graft, when present) is next examined for any abnormalities. Flow velocity and waveforms are obtained at the distal endovascular graft termination and in the outflow vessel distal to the graft. For these and all other velocity measurements, typical procedures are followed: The Doppler angle is maintained at 60 degrees (preferably, or less if necessary), and the angle cursor is aligned so that it is parallel to the vessel wall. The distal end of the endovascular graft is usually attached to the surrounding artery wall by the supporting stent of the endovascular graft but otherwise may be sutured endoluminally in the setting of a nonsupported endovascular graft.[36]

To this point, the ultrasound examination has focused principally on the endovascular graft. The focus next is turned to the surrounding aneurysm (perigraft sac). Special attention is directed to the detection of any flow outside the endovascular graft (endoleak), to measuring the size of the surrounding aneurysm, and to assessing for the presence and evolution of clot formation within the aneurysm sac. A moderately rapid longitudinal sweep (color flow cineangio) of the endovascular graft and adjacent inflow and outflow vessels is then performed and recorded for review by the interpreting physician.

Finally, a worksheet is completed, and a diagram detailing the anatomy of the endovascular graft, adjacent vessels, flow velocities, waveforms, and the site(s) of any abnormalities that are detected is created as a reference for follow-up studies. Ideally, the same examiner performs the follow-up studies; however, a well-documented study can avoid the problems of interexaminer or intraexaminer variability that may be encountered on serial study evaluations.

ENDOLEAK DETECTION

Computed tomography is considered by many to be the gold standard for the detection of endoleak following endovascular AAA repair. In skilled hands, however, color Doppler ultrasound is an accurate, cost-effective, noninvasive method to evaluate and follow endovascular grafts that can serve as a valuable adjunct (and in some instances be superior) to CT. Because of its obvious advantages, color Doppler is now being advocated by many as the test of choice to *screen* for endoleak and follow aneurysm size serially.

Computed tomography is fundamentally a static imaging system that requires some precision in the timing of contrast injection to obtain optimal diagnostic results. Several studies have demonstrated the superiority of color Doppler ultrasound over CT for identifying small, low-flow, type 2, side branch leaks and for documenting the source and outflow of an endoleak.[3,6,8,9,10] These studies conclude that side branch endoleak is more readily detected with color Doppler because it is a real-time imaging modality; that is, there is no dilution of contrast material and no need to obtain delayed images. However, special care must be taken to adjust the pulse repetition frequency (PRF)/velocity range and color flow gain of the ultrasound equipment to allow for detection of the very-low-flow rates that exist in the aneurysm sac in association with type 2 endoleak.

Both CT and color Doppler confirm the diagnosis of endoleak by identifying the presence of contrast or color flow outside of the endovascular graft but inside the aneurysm sac (Fig. 30–9). Side branch endoleaks fill the aneurysm sac in a retrograde manner (via patent collaterals) and may fill the aneurysm sac slowly, which is a problem for CT, since the time delay after contrast injection may be insufficient to detect these leaks. This is not a problem for color Doppler imaging, which visualizes the leak directly, without the need for a contrast agent. The use of color flow Doppler imaging is essential for confirming or excluding the presence of endoleak. When an aneurysm is successfully treated, the blood within its sac tends to clot. These areas of thrombus are generally easy to visualize on the B-mode image. The examiner, however, must be suspicious for the presence of endoleak when echolucent areas are present within the aneurysm sac (Fig. 30–10). Such lucent areas must be interrogated thoroughly, as they may represent fluid blood within the sac that communicates with the arterial circulation (endoleak). In the early postoperative period, the movement of nonclotted blood within the aneurysm sac, caused by the pulsatile wall motion of the adjacent endovascular graft, may create color artifacts that mimic a true endoleak. We refer to this phenomenon as a pseudoleak (Fig. 30–11). Therefore, one must avoid the temptation to report an

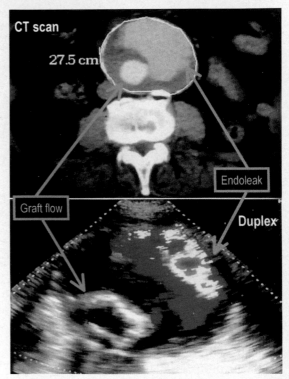

FIGURE 30–9. The upper panel is a computed tomographic (CT) scan with contrast that shows a large type Ia endoleak that arises from the proximal attachment site. Contrast is seen both in the endovascular graft (graft flow) and within the aneurysm sac. The *lower panel* is a duplex scan image of the same patient. The indwelling endovascular graft is seen in the lower left of the aneurysm sac (graft flow). Color is seen within both the endovascular graft and the aneurysm sac. Note how closely the duplex image resembles the CT scan.

endoleak based solely on the presence of color flow within the aneurysm sac. True endoleaks typically produce a uniform color Doppler appearance and are most times reproducible. In order to reduce false-positive findings, the technologist must take special care to correctly adjust the pulse repetition frequency and color flow gain settings throughout the course of the ultrasound examination. The use of spectral Doppler also can be helpful in this situation. Endoleak should yield Doppler waveforms that are reproducible, similar to the flow patterns seen within the peripheral circulation and synchronous with the patient's cardiac cycle. Spectral Doppler may also play a role in predicting endoleak thrombosis or persistence. A study by Carter and associates[37] revealed that endoleak with

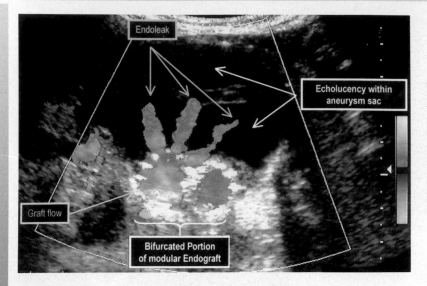

FIGURE 30–10. Type III endoleak. The flow in the aneurysm sac results from a defect at the junction of two limbs of a modular endovascular graft. Although thrombus has started to form, there are significant areas of echolucency within the aneurysm sac suggesting the presence of endoleak and confirmed by the color flow image.

very attenuated, monophasic, or bidirectional (to and fro) Doppler waveforms in the source vessel tended to occlude spontaneously, whereas the presence of normal, biphasic peripheral flow waveforms in the source vessel portended endoleak persistence. However, the number of patients in this study was small, and these preliminary results have not yet correlated with our experience.

As noted previously, a thorough examination to determine the presence of endoleak includes not only visualization of the endovascular graft attachment sites and the graft body but also visualization and interrogation of the *entire* AAA sac, in both the long and short axes. Thorough assessment also requires color Doppler interrogation of all potential leak sites suggested by the preoperative, intraoperative, and postoperative imaging studies. It is critical, therefore, that the vascular technologist be cognizant of the results of any preoperative imaging studies, the sites for potential endoleak, and

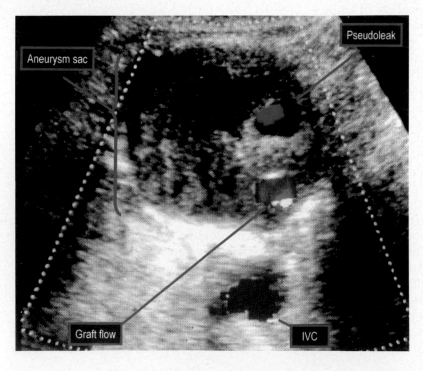

FIGURE 30–11. Cross-sectional color Doppler image of a pseudoleak. An area of color is seen within the aneurysm sac that results from movement of residual fluid blood in response to pulsations of the nearby endovascular graft. Thrombus has filled the remainder of the sac. No endoleak source was identified, and the Doppler signal at the area of color was atypical and not consistently reproducible. This patient had a computed tomographic scan that was endoleak negative.

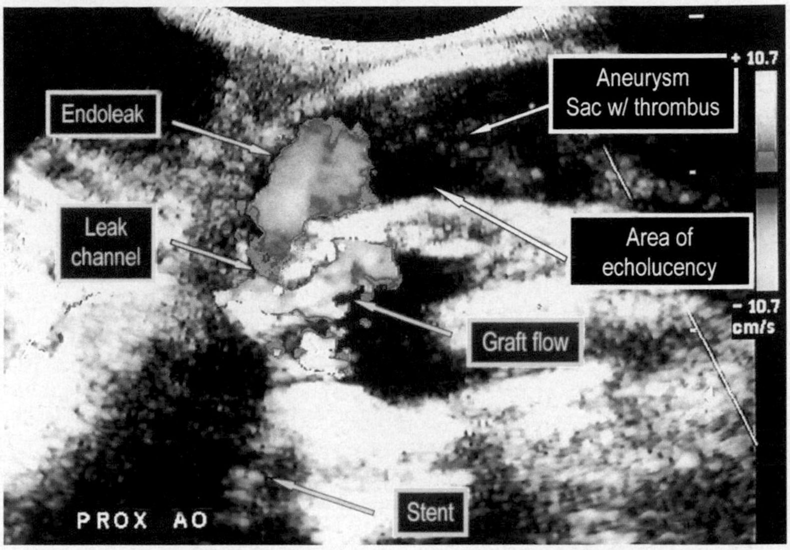

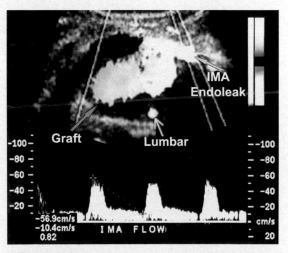

FIGURE 30–12. Type Ia endoleak. (Long-axis image at the level of the proximal aortic attachment site [PROX AO]). Flow is entering the aneurysm sac through a channel at the proximal attachment site. Note the area of echolucency near the endoleak flow.

the details of the surgical procedure, including any problems that occurred intraoperatively, preoperatively, or during intraoperative supplemental procedures.

In our opinion, definitive identification of a flow source is the most important feature in the confirmation of true endoleak. It is important to examine the entire intra-aneurysm sac portion of the endovascular graft body, identify patent side branches, and document the direction of flow within the side branches in an attempt to identify the source of endoleak flow. Endoleak flow can originate from proximal or distal endovascular graft attachment sites (type 1), through the endovascular graft itself (types 3 or 4), or from patent aortic branches (side branch or type 2 endoleak). Potential endoleak source branches include the lumbar arteries, the inferior mesenteric artery, the hypogastric arteries, and accessory renal arteries that communicate with the aneurysm.[24] The inferior mesenteric artery (IMA) is typically found sonographically anterior and to the left of the aneurysm sac. The lumbar arteries are located posterior to the aneurysm sac, and accessory renal arteries may be seen at any location (Figs. 30–12 to 30–15). In the absence of detectable flow within the sac, flow seen in the IMA or lumbar arteries adjacent to the aneurysm sac is diagnostic of endoleak, as these vessels should occlude after deployment of the endovascular graft.

If these vessels are patent, the flow direction must be assessed to determine whether the vessels are afferent or efferent channels relative to the aneurysm sac (Fig. 30–16).

ANEURYSM SIZE

After endovascular AAA repair, aneurysms that have been totally excluded from the circulation usually decrease in size or

FIGURE 30–13. Type 2 endoleak. In this patient with a bifurcated endovascular graft, the inferior mesenteric artery (IMA) is seen in the upper right of the ultrasound image and is the channel for outflow. A lumbar artery posteriorly is the afferent tract. The sample volume placed within the lumen of the IMA yields a negative Doppler shift, confirming that the IMA is the outflow tract.

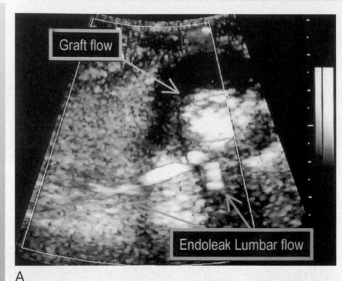

A

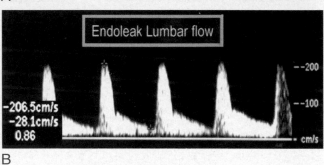

B

FIGURE 30–14. Combination endoleak. *A*, This patient has inflow from a proximal attachment site defect (type Ia), not seen in this image, and outflow via multiple patent lumbar arteries (type 2). *B*, Because of direct aortic inflow, velocity in the lumbar artery is in excess of 200 cm/sec.

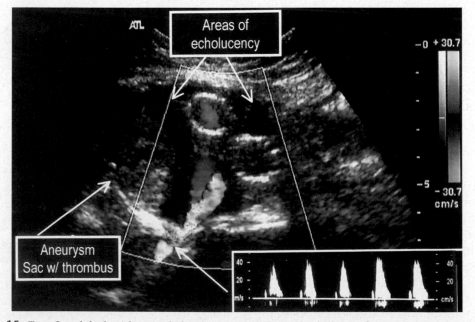

FIGURE 30–15. Type 2 endoleak with a single lumbar artery acting as both the outflow and inflow tracts. The corresponding spectral waveform is on the bottom right of the image. The spectral waveform captured in the lumbar artery in systole yields a positive Doppler shift; the color flow image of the sac shows evidence of flow in both directions simultaneously.

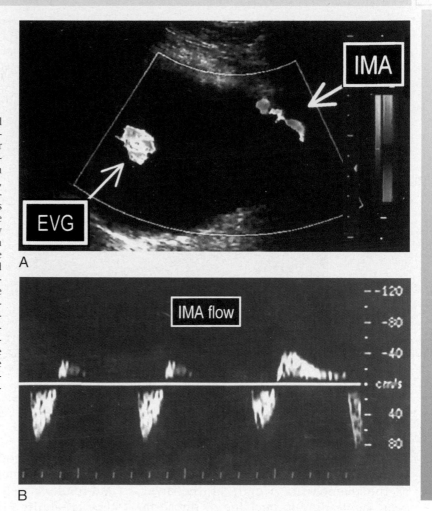

FIGURE 30–16. A cross-sectional image of an abdominal aortic aneurysm after endovascular graft repair with a type 2 endoleak. *A,* Blood flow is seen within the endovascular graft (EVG), as well as in the inferior mesenteric artery (IMA), which is clearly patent and perfusing the aneurysm sac (although flow within the sac is not shown in this image). In this case, the IMA acts as both inflow and outflow channel. *B,* This phenomenon is reflected in the spectral waveform, showing to-and-fro flow similar to a pseudoaneurysm tract. The waveform is strikingly different (velocity and morphology) from the spectral waveform seen in Figure 30–15. The prognostic significance of a to-and-fro flow pattern is unknown.

remain stable (Fig. 30–17). Conversely, AAAs with a documented endoleak often increase in size. Therefore, it is critical to measure AAA sac size in at least two locations along the length of the aneurysm. A transverse sweep of the aneurysm sac is performed to determine the site of its maximal diameter. With the scan plane aligned with the short axis of the vessel, the outer-to-outer diameter of the aneurysm sac is measured in the anteroposterior and transverse planes, and an image is obtained recording the measurements (Fig. 30–18). The image plane is then oriented with the long axis of the aneurysm, and the maximum anteroposterior dimension is again measured and recorded. Review of previous imaging studies (CT or ultrasound) is recommended to ensure that the location of the current measurements corresponds with those

obtained previously, although comparison of CT and ultrasound measurements is not recommended.[38] Any patient with a significant increase in aneurysm size (>0.5 cm) detected with ultrasound during the follow-up period should be suspected of having endoleak, even if no leak can be demonstrated, and further imaging with CT or contrast arteriography should be performed as indicated.

ENDOVASCULAR GRAFT DEFORMITY AND NATIVE ARTERY COMPLICATIONS

Kinking of the endovascular graft body within the aneurysm sac may occur in the late postoperative period, despite not having been present in the perioperative

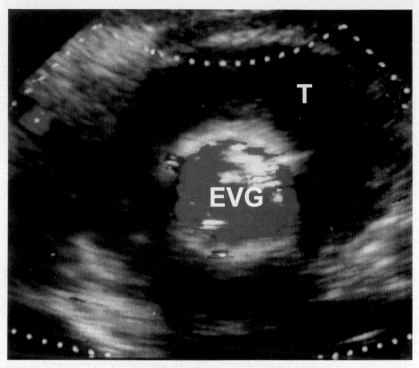

FIGURE 30–17. Uncomplicated endovascular graft. This cross-sectional color Doppler image shows complete exclusion after endovascular graft (EVG) repair. Color flow is seen only within the indwelling endovascular graft. The *T* seen above the endovascular graft connotes thrombus that has completely filled the residual aneurysm sac.

or early postoperative period. The cause of such kinking may be continued growth of the diameter or length of the aneurysm sac, leading to buckling of the aorta. Morphologic alterations of this sort can lead to significant conformational changes of the sac and indwelling endovascular graft and subsequent disassociation or kinking of the endovascular graft limb(s). Possible consequences include lower extremity ischemia due to kinking and decreased flow or endoleak due to disassociation of the endovascular graft limbs. When the aorta is effectively excluded and shrinks in diameter or length, the endovascular graft is subjected to stress, especially at limb junctions and at the proximal and/or distal attachment sites. The consequence, once again, may be endoleak.

Endovascular graft deformation, in the form of extrinsic graft compression, twisting (torsion), or kinking can lead to stenosis or thrombosis of the distal endovascular graft limb(s), potentially causing lower extremity ischemia. The superiority of ultrasound for demonstrating these problems has been documented in several studies[2,39] and results largely from the dynamic, real-time capabilities of ultrasound, as opposed to arteriography or CT.

Extrinsic endovascular graft compression is sometimes caused by atherosclerotic plaque in the wall of the artery that surrounds the endovascular graft, but is usually due to tortuosity of the endovascular graft. Because these stenotic lesions have been excluded from the arterial circulation, they are residual and may not progress. They are followed, however, per our endovascular graft surveillance protocol in the setting of aortoiliac arterial occlusive disease.[2] Hemodynamically significant atherosclerotic plaques cause focal increases in flow velocity along the iliofemoral limb of the endovascular graft. When deemed to be flow limiting on the basis of spectral Doppler findings (see Chapter 18), they are treated with balloon angioplasty, with or without stenting. Kinks and twists are often due to severe vessel tortuosity or graft redundancy (excessive graft length) and

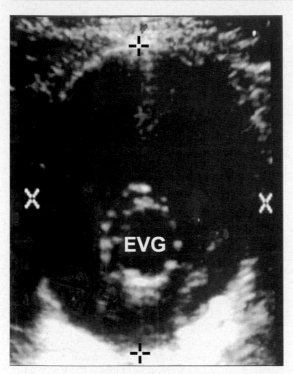

FIGURE 30–18. Aneurysm measurement. Transverse image of a large (7.16 cm anteroposterior × 7.47 cm transverse) abdominal aortic aneurysm with an indwelling endovascular graft (EVG). Note the cursors on the anteroposterior and lateral walls. Aortic aneurysm size should be measured at the level of maximal aneurysm size and/or at the proximal and mid aorta.

may cause hemodynamically significant flow reduction.

Another endovascular graft follow-up consideration is iatrogenic trauma to the distal vessels secondary to arterial manipulations performed through tortuous and diseased vessels and/or endovascular graft deployment itself. Such trauma may cause various complications, including dissection, intramural or extramural hematoma, pseudoaneurysm, arteriovenous fistula, and emboli to the lower extremities. The ultrasound findings associated with these complications are described in Chapter 20.

PERSONAL COMMENTARY

Although there continues to be controversy regarding the accuracy and utility of color Doppler sonography for aortic endovascular graft assessment,[31] we feel that color Doppler can effectively detect the presence of endoleak and monitor aneurysm size, both essential components for follow-up after endovascular AAA repair. Color Doppler endovascular graft evaluation is a technically challenging endeavor that should be reserved for senior-level technologists. These individuals must be facile with ultrasound technique, have accrued the considerable skill required to scan the deep structures of the abdomen, and have extensive knowledge of the endovascular exclusion of abdominal aortic aneurysms and associated complications. In addition, there must be a commitment to endovascular graft evaluation on the part of the technologist, the interpreting physician, and the institution. The major weaknesses of the majority of the negative literature reports concerning color Doppler endovascular graft assessment can be traced to a lack of commitment to the education of the technologist, a lack of appropriate time allocation for performing the examinations, and opposition to investment of funds for the high-end, state-of-the-art equipment necessary to adequately image aortic endovascular grafts. Those facilities that have made these commitments have had excellent results using color Doppler in this setting.

Another important factor standing in the way of the color Doppler ultrasound technique is a lack of standardization of the endovascular graft examination protocol, such as we see in other areas of vascular ultrasound (e.g., lower extremity venous and cerebrovascular testing), where color Doppler is proven to be extremely accurate and has been widely accepted as the diagnostic "gold standard." With the increasing prevalence of the endovascular technique, and the continued sharing of common experiences among vascular laboratories around the country, we feel that this weakness can be overcome. In addition, the Society for Vascular Ultrasound has recently published examination guidelines that should further decrease the variability seen in the performance of this examination.[40]

Finally, the addition of ultrasound contrast agents to the color Doppler examination has been shown to increase the sensitivity of ultrasound to the detection of endoleak.[3,41] Although not currently approved for widespread use in the United States, the use of this adjunctive method and advances in ultrasound technology, such as tissue harmonic imaging, promise to add to the utility of color Doppler ultrasound for the detection of endoleak.

CONCLUSIONS

This chapter characterizes the complications associated with endovascular AAA repair and demonstrates the effectiveness of color Doppler sonography for evaluation of these procedures. As with the entire field of endovascular surgery, imaging techniques and recommendations regarding endovascular graft use are evolving rapidly. Although contrast arteriography and spiral CT are important methods for endovascular graft evaluation, we feel that a combination of examinations is superior to any single test. In centers of excellence, color Doppler is an important noninvasive adjunctive study and may decrease the required frequency for more expensive studies, such as CT, thus allowing color Doppler to be the principal screening modality in the postoperative period for endoleak detection and surveillance after endovascular exclusion of abdominal aortic aneurysms. Finally, because of its noninvasive nature, patient compliance and satisfaction may also be improved by the use of ultrasound.

Acknowledgments. The authors wish to acknowledge Reese A. Wain, MD; William D. Suggs, MD; Takao Ohki, MD; N. Gargiulo, MD; Joshua Cruz, RVT; and Frank J. Veith, MD, for their contributions to this manuscript.

References

1. Berdejo GL, Del Valle WN, Lyon RT, Veith FJ: Value of color Doppler ultrasonography in the planning and assessment of endovascular stented grafts for traumatic arterial injuries [abstract]. J Vasc Tech 20:178, 1996.
2. Berdejo GL, Lyon RT, Del Valle WN, et al: Color Doppler ultrasonography for the evaluation of endovascular PTFE stented grafts for occlusive disease. J Vasc Tech 21:11–15, 1997.
3. Heilberger P, Schunn C, Ritter W, et al: Postoperative color flow duplex scanning in aortic endografting. J Endovascular Surg 4:262–271, 1997.
4. Johnson BL, Harris EJ Jr, Fogarty TJ, et al: Color duplex evaluation of endoluminal aortic stent grafts. J Vasc Tech 22:97–104, 1998.
5. Berdejo GL, Lyon RT, Ohki T, et al: Color duplex ultrasound evaluation of transluminally placed endovascular grafts for aneurysm repair. J Vasc Technol 22:201–207, 1998.
6. Sato DT, Goff CD, Gregory RT, et al: Endoleak after aortic stent graft repair: Diagnosis by color duplex ultrasound vs. CT scan. J Vasc Surg 28:657–663, 1998.
7. Lyon RT, Berdejo GL, Veith FJ: Ultrasound imaging techniques for evaluation of endovascular stented grafts. In Parodi JC, Veith FJ, Marin ML (eds): Endovascular Grafting Techniques. Media, PA, Williams & Wilkins, 1999.
8. Wolf YG, Johnson BL, Hill BB, et al: Duplex ultrasonography vs. CT angiography for postoperative evaluation of endovascular abdominal aortic aneurysms repair. J Vasc Surg 32:1142–1148, 2000.
9. Zanetti S, DeRango P, et al: Role of duplex scan in endoleak detection after endoluminal aortic repair. Eur J Vasc Endovasc Surg 19:531–535, 2000.
10. Parent FN, Meier GH, Parker FM, et al: The incidence and natural history of type I and II endoleak: A 5-year follow-up assessment with color duplex ultrasound scan. J Vasc Surg 35:474–481, 2002.
11. Matsumura JS, Moore WS: Clinical consequences of periprosthetic leak after endovascular repair of abdominal aortic aneurysm. J Vasc Surg 27:606–613, 1998.
12. Matsumura JS, Pearce WH, McCarthy WJ, Yao GS: Reduction in aortic aneurysm size: Early results after endovascular graft placement. J Vasc Surg 25:113–123, 1997.
13. Gilling-Smith G, Brennan J, Harris P, et al: Endotension after endovascular aneurysm repair: Definition, classification and strategies for surveillance and intervention (review). J Endovasc Surg 6:305–307, 1999.
14. White GH, May J: How should endotension be defined? History of a concept and evolution of a new term. J Endovasc Ther 7:435–438; discussion 439–440, 2000.
15. Gilling-Smith G, Martin J, Sudhindran S, et al: Freedom from endoleak after endovascular aneurysm repair dos not equal treatment success. Eur J Vasc Endovasc Surg 19:421–425, 2000.
16. Parodi JC, Palmaz JC, Barone HD: Transfemoral intraluminal graft implantation for abdominal

aortic aneurysms. Ann Vasc Surg 5:491–499, 1991.

17. Veith FJ, Abbott WM, Yao JST, et al: Guidelines for development and use of transluminally placed endovascular prosthetic grafts in the arterial system. J Vasc Surg 21:670–685, 1995.

18. Marin ML, Veith FJ, et al: Transfemoral endovascular stented graft treatment of aorto-iliac and femoropopliteal occlusive disease for limb salvage. Am J Surg 168:156–162, 1994.

19. Panetta TF, Marin ML, Veith FJ: Endovascular stent grafts in the management of vascular trauma. In Veith FJ (ed): Current Critical Problems in Vascular Surgery, Vol 6. St Louis, MO, Quality Medical Publishing, Inc., 1994.

20. Lipsitz EC, Ohki T, Veith FJ: Overview of techniques and devices for endovascular abdominal aortic aneurysm repair [review]. Semin Interv Cardiol 5:21–28, 2000.

21. Zarins CK, White RA, Moll FL, et al: The AneuRx stent graft: Four year results and worldwide experience 2000 [review]. J Vasc Surg 33(2 Suppl):S135–S145, 2001.

22. Moore WS, Rutherford RB: Transfemoral endovascular repair of abdominal aortic aneurysms: Results of the North American EVT Phase 1 Trial. J Vasc Surg 23:543–553, 1996.

23. Greenberg R; Zenith Investigators: The Zenith AAA endovascular graft for abdominal aortic aneurysms: Clinical update. Semin Vasc Surg 16:151–7, 2003.

24. Wain RA, Marin ML, Ohki T, et al: Endoleaks after endovascular graft treatment of aortic aneurysms: Classification, risk factors and outcome. J Vasc Surg 27:69–80, 1998.

25. White GH, Yu W, May J: Endoleak—a proposed new terminology to describe incomplete aneurysm exclusion by an endoluminal graft. J Endovasc Surg 3:124–125, 1996.

26. Zarins CK, White RA, Fogarty TJ: Aneurysm rupture after endovascular repair using AneuRx stent graft. J Vasc Surg 31:960–970, 2000.

27. Chuter TA, Risberg B, Hopkinson BR, et al: Clinical experience with a bifurcated endovascular graft for abdominal aortic aneurysm repair. J Vasc Surg 24:655–666, 1996.

28. White GH, Yu W, May J: Endoleak following endoluminal repair of AAA: Diagnosis, significance and management [abstract]. J Endovasc Surg 3:339–340, 1996.

29. Zarins CK, White RA, Fogarty TJ: Aneurysm rupture after endovascular repair using the AneuRx stent graft. J Vasc Surg 31:960–970, 2000.

30. Lumsden AB, Allen RC, Chaikoff EL: Delayed rupture of aortic aneurysms following endovascular stent grafting. Am J Surg 170:174–178, 1995.

31. Raman KG, Missig-Carroll N, Richardson T, et al: Color flow duplex ultrasound scan versus computed tomographic scan in the surveillance of endovascular aneurysm repair. J Vasc Surg 38:645–651, 2003.

32. McLafferty RB, McCrary BS, Mattos MA, et al: The use of color flow duplex scan for the detection of endoleaks. J Vasc Surg 36:100–104, 2002.

33. Chuter T, DeWeese JA: Treatment of abdominal aortic aneurysm by endovascular grafting. In Ernst CB, Stanley JC (eds): Current Therapy in Vascular Surgery, 3rd ed. St. Louis, MO, Mosby, pp 265–270.

34. May J, White GH, Harris JP: Devices for aortic aneurysm repair. Surg Clin North Am 79:507–527, 1999.

35. Cramer MM: Color flow duplex examination of the abdominal aorta: Atherosclerosis, aneurysm and dissection. J Vasc Tech 19:249–260, 1995.

36. Wain RA, Lyon RT, Veith FJ, et al: Alternative techniques for management of distal anastomoses of aortofemoral and iliofemoral endovascular grafts. J Vasc Surg 32:307–314, 2000.

37. Carter KA, Nelms CR, Bloch PHS, et al: Doppler waveform assessment of endoleak following repair of abdominal aortic aneurysm: Predictors of endoleak thrombosis. J Vasc Tech 24:119–122, 2000.

38. Sprouse RL, Meier GH, LeSar CJ, et al: Comparison of abdominal aortic aneurysm diameter measurements obtained with ultrasound and computed tomography: Is there a difference? J Vasc Surg 38:466–472, 2003.

39. Lyon RT, Veith FJ, Berdejo GL, et al: Utility of operative intravascular ultrasound for the assessment of endovascular procedures. Proceedings of the Joint Annual Meeting of the Society for Vascular Surgery/North American Chapter, International Society for Cardiovascular Surgery, Boston, June 1–4, 1997.

40. Examination performance guidelines. "Members Only" section of the Society for Vascular Ultrasound website, www.svunet.org.

41. Bendick PJ, Zelenock GB, Bove PG, et al: Duplex ultrasound imaging with an ultrasound contrast agent: The economic alternative to CT angiography for aortic stent graft surveillance. Vasc Endovascular Surg 37:165–170, 2003.

Ultrasound Assessment of the Splanchnic (Mesenteric) Arteries

John S. Pellerito, MD

Color and pulsed Doppler evaluation of the splanchnic arteries is performed to evaluate for insufficiency of intestinal blood flow in patients presenting with abdominal pain. This examination is frequently requested for patients whose abdominal pain is unexplained or atypical. The concern is that decreased blood flow to the bowel could be the cause of the patient's symptoms. This examination includes the evaluation of the abdominal aorta, celiac, superior mesenteric (SMA), and inferior mesenteric (IMA) arteries. Like the examination of the renal arteries, these studies are technically challenging and rely on operator experience and expertise. In this chapter, we will review all the technical tips, tricks, and insights that allow for the successful evaluation of the splanchnic arteries.

ANATOMY AND PHYSIOLOGY

The splanchnic, or mesenteric, arteries comprise the celiac, superior mesenteric, and inferior mesenteric arteries (Fig. 31–1). All three vessels arise from the abdominal aorta. The celiac artery is the first major branch of the abdominal aorta. The SMA is located just inferiorly to the celiac artery. On occasion, the celiac and SMA may share a common origin or trunk. The renal arteries are the next major branches of the abdominal aorta and arise laterally, toward the kidneys. The IMA is identified just below the renal arteries and originates at the left anterolateral aspect of the abdominal aorta. The IMA can be identified in the majority of patients studied for mesenteric insufficiency.

The celiac and superior mesenteric arteries supply blood to the duodenum and small bowel. The superior mesenteric and inferior mesenteric arteries supply the colon and proximal rectum. A rich collateral network exists between the different mesenteric vessels. The major collateral circuits include the pancreaticoduodenal arcade, the arc of Riolan, and the marginal artery of Drummond. The pancreaticoduodenal arcade permits collateral flow between the celiac and SMA, whereas the arc of Riolan and marginal artery of Drummond link the SMA and IMA.

Mesenteric ischemia is related to acute or chronic compromise of the blood supply to the small and large intestines. Acute mesenteric ischemia, or thrombosis, can be a life-threatening condition, which requires immediate diagnosis and intervention. This is considered a surgical emergency, and an arteriogram or a computed tomographic or magnetic resonance angiogram is performed for diagnosis. The cause of thrombosis is usually embolic occlusion of one or more mesenteric arteries. Patients typically present with an acute syndrome of sudden onset of abdominal pain with abdominal distention, fever, dehydration, and acidosis. These patients do not typically present to the vascular laboratory or ultrasound suite for evaluation due to the severity of their symptoms and the urgency of the condition.

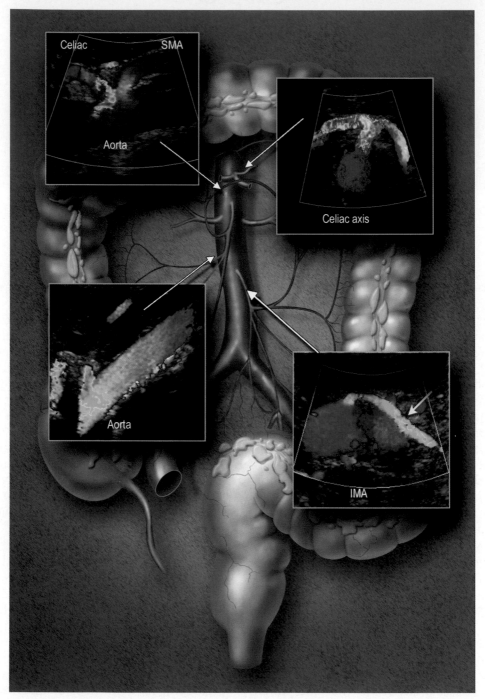

FIGURE 31–1. Montage with normal color flow images of the aorta, celiac axis, superior mesenteric artery (SMA), and inferior mesenteric artery (IMA).

Patients with suspected *chronic* mesenteric ischemia classically present with abdominal pain apparently related to recent ingestion of a meal. Patients typically complain of postprandial pain, bloating, weight loss, and diarrhea. They may describe a "fear of food," as they experience pain after meals. They may change their diet or eating habits to more frequent, smaller meals to avoid discomfort. In some cases, this change of eating habits is not recognized by the patient, who notes only weight loss. Other patients have a confusing clinical picture with vague symptoms of pain that may or may not be related to meals. Chronic mesenteric ischemia should be considered in elderly patients with unexplained abdominal pain and weight loss. Evaluation of the mesenteric arteries is helpful to work through the differential diagnosis in this group of patients with an unclear etiology for their clinical symptoms.

Collateral flow through the gastroduodenal artery, the marginal arteries, and the arc of Riolan usually allows adequate mesenteric circulation in the presence of atherosclerotic disease of the splanchnic arteries. In general, severe compromise (>70% stenosis or occlusion) of at least two of the three mesenteric arteries is required for symptoms of mesenteric ischemia to be present. Mesenteric stenosis or occlusion of a single vessel does not usually produce symptoms in light of a patent collateral network. The "two-vessel rule" holds in most patients and is utilized clinically for the diagnosis of chronic mesenteric ischemia.[1]

The celiac artery supplies blood to the low-resistance vascular beds of the liver, spleen, and stomach via the hepatic, splenic, and left gastric branches. Pulsed Doppler demonstrates low-resistance flow in the celiac artery, with high end-diastolic velocities (Fig. 31–2). This low-resistance flow pattern relates to the need for continuous forward flow in both systole and diastole to supply the high oxygen demands of the liver and spleen throughout the cardiac cycle. This flow pattern is similar to the low-resistance signals seen in the renal and internal carotid arteries. The celiac artery low-resistance flow pattern is not dependent on food intake. In other words, there is no significant change in peak systolic or end-diastolic velocities obtained from the celiac artery after a meal.

The superior and inferior mesenteric arteries supply the high-resistance vascular beds of the small intestine and colon. Pulsed Doppler examination reveals high impedance flow with low diastolic velocities in the fasting state (see Fig. 31–2). This is due to the relative vasoconstriction of the splanchnic branch vessels prior to a meal,

when the bowel is empty and quiescent. After a meal, there is an increase in mesenteric arterial blood flow to assist digestion. Vasodilation of the mesenteric branches allows increased blood flow to the intestines. Moneta and colleagues[2] showed that both peak systolic and end-diastolic velocities increase after a meal. The authors described at least doubling of the end-diastolic velocity in the SMA after eating. They found the greatest increase in flow after a meal that includes fat, carbohydrate, and protein, and they concluded that this provocative test provides a mechanism for evaluating the reactivity of the splanchnic circulation. The presence of increased flow velocities after a meal was used to infer the adequacy of the splanchnic blood supply in their studies.

Although duplex ultrasound examinations of the mesenteric arteries can be performed before and after a meal to identify physiologic changes in blood flow, there appears to be significant variability in the response to food. Healy and associates[3] found that postprandial duplex studies were not dependable and did not improve diagnostic accuracy in their series of patients. We no longer routinely perform pre- and postprandial duplex examinations of the mesenteric vessels because we found these examinations to be less reliable for the diagnosis of stenosis, as compared with other direct measurements.

TECHNIQUE

The duplex and color Doppler examination of the mesenteric arteries usually includes the evaluation of the proximal abdominal aorta as well as the ostia and proximal portions of the celiac, SMA, and IMA. The distal segments of the mesenteric arteries cannot be seen with ultrasound. Most atherosclerotic lesions typically occur at the ostia of these vessels, and this is the main focus of investigation.

In preparation for our abdominal Doppler studies, we ask our patients to fast for at least 12 hours. This reduces the amount of scatter and attenuation from intraabdominal bowel gas. Fasting also avoids

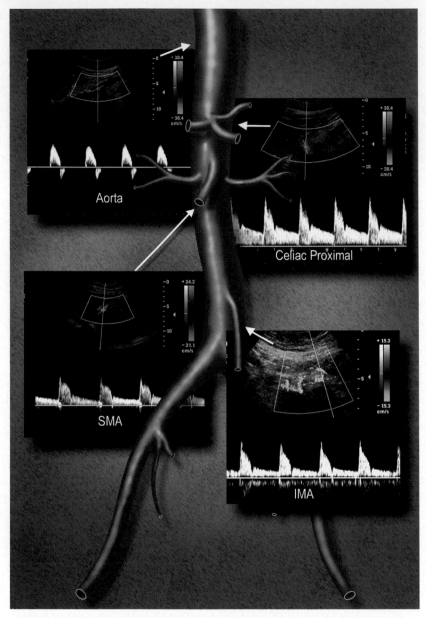

FIGURE 31-2. Montage of normal Doppler waveforms. IMA, inferior mesenteric artery; SMA, superior mesenteric artery.

the elevated velocities noted in the post-prandial state, which can be confused with stenotic flow. We give no medication prior to examination. With the patient in the supine position, we start by placing the transducer just below the xiphoid process to visualize the abdominal aorta and celiac artery. We can usually obtain all required data from an anterior approach with the patient supine. Occasionally, we will turn the patient to a decubitus or oblique posi-tion to view the aorta, celiac, and SMA through the liver. We ask the patient to either breath-hold or breathe quietly dur-ing the examination to obtain adequate Doppler spectral samples.

Mesenteric Doppler studies should be per-formed on modern ultrasound instruments with high-quality color and power Doppler imaging and with sensitive pulsed Doppler capability. Most studies are performed with low-frequency transducers in the 2- to 5-

MHz range. We also routinely employ harmonic imaging to improve resolution and decrease noise in the image. It has been noted in the literature that studies performed by experienced vascular technologists, sonographers, or sonologists provide the best results.[4] Indeed, we have noted that our finest abdominal vascular studies are performed by sonographers and physicians with at least 1 year of experience with abdominal Doppler examinations and a working knowledge of Doppler physics. The learning curve for these examinations depends on the technical ability, motivation, and patience of the examiner. It is clear that a steady volume of abdominal Doppler studies is required to gain proficiency with these examinations. It is also clear that experience with these studies allows the examiner to determine, in short order, whether a successful study will be obtained in any given patient. It should be obvious in most cases whether excessive bowel gas, shortness of breath, large body size, or severe atherosclerotic disease will preclude a complete study. This is usually determined within the first 10 minutes of examination.

The experienced examiner employs a number of technical shortcuts to improve visualization of the abdominal vessels and the detection of significant lesions. Optimization of gray-scale and color Doppler parameters assists in the visualization of vessel walls, the detection of atherosclerotic plaque, and assessment of the residual lumen. The color Doppler gain, pulse repetition frequency, and wall filter are adjusted such that laminar flow in the normal segment of the aorta and branch vessel has a homogeneous color flow pattern (Fig. 31–3). These adjustments should be tailored to each patient, as mesenteric arterial velocities vary widely. Proper adjustment of the color Doppler parameters aids in the observation of vessel patency and visualization of normal flow in the vessel. Equally important, correct instrument adjustment permits the examiner to screen the vessel quickly for flow abnormalities and to detect color aliasing and color bruit artifacts that occur with significant flow disturbance (Fig. 31–4). Demonstration of these color flow changes

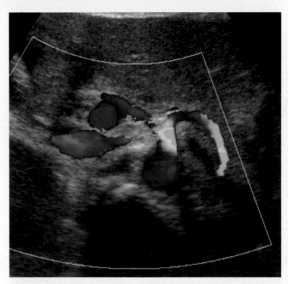

FIGURE 31–3. Color Doppler image of the celiac axis demonstrates normal homogeneous color flow pattern.

increases the sensitivity for stenosis and decreases the time of examination.

Pulsed Doppler waveforms are obtained with a small sample volume (1.5 to 3 mm) to ensure that velocity information is derived from the vessel of interest and not from adjacent structures. Angle correction is always performed for correct Doppler analysis. Most studies are performed at constant 60-degree angles to provide consistency in Doppler measurements. A 60-degree angle of insonation may be difficult to obtain in the celiac artery, since the artery projects toward the probe at a 0- to 30-degree angle. In many cases, a lower Doppler angle is used for celiac artery velocity measurement. This should be noted in the report or patient's chart so that the same angle can be used on follow-up evaluations. Most spectral samples are obtained from a sagittal projection of the aorta and mesenteric vessels.

EXAMINATION PROTOCOL

Our protocol includes the initial evaluation of the abdominal aorta with gray-scale and color Doppler to assess for the presence or absence of plaque, luminal narrowing, and aneurysm (Fig. 31–5). Pulsed Doppler samples are obtained from the abdominal

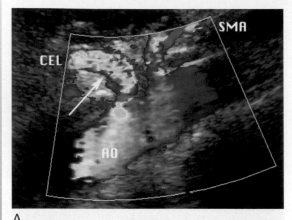

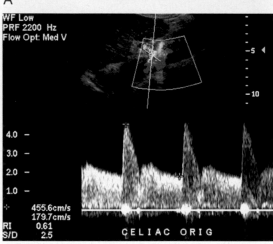

FIGURE 31–4. *A,* Color Doppler image demonstrates aliasing artifact (*arrow*) in the proximal celiac artery (CEL) consistent with stenosis. Note the normal color flow patterns in the aorta (AO) and superior mesenteric artery (SMA). *B,* Pulsed Doppler evaluation at the site of aliasing in the celiac artery demonstrates high-velocity (456 cm/sec) flow, confirming the presence of a high-grade stenosis.

DIAGNOSTIC CRITERIA

The range of normal blood flow velocity in the celiac artery is quite small: from 98 to 105 cm/sec.[5] Much wider normal ranges are reported in the SMA (97 to 142 cm/sec) and in the IMA (93 to 189 cm/sec).[5]

A review of the literature reveals that many different criteria have been proposed for the diagnosis of splanchnic artery stenosis and no consensus has been reached regarding the optimal Doppler criteria for the diagnosis of significant mesenteric artery stenosis. The most popular and widely accepted criteria are based on PSV measurements of the mesenteric arteries, as reported by Moneta and colleagues.[6] In a retrospective review of mesenteric duplex examinations and arteriograms in 34 patients, these authors showed that a PSV greater than or equal to 200 cm/sec in the

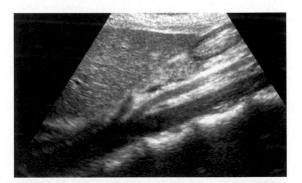

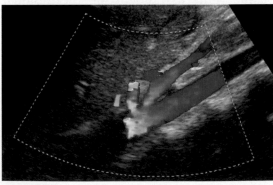

FIGURE 31–5. *A,* Sagittal gray-scale image of the abdominal aorta demonstrates normal-caliber vessels without significant atherosclerotic changes. *B,* Color Doppler evaluation of the abdominal aorta and branch vessels demonstrates normal laminar flow without color flow abnormalities.

aorta at the level of the mesenteric arteries. This measurement provides a baseline velocity for comparison with the mesenteric artery peak systolic velocities. Peak velocity measurements are also obtained from the origin and visualized segments of the celiac, SMA, and IMA. In practice, the sample volume is passed from the abdominal aorta into the ostium and proximal segment of each artery, in search of the highest peak systolic velocity (PSV) and signs of post-stenotic turbulence and bruit (Fig. 31–6). Remember, the highest velocity measurement will be obtained within the stenosis.

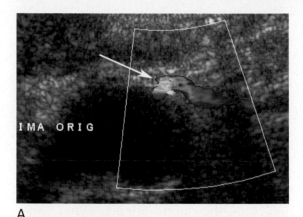

A

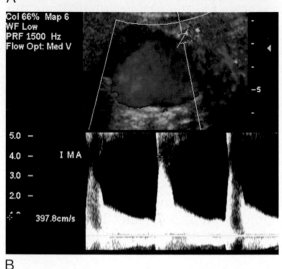

B

FIGURE 31–6. *A,* Color Doppler image demonstrates focal color aliasing (*arrow*) at the origin of the inferior mesenteric artery (IMA). *B,* Pulsed Doppler sampling of the origin of the IMA reveals markedly elevated peak systolic velocity (398 cm/sec) consistent with severe stenosis.

celiac artery and a PSV greater than or equal to 275 cm/sec in the SMA were predictive of stenosis of 70% or more. Sensitivity, specificity, and positive predictive values for the SMA were 89%, 92%, and 80%, respectively; and 75%, 89%, and 85% for the celiac artery. Similar values were not obtained for the IMA, which was not assessed in that study. Moneta and associates found that end-diastolic velocities and velocity ratios did not offer any advantage over arterial PSV measurements. A follow-up prospective study of 100 patients by Moneta and colleagues[7] supported the authors' initial results and suggested that duplex evaluation

may be clinically useful as a screening examination to detect celiac and SMA stenosis. In a study of 82 patients, Lim and associates[8] confirmed the value of the Moneta criteria for the detection of mesenteric stenosis with an overall sensitivity of 100% and specificity of 87% for the celiac artery and 98% specificity for the SMA.

Bowersox and coworkers[9] concluded that an end-diastolic velocity greater than 45 cm/sec was the best indicator of hemodynamically significant SMA stenosis (considered ≥ 50% diameter reduction). In this series, elevated PSV was less sensitive but more specific for severe SMA stenosis. Other investigators have also noted that the end-diastolic velocity was the more accurate parameter for the detection of significant mesenteric stenosis. Zwolak and colleagues[10] published a series of 243 mesenteric scans with 46 correlative angiograms. Perko and associates[11] studied 39 patients with duplex ultrasonography and arteriography. Both investigators concluded that the end-diastolic velocity was the superior threshold value for identification of SMA and celiac stenosis. They also considered a stenosis with diameter reduction greater than or equal to 50% as clinically significant.

It is interesting to note that the studies discussed previously did not include the inferior mesenteric artery in their investigations. This is pertinent in light of the fact that most clinicians follow the "two-vessel rule" in the diagnosis of chronic mesenteric ischemia. A complete study requires identification and Doppler analysis of all three mesenteric arteries. It is imperative to visualize the IMA to exclude mesenteric insufficiency when a significant stenosis or occlusion is identified in the celiac artery or SMA.

Recent studies have shown that the IMA is readily visible in most patients, and adequate Doppler waveforms can be obtained that allow calculation of the PSV, end-diastolic velocity, and resistive index. Mirk and coworkers[12] visualized the IMA in 88.8% of studies in 116 patients. Denys and associates[13] were successful in demonstrating the IMA in 92% of cases in their study of 100 consecutive fasting adults. PSV and resistive index measurements differed among the studies. The PSV of the IMA ranged from 93 to 189 cm/sec in normal patients. Erden and colleagues[14] showed that the PSV varies with the degree of collateral flow through the IMA when there is occlusive disease of the abdominal aorta and other mesenteric vessels. Increases in IMA PSV up to 190 cm/sec were seen in patients with occlusion of the celiac, SMA, and common iliac arteries.

We also utilize velocity ratios for the diagnosis of mesenteric artery stenosis, similar to the renal-aortic ratio (RAR) used to diagnose renal artery stenosis. The PSV at the site of the stenosis in the mesenteric artery is divided by the PSV in the abdominal aorta. The normal mesenteric-aortic ratio is usually slightly greater than 1.0. In general, the mesenteric-aortic ratio associated with hemodynamically significant stenosis is greater than 3.0. We find this ratio particularly useful in patients with abnormally high or low velocities in the aorta and branch vessels. Low-velocity flow is seen in patients with poor cardiac function and diffuse atherosclerotic disease. Significant stenosis may be present with lower velocities, sometimes less than 200 cm. A mesenteric-aortic ratio greater than 3.0 suggests severe stenosis even when PSVs in the stenosis are lower than anticipated. Conversely, elevated velocities may occur in patients without underlying stenosis. This is seen especially in young adults and children with high cardiac output or increased metabolic state. Although elevated velocities are detected in these patients, there is no focal elevation of velocity or significant increase in the mesenteric-aortic ratio to suspect significant disease. Validation of the mesenteric-aortic ratio is based on our experience and a recent retrospective review of more than 1000 abdominal Doppler studies performed at our institution.

Variability in PSV measurement is one reason why there is confusion and controversy regarding the evaluation of the mesenteric arteries. A review of recent papers shows a range of normal SMA PSV from 103 to 197 cm/sec. Rizzo and coworkers[15] showed that varying the angle of insonation from 0 to 80 degrees produces marked increases in SMA PSV in normal volunteers. They found that for the SMA, 70-degree and 80-degree angles produced 16% and 120% increases, respectively, in PSV. Because estimation of PSV is inversely proportional to the cosine of the angle of insonation, accurate measurement is dependent on precise Doppler angle correction. Errors in angle correction will result in changes in velocity calculation, particularly at higher angles. This phenomenon, they noted, also occurs in other arterial systems, including the carotid arteries. Other issues are related to the technical limitations and appropriate diagnostic criteria. These concerns have been fueled by conflicting reports in the literature, which either advocate or refute the ability of Doppler ultrasound to contribute to the evaluation of the abdominal arteries. Newer modalities, including computed tomographic angiography and magnetic resonance angiography, have demonstrated high accuracies in the noninvasive evaluation of the mesenteric arteries. For these reasons, it is important to review the techniques and features that improve the quality and diagnostic accuracy of mesenteric Doppler studies.

KEYS TO SUCCESSFUL EXAMINATION

The keys to a successful abdominal Doppler examination include adequate patient preparation, modern ultrasound equipment, examiner experience, proven diagnostic criteria, and correlation with confirmatory studies, when available. We schedule the majority of our patients for morning ultrasound evaluation, following an overnight fast. Abdominal Doppler studies are usually performed by our most experienced sonographers. They choose to perform these examinations on our best Doppler units. Our junior sonographers and trainees observe and perform these studies with supervision by the more experienced senior technologists.

My experience with Doppler studies, including mesenteric arterial examinations, has prompted me to develop a practical approach to the interpretation of abdomi-

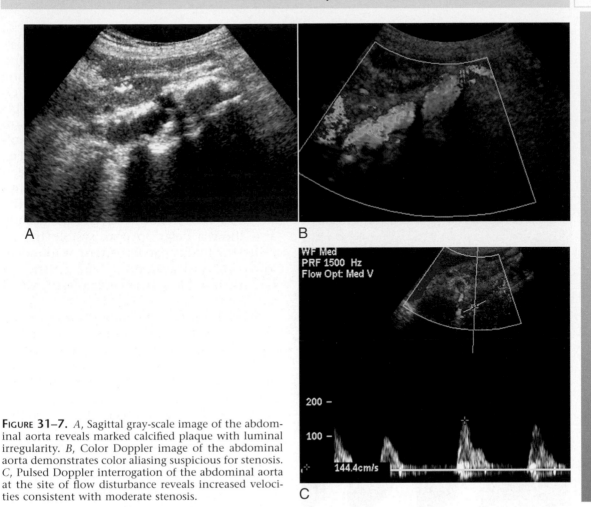

FIGURE 31–7. *A,* Sagittal gray-scale image of the abdominal aorta reveals marked calcified plaque with luminal irregularity. *B,* Color Doppler image of the abdominal aorta demonstrates color aliasing suspicious for stenosis. *C,* Pulsed Doppler interrogation of the abdominal aorta at the site of flow disturbance reveals increased velocities consistent with moderate stenosis.

nal Doppler. Similar to other Doppler examinations, significant arterial occlusive disease is usually associated with gray-scale, color, and pulsed Doppler abnormalities. Gray-scale evaluation should disclose atherosclerotic plaque or thrombus at the site of stenosis or occlusion (Fig. 31–7). The absence of plaque, wall thickening, or thrombus reduces the likelihood of a stenotic lesion in the visualized segment of the vessel.

Color Doppler is extremely useful in the diagnosis of stenosis and occlusion. Luminal narrowing, color flow aliasing, and the presence of collateral vessels are important color Doppler findings in arterial stenosis (Fig. 31–8). A search for these findings with color and power Doppler imaging facilitates the diagnosis of stenosis. The absence of color flow in the vessel leads to the diag-

nosis of arterial occlusion. This is confirmed by the absence of arterial signals during pulsed Doppler interrogation.

Reversal of flow and the presence of color bruit are additional signs of significant disease of the mesenteric circulation. Reversal of flow in the hepatic and gastroduodenal arteries is seen with celiac artery occlusion. Similarly, reversal of flow in the SMA is seen with occlusion at the origin of this vessel. The presence of a color bruit increases suspicion for significant stenosis (Fig. 31–9). Bruit artifacts are also associated with arteriovenous fistula and pseudoaneurysms. Color bruit artifacts are produced by low-level frequency shifts. These frequency shifts occur when high-velocity jets induce vibrations in the tissues surrounding the lesion or stenosis. Pulsed Doppler sampling at the site of the bruit usually

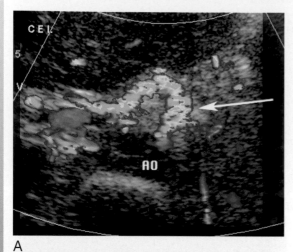

A

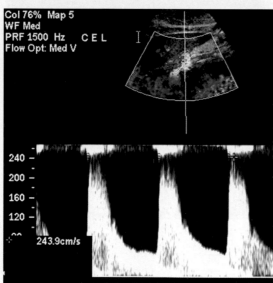

B

FIGURE 31–8. A, Color flow aliasing (*arrow*) allows rapid identification of stenosis in the proximal celiac artery. B, Pulsed Doppler evaluation of the proximal celiac (CEL) artery demonstrates increased velocities consistent with stenosis.

demonstrates elevated peak systolic velocities.

Pulsed Doppler is essential in the identification and characterization of stenosis and occlusion. Pulsed Doppler demonstrates elevated velocities and post-stenotic turbulence, diagnostic of a hemodynamically significant lesion (Fig. 31–10). In most patients, PSVs greater than 200 cm/sec are associated with stenosis. In addition to sampling the site of stenosis, it is important to sample the post-stenotic region. A post-

stenotic signal confirms the presence of a pressure-reducing lesion. In the post-stenotic zone, the systolic jet dissipates into eddy currents, with red blood cells moving in different directions at different velocities. This is termed *post-stenotic turbulence* and is recognized as a lower-velocity waveform with irregular borders, usually with a simultaneous bidirectional pattern (see Fig. 31–10). This "shaggy" waveform is seen within 1 to 2 cm distal to the stenosis and dissipates with increasing distance from the stenosis. Post-stenotic waveforms usually also show a delay to peak systole that is called the tardus-parvus pattern. A rounded, low-velocity waveform, characteristic of tardus-parvus flow, is a marker of a proximal stenosis or occlusion (Fig. 31–11).

In addition to the demonstration of elevated velocities and post-stenotic turbulence, we also utilize the mesenteric/aortic PSV ratio as a diagnostic criterion, as described previously. In most patients, abnormalities are seen with gray-scale, color, and pulsed Doppler when a significant mesenteric occlusive lesion is present. In other words, findings of plaque on gray-scale, narrowing and aliasing on color Doppler, and elevated velocities and ratios with post-stenotic turbulence are typical of a high-grade lesion. Further investigation is warranted when there is discordance between gray-scale, color, and pulsed

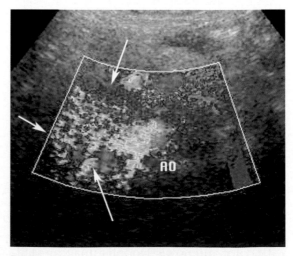

FIGURE 31–9. Marked color bruit artifact (*arrows*) is noted in the region of the celiac artery origin consistent with severe stenosis. AO, aorta.

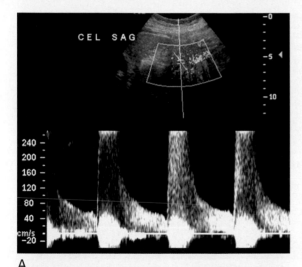

FIGURE 31–10. *A*, Spectral analysis of the region of flow disturbance in the celiac (CEL) artery demonstrates markedly elevated peak systolic velocities consistent with significant stenosis. SAG, sagittal. *B*, Pulsed Doppler sampling of the post-stenotic region reveals lower-velocity flow with irregular borders and a bidirectional flow pattern.

Doppler findings. We recommend other noninvasive tests, including computed tomographic or magnetic resonance angiography for the difficult cases in which the study is indeterminate and intervention is not immediately indicated.

Several pitfalls should be considered in the evaluation of the mesenteric arteries. Doppler insonation of the mesenteric vessels, especially the celiac artery, can be challenging due to vessel tortuosity. It may not be possible to maintain a constant angle of insonation in these vessels. Increasing Doppler angles can produce spuriously increased velocity measurements. It should also be remembered that there is a wide range of normal velocities in the splanchnic vessels.

As noted previously, low mesenteric arterial velocities may be seen in elderly patients and patients with poor cardiac output, even with significant mesenteric disease. Conversely, elevated velocities are commonly seen in younger patients in the absence of significant mesenteric stenosis. Velocity ratios tend to work better than PSV criteria in these patients who have baseline velocities outside the normal range. Elevated velocities may also be noted in vessels serving as major collateral channels.

An interesting phenomenon is the median arcuate ligament syndrome. This is a potential pitfall for celiac artery stenosis, as increased velocities are noted in the celiac artery during expiration (Fig. 31–12). The median arcuate ligament is a leaflet of the diaphragm, which crosses and compresses the superior aspect of the celiac artery in expiration. Increased velocities are noted in the celiac artery during compression by the median arcuate ligament. There is an immediate decrease in PSV with deep inspiration,

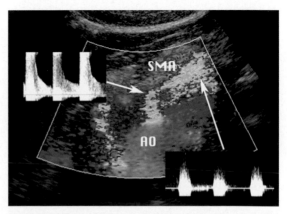

FIGURE 31–11. This montage of waveforms shows high-velocity continuous flow at the site of superior mesenteric artery (SMA) stenosis (*short arrow*) and low-velocity, rounded (tardus parvus) waveforms (*long arrow*) in the post-stenotic zone. Note the abnormal turbulent color flow pattern in the SMA. AO, aorta.

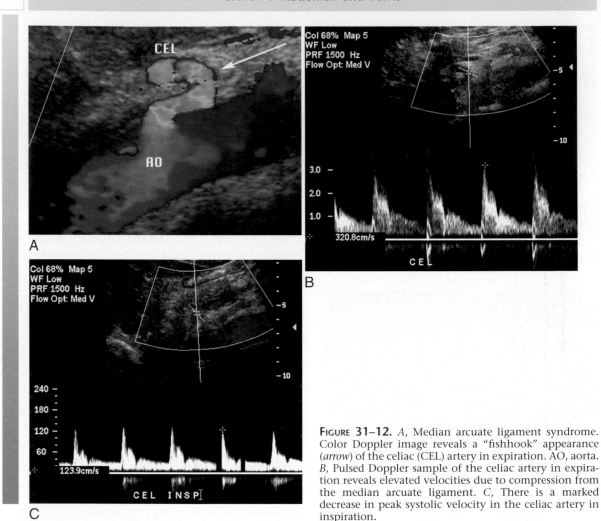

FIGURE 31–12. *A,* Median arcuate ligament syndrome. Color Doppler image reveals a "fishhook" appearance (*arrow*) of the celiac (CEL) artery in expiration. AO, aorta. *B,* Pulsed Doppler sample of the celiac artery in expiration reveals elevated velocities due to compression from the median arcuate ligament. *C,* There is a marked decrease in peak systolic velocity in the celiac artery in inspiration.

as compression of the celiac artery is relieved.

CONCLUSIONS

Doppler ultrasound has proven value in the detection of mesenteric artery stenosis and occlusion. Proper patient preparation and the use of sensitive Doppler equipment are necessary to start the investigation. Operator experience and knowledge of technical shortcuts increase accuracy and decrease the time of the examination. Finally, the use of proven diagnostic criteria and correlation with confirmatory studies are also keys to diagnostic success.

Acknowledgments. I would like to thank Saiedeh "Nanaz" Maghoul for her excellent images and James Cooper for his wonderful illustrations.

References

1. Baxter BT, Pearce H: Diagnosis and surgical management of chronic mesenteric ischemia. In Strandness DE, Van Brida A (eds): Vascular Diseases Surgical and Interventional Therapy, 1st ed. New York, Churchill Livingstone Publishers, 1994, pp 795–802.
2. Moneta GL, Taylor DC, Helton WS, et al: Duplex ultrasound measurement of postprandial intestinal blood flow: Effect of meal composition. Gastroenterology 95:1294–1301, 1988.

3. Healy DA, Neumyer MM, Atnip RG, Thiele BL: Evaluation of celiac and mesenteric vascular disease with duplex ultrasonography. J Ultrasound Med 11:481–485, 1992.

4. Nicoloff AD, Williamson WK, Moneta GL, et al: Duplex ultrasonography in evaluation of splanchnic artery stenosis. Surg Clin North Am 77:339–355, 1997.

5. Jager K, Bollinger A, Valli C, Ammann R: Measurement of mesenteric blood flow by duplex scan. J Vasc Surg 3:462–469, 1986.

6. Moneta GL, Yeager RA, Dalman R, et al: Duplex ultrasound criteria for diagnosis of splanchnic artery stenosis or occlusion. J Vasc Surg 14:511–520, 1991.

7. Moneta GL, Lee RW, Yeager RA, et al: Mesenteric duplex scanning: A blinded prospective study. J Vasc Surg 17:79–86, 1993.

8. Lim HK, Lee WJ, Kim SH, et al: Splanchnic arterial stenosis or occlusion: Diagnosis at Doppler US. Radiology 211:405–410, 1999.

9. Bowersox JC, Zwolak RM, Walsh DB, et al: Duplex ultrasonography in the diagnosis of celiac and mesenteric artery occlusive disease. J Vasc Surg 14:780–788, 1991.

10. Zwolak RM, Fillinger MF, Walsh DB, et al: Mesenteric and celiac duplex scanning: A validation study. J Vasc Surg 27:1078–1088, 1998.

11. Perko MJ, Just S, Schroeder TV: Importance of diastolic velocities in the detection of celiac and mesenteric artery disease by duplex ultrasound. J Vasc Surg 26:288–293, 1997.

12. Mirk P, Palazzoni G, Cotroneo AR, et al: Sonographic and Doppler assessment of the inferior mesenteric artery: Normal morphologic and hemodynamic features. Abdom Imaging 23:364–369, 1998.

13. Denys AL, Lafortune M, Aubin B, et al: Doppler sonography of the inferior mesenteric artery: A preliminary study. J Ultrasound Med 14:435–439, 1995.

14. Erden A, Yurdakul M, Cumhur T: Doppler waveforms of the normal and collateralized inferior mesenteric artery. Am J Roentgenol 171:619–627, 1998.

15. Rizzo RJ, Sandager G, Astleford, P, et al: Mesenteric flow velocity variations as a function of angle of insonation. J Vasc Surg 11:688–694, 1990.

Chapter 32

Ultrasound Assessment of the Hepatic Vasculature

WILLIAM J. ZWIEBEL, MD

Vascular disorders of the liver are of considerable interest to ultrasound practitioners because the liver vessels are effectively imaged with ultrasound in a high percentage of patients. As a result, ultrasound is widely used for clinical assessment of hepatic vascular disorders. This chapter considers the sonographic assessment of portal hypertension, intrahepatic portosystemic shunts, portal vein occlusion, and hepatic vein occlusion. Although sonography is an important method for assessing hepatic vessels before and after liver transplantation, this subject is not included here. Liver transplantation is performed in relatively few specialized centers; therefore, a discussion of liver transplantation is beyond the scope of this introductory text.

PORTAL HYPERTENSION

The term *portal hypertension* refers to elevated pressure in the portal venous system; specifically, a pressure gradient from the portal vein to the hepatic veins or inferior vena cava of 10 mm Hg or greater. The most common cause of portal hypertension in Western countries is sinusoidal obstruction due to cirrhosis, which, in turn, is most often caused by excessive alcohol consumption or chronic active hepatitis. The sinusoids of the liver are analogous to capillaries in other tissues. Other sinusoidal causes of portal hypertension include primary biliary cirrhosis and the sinusoidal form of the Budd-Chiari syndrome (discussed later). Presinusoidal portal hyper-

tension refers to obstruction prior to entry of blood into the sinusoids and includes causes such as portal vein occlusion, schistosomiasis, and hepatic fibrosis (from various causes). Postsinusoidal causes of portal hypertension include chronic right heart failure, hepatic vein occlusion, and inferior vena cava (IVC) occlusion.[1-56]

Advances in ultrasound instrumentation have made direct, noninvasive interrogation of portal vein flow possible. Furthermore, ultrasound examination of the portal venous system (portal vein, splenic vein, and superior mesenteric vein) is successful in 93% to 95% of patients.[8,57] Certain ultrasound parameters have been identified that permit sonographic diagnosis of portal hypertension. These include (1) portal vein diameter; (2) response of the portal, splenic, or superior mesenteric veins to respiration; (3) portal flow direction; (4) portal flow velocity and waveforms; (5) spleen size; and (6) the presence of portosystemic collaterals. Each of these diagnostic findings is discussed in turn.

Portal Vein Diameter

In normal individuals (Fig. 32–1), the portal vein diameter does not exceed 13 mm in quiet respiration, measured where the portal vein crosses anterior to the IVC.[6,12-21] Respiration and patient position greatly affect the size of the portal vein and its tributaries; therefore, diagnostic measurements must be standardized by examining the patient in the supine position and in a state of quiet respiration. Under these

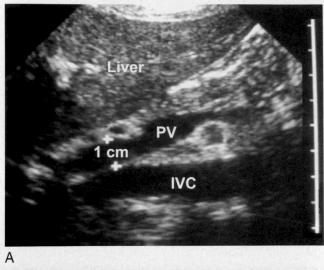

A

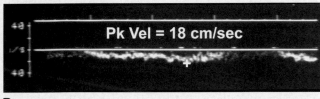

B

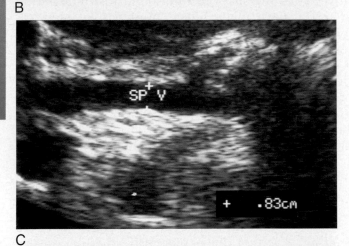

C

FIGURE 32–1. Normal portal vein features. *A*, The portal vein (PV) is measured where it crosses anterior to the inferior vena cava (IVC). With the patient supine and breathing quietly, the portal vein diameter (*cursors*) does not normally exceed 13 mm. *B*, Portal flow velocity undulates slightly in response to cardiac pulsation and respiration. Peak velocity (Pk Vel) is 18 cm/sec in this normal individual. In the same subject, the diameter of the splenic vein (SP V) increases more than 70% from quiet respiration (*C*) to deep inspiration (*D*).

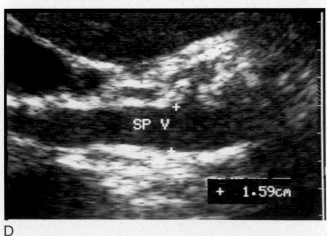

D

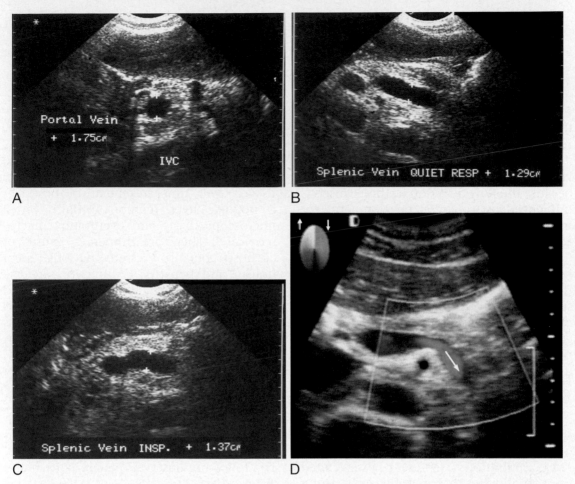

FIGURE 32–2. Features of portal hypertension. *A,* In this 48-year-old patient with alcohol-induced liver disease, the portal vein diameter (*cursors*) is 18 mm with the patient supine and breathing quietly. IVC, inferior vena cava. The diameter of the splenic vein increases only 6% from quiet respiration (*B*) to deep inspiration (*C*). *D,* In another patient with portal hypertension, splenic vein flow (*arrow*) is reversed (toward the spleen). (The spleen is not visible in this view.)

circumstances, a portal vein diameter exceeding 13 mm (Fig. 32–2*A*) indicates portal hypertension with a high degree of specificity (100% reported) but with low sensitivity (45%–50%).[20,21] Sensitivity is increased by evaluating the response of the splenic or superior mesenteric veins to respiratory maneuvers. In normal individuals, the diameter of these veins increases by 70% to 100% from quiet respiration to deep inspiration (see Fig. 32–1*C* and *D*). An increase of less than 70% (see Fig. 32–2*B* and *C*) indicates portal hypertension with reported sensitivity of about 80% and high specificity.[21] To understand the absence of respiratory response in portal hypertension, consider that elevated portal pressure has maximized portal vein distention. As a result, little or no additional distention occurs when the portal vein outflow is indirectly restricted by sustained inspiration.

Portal Flow Direction and Velocity

In normal individuals, portal flow is hepatopedal (toward the liver) throughout the entire cardiac cycle. Mean flow velocity is about 15 to 18 cm/sec,[15,16,22–24] but the normal range is wide. Portal flow velocity varies with cardiac activity and respiration, giving the portal waveform an undulating appearance (see Fig. 32–1*B*).

With the development of portal hypertension, portal flow velocity may decrease and velocity fluctuations may disappear (i.e., flow becomes continuous). Ultimately, as portal pressure increases, portal vein flow may become to and fro (biphasic), or the flow direction may reverse (hepatofugal flow) (see Fig. 32–2D). Concomitant flow reversal may occur in the splenic vein.

Flow reversal in the portal or splenic veins is a variable finding in portal hypertension, because the flow direction in these vessels is influenced by collateral development. For instance, if splenorenal collaterals are the primary mode of portal decompression, flow may reverse in the portal vein. If, however, a large umbilical vein collateral is the primary mode of decompression, splenic and portal vein flow may remain normal (hepatopedal), because the diverting collateral (the umbilical vein) originates in the left portal system. For the same reason, it is possible for flow to be simultaneously reversed in the right portal vein and normally directed in the left portal vein.

When portal hypertension results from right heart failure, pulsations may be present in the portal vein Doppler signal. These pulsations represent exaggerated right atrial pulses that are sufficiently strong to penetrate the hepatic sinusoids and appear in the portal vein.[22,23]

Increased Hepatic Artery Flow

Under normal circumstances, the liver receives about 70% of its blood supply from the portal vein and 30% via the hepatic artery. When portal hypertension is caused by cirrhosis, hepatic artery flow may increase substantially as compensation for diminished portal vein flow. Ultimately, the bulk of liver blood flow is provided by the hepatic artery, which is visibly enlarged on color flow examination and shows substantially increased blood flow on Doppler interrogation. Unfortunately, the hepatic artery does not have the capacity to make up for the loss of portal vein flow, and persistent hepatic ischemia develops, representing a significant cause of ongoing hepatocyte damage and progression of fibrotic scarring.

Cirrhotic Liver Morphology

Imaging findings that indicate the presence of cirrhoisis also indicate the presence of portal hypertension, for by the time cirrhosis is evident, substantial sinusoidal flow obstruction is invariably present. Cirrhosis[58] is the nonspecific, end-stage manifestation of hepatocyte injury, which leads, ultimately, to tissue necrosis, fibrosis, and attempted regeneration of liver tissue. Over time, regeneration produces a nodular liver texture, initially on a microscopic basis and eventually, macroscopically. There are numerous causes of cirrhosis, but in Western nations, alcoholism and hepatitis C infection are the principal etiologies. In Asia, Africa, and most developing countries, viral hepatitis is the usual cause. Cirrhosis is classified as *micronodular* or *macronodular*, depending on the size of regenerative nodules present. Macronodular cirrhosis is simply an advanced stage that has gone beyond the micronodular form.

Cirrhosis may be diagnosed with ultrasound only when specific findings are identified,[58–65] as illustrated in Figure 32–3. The following observations are particularly noteworthy:

1. Ultrasound is not sensitive for the presence of cirrhosis. Biopsy-definable cirrhosis (and associated portal hypertension) is frequently present in livers that look absolutely normal on ultrasound examination. It is only when morphological changes occur in the liver or portal hypertension is evident that ultrasound can confirm the existence of cirrhosis.

2. Ultrasound attenuation by the cirrhotic liver is *similar* to that of the normal hepatic parenchyma. The cirrhotic liver may have a slightly more coarse texture than a normal liver, but it is not strongly echogenic and is easily penetrated by the ultrasound beam. High parenchymal echogenicity and marked ultrasound attenuation are signs of fatty infiltration of the liver (also called steatosis). This condition can be superimposed on cirrhotic changes but is not a manifestation of cirrhosis, per se.

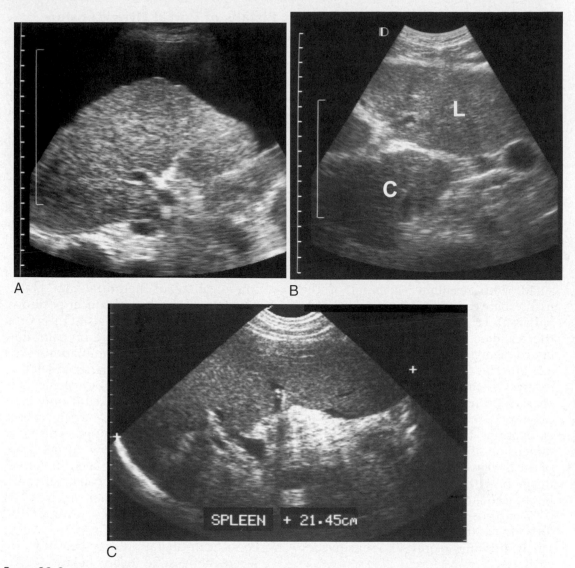

FIGURE 32–3. Morphologic findings associated with cirrhosis. *A,* The liver surface is nodular, and a large amount of ascites (*black area*) surrounds the liver. *B,* The left (L) and caudate (C) lobes of the liver are enlarged. *C,* The spleen is enlarged.

3. In patients with advanced cirrhosis, the texture of the liver is more coarse than normal, and the surface is irregular because of the presence of regenerative nodules. Surface nodularity is most easily detected when ascites surrounds the liver and highlights its surface (see Fig. 32–3*A*). Even fine surface nodularity is abnormal and confirms the diagnosis of cirrhosis.[59] Furthermore, as stated previously, the presence of nodularity or other specific findings of cirrhosis clearly indicates sinusoidal obstruction and the presence of portal hypertension.

4. Large regenerative nodules may occasionally be visualized with ultrasound as discrete, rounded structures within the liver parenchyma.[62–65] These nodules are either isoechoic or slightly hypoechoic relative to the surrounding hepatic tissue. Regenerative nodules are extremely numerous in cirrhotic livers, yet their visualization with ultrasound is *rare*. Therefore, a regenerative nodule should not be the first thought when a discrete lesion is seen in a cirrhotic liver. Instead, the sonologist should think of neoplasia and particularly of hepatocellular carcinoma.

5. The number of visible portal or hepatic veins is reduced in cirrhotic livers, in proportion to the severity of disease. The loss of visible vessels appears to be a compressive phenomenon related to hepatic fibrosis, but the exact etiology is unknown.

6. As suggested by previous statements, portal hypertension is a frequent concomitant finding in cirrhosis. The presence of portal hypertension confirms the diagnosis of cirrhosis, unless there is clinical or imaging evidence for other causes of portal hypertension.

7. Severe, end-stage cirrhosis is accompanied by shrinkage of the liver in a characteristic pattern: 1) The right lobe is small, with resultant widening of the fissure between the right and left lobes (adjacent to the gall bladder); and 2) the caudate and left lobes are enlarged owing to regeneration[59–61] (see Fig. 32–3B). The cause of these morphologic changes is not known for certain. Cirrhosis (and portal hypertension) may be diagnosed in some patients simply by comparing the maximum transverse dimension of the caudate and right lobes of the liver, using a transverse ultrasound image just below the portal bifurcation. If the caudate/right lobe ratio exceeds 0.65, cirrhosis may be diagnosed with 90% to 100% certainty.[58,61] Unfortunately, this ratio is only 43% sensitive for cirrhosis.[61]

Splenomegaly

An important manifestation of portal hypertension is splenomegaly (see Fig. 32–3C). The size of the spleen does not correlate well with the level of portal pressure, and splenomegaly may be caused by numerous conditions in addition to portal hypertension. Nonetheless, splenomegaly commonly accompanies portal hypertension and is a noteworthy finding.[1,2] The spleen is best measured in a coronal plane. A maximal cephalocaudal measurement exceeding 13 cm indicates enlargement with a high degree of reliability.[66]

Pitfalls of Portal Hypertension Assessment

Ultrasound is a useful method for evaluating the portal venous system and for confirming the diagnosis of portal hypertension, but it is not a perfect method, as indicated by the following diagnostic pitfalls.

1. Most importantly, the absence of the findings described previously *does not exclude* portal hypertension, nor does it exclude the presence of cirrhosis.

2. The direction of flow in the portal vein may be ambiguous or may spuriously appear to be reversed for technical reasons. Abnormal flow direction, therefore, should be confirmed with several interrogations of the portal vein, preferably from different transducer positions.

3. When flow is very sluggish, the portal vein may appear occluded on color flow or spectral Doppler examination, even though it is patent, as discussed later.

4. Splenic vein occlusion or splenic flow reversal may be overlooked if only hilar branches are visualized and the splenic vein per se is not examined. This error occurs because blood flow, of necessity, must exit the spleen, even if subsequently channeled into collateral veins. Hence, flow in the hilar branches is always normally directed, even if the splenic vein is occluded.

5. Portal vein dilatation may be caused by severe congestive heart failure (CHF), because of transmission of back pressure from the right atrium through the hepatic sinusoids to the portal circulation.[25,26] Such dilation may be attributed mistakenly to cirrhosis. Two findings help to identify CHF: Portal flow is often markedly pulsatile, and the IVC is dilated. Neither of these findings is a feature of portal hypertension related to liver disease.

PORTOSYSTEMIC VENOUS COLLATERALS

Portosystemic venous collaterals[2,3,6,27–49] are important findings, for in most cases, their

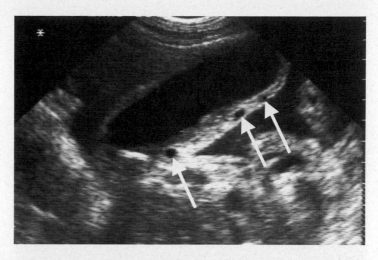

FIGURE 32–6. Gallbladder wall collateral. A longitudinal sonogram in a patient with cirrhosis shows large varices (*arrows*) within the gallbladder wall. Flow in these vessels was visualized on a computed tomogram (not shown). Ascites surrounds the gallbladder.

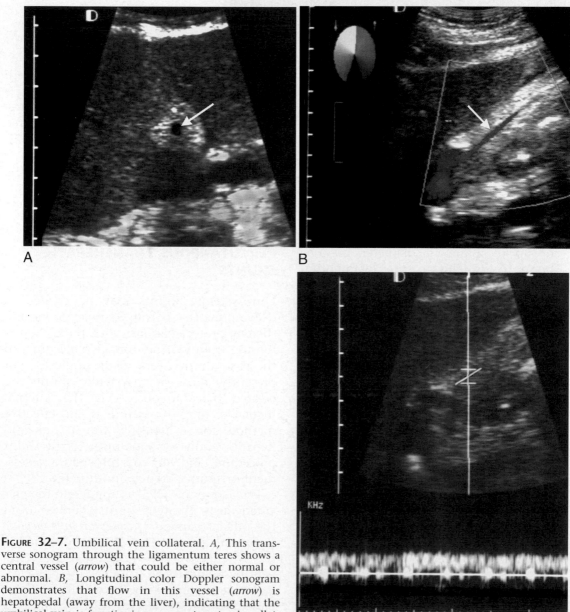

FIGURE 32–7. Umbilical vein collateral. *A,* This transverse sonogram through the ligamentum teres shows a central vessel (*arrow*) that could be either normal or abnormal. *B,* Longitudinal color Doppler sonogram demonstrates that flow in this vessel (*arrow*) is hepatopedal (away from the liver), indicating that the umbilical vein is functioning as a portosystemic collateral. *C,* Continuous flow away from the liver is confirmed with the Doppler spectrum.

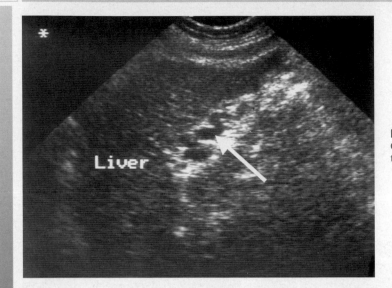

FIGURE 32–8. Left gastric collaterals. Collateral veins (*arrow*) are seen dorsal to the left lobe of the liver.

4 mm, whereas, a diameter exceeding 7 mm is evidence of an abnormal portal/systemic pressure gradient (exceeding 10 mm Hg). Hepatofugal coronary vein flow also indicates an abnormal portosystemic pressure gradient.[36,42,69]

3. *Umbilical vein** collateral flow, which begins in the area of the ligamentum teres, is an important feature of portal hypertension, for it carries a diagnostic specificity of 100%.[47,48] An artery or vein of up to 2 mm in diameter may be present normally in the ligamentum teres; therefore, *the mere presence of a vessel in the ligamentum teres does not imply umbilical vein collateralization.*[43–48] The diagnosis of collateral flow requires documentation of venous flow *away from* the liver (see Fig. 32–5). It should be noted, however, that flow sometimes is away from the liver in a normal ligamentum teres vein, but in such cases, the velocity does not exceed 5 cm/sec.[44–46,70]

4. Portosystemic collaterals may develop in response to venous occlusive disease unrelated to portal hypertension. The most common example is splenic vein occlusion, which is the most likely diagnosis when large splenosystemic collaterals are detected[49] (see Fig. 32–9).

Differentiation between splenic vein thrombosis and portal hypertension is generally not a problem, because the presence or absence of a patent splenic vein can usually be documented with color flow examination.

5. Large portosystemic collaterals at the esophagogastric junction may be mistaken for neoplastic masses if color flow examination is not performed.[32]

PERCUTANEOUS TRANSHEPATIC SHUNTS

Portosystemic shunts may be created to decompress the portal venous system and thereby protect patients with portal hypertension from gastroesophageal bleeding. In the past, shunts were made surgically, but presently, most portosystemic shunts are created percutaneously, via the internal jugular vein. Ultrasound is an effective method for evaluating the portal and hepatic venous systems prior to the shunt procedure and for postprocedure assessment of shunt patency and function.[2,6,50–56]

The acronym "TIPS" is applied to the percutaneously created shunts, derived from the official name: *Transjugular Intrtahepatic Portocaval Shunt.* The TIPS procedure is highly effective for reducing ascites, preventing hemorrhage from gastroesophageal varices, and improving the quality of life of patients with severe cirrhosis,[70–74] but TIPS shunts are subject to a high rate of stenosis

*Whether this is a recanalized portion of the umbilical vein or a paraumbilical vein is subject to debate.[46–48,66]

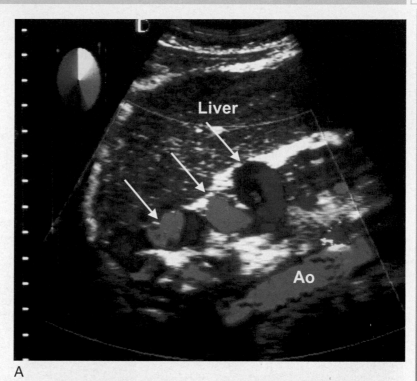

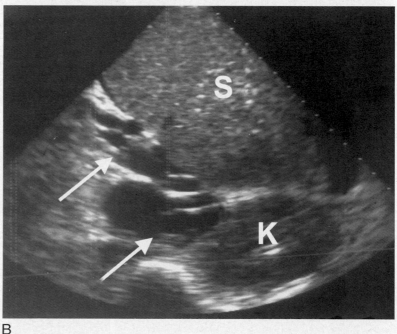

FIGURE 32–9. Splenic collaterals. *A,* Large, tortuous collateral veins (*arrows*) are seen in the vicinity of the gastroesophageal junction on this longitudinal scan through the left lobe of the liver. These collaterals arise from the splenic hilum (not seen on this image). Ao, aorta. *B,* In this patient with congenital hepatic fibrosis, large splenorenal collateral veins (*arrows*) are seen to extend from the inferior end of the spleen (S) toward the left kidney (K).

or occlusion, which can result in recurrent hemorrhage and reaccumulation of ascites. Primary TIPS patency (i.e., without intervention either to preserve or restore patency) ranges from 23% to 66% at 1 year.[75–78] With intervention for thrombosis or occlusion (balloon angioplasty and thrombolysis), the 1-year patency rate is increased to about 85%.[63] The importance of postprocedure shunt surveillance to detect stenosis is obvious from these statistics. Occlusion or stenosis occurring within the first or second week after the TIPS procedure is the result of thrombosis and may be related to technical problems with the TIPS procedure. Occlusion or stenosis occurring later results from pseudointimal (neointimal) hyperplasia; in essence, fibrous tissue proliferation in the stent wall.

The terms *stent* and *shunt* are a little confusing. The shunt is the channel created between the portal and hepatic vein, while the stent is the device used to create the shunt and keep it open. The metallic stents used to create TIPS shunts are readily seen and evaluated with ultrasound[58,57] (Fig. 32–10), and for that reason, sonography is

the primary method for TIPS follow-up. The goal of ultrasound examination is to confirm that the shunt is patent and to search for stenosis. The following examination protocol has been recommended for TIPS assessment.[66]

Before the Procedure

In preparation for the TIPS procedure, a scan is performed to document patency and

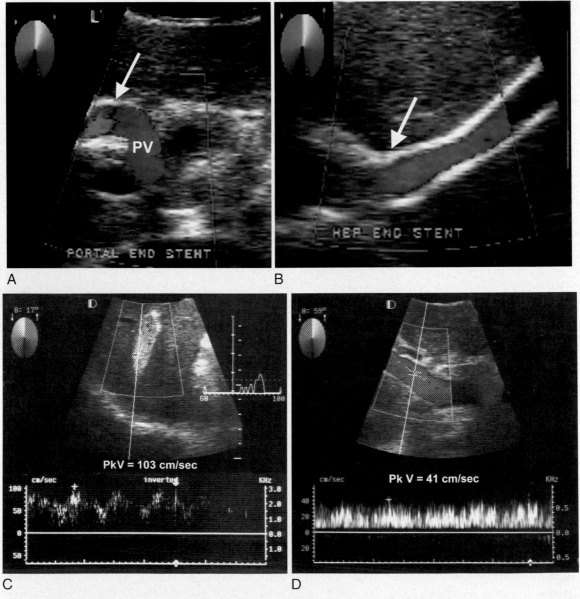

FIGURE 32–10. Normally functioning Transjugular Intrtahepatic Portocaval Shunt (TIPS). *A,* Color-Doppler image of the portal end of the shunt (*arrow*). PV, portal vein. *B,* Color Doppler view of the hepatic (Hep) vein end of the shunt (*arrow*) near the right atrium. *C,* Typical mid-shunt Doppler signal. Peak velocity (Pk V) is 103 cm/sec. *D,* A large volume of portal blood flow is indicated by a portal vein velocity (Pk V) of 41 cm/sec.

flow direction in the portal, splenic, and superior mesenteric veins and to confirm that the hepatic veins and the internal jugular vein (insertion site) are patent. It is also important to note whether the portal vein bifurcates within or outside of the hepatic parenchyma. The latter configuration, though uncommon, increases the risk of perforation of the portal vein during the procedure. Finally, the liver is examined for mass lesions, possibly representing hepatoma, the presence of which would influence the decision to create the shunt.

After the Procedure

Space limitations do not permit description of the TIPS procedure. Suffice it to say that the completed shunt typically extends from the right portal vein to the middle or right hepatic vein. After the TIPS procedure, the shunt is scanned within the first 24 hours to document patency and establish baseline flow velocities in the shunt and the portal vein. Follow-up examinations are then conducted at the discretion of the interventional radiologist (typically at 3 months and then at 6-month intervals thereafter). Regular follow-up is advisable, for reasons mentioned previously.

Normal shunt findings include the following:

1. The proximal and distal ends of the stent are squarely positioned in the hepatic and portal veins, respectively (as opposed to partially within the vein and partially embedded in the liver parenchyma). The ends of the stent may protrude slightly into the portal or hepatic vein.
2. On color flow examination, blood flow "fills" the stent from wall to wall (no filling defect).
3. Doppler flow signals are monophasic and slightly pulsatile.
4. Moderate spectral broadening (turbulence) is the norm.
5. Peak systolic velocity in the shunt is at least 50 to 60 cm/sec[79,80-82] and normally ranges from 90 to 120 cm/sec.[80,83,84]
6. Flow velocity is similar throughout the shunt.
7. Portal vein flow is hepatopedal. (Note: Flow may be reversed in the right or left portal vein branches in a normally functioning shunt.)
8. Main portal vein flow velocity is substantially increased, as compared with preshunt values (peak velocity at least 30 cm/sec, with a typical shunt range of 37–47 cm/sec).[80,83-88]

Shunt Stenosis

The most common location for shunt stenosis (Fig. 32–11) is in the hepatic vein branch immediately adjacent to the proximal end of the stent, but stenosis can also occur at other locations in the shunt or diffusely throughout it. Shunt stenosis often can be diagnosed directly with ultrasound through detection of *localized* high-velocity flow and severe turbulence. Stenosis-related velocities as high as 400 cm/sec have been reported.[72] Shunt stenosis is also indicated by generalized reduced flow velocity *throughout* the stent, as compared with baseline values. A shunt velocity of less than 50 or 60 cm/sec (at any location) highly suggests shunt malfunction and warrants close investigation of the shunt.[81-83,86,87] A further indicator of shunt stenosis is a change in velocity exceeding 100 cm/sec from a normal part of the shunt to a narrowed area.

A drop in portal vein flow velocity from the postprocedure baseline is highly suggestive of shunt malfunction.[83,85-87] This stands to reason, as the shunt is a direct communication between the portal and systemic systems. Portal vein flow should be at a high volume (and velocity) if the shunt is patent. As noted previously, a portal vein flow velocity less than 30 cm/sec is of great concern.

Shunt Occlusion

Shunt occlusion is indicated by absence of flow in the shunt and return of portal flow velocity and direction to preprocedure status. Caution is advised in assessing the apparently occluded shunt, as *low-flow*

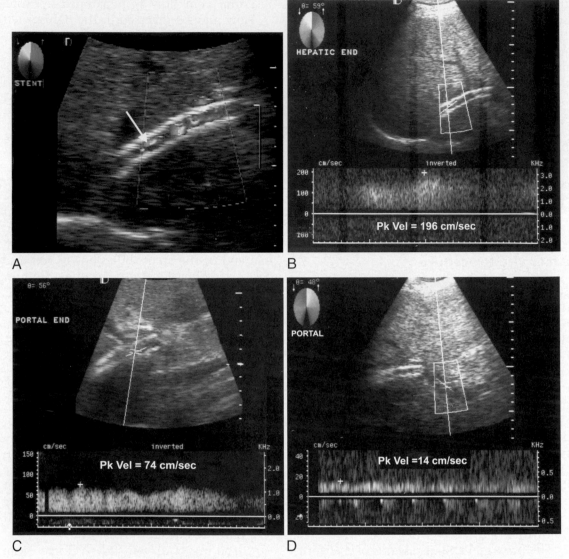

FIGURE 32-11. Transjugular Intrahepatic Portocaval Shunt (TIPS) stenosis. *A,* Near the hepatic vein end, the lumen of the shunt appears narrowed (*arrow*), and flow appears turbulent. *B,* The peak velocity (Pk Vel) in the narrowed segment is 196 cm/sec. This is more than 100 cm/sec greater than the portal end (*C*), which is 74 cm/sec. *D,* Portal vein velocity is low (Pk Vel only 14 cm/sec).

velocity in a highly stenosed shunt may be difficult to detect with ultrasound. If flow is not detected with color flow imaging, try spectral Doppler (which generally is more sensitive) before concluding that the shunt is occluded. In my opinion, shunt occlusion should be confirmed angiographically, as a "trickle" of flow may be present that cannot be detected with ultrasound. A highly stenosed or recently occluded shunt may be returned to patency, whereas a more chronically occluded shunt cannot be repaired by any means.

TIPS Summary

Normal and abnormal TIPS Doppler values are listed in Table 32-3.

PORTAL VEIN OCCLUSION

Pathology

Portal vein occlusion[2,4–6,10,67–116] is principally caused by thrombosis or tumor invasion. Thrombosis may be precipitated by

Table 32–3. Normal and Abnormal Doppler Parameters for Tips Shunts

Normal

1. Pulsatile flow in shunt
2. Peak systolic shunt velocity:
   At least 50–60 cm/sec
   Range 90–120 cm/sec
3. Velocity similar at portal and hepatic ends of shunt
4. Portal and splenic vein flow hepatopedal
5. Portal vein velocity:
   Substantially greater than preshunt value
   At least 30 cm/sec
   Range 37–47 cm/sec

Abnormal

1. Localized high velocity (stenosis) and flow disturbance (poststenosis)
2. Increase in velocity from one point to another in the shunt of more than 100 cm/sec
3. Visible diffuse narrowing with or without high velocity
4. Generalized low velocity throughout shunt (less than 50 cm/sec)
5. Continuous (nonpulsatile) flow in shunt
6. Decrease in portal vein velocity from post-procedure baseline
7. Portal vein velocity less than 30 cm/sec
8. Hepatofugal or to-and-fro portal or splenic vein flow
9. Absence of flow in shunt

stagnant portal flow in patients with cirrhosis. Other causes include hypercoagulable states, surgery, and intraperitoneal inflammatory processes, such as pancreatitis and appendicitis. With pancreatitis, the peripancreatic inflammatory process extends to the portal and splenic veins and causes phlebitis, predisposing them to thrombose. In appendicitis, bacteria shed into the portal system causes portal phlebitis, which in turn causes thrombus to form. Tumor invasion of the portal vein occurs most frequently with hepatocellular carcinoma and pancreatic carcinoma.[88,91–94,101,103–107]

Portal vein occlusion is usually permanent, but recanalization occurs in some cases of thrombosis. More frequently, portal flow is reestablished via cavernous transformation (discussed later). If portal flow is not adequately reestablished, decompression of the portal system occurs via spontaneous portosystemic collaterals (see Fig. 32–4).

Acute Findings

The main portal vein is seen on 97% of upper abdominal sonograms[96,97]; therefore, when a normal-appearing portal vein is not *readily* seen, portal vein occlusion should come to mind.[2,6,70,72–80,89,90] The most important findings that corroborate the diagnosis are absence of portal flow, accompanied by echogenic material within the portal vein lumen. Occluding material, whether thrombus or tumor, is generally low or moderate in echogenicity. Recently formed thrombus may be so slightly echogenic as to be overlooked, in the absence of color flow examination. Blood flow may be absent in an occluded portal vein, or a trickle of flow may be seen around the occluding material. Color flow distinguishes between portal vein tumor and thrombus through the detection of tiny tumor blood vessels within the occluded vein (with pulsatile arterial flow) in cases of portal vein tumor extension. Blood vessels do not occur within thrombus. If the portal vein is only partially blocked (Fig. 32–12A), increased flow velocity and disturbed flow may be apparent at the site of obstruction.

The occluding material frequently dilates the portal vein and its branches noticeably (see Fig. 32–12B). Massive dilatation, with a portal vein diameter exceeding 23 mm, suggests tumor, but this is not specific.[107] Thrombus may extend into the splenic or superior mesenteric veins (see Fig. 32–12C), and these tributaries should be evaluated to confirm the extent of occlusion. Patent segments of the portal system distal* to an occluded portal vein are often dilated. Low-velocity, continuous flow, rather than the normal phasic flow pattern, may be present in these segments. Intrahepatic collateral vessels may develop following portal

*The terms *distal* and *proximal* are used with respect to the heart. *Proximal* means closer to the heart, and *distal* means farther from the heart.

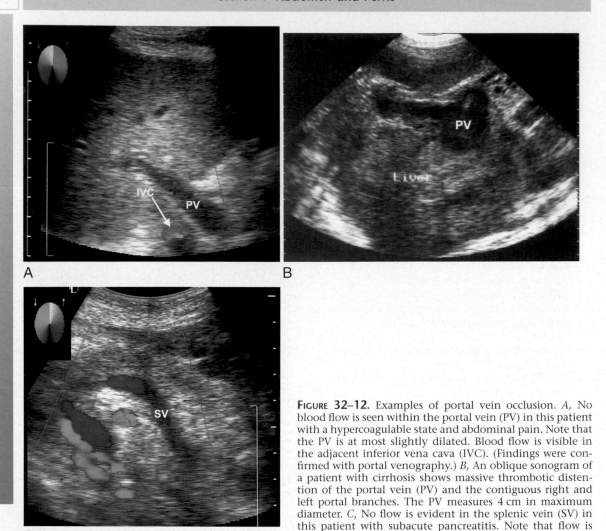

FIGURE 32–12. Examples of portal vein occlusion. *A,* No blood flow is seen within the portal vein (PV) in this patient with a hypercoagulable state and abdominal pain. Note that the PV is at most slightly dilated. Blood flow is visible in the adjacent inferior vena cava (IVC). (Findings were confirmed with portal venography.) *B,* An oblique sonogram of a patient with cirrhosis shows massive thrombotic distention of the portal vein (PV) and the contiguous right and left portal branches. The PV measures 4 cm in maximum diameter. *C,* No flow is evident in the splenic vein (SV) in this patient with subacute pancreatitis. Note that flow is visible in other vessels at an equal depth.

vein occlusion, connecting one portal segment with another, and these may be visualized sonographically.[111] Finally, blood flow may be reversed in the splenic or superior mesenteric veins when the portal vein is occluded.

Chronic Findings

If portal vein thrombosis persists without substantial lysis, the portal vein undergoes fibrosis and may vanish from a sonographic perspective. Cavernous transformation of the portal vein is the principal manifestation of chronic portal vein thrombosis. In this condition, a tangle of tortuous collat-

eral veins are seen along the usual course of the portal vein (Fig. 32–13). These collaterals develop within 6 to 20 days after acute occlusion.[111] The uninitiated sonographer may mistake these vessels for other pathology, including biliary dilatation. Color flow ultrasound examination should prevent such errors, however, by demonstrating venous flow in the collateral vessels. A secondary sign of chronic portal vein occlusion is the development of portosystemic collaterals. These are identical in location and appearance to those described previously (see Table 32–2 and Fig. 32–4). Intrahepatic collaterals may also develop.[111] Lobar atrophy may occur if only a portion of the intrahepatic portal system is occluded, but

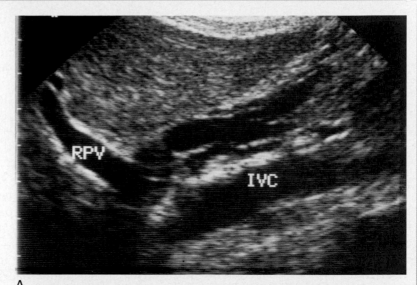

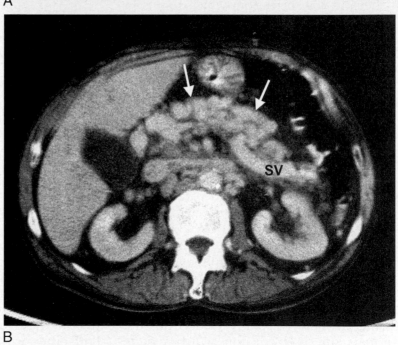

FIGURE 32–13. Cavernous transformation of the portal veins. *A,* An irregular tangle of vessels is seen at the porta hepatis in this patient with a remote history of portal vein thrombosis caused by abdominal sepsis. IVC, inferior vena cava; RPV, right portal vein. *B,* Contrast-enhanced computed tomography in the same patient shows a large tangle of collateral veins *(arrows)* in the vicinity of the pancreas that eventually coalesce as the splenic vein (SV).

this usually occurs when concomitant biliary obstruction is present.[11]

It is reasonable to assume that portal vein thrombosis is a devastating, deadly occurrence, but this clearly is not always the case. If adequate collateralization is established, flow to the liver may be satisfactory and no long-term consequences may occur. However, some patients will suffer gastroesophageal bleeding (possibly life threatening) due to collateralization,

especially when gastroesophageal collaterals develop.

Diagnostic Accuracy

The sonographic diagnosis of portal vein occlusion is highly accurate (sensitivity 89%–100% and specificity 96%–100%).[99–106,109,116] Although diagnostic errors are uncommon, three pitfalls are particularly noteworthy. First, recently formed thrombus that is virtually anechoic may be undetected if color flow sonography is not used, as noted previously. Second, patients with portal hypertension may have low-velocity or to-and-fro portal flow that is difficult to detect with Doppler ultrasound, causing a false-positive impression of occlusion. Third, an inadequate Doppler angle may preclude detection of portal flow, leading to a false-positive diagnosis.

HEPATIC VEIN OCCLUSION

A second venous occlusive disorder of the liver that may be detected sonographically is hepatic vein occlusion, which results in a clinical complex called the *Budd-Chiari syndrome*.[2,5,114–133]

Pathology

The term *Budd-Chiari syndrome* refers to clinical and histologic abnormalities occurring in response to acute obstruction of hepatic vein flow.[82–85] The clinical abnormalities are hepatomegaly (a result of congestion), abdominal pain (a result of hepatomegaly), abrupt development of ascites, and hepatocellular dysfunction (evidenced by biochemical tests). The histologic findings specific for Budd-Chiari syndrome are centrizonal sinusoidal distention and pooling of blood in the sinusoids.

The causes of Budd-Chiari syndrome are numerous and vary in relation to the primary site of obstruction, which may be sinusoids, at the hepatic vein level, or in the IVC. The following imaging ramifications of these locations are noteworthy:

1. With sinusoidal occlusion,* the major hepatic veins may remain patent or may become occluded *secondarily* as a result of sluggish blood flow. Ultrasound can only diagnose the sinusoidal form of Budd-Chiari syndrome when the hepatic veins undergo secondary thrombosis. Fortunately, the sinusoidal form of hepatic vein occlusion is rare, limiting the potential for false-negative diagnoses.

2. *Primary* hepatic vein occlusion is readily detected with ultrasound. Such occlusion results from either thrombosis or tumor invasion of the hepatic veins. Thrombosis is often related to cirrhosis (20% of cases)[83] or hypercoagulable disorders. Neoplastic invasion is most commonly seen with hepatoma.

3. Stenosis or occlusion of the IVC *cephalad to* the hepatic veins causes Budd-Chiari syndrome by inducing hepatic vein congestion (back-pressure) or secondary hepatic vein thrombosis. IVC obstruction may have a variety of causes, including congenital stenosis or occlusion,† thrombosis from hypercoagulable states, and neoplastic invasion. Obstruction of the IVC is readily detected with ultrasound.

4. Finally, a Budd-Chiari–like syndrome may occur with excessive right atrial pressure, as seen with severe congestive heart failure or cardiac tamponade from pericardial effusion.

Therapy

Certain cases of IVC occlusion are amenable to surgery, but in the past, no treatment was available for primary hepatic vein occlusion. More recently, TIPS has proved effective for cases of thrombotic occlusion, in both the acute and the more chronic states.[131,132] It is likely that TIPS will be used more commonly to treat hepatic venoocclusive disease in the future.

The ultrasound findings associated with hepatic vein obstruction fall into three categories: (1) direct manifestations of hepatic vein or IVC occlusion, (2) secondary morphologic changes in the liver, and (3) secondary extrahepatic findings.

---

*Centrilobular venous occlusion is sometimes referred to by the confusing term *venoocclusive disease of the liver.*

†This rare condition is attributed to congenital causes; nevertheless, Budd-Chiari syndrome frequently does not occur until the fifth decade of life (40 yr or older).

Direct Ultrasound Findings

The principal direct ultrasound manifestation of hepatic vein obstruction[2,5,6,113,118-132] (Fig. 32–14) is the presence of echogenic intraluminal material (thrombus or tumor) accompanied by absence of hepatic vein flow (see Fig. 32–14). If the hepatic vein is narrowed but not completely blocked, focal elevated velocity and poststenotic turbulence may be seen.

Frequently, proximal portions of the hepatic veins (deep within the liver) remain patent, while distal regions (near the IVC) are occluded. Continuous flow (see Fig. 32–14D), to-and-fro flow, or reversed flow patterns (rather than the normal, hepatofugal, pulsatile flow pattern) may be seen in portions of the hepatic veins that remain patent deep within the liver. A characteristic finding in these cases is *bicolor* flow, in which one branch of a hepatic vein is blue and another is red. In such cases, the flow direction is normal in one branch and reversed in the other branch, which serves as a collateral channeling blood to other hepatic veins or, indirectly, to the systemic circulation. Intrahepatic collaterals are commonly present in cases of hepatic vein occlusion and may be visualized sonographically as conduits that do not follow the usual course of hepatic vessels. They may connect one hepatic vein branch with another or may connect a hepatic vein with a portal or systemic vein. They may also be seen in a subcapsular location. It has been stated that intrahepatic collateralization is specific for hepatic vein occlusion. This is incorrect, as intrahepatic collateralization can also be seen in cirrhotic livers and even in cases of severe hepatic congestion in which the hepatic veins are patent.[131]

Secondary portal blood flow abnormalities, caused by back-pressure, also may be detected in cases of hepatic vein occlusion. These changes include biphasic or reversed portal flow, decreased flow velocity, or even portal vein thrombosis.

When IVC occlusion causes the Budd-Chiari syndrome,[2,5,6,114-118,121-124,126,127] occluding material (thrombus or tumor) is seen within the IVC lumen (see Fig. 32–14). If the IVC is stenotic but not occluded, high flow velocity and turbulence may be seen in the stenotic area. Distal portions of the IVC, as well as the iliac veins, typically remain patent. These vessels are dilated, and they demonstrate flow abnormalities that may include flow reversal, a continuous flow pattern, and absence of the normal Valsalva response.

The occluding material in the IVC generates low-level echogenicity regardless of whether it is tumor or thrombus. Color flow examination may differentiate between tumor and thrombus through visualization of tumor vessels within the occluding material. (See previous discussion concerning portal vein occlusion.) The presence of a solid liver mass also favors neoplastic obstruction.

The hepatic veins usually become occluded secondarily in patients with IVC obstruction, either from stasis-related thrombosis or from tumor extension (see Fig. 32–14). In some patients, however, the hepatic veins remain patent, and low-velocity antegrade flow is present in the hepatic veins, accompanied by *retrograde* flow in the nonobstructed portions of the IVC.

Secondary Morphologic Changes

Striking morphologic changes may occur in the liver in association with hepatic vein obstruction. Acutely, the portions of the liver subtended by obstructed veins are enlarged (swollen) and hypoechoic (see Fig. 32–14B). In the subacute and chronic phases, the affected areas become fibrotic and shrink in size, and these areas may be relatively echogenic, as compared with normal hepatic parenchyma. The caudate or left lobes of the liver may undergo striking compensatory enlargement, because these portions of the liver are relatively spared from the effects of venous back-pressure.

Secondary Extrahepatic Manifestations

Ascites, pleural effusion, and gallbladder edema are commonly seen in the acute

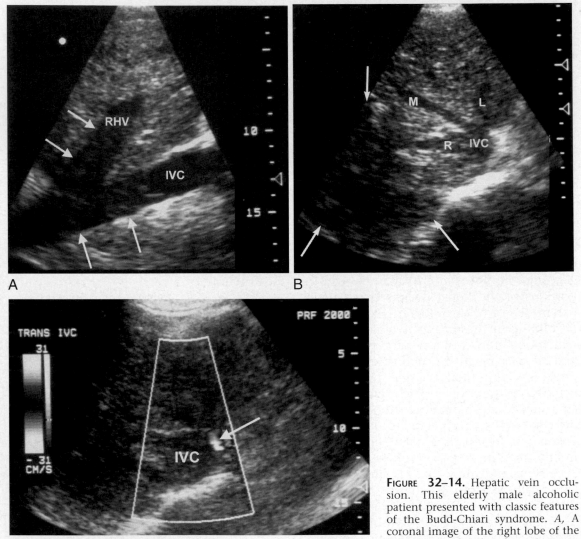

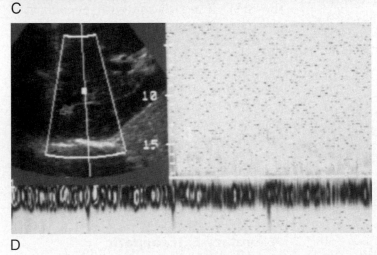

Figure 32–14. Hepatic vein occlusion. This elderly male alcoholic patient presented with classic features of the Budd-Chiari syndrome. *A,* A coronal image of the right lobe of the liver shows a faintly echogenic tumor (*arrows*) within the dilated right hepatic vein (RHV) and the inferior vena cava (IVC). *B,* A transverse scan shows the tumor-filled right hepatic vein (R) and IVC. A poorly defined hypoechoic area (*arrows*), representing hepatic edema, is seen in the posterior portion of the right hepatic lobe. The middle (M) and left (L) hepatic veins are patent, but this is not apparent on this gray-scale image. *C,* Blood flow from the middle and left hepatic veins passes through a narrow residual lumen (*arrow*) between the tumor mass and the wall of the IVC. (Black and white representation of a transverse color Doppler image.) *D,* Doppler flow signals in the middle and left hepatic veins are continuous, consistent with significant obstruction.

stage of Budd-Chiari syndrome. Spleno-megaly and portosystemic collaterals may be evident in chronic cases, in relation to persistent portal hypertension. With IVC obstruction, lower extremity edema is present in both the acute and subacute stages.

Hepatic Vein Nonvisualization

Nonvisualization or poor visualization of the hepatic veins is a diagnostic problem when the Budd-Chiari syndrome is suspected. In some cases, poorly seen or non-visualized veins may actually be patent and normal. In other cases, a patent hepatic vein may be seen deep within the liver, yet the same vein is obstructed proximally near the diaphragm. *In the author's opinion, the Budd-Chiari syndrome can be excluded only when the patency of the major hepatic veins can be confirmed unequivocally.* If the hepatic veins cannot be seen clearly from the IVC to deep within the liver, no comment can be made with respect to their patency or the presence of Budd-Chiari syndrome, unless secondary findings, such as intrahepatic shunts, are seen. It is easy to locate and follow the hepatic veins in a healthy individual, but this task may be difficult or impossible in a patient with cirrhosis or steatosis.

References

1. Sherlock S, Dooley J: Diseases of the Liver and Biliary System, 9th ed. London, Blackwell Scientific Publications, 1993.
2. Koslin DB, Mulligan SA, Berland LL: Duplex assessment of the splanchnic vasculature. Semin Ultrasound CT MR 13:34–39, 1992.
3. Zwiebel WJ, Fruechte D: Basics of abdominal and pelvic duplex: Instrumentation, anatomy, and vascular Doppler signatures. Semin Ultrasound CT MR 13:3–21, 1992.
4. Ralls PW: Color Doppler sonography of the hepatic artery and portal venous system. Am J Roentgenol 155:517–525, 1990.
5. Becker CD, Cooperberg PL: Sonography of the hepatic vascular system. Am J Roentgenol 150:999–1005, 1988.
6. Bolondi L, Mazziotti A, Arienti V, et al: Ultrasonographic study of portal venous system in portal hypertension and after portosystemic shunt operations. Surgery 95:261–269, 1984.
7. Taylor KJW, Burns PN: Duplex Doppler scanning in the pelvis and abdomen. Ultrasound Med Biol 11:643–658, 1985.
8. Patriquin H, Lafortune M, Burns PN, Dauzat M: Duplex Doppler examination in portal hypertension: Technique and anatomy. Am J Roentgenol 149:71–76, 1987.
9. Zierler BK, Horn JR, Bauer LA, et al: Hepatic blood flow measurements by duplex ultrasound: How to minimize variability. J Vasc Technol 15:16–22, 1991.
10. Parvey HR, Eisenberg RL, Giyanani V, Krebs CA: Duplex sonography of the portal venous system: Pitfalls and limitations. Am J Roentgenol 152:765–770, 1989.
11. Bolondi L: The value of Doppler US in the study of hepatic hemodynamics (consensus conference report, Bologna, Italy, 12 Sept 1989). J Hepatol 10:353–355, 1990.
12. Strohm VWD, Wehr B: Korrelation zwischen Lebervenverchylubfrick und sonographich bestimmtem Durchmesser von Pfortader und Milz bei Leberkranken. Z Gastroenterol 17:695–703, 1979.
13. Rahim N, Adam EJ: Ultrasound demonstration of variations in normal portal vein diameter with posture. Br J Radiol 58:313–314, 1985.
14. Weinreb J, Kumari S, Phillips G, Pochaczevski R: Portal vein measurements by real-time sonography. Am J Roentgenol 139:497–499, 1982.
15. Rabinovici N, Narot N: The relationship between respiration, pressure and flow distribution in the vena cava and portal and hepatic veins. Surg Gynecol Obstet 151:753–763, 1980.
16. Moriyasu F, Ban N, Nishida O, et al: Clinical application of an ultrasonic duplex system in the quantitative measurement of portal blood flow. J Clin Ultrasound 14:579–588, 1986.
17. Zoli M, Dondi C, Marchesini G, et al: Splanchnic vein measurements in patients with liver cirrhosis: A case-control study. J Ultrasound Med 4:641–646, 1985.
18. Goyal AK, Pokharna DS, Sharma SK: Ultrasonic measurements of portal vasculature in diagnosis of portal hypertension. A controversial subject reviewed. J Ultrasound Med 9:45–48, 1990.
19. Cottone M, D'Amico G, Maringhini A, et al: Predictive value of ultrasonography in the screening of non-ascitic cirrhotic patients with large varices. J Ultrasound Med 5:189–192, 1965.
20. Bolondi L, Gamrolfi L, Arienti V, et al: Ultrasonography in the diagnosis of portal hypertension: diminished response of portal vessels to respiration. Radiology 142:167–172, 1982.

21. Bolondi L, Mazziotti A, Arienti V, et al: Ultrasonographic study of portal venous system in portal hypertension and after portosystemic shunt operations. Surgery 95:261–269, 1984.

22. Moriyasu F, Ban N, Nishida O, et al: Portal hemodynamics in patients with hepatocellular carcinoma. Radiology 161:707–711, 1986.

23. Moriyasu F, Nishida O, Ban N, et al: "Congestion index" of the portal vein. Am J Roentgenol 146:735–739, 1986.

24. Gaiani S, Bolondi L, Li Bassi S, et al: Effect of meal on portal hemodynamics in healthy humans and in patients with chronic liver disease. Hepatology 9:815–819, 1989.

25. Hosoki T, Arisawa J, Marukawa T, et al: Portal blood flow in congestive heart failure: Pulsed duplex sonographic findings. Radiology 174:733–736, 1990.

26. Duerinckx A, Grant EG, Perrella RR, et al: The pulsatile portal vein in cases of congestive heart failure: Correlation of duplex Doppler findings with right atrial pressures. Radiology 176:655–658, 1990.

27. DeCandio G, Campstelli A, Mosca F, et al: Ultrasound detection of unusual spontaneous portosystemic shunts associated with uncomplicated portal hypertension. J Ultrasound Med 4:297–305, 1985.

28. Patriquin H, Tessier G, Grignon A, Boisvert J: Lesser omental thickness in normal children: Baseline for detection of portal hypertension. Am J Roentgenol 145:693–696, 1985.

29. Neumaier CE, Cicco GR, Derchi LE, Biggi E: The patent ductus venosus: An additional ultrasonic finding in portal hypertension. J Clin Ultrasound 11:231–233, 1983.

30. West MS, Garra BS, Horii SC, et al: Gallbladder varices: Imaging findings in patients with portal hypertension. Radiology 179:179–182, 1991.

31. Marchal GF, Van Holsbeeck M, Tschibwabwa-Ntumba E, et al: Dilatation of the cystic veins in portal hypertension: Sonographic demonstration. Radiology 154:187–189, 1985.

32. Brady TM, Gross BH, Glazer GM, Williams DM: Adrenal pseudomasses due to varices: Angiographic-CT-MRI-pathologic correlations. Am J Roentgenol 145:301–304, 1985.

33. Di Candio G, Campatelli A, Mosca F, et al: Ultrasound detection of unusual spontaneous portosystemic shunts associated with uncomplicated portal hypertension. J Ultrasound Med 4:297–305, 1985.

34. Jüttner H-U, Jenney JM, Ralls PW, et al: Ultrasound demonstration of portosystemic collaterals in cirrhosis and portal hypertension. Radiology 142:459–463, 1982.

35. Dökmeci AK, Kimura K, Matsutani S, et al: Collateral veins in portal hypertension: Demonstration by sonography. Am J Roentgenol 137:1173–1177, 1981.

36. Dach JL, Hill MC, Palaez JC, et al: Sonography of hypertensive portal venous system: Correlation with arterial portography. Am J Roentgenol 137:511–517, 1981.

37. Mori H, Hayashi K, Fukuda T, et al: Intrahepatic portosystemic venous shunt: Occurrence in patients with and without liver cirrhosis. Am J Roentgenol 149:711–714, 1987.

38. Sie A, Johnson MB, Lee KP, Ralls PW: Color Doppler sonography in spontaneous splenorenal portosystemic shunts. J Ultrasound Med 10:167–169, 1991.

39. Subramanyam BR, Balthazar EJ, Raghavenadra BN, Lefleur RS: Sonographic evaluation of patients with portal hypertension. Am J Gastroenterol 78:369–373, 1983.

40. Subramanyam BR, Balthazar EJ, Madamba MR, et al: Sonography of porto-systemic collaterals in portal hypertension. Radiology 146:161–166, 1983.

41. Takayasu K, Moriyama N, Shima Y, et al: Sonographic detection of large spontaneous splenorenal shunts and its clinical significance. Br J Radiol 57:565–570, 1984.

42. Lafortune M, Marleau D, Breton G, et al: Portal venous system measurements in portal hypertension. Radiology 151:27–30, 1984.

43. Schabel S, Rittenberg GM, Javid LH, et al: The "Bull's-Eye" falciform ligament: A sonographic finding of portal hypertension. Radiology 136:157–159, 1980.

44. Saddekni S, Hutchinson DE, Cooperberg PL: The sonographically patent umbilical vein in portal hypertension. Radiology 145:411–443, 1982.

45. Aagaard J, Jensen LI, Sørensen TIA, et al: Recanalized umbilical vein in portal hypertension. Am J Roentgenol 139:1107–1109, 1982.

46. Lafortune M, Constantin A, Breton G, et al: The recanalized umbilical vein in portal hypertension: A myth. Am J Roentgenol 144:549–553, 1985.

47. Gibson RN, Gibson PR, Donlan JD, Clunie DA: Identification of a patent paraumbilical vein by using Doppler sonography: Importance in the diagnosis of portal hypertension. Am J Roentgenol 153:513–516, 1989.

48. Mostbeck GH, Wittich GR, Herold C, et al: Hemodynamic significance of the paraumbilical vein in portal hypertension: Assessment with duplex US. Radiology 170:339–342, 1989.

49. Marn CS, Glazer GM, Williams DM, Francis IR: CT-angiographic correlation of collateral venous pathways in isolated splenic vein occlusion: New observations. Radiology 175:375–380, 1990.

50. Rice S, Lee KP, Johnson MB, et al: Portal venous system after portosystemic shunts or endoscopic sclerotherapy: Evaluation with Doppler sonography. Am J Roentgenol 156:85–89, 1991.

51. O'Connor SE, LaBombard E, Musson AM, Zwolak RM: Duplex imaging of distal splenorenal shunts. J Vasc Technol 15:28–31, 1991.

52. Chezmar JL, Bernardino ME: Mesoatrial shunt for the treatment of Budd-Chiari syndrome: Radiologic evaluation in eight patients. Am J Roentgenol 149:707–710, 1987.

53. Lafortune M, Patriquin H, Pomier G, et al: Hemodynamic changes in portal circulation after portosystemic shunts: Use of duplex sonography in 43 patients. Am J Roentgenol 149:701–706, 1987.

54. Patriquin H, Lafortune M, Weber A, et al: Surgical portosystemic shunts in children: Assessment with duplex Doppler US. Radiology 165:25–28, 1987.

55. Grant EG, Tessler FN, Gomes AS, et al: Color Doppler imaging of portosystemic shunts. Am J Roentgenol 154:393–397, 1990.

56. Bolondi L, Gaiani S, Mazziotti A, et al: Morphological and hemodynamic changes in the portal venous system after distal splenorenal shunt: An ultrasound and pulsed Doppler study. Hepatology 8:652–657, 1988.

57. Yeh H-C, Stancato-Pasik A, Ramos R, Rabinowitz JG: Paraumbilical venous collateral circulations: Color Doppler ultrasound features. J Clin Ultrasound 24:359–366, 1996.

58. Harbin WP, Robert NJ, Ferrucci JT: Diagnosis of cirrhosis based on regional changes in hepatic morphology. Radiology 135:273–283, 1980.

59. Di Lelio A, Cestari C, Lomazzi A, Beretta L: Cirrhosis: Diagnosis with sonographic study of the liver surface. Radiology 172:389–392, 1989.

60. Gore RM, Ghahremani GG, Joseph AE, et al: Acquired malposition of the colon and gallbladder in patients with cirrhosis: CT findings and clinical implications. Radiology 171:739–742, 1989.

61. Giorgio A, Amoroso P, Lettieri G, et al: Cirrhosis: Value of caudate to right lobe ratio in diagnosis with US. Radiology 161:443–445, 1986.

62. Freeman MP, Vick CW, Taylor KJW, et al: Regenerating nodules in cirrhosis: Sonographic appearance with anatomic correlation. Am J Roentgenol 146:533–536, 1986.

63. Day DL, Letourneau JG, Allan BT, et al: Hepatic regenerating nodules in hereditary tyrosinemia. Am J Roentgenol 149:391–393, 1987.

64. Murakami T, Kuroda C, Murakawa T, et al: Regenerating nodules in hepatic cirrhosis: MR findings with pathologic correlation. Am J Roentgenol 155:1227–1231, 1990.

65. Giorgio A, Francica G, de Stefano G, et al: Sonographic recognition of intraparenchymal regenerating nodules using high-frequency transducers in patients with cirrhosis. J Ultrasound Med 10:355–359, 1991.

66. Senecal B: Sonographic anatomy of the normal spleen, normal anatomic variants, and pitfalls. In Bruneton JN (ed): Ultrasonography of the Spleen. Berlin, Springer-Verlag, 1988, pp 1–13.

67. Bach AM, Hann LE, Brown KT, et al: Portal vein evaluation with US: Comparison to angiography combined with CT arterial portography. Radiology 201:149–154, 1996.

68. Schmassmann A, Zuber M, Livers M, et al: Recurrent bleeding after variceal hemorrhage: Predictive value of portal venous duplex sonography. Am J Roentgenol 160:41–47, 1993.

69. Morin C, Lafortune M, Pomier G, et al: Patent paraumbilical vein: Anatomic and hemodynamic variants and their clinical importance. Radiology 185:253–256, 1992.

70. Casarella WJ: Transjugular intrahepatic portosystemic shunt: A defining achievement in vascular and interventional radiology. Radiology 196:305, 1995.

71. Nazarian GK, Ferral H, Bjarnason H, et al: Effect of transjugular intrahepatic portosystemic shunt on quality of life. Am J Roentgenol 167:963–969, 1996.

72. Ochs A, Rossle M, Haag K, et al: The transjugular intrahepatic portosystemic stent-shunt procedure for refractory ascites. N Engl J Med 332:1192–1197, 1995.

73. Polak JF: Transjugular intrahepatic portosystemic shunt: Building on experience. Radiology 196:306–307, 1995.

74. Coldwell DM, Ring EJ, Rees CR, et al: Multicenter investigation of the role of transjugular intrahepatic portosystemic shunt in management of portal hypertension. Radiology 196:335–340, 1995.

75. Kerlan RK Jr, LaBerge JM, Gordon RL, Ring EJ: Transjugular intrahepatic portosystemic shunts: Current status. Am J Roentgenol 164:1059–1066, 1995.

76. Ducoin H, El-Khoury J, Rosseau H, et al: Histopathologic analysis of transjugular intrahepatic portosystemic shunts. Hepatology 25:1064–1069, 1997.

77. Sterling KM, Darcy MD: Stenosis of transjugular intrahepatic portosystemic shunts: Presentation and management. Am J Roentgenol 168:239–244, 1997.

78. Nazarian GK, Ferral H, Castañeda-Zúñiga WR, et al: Development of stenoses in transjugular intrahepatic portosystemic shunts. Radiology 192:231–234, 1994.

79. Chong WK, Malisch TW, Mazer MJ, et al: Transjugular intrahepatic portosystemic shunts: US assessment with maximum flow velocity. Radiology 189:789–793, 1993.

80. Foshager MC, Ferral H, Nazarian GK, et al: Duplex sonography after transjugular intrahepatic portosystemic shunts (TIPS): Normal hemodynamic findings and efficacy in predicting shunt patency and stenosis. Am J Roentgenol 165:1–7, 1995.

81. Feldstein VA, Patel MD, LaBerge JM: Transjugular intrahepatic portosystemic shunts: Accuracy of Doppler US in determination of patency and detection of stenoses. Radiology 201:141–147, 1996.

82. Dodd GD III, Zajko AB, Orons PD, et al: Detection of transjugular intrahepatic portosystemic shunt dysfunction: Value of duplex Doppler sonography. Am J Roentgenol 164:1119–1124, 1995.

83. Kanterman RY, Darcy MD, Middleton WD, et al: Doppler sonography findings associated with transjugular intrahepatic portosystemic shunt malfunction. Am J Roentgenol 168:467–472, 1997.

84. Surratt RS, Middleton WD, Darcy MD, et al: Morphologic and hemodynamic findings at sonography before and after creation of a transjugular intrahepatic portosystemic shunt. Am J Roentgenol 160:627–630, 1993.

85. Haskal ZJ, Carroll JW, Jacobs JE, et al: Sonography of transjugular intrahepatic portosystemic shunts: Detection of elevated portosystemic gradients and loss of shunt function. J Vasc Interv Radiol 8:549–556, 1997.

86. Murphy TP, Beechman RP, Kim HM, et al: Long-term follow-up after TIPS: Use of Doppler velocity criteria for detecting elevation of the portosystemic gradient. J Vasc Interv Radiol 9:275–281, 1998.

87. Bodner G, Peer S, Fries D, et al: Color and pulsed Doppler ultrasound findings in normally functioning transjugular intrahepatic portosystemic shunts. Eur J Ultrasound 12:131–136, 2000.

88. Grendell JH, Ockner RK: Mesenteric venous thrombosis. In Sleisinger MH, Fordtran JS (eds): Gastrointestinal Disease. Philadelphia, WB Saunders, 1983, pp 1557–1558.

89. Wachsberg RH, Simmons MZ: Coronary vein diameter and flow direction in patients with portal hypertension: Evaluation with duplex sonography and correlation with variceal bleeding. Am J Roentgenol 162:637–641, 1994.

90. Khedkar N, Traverso L, Walat S, et al: Transjugular intrahepatic portosystemic shunt (TIPS) duplex imaging. J Vasc Technology 17:192, 1993.

91. Johnson CC, Baggenstoss AH: Mesenteric vascular occlusion: Study of 99 cases of occlusion of veins. Mayo Clin Proc 24:628–636, 1949.

92. North JP, Wollenman OJ: Venous mesenteric occlusion in course of migratory thrombophlebitis. Surg Gynecol Obstet 95:665–671, 1952.

93. Babcock DS: Ultrasound diagnosis of portal vein thrombosis as a complication of appendicitis. Am J Roentgenol 133:317–319, 1979.

94. Verbanck JJ, Rutgeerts LJ, Haerens MH, et al: Partial splenoportal and superior mesenteric venous thrombosis. Gastroenterol 86:949–952, 1984.

95. Papanicolaou N, Harmatz P, Simeone JF, et al: Sonographic demonstration of reversible portal vein thrombosis following splenectomy in an adolescent. J Clin Ultrasound 12:575–577, 1984.

96. Merritt CBR: Ultrasonographic demonstration of portal vein thrombosis. Radiology 133:425–427, 1979.

97. Marx M, Scheible W: Cavernous transformation of the portal vein. J Ultrasound Med 1:167–169, 1982.

98. Subramanyam BR, Balthazar EJ, Lefleur RS, et al: Portal venous thrombosis: Correlative analysis of sonography, CT, and angiography. Am J Gastroenterol 79:773–776, 1984.

99. Kauzlaric D, Petrovic M, Barmeir J: Sonography of cavernous transformation of the portal vein. Am J Roentgenol 142:383–384, 1984.

100. Weltin G, Taylor KJW, Carter AR, Taylor CR: Duplex Doppler: Identification of cavernous transformation of the portal vein. Am J Roentgenol 144:999–1001, 1985.

101. Gansbeke FV, Avni EF, Delcour C, et al: Sonographic features of portal vein thrombosis. Am J Roentgenol 144:749–752, 1985.

102. Tessler FN, Gehring BJ, Gomes AS, et al: Diagnosis of portal vein thrombosis: Value of color Doppler imaging. Am J Roentgenol 157:293–296, 1991.

103. Wang L-Y, Lin Z-Y, Chang W-Y, et al: Duplex pulsed Doppler sonography of portal vein thrombosis in hepatocellular carcinoma. J Ultrasound Med 10:265–269, 1991.

104. Subramanyam BR, Balthazer EJ, Hilton S, et al: Hepatocellular carcinoma with venous invasion. Radiology 150:793–796, 1984.

105. Atri M, de Stempel J, Bret PM, Illescas FF: Incidence of portal vein thrombosis complicating liver metastasis as detected by duplex ultrasound. J Ultrasound Med 9:285–289, 1990.

106. Tanaka K, Numata K, Okazaki H, et al: Diagnosis of portal vein thrombosis in patients with hepatocellular carcinoma: Efficacy of color Doppler sonography compared with angiography. Am J Roentgenol 160:1279–1283, 1993.

107. Tublin ME, Dodd GD, Baron RL: Benign and malignant portal vein thrombosis: Differentiation by CT characteristics. Am J Roentgenol 168:719–723, 1997.

108. Blum U, Haag K, Rössle M, et al: Noncavernomatous portal vein thrombosis in hepatic cirrhosis: Treatment with transjugular intrahepatic portosystemic shunt and local thrombolysis. Radiology 195:153–157, 1995.

109. Chawla Y, Dilawari JB, Katariya S: Gallbladder varices in portal vein thrombosis. Am J Roentgenol 162:643–645, 1994.

110. Furuse J, Matsutani S, Yoshikawa M, et al: Diagnosis of portal vein tumor thrombus by pulsed Doppler ultrasonography. J Clin Ultrasound 20:439–448, 1992.

111. De Gaetano AM, Lafortune M, Patriquin H, et al: Cavernous transformation of the portal vein: Patterns of intrahepatic and splanchnic collateral circulation detected with Doppler sonography. Am J Roentgenol 165:1151–1155, 1995.

112. Hann LE, Getrajdman GI, Brown KT, et al: Hepatic lobar atrophy: Association with ipsilateral portal vein obstruction. Am J Roentgenol 167:1017–1021, 1996.

113. Pollard JJ, Nebesar RA: Altered hemodynamics in the Budd-Chiari syndrome demonstrated by selective hepatic and selective splenic angiography. Radiology 89:236–243, 1967.

114. Chopra S: Budd-Chiari syndrome and veno-occlusive disease. In Disorders of the Liver. Philadelphia, Lea & Febiger, 1988.

115. Stanley P: Budd-Chiari syndrome. Radiology 170:625–627, 1989.

116. Hommeyer SC, Teefey SA, Jacobson AF, et al: Venocclusive disease of the liver: Prospective study of US evaluation. Radiology 184:683–686, 1992.

117. Cho KY, Geisinger KR, Shields JJ, Forrest ME: Collateral channels and histopathology in hepatic vein occlusion. Am J Roentgenol 139:703–709, 1982.

118. Murphy FB, Steinberg HV, Shires GT, et al: The Budd-Chiari syndrome: A review. Am J Roentgenol 147:9–15, 1986.

119. Mathieu D, Vasile N, Menu Y, et al: Budd-Chiari syndrome: Dynamic CT. Radiology 165:409–413, 1987.

120. Harter LP, Gross BH, St Hilaire J, et al: CT and sonographic appearance of hepatic vein obstruction. Am J Roentgenol 139:176–178, 1982.

121. Baert AL, Fevery J, Marchal G, et al: Early diagnosis of Budd-Chiari syndrome by computed tomography and ultrasonography: Report of five cases. Gastroenterology 84:587–595, 1983.

122. Makuuchi M, Hasegawa H, Yamazaki S, et al: Primary Budd-Chiari syndrome: Ultrasonic demonstration. Radiology 152:775–779, 1984.

123. Menu Y, Alison D, Lorphelin J-M, et al: Budd-Chiari syndrome: US evaluation. Radiology 157:761–764, 1985.

124. Grant EG, Perrella R, Tessler FN, et al: Budd-Chiari syndrome: The results of duplex and colour Doppler imaging. Am J Roentgenol 152:377–381, 1989.

125. Brown BP, Abu-Yousef M, Farner R, et al: Doppler sonography: A noninvasive method for evaluation of hepatic veno-occlusive disease. Am J Roentgenol 154:721–724, 1990.

126. Hosoki T, Kuroda C, Tokunaga K, et al: Hepatic venous outflow obstruction: Evaluation with pulsed duplex sonography. Radiology 170:733–737, 1989.

127. Takayasu K, Moriyama N, Muramatsu Y, et al: Intrahepatic venous collaterals forming via the inferior right hepatic vein in 3 patients with obstruction of the inferior vena cava. Radiology 154:323–328, 1985.

128. Cho O-K, Koo J-H, Kim Y-S, et al: Collateral pathways in Budd-Chiari syndrome: CT and venographic correlation. Am J Roentgenol 167:1163–1167, 1996.

129. Kane R, Eustace S: Diagnosis of Budd-Chiari Syndrome: Comparison between sonography and MR angiography. Radiology 195:117–121, 1995.

130. Millener O, Grant EG, Rose S, et al: Color Doppler imaging findings in patients with Budd-Chiari Syndrome: Correlation with venographic findings. Am J Roentgenol 161:307–312, 1993.

131. Middleton MA, Middleton WD: Intrahepatic venous collaterals in a patient with congestive heart failure. J Ultrasound Med 13:479–481, 1994.

132. Blum U, Rössle M, Haag K: Budd-Chiari syndrome: Technical, hemodynamic, and clinical results of treatment with transjugular intrahepatic portosystemic shunt. Radiology 197:805–811, 1995.

133. Singh V, Sinha SK, Nain CK, et al: Budd-Chiari syndrome: Our experience of 71 patients. J Gastroenterol Hepatol 15:550–554, 2000.

Chapter 33

Ultrasound Assessment of Native Renal Vessels and Renal Allografts

JOHN S. PELLERITO, MD, AND WILLIAM J. ZWIEBEL, MD

This chapter concerns duplex ultrasound assessment of the renal arteries and veins. Native renal vessels, including renal artery stenosis and occlusion, renal vein thrombosis, and tumor invasion of the renal veins, are considered first. Renal allografts, including postoperative vascular complications and allograft rejection, are then considered.

ANATOMY

Both renal arteries arise from the proximal abdominal aorta just below the origin of the superior mesenteric artery, which serves as a handy reference point (Fig. 33–1). The right renal artery arises at an anterolateral location and passes posterior to the inferior vena cava (IVC). It is the only major vessel posterior to the IVC. The left renal artery generally arises from the lateral or posterolateral aspect of the aorta. Duplicate main renal arteries and polar accessory renal arteries occur in approximately 12% to 22% of patients.[1-8] Polar accessory renal arteries may arise from the aorta or the iliac arteries and usually go unrecognized with ultrasound. Even duplicated main renal arteries may be overlooked sonographically.[1-5,9-15] The right renal vein is located anterior to the right renal artery. The left renal vein lies *between* the superior mesenteric artery and the aorta (as opposed to the splenic vein, which lies *anterior* to the superior mesenteric artery). The left renal vein may normally be quite large in a supine individual.

PRINCIPLES OF EXAMINATION

Duplex ultrasound evaluation of native renal vessels is a technically difficult examination. Most sonographers are initially frustrated by difficulties with locating and following the renal arteries and with obtaining Doppler signals from these vessels. With a little patience, however, a sonographer can become adept at this study and perform the examination in a reasonable period of time. Literature reports indicate that as many as 95% of main renal arteries can be adequately examined in adult patients.[9-11,14,16] The key to the renal Doppler examination is accurate demonstration of the vascular anatomy. This requires an understanding of renal vascular anatomy as well as the ability to recognize normal and abnormal Doppler waveforms.

Several imaging modalities are available to evaluate the renal vessels. Catheter angiography remains the "gold standard" examination but is limited by its invasive nature as well as the fact that it exposes patients to iodinated contrast material and radiation. Multidetector computed tomographic angiography and contrast-enhanced magnetic resonance angiography (MRA) are less invasive alternatives to angiography. Both techniques have proven valuable in the demonstration of renal arterial disease. Computed tomographic angiography offers higher resolution than MRA but also requires iodinated contrast material and is contraindicated in

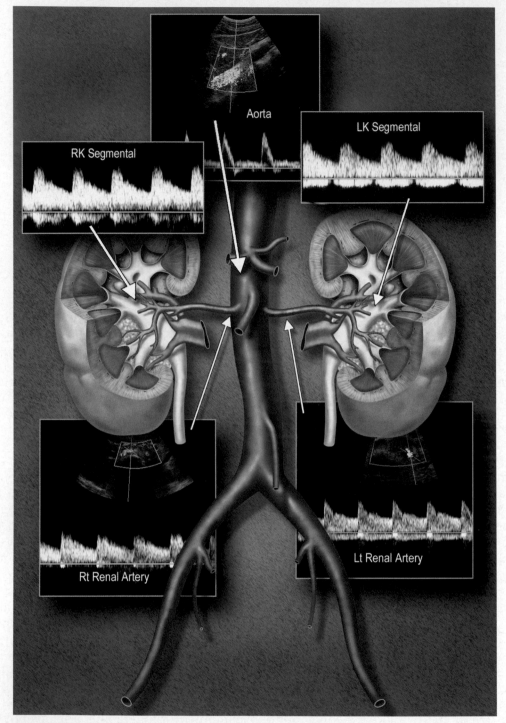

Figure 33–1. Renal artery anatomy with montage of normal Doppler waveforms. LK, left kidney; RK, right kidney.

patients with renal insufficiency. MRA also requires intravenous contrast injection and in addition is expensive and cannot be performed on claustrophobic patients. Computed tomographic angiography and MRA provide only anatomic information, but pressure measurements may be obtained with catheter arteriography. Compared with these modalities, Doppler sonography is inexpensive and noninvasive and does not require contrast material. Doppler examination also provides physiologic as well as anatomic information. Thus, Doppler can determine the hemodynamic significance of a lesion and can assess the need for intervention. Doppler examination also plays a complementary role to computed tomography and MRA and can clarify uncertain or indeterminate computed tomographic or magnetic resonance imaging diagnoses.

There are several key elements to a successful abdominal Doppler examination. Adequate patient preparation is important to reduce the amount of bowel gas, which produces scatter and attenuates the ultrasound beam. We recommend a 12-hour fast prior to examination. We prefer to schedule our renal Doppler studies in the morning, before patients have breakfast to improve visualization of the vascular structures. We do not give any medication prior to the study. The examination is performed on a modern ultrasound unit, offering adequate gray-scale imaging as well as sensitive color, power, and pulsed Doppler modalities. We routinely utilize harmonic imaging during our investigations to improve resolution and decrease artifacts. The technical success of each study is also influenced by the degree of operator experience. We have had tremendous success by training dedicated sonographers and sonologists in the techniques required to perform complete renal Doppler studies in a timely manner. The best examiners share several characteristics: motivation, patience, and commitment to succeed. The learning curve is variable, requiring months to a year of experience, depending on the volume of cases performed.

TECHNIQUE

Color flow imaging is an integral component of renal artery ultrasound examination. Color flow imaging is used to locate the renal arteries and detect flow disturbances that indicate stenosis. However, when used alone, this modality may give a false impression of renal artery stenosis, because atherosclerotic plaques can cause flow disturbances in vessels that are not significantly stenotic. Pulsed Doppler spectral analysis must be used in conjunction with color flow imaging, as it provides quantitative information through the measurement of blood flow velocity in areas of stenosis.

There are a number of technical shortcuts that increase the likelihood of identifying both renal arteries in their entirety and decreasing the time of the examination. The first step is to optimize the color and pulsed Doppler parameters so as to improve renal artery visualization as well as the conspicuity of flow-reducing lesions. Adjustment of the color Doppler parameters, including color gain, pulse repetition frequency (color velocity scale), and wall filter, is achieved in areas of laminar flow, in either the aorta or a normal segment of a renal artery. Proper color Doppler adjustment allows the examiner to "screen" the vessel quickly for stenosis, as elevated velocities in stenotic regions then produce a color aliasing artifact that is readily apparent. The examiner can then place the Doppler sample volume at the site of flow disturbance to determine the highest peak systolic velocity.

In addition to optimization of the color Doppler parameters, the experienced sonographer utilizes all available acoustic windows to obtain velocity information from the renal arteries. When possible, the renal arteries are visualized directly from an anterior abdominal approach, but this may not be feasible due to artifacts and attenuation from bowel gas or obesity. When the anterior abdominal approach fails, we utilize additional soft tissue windows to visualize the deep abdominal vessels. The patient is positioned in an oblique or decubitus position, and sound is transmitted to the renal arteries and aorta through the kidneys and liver. It is possible to obtain all the necessary color flow views and spectral Doppler samples from the renal arteries in the decubitus position.

The spectral Doppler examination is performed with a small sample volume so as to obtain flow information from only the vessel of interest. Pulsed Doppler sampling is performed with angles of 60 degrees or less. We never use angles of greater than 60 degrees, because this artifactually increases

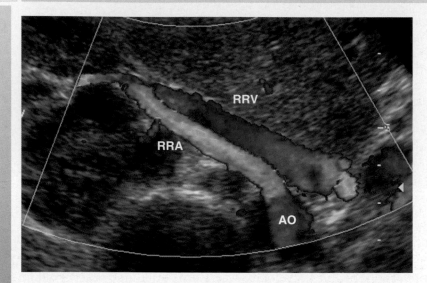

FIGURE **33–2.** Color Doppler image displays the entire right renal artery (RRA) from the aorta (AO) to the renal hilum. Note the anterior liver parenchyma serves as an acoustic window. RRV, right renal vein.

the peak systolic velocity measurement. The pulse repetition frequency (PRF) is adjusted so that the waveforms are large and easy to read but without causing aliasing.

The protocol for our renal artery Doppler examination includes complete evaluation of the kidneys. Left and right decubitus patient positions are preferred for the kidney examination (left decubitus for the right kidney and vice versa). We note the echogenicity and thickness of the renal parenchyma and measure the kidney length. We also assess the kidneys for atrophy, scarring, hydronephrosis, calculi, or masses. We identify occult renal cell carcinomas each year during renal Doppler examinations.

We next perform a longitudinal survey of the abdominal aorta from the celiac artery to the iliac bifurcation and evaluate the amount of atherosclerotic plaque. This is done with both gray-scale and color flow Doppler. Gray-scale evaluation is important to assess for irregular plaque and ostial lesions (i.e., at the origin of the aortic branches), which may be obscured by color flow blooming.* The presence of significant atherosclerotic plaque should increase the suspicion for possible ostial renal artery disease, particularly in elderly or diabetic

Blooming refers to the tendency of the color flow Doppler image to extend beyond the vascular lumen, obscuring adjacent structures, including atherosclerotic plaque and the vessel wall.

patients. Conversely, the absence of plaque in the aorta decreases the likelihood of atherosclerotic renal artery stenosis. We also look for flow abnormalities at the origin of the celiac and superior mesenteric arteries that indicate significant stenosis. The size and location of abdominal aortic aneurysms are noted. Finally, angle-corrected peak systolic velocity measurements are obtained from the abdominal aorta at the level of the renal arteries. These aortic velocity measurements are used to determine the renal artery–to–aorta velocity ratio, as discussed later.

Our protocol for the evaluation of renal arterial disease includes the direct examination of both renal arteries as well as sampling of the segmental branches in both renal hila. When possible, we locate the origin of the renal arteries on transverse images of the aorta using an anterior transducer approach.[17] We begin at the celiac axis or the superior mesenteric artery, because these are easily located, and move slightly caudad along the aorta until the origin of each renal artery is seen. The right renal artery is often easier to identify than the left and is relatively easy to follow to the renal hilum (Fig. 33–2). The left renal artery is harder to follow all the way to the kidney from an anterior approach. The distal portion of the left renal artery may be seen by positioning the patient in a *right* lateral decubitus position and scanning from a *left*

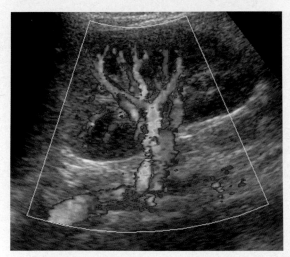

FIGURE 33–3. Color Doppler scan through the left kidney, obtained in the right lateral decubitus position, allows complete visualization of the left renal artery.

posterolateral transducer approach,[18] using the left kidney as an acoustic window (Fig. 33–3). An analogous approach can be used to visualize the distal right renal artery and its branches, with the patient in a *left* lateral decubitus position. In children, both renal arteries can sometimes be viewed simulta-neously from a coronal approach through the left kidney. Transverse and sagittal sweeps of the abdominal aorta and kidneys are performed to identify duplicate renal arteries. These arteries may arise from the inferior aorta or iliac arteries and can be followed to the renal hilum or either pole of the kidney (Fig. 33–4).

Each renal artery should be examined with color flow imaging from its origin to the hilum of the kidney, including the main hilar branches (if possible). Look for areas of high-velocity flow, indicated by color shifts or aliasing, as well as turbulence-related flow disturbances, as these may be related to stenosis (Fig. 33–5). Interrogate these areas with spectral Doppler analysis. If there are no areas of abnormal flow, obtain peak systolic velocity measurements from the origin, proximal, mid-, and distal segments of each renal artery. Finally, waveforms are also obtained from the segmental arteries in the upper, mid-, and lower poles of each kidney. Thus, at least seven waveforms are captured from each side. It is important to obtain clean, crisp waveforms with well-defined borders for analysis (Fig. 33–6). This

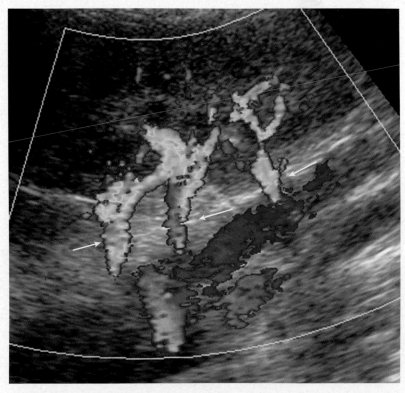

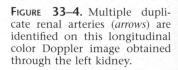

FIGURE 33–4. Multiple duplicate renal arteries (*arrows*) are identified on this longitudinal color Doppler image obtained through the left kidney.

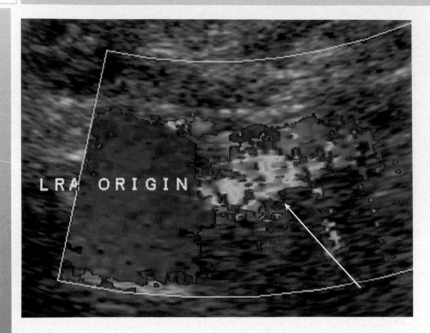

FIGURE 33–5. Focal color aliasing (*arrow*) represents high velocity flow at the site of stenosis at the origin of the left renal artery (LRA).

is accomplished by adjusting the spectral display so that the waveforms are large and easily measured.[19] This allows the examiner to readily determine the peak systolic velocity, acceleration time or index, and the resistive index (RI)* and facilitates side-to-side waveform comparison.

Our philosophy on renal artery duplex ultrasound examination is quite pragmatic. We limit the amount of time allotted for our renal Doppler studies. In our experience, a complete renal artery Doppler examination can be performed in as little as 20 minutes, with the examinations completed within 40 minutes. We never exceed 60 minutes. Experienced examiners can assess a patient pretty quickly and determine if the study can be completed in a timely manner. Studies on difficult patients who cannot cooperate or are not "sonogenic" are aborted promptly, and an alternative study is recommended for further evaluation. It is also important to recognize that atherosclerotic renal artery disease is far and away the most common etiology of significant renal artery stenosis, and these lesions occur at the origin and proximal segments of the renal artery. We pay close attention to these seg-

ments in our elderly patients who are apt to have atherosclerotic obstructive lesions.[10,14] In younger adults, it is more important to see the entire renal artery, as these patients are more likely to have fibromuscular hyperplasia, which can affect the distal renal artery or the segmental branches.[13,20]

The technical difficulties associated with renal artery examination may be eased substantially by the use of ultrasound contrast (echo-enhancing) agents, which greatly increases the visibility of blood vessels. In addition to reducing examination time, the use of these agents may enhance ultrasound visualization of multiple renal arteries and hilar branches. Ultrasound contrast agents are already approved in the United States for echocardiography and should be approved by the Food and Drug Administration for abdominal Doppler studies concurrent with the publication of this textbook. Please see Chapter 4 for further details.

VASCULAR DISORDERS

Renal Artery Stenosis

Stenosis, or occlusion of a main renal artery or an accessory renal artery, may cause renal ischemia, which in turn triggers the renin-angiotensin mechanism and causes hypertension. Renal artery stenosis can also cause

---

*This parameter is not used for diagnosis of renal artery stenosis, but pulsatility may be elevated in parenchymal renal disease and urinary tract obstruction. The RI may also play a role in predicting response to revascularization.

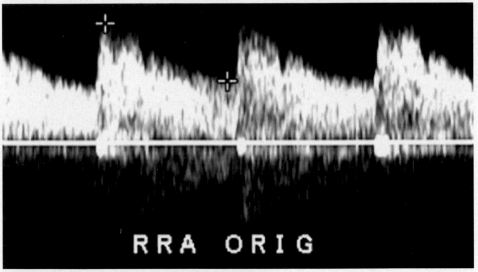

RRA ORIG

A

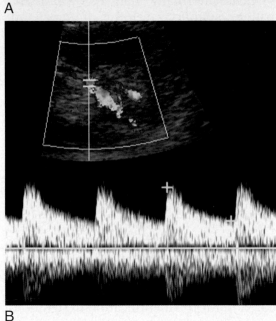

B

FIGURE 33–6. *A*, Normal Doppler waveform obtained at the origin of the right renal artery (RRA ORIG) demonstrates a low resistance flow pattern with a rapid systolic upstroke. *B*, Waveforms obtained from a segmental artery branch, at the renal hilum, demonstrate normal waveform shape and acceleration.

or contribute to renal insufficiency by inducing renal parenchymal damage. The threshold level of renal artery stenosis that produces hypertension or ischemic damage is uncertain and probably varies from one patient to another. From a hemodynamic perspective, renal artery obstruction is considered hemodynamically significant (or flow reducing) when the lumen diameter is narrowed by 50% to 60%.

It is estimated that 10% of the United States population has hypertension, and 3% to 5% of this group has renal arterial disease.[1,21] Although the latter percentages are small, renal artery disease represents the most common *correctable* cause of hypertension.[21] More recently, clinical interest has focused on the potential role of renal ischemia in the etiology of chronic renal insufficiency.[22,23] Once again, the potential correctability of renal artery stenosis has been stressed. Few kidney diseases can be cured, and it is understandable that clinicians should be keenly interested in a potentially curable disorder such as renal artery stenosis. Does this mean, however, that we should seek to diagnose renal artery disease in every patient with hypertension or renal insufficiency? To do so could be expensive and not cost-effective.[24] Furthermore, intervention for renal artery disease may be risky (e.g., arterial occlusion or rupture) and is not always successful. Considering these points, we believe that renal artery stenosis should be sought in the following selected groups of patients: (1) young patients with severe hypertension; (2) patients with rapidly accelerating hypertension or malignant hypertension; (3) patients with hypertension that is difficult to control despite a suitable treatment program; (4) patients with concomitant hypertension and deteriorating renal function; and (5) patients with renal insufficiency and discrepant kidney size (inferring renal artery stenosis).[1,21–24]

Doppler Renal Artery Evaluation

As noted previously, color flow imaging is used to identify flow abnormalities that *may* be stenosis related, but spectral Doppler measurements provide quantitative data that are essential for determining the severity of stenosis.[1–51] The following general comments about Doppler diagnosis of renal artery stenosis are noteworthy:

1. The principal ultrasound criterion for renal artery stenosis is Doppler-detected flow velocity elevation in the stenotic portion of the vessel.[1,13,14,16,20,29,30] Flow velocity is increased in proportion to the severity of luminal narrowing; therefore, spectral Doppler measurements can be used to approximate stenosis severity. Narrowed areas detected with color flow imaging must be carefully surveyed with the Doppler sample volume to ensure that the maximum flow velocity is identified.

2. Accurate assignment of the Doppler angle is essential for reliable measurement of stenosis-related velocity elevation, and a Doppler-to-vessel angle of 60 degrees or less is mandatory to ensure that velocity information is accurate.

3. Major stenoses are accompanied by post-stenotic flow disturbance (turbulence). Although disturbed flow is a useful beacon for the presence of stenosis, it is neither quantitative nor specific. Disturbed flow may occur without significant stenosis.

4. Arterial waveforms within the kidney (segmental or interlobar arteries) may be scrutinized for evidence of damping, which is a downstream manifestation of renal artery stenosis. The most important downstream findings are the absence of an early systolic peak, a prolonged systolic acceleration time, or a reduced acceleration index.[6,19,29,31–35]

Diagnostic Criteria

Blood flow in the renal artery and its branches normally has a low-resistance pattern; systolic waveforms are broad, and forward flow is present throughout diastole. The peak systolic velocity in normal renal arteries ranges from 74 to 127 cm/sec in both adults and children.[17,20,36,37] Numerous Doppler velocity criteria have been used in attempts to diagnose hemodynamically significant renal artery stenosis (defined generally as $\geq 50\%$ to 60% diameter reduction).* The most universally accepted Doppler criteria are (1) peak systolic velocity in the stenosis of 180 to 200 cm/sec or greater and (2) a renal/aortic ratio (RAR) exceeding 3.3 or 3.5.[1–3,10–12,16,20] The latter is the ratio of peak systole in the stenotic portion of the renal artery divided by peak systole in the aorta at the renal artery level (Fig. 33–7). The renal/aortic ratio has become our primary criterion for the identification of significant renal artery stenosis. In theory, the renal/aortic ratio compensates for hemodynamic variability between patients. Younger patients tend to have higher normal peak systolic velocity flow in the aorta and branch vessels that can exceed 180 cm/sec without stenosis. Elderly patients, particularly patients with severe cardiac disease and poor cardiac output, may demonstrate lower peak systolic velocities, even in regions of stenosis. Some authors have found peak systolic velocity measurements, used alone, to be more accurate than the renal/aortic ratio.[3] Doppler assessment of the renal arteries is

*See references 1–5, 13, 15, 17, 19, 21, 32, 34, 35, 38–43

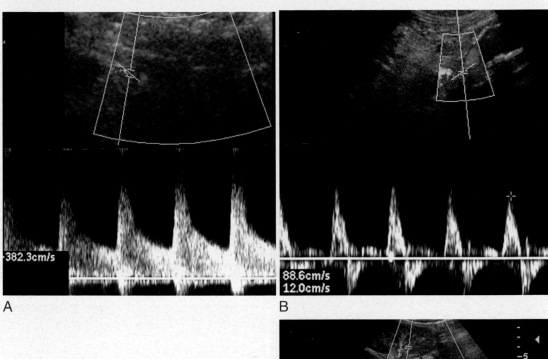

FIGURE 33–7. *A*, Renal artery stenosis. Pulsed Doppler interrogation of the right renal artery, at the site of color aliasing, reveals elevated peak systolic velocities. (PSV = 382.3 cm/sec.) *B*, Pulsed Doppler sampling of the aorta, at the level of the renal arteries, reveals a peak systolic velocity of 88.6 cm/sec. The renal-aortic ratio = 4.3, consistent with significant renal artery stenosis. *C*, Renal hilar sampling reveals characteristic damping ("tardus parvus") of the segmental artery waveform. Note the absence of the early systolic peak, rounded contour and prolonged systolic acceleration time. (LP, lower pole; RK, right kidney, SEG, segmental artery).

also valuable following revascularization with angioplasty, bypass, or stent placement. Measurement of renal artery peak systolic velocity is used to assess residual or recurrent stenosis after therapy. There is a reduction in peak systolic velocity in the stenotic region following successful angioplasty and stent placement. Hilar waveforms will also return to normal appearance after successful treatment (Fig. 33–8).

Damping of *intrarenal* arterial signals is also a valuable criterion for diagnosis of renal artery stenosis. Damping is defined numerically with the acceleration index or the acceleration time. Both of these measures reflect the rate of systolic acceleration,

which is slower than normal, downstream from a hemodynamically significant stenosis. An acceleration index less than 300 cm/sec or an acceleration time exceeding 0.07 second is considered abnormal and suggests a 60% or greater renal artery stenosis.[1,2,6,14,19,31,34,43] Some authors use an acceleration time of 0.10 or 0.12 second as the cutoff for significant stenosis, which increases specificity.[1,2,43]

It has been suggested that the downstream effects of renal artery stenosis can be diagnosed merely by visual inspection of the shape of the segmental or interlobar Doppler waveforms.[19,29,43] Either the initial systolic peak is absent or the systolic peak is

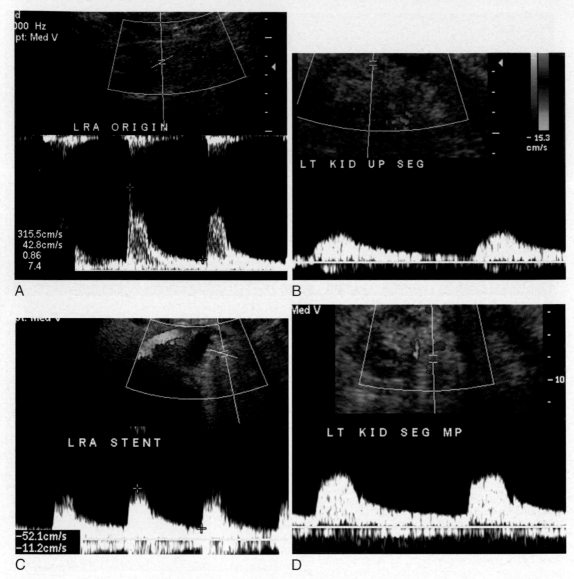

FIGURE 33–8. *A,* Elevated velocities are detected at the origin of the left renal artery (LRA ORIG) consistent with significant stenosis in this patient with hypertension. *B,* Typical tardus waveforms (delayed upstroke and rounded contour) are obtained from the left upper pole segmental artery in the left kidney (LT KID UP SEG). *C,* Following renal artery stent placement, peak systolic velocities in the left renal artery (LRA) return to the normal range. (PSV = 52.1 cm/sec.) *D,* Pulsed Doppler waveforms obtained from the left midpole segmental artery demonstrate a return to normal appearance with normal upstroke (acceleration) and waveform shape. (LT KID, left kidney; MP, midpole; SEG, segmental artery).

grossly rounded in patients with severe ipsilateral stenosis, as illustrated in Figures 33–7 and 33–8. However, the diagnostic accuracy of hilar waveform evaluation has been questioned, as discussed later.

Reported Results

Wide ranges of sensitivity (0%–98%) and specificity (37%–99%) have been reported

for *direct* duplex detection of renal artery stenosis, based on either an elevated systolic velocity in the renal artery or an abnormal renal/aortic ratio.[1,11,12,14,19,30,32,38–41,44–46] The disparate results of these studies are a reflection of selection bias, examiner experience, and statistical methods. For instance, several of the more successful studies were potentially biased because most or all of their patients were elderly individuals who, for the most part, have atherosclerotic stenoses at the renal artery origins. Because the origins of the renal arteries are the portions most easily visualized with ultrasound, greater accuracy may be expected in this population than in younger individuals who may have more distal renal artery disease.[10–12,16] In addition, some studies included only successful Doppler examinations in statistical tabulation, whereas other studies included all examinations, regardless of the level of success or experience.

Despite the spread of reported results, it appears that *direct* duplex examination of the renal arteries is reasonably effective for diagnosis of clinically significant renal artery stenosis. With experience and good technique, the examiner is likely to attain sensitivity and specificity levels for adult patients in the vicinity of 90% for 60% or greater (diameter) stenosis in the proximal 4 cm (or so) of the main renal arteries. Diagnostic accuracy for distal renal artery and segmental branch lesions may not be as good as that for more proximal stenoses, as discussed later.

Duplicate Artery Problems

In hypertensive patients, the documentation or exclusion of renovascular etiology requires the assessment of the main renal artery, whether single or duplicate, and segmental arteries in the renal hilum. We use the term *duplicate main renal arteries* in reference to arteries that enter the renal hilum and supply segmental branches. Stenoses in duplicated main renal arteries can clearly cause hypertension and possibly renal insufficiency, in contrast to stenoses in small polar accessory arteries that are thought to rarely cause hypertension and are probably not a significant cause of renal insufficiency.[1,4,6–8,17] In medical literature reports, duplicate main renal arteries and polar accessory arteries are frequently called *accessory renal arteries*, which we feel is unfortunate, as they probably have considerably different importance from a clinical perspective.

Angiographic studies show that 12% to 22% of kidneys are supplied by more than one renal artery. Kliewer and associates[5] found that 15% of kidneys had double main renal arteries, and 13% had accessory arteries (usually at the poles of the kidney). Accessory arteries usually arise from the aorta but may also arise from the iliac arteries.

Unfortunately, the detection rate for multiple renal arteries with duplex ultrasound (including color flow imaging) seems to be quite poor. Hélénon and colleagues[13] reported detecting 30% of duplicate renal arteries with ultrasound, but they did not say whether these were double main renal arteries or polar arteries. They failed to detect 25% of main renal arteries, which apparently included some duplicate arteries. Melany and coworkers[15] visualized several duplicate main renal arteries with ultrasound contrast enhancement but failed to see three polar accessory arteries. In the literature reports of which we are aware, there is no clear indication of how reliably ultrasound visualizes duplicate main renal arteries, but there is some evidence that failure to detect these arteries adversely affects ultrasound accuracy.[2–5,9,11–13] In the study by Hansen and associates,[11] duplex ultrasound sensitivity for 60% (diameter) stenosis was 98% for single main renal arteries but only 67% for all renal arteries, including duplicate vessels.

It appears that polar accessory renal arteries rarely cause hypertension or significant ischemia; hence, one could argue that their visualization is unimportant. Duplicated main renal arteries, however, can be repaired, and their detection *is* clinically significant. The following scenario is easily envisioned: A normal renal artery is seen sonographically, but a second stenotic renal artery, the actual source of renal ischemia and hypertension, is overlooked. This limitation of sonography should be kept in mind, and a diligent search should be made for duplicate main renal arteries.

Segmental Branch Problems

As noted previously, atherosclerotic obstruction tends to occur at or near the origin of the main renal arteries and is detected quite easily with color flow sonography. Fibro-muscular hyperplasia, however, can occur at any location from the origin of the vessel to the hilar segmental branches and may involve multiple branches. Statistical details are limited, but our experience and others suggest that duplex results are poorer for segmental branch stenoses than they are for the main renal artery.[5,13,20] For instance, Hélénon and colleagues[13] reported a sensitivity level of only 60% for hilar branch stenoses, and Kliewer and associates[5] reported missing three branch vessel stenoses with duplex examination. Stenoses in hilar branch vessels can be repaired with angioplasty,[47] so their detection in hypertensive patients is important. For this reason, we advise careful assessment of younger hypertensive patients who might have fibromuscular hyperplasia, and the use of angiographic procedures when hilar branch visualization is suboptimal.[2–8,13]

Intrarenal Waveform Assessment

An ideal survey method for renal artery stenosis would be accurate, quick, and easy. This is the appeal of *indirect* diagnosis of renal artery stenosis through the detection of damped Doppler waveforms in segmental or interlobar arteries within the kidney. For an experienced sonographer, the acquisition of intrarenal arterial Doppler signals is relatively easy, and, therefore, the examination is brief and successful in most individuals.

It has long been recognized that renal artery stenosis can cause pulsus tardus and parvus changes in intrarenal arterial flow signals.[48,49] It would be very convenient to simply look for these flow changes in the kidneys and thereby diagnose renal artery stenosis without the arduous task of finding and directly evaluating the renal arteries. Unfortunately, the accuracy of this diagnostic method is questionable. Several literature reports (based on acceleration time, acceleration index, and waveform shape changes) were promising, with sensitivity ranging from 89% to 95% and specificity ranging from 83% to 97% for main renal artery stenoses exceeding 60% or 70% diam-

eter reduction.[2,19,31,34] But other literature reports, based on the same Doppler parameters, indicate poor results ranging from moderate accuracy to complete absence of correlation between Doppler and angiographic findings.[5,6,13,29,33,44,50] Because of these unfavorable results, this technique for diagnosis of renal artery stenosis has been largely abandoned as the sole diagnostic measure.

The question, then, is why doesn't intrarenal Doppler work? To begin with, it appears that intrarenal waveform findings are more accurate for high-grade renal artery stenoses exceeding 70% diameter reduction,[2,5,33] but even at high levels of stenosis, some patients do not have appreciable waveform damping. This is because the shape of intrarenal arterial waveforms is affected by multiple factors, including the stiffness (compliance) of the arteries, the resistance of the microcirculation, and inflow phenomena, such as renal artery stenosis.[50,51] In a patient with generalized arterial stiffness and/or high resistance in the microvasculature from parenchymal renal disease (e.g., diabetes-related nephropathy), the damping effects of a main renal artery stenosis may be obliterated (Fig. 33–9). To make matters worse, damped intrarenal waveforms can occasionally be seen in the absence of significant renal artery stenosis in patients with aortic stenosis or aortic occlusion.

Because intrarenal Doppler waveform analysis has not been consistently accurate, we do not recommend the exclusive use of hilar waveform analysis for the diagnosis of renal artery stenosis. However, we do not ignore intra-arterial waveform findings either. We evaluate acceleration and waveform shape in intrarenal arteries in conjunction with direct renal artery interrogation. The detection of abnormal waveforms, when present, confirms the hemodynamic significance of a main renal artery stenosis. Furthermore, damped intrarenal arterial signals may indicate occult stenosis or occlusion in the main renal artery, a duplicated renal artery, or a segmental artery. This is a particularly important finding when the direct examination is technically limited.

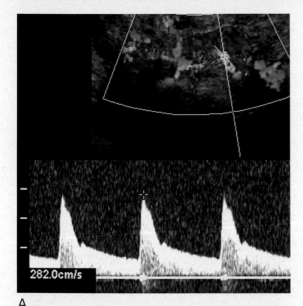

A

B

FIGURE 33–9. *A,*Elevated velocities (PSV = 282 cm/sec) are identified in the left renal artery consistent with significant stenosis, confirmed with magnetic resonance angiography. *B,* Hilar waveforms obtained from the left kidney are normal in appearance. This is a false-negative finding obtained by indirect arterial sampling.

zation. Radermacher and colleagues[52] found that a renal RI greater than 0.8 reliably identifies patients with renal artery stenosis that are not likely to respond to revascularization. In their series of 5950 patients with hypertension, an RI greater than 0.8 before therapy was a strong predictor of worsening renal function and a lack of improvement in blood pressure, despite correction of renal artery stenosis. Elevation of the RI results from accentuated microvasculature resistance, which in turn indicates the presence of generalized renal parenchymal disease, as discussed later.

Doppler Waveform Abnormalities in Nonvascular Renal Disease

Flow resistance within the renal parenchyma may be increased by a variety of pathologic processes, including urinary tract obstruction and a host of acute and chronic parenchymal disorders, including renal vein obstruction, glomerulosclerosis, acute tubular necrosis, and pyelonephritis.[53,54] All of these conditions are associated with increased flow resistance in the microvasculature of the kidney, which causes the Doppler waveforms to exhibit *increased pulsatility.* This may be evident on visual inspection of waveforms or through pulsatility measures such as the pulsatility index or RI. In normal kidneys, a large amount of diastolic blood flow is evident on visual inspection of the intrarenal Doppler signals, and the RI in segmental or intralobar arteries does not exceed 0.7.

An increase in vascular resistance (and pulsatility) in renal pathology is an interesting finding, but it is of limited diagnostic value because it is multifactorial in origin. Increased pulsatility is of greatest diagnostic value when it is seen unilaterally, for in such cases, it implies an acute process such as urinary tract obstruction or renal vein obstruction on the side with high pulsatility. High pulsatility may be apparent before significant urinary tract dilation occurs.[53,54]

Although the RI, as measured in intrarenal arteries, is not reliable for diagnosing renal artery stenosis, for reasons given previously, it appears to have value in predicting the outcome of renal revasculari-

Renal Artery Occlusion

Renal artery occlusion is diagnosed on the basis of the following findings: (1) absence of a visible main renal artery; (2) markedly reduced kidney size (smaller than 9 cm in length); and (3) either absence of detectable intrarenal blood flow or very-low-amplitude, damped intrarenal flow signals.[1,3,10,16]

Diagnostic accuracy for renal artery occlusion is predicated on reasonable color flow and spectral Doppler sensitivity at the level of the renal artery or kidney. That is, flow should be readily detected in other vessels at a similar depth or in the contralateral kidney before it is concluded that a renal artery is occluded. Although relatively few data exist in the medical literature, it appears that duplex diagnosis of renal artery occlusion is reasonably accurate. Thirty-eight of 41 occluded arteries were correctly diagnosed in three published series, for an overall accuracy rate of 93%.[3,10,16]

False-positive diagnosis of renal artery occlusion can occur when visualization of the main renal artery is poor or the kidney is small for reasons other than arterial occlusion. False-negative results are caused by collateralization, which may occur via capsular or adrenal branches, and duplicate renal arteries. In the collateralized kidney, flow signals may well be present in the kidney parenchyma or in the renal hilum despite renal artery occlusion. Doppler waveforms may even be normal in the kidney in some cases, although tardus parvus waveforms are typically seen.

Renal Vein Thrombosis

Renal vein thrombosis appears to be an underdiagnosed vascular disease because of the nonspecificity of clinical and radiographic findings.[55-57] Acute renal vein thrombosis usually presents with pain and hematuria, and it may occasionally cause thromboembolic complications, such as pulmonary embolism. Chronic renal vein thrombosis may be asymptomatic or may present with the nephrotic syndrome, hematuria, or renal failure.

The renal vein may be blocked by intraluminal tumor or thrombus formation or by extrinsic compression (possibly accompanied by secondary venous thrombosis). Associated or predisposing conditions include preexisting renal disease, renal cell carcinoma, hypercoagulable state, vena caval or ovarian vein thrombus (with extension to the renal veins), abdominal surgery, trauma, and dehydration. Primary renal disease is the most common predisposing factor, particularly the nephrotic syndrome and membranous glomerulonephritis.[57] Extrinsic retroperitoneal causes of renal vein thrombosis include acute pancreatitis, lymph node enlargement from a host of tumors, and retroperitoneal fibrosis. These conditions generally cause extrinsic compression of the vascular pedicle, predisposing to thrombosis.[55]

Renal vein thrombosis typically induces ischemic parenchymal damage in the kidney and acute renal failure.[55-57] The long-term effects of renal vein thrombosis are varied. The potential exists for recanalization of the renal vein or the development of venous collaterals, and, in some cases, the kidney returns to a normal sonographic appearance. If the kidney is severely damaged, however, chronic changes become evident, including diminished kidney size and increased echogenicity (secondary to fibrosis).

The most easily detected ultrasound findings in *acute* renal vein occlusion[58-65] are kidney enlargement and altered parenchymal echogenicity, both of which are caused by parenchymal edema and in some cases by hemorrhage. Changes in echogenicity may include the following: (1) hypoechoic cortex with decreased corticomedullary differentiation, (2) hyperechoic cortex with preservation of corticomedullary differentiation, and (3) mottled heterogeneity accompanied by the loss of normal intrarenal architecture. In some cases, echogenic linear streaks of unknown origin course through the renal parenchyma. These streaks are thought to be pathognomonic for renal vein thrombosis.[60,61]

Kidney enlargement and altered parenchymal echogenicity are nonspecific findings, and the conclusive diagnosis of renal vein thrombosis depends on the direct identification of thrombus in the renal vein. With acute thrombosis, the renal vein is invariably enlarged, and Doppler signals are absent. A small trickle of flow may be present around the clot, and this may produce low-velocity, continuous Doppler signals (lacking respirophasic variation). Recently formed thrombus is hypoechoic and in some cases appears anechoic. As a result, the thrombus may not be readily seen with gray-scale sonography and is detectable only with color flow imaging (Fig. 33–10). Two additional pitfalls are noteworthy. First, venous flow may be present within the kidney itself, even though the renal vein is occluded, because large hilar collaterals may develop quickly. Second, very sluggish renal vein flow (as a result of more proximal obstruction or congestion) may mimic thrombosis, because the Doppler signal may be difficult to detect at very slow flow rates.

Renal Vein Tumor Extension

Tumor extension into the renal vein is most commonly associated with renal cell carcinoma, although renal lymphoma, transitional cell carcinoma, and Wilms' tumor can also propagate along the renal veins. Venous invasion is common in renal cell carcinoma, with gross involvement of the main renal vein occurring in 21% to 35% of patients with large tumors and inferior vena cava tumor extension in 5% to 10% of patients.[64,65] Vena caval invasion is approximately three times more common in right-sided tumors than those on the left because of the shorter length of the right renal vein.[64,65] Preoperative diagnosis of venous tumor extension significantly influences surgical therapy. If no tumor is present, routine ligation of the renal vein may be performed through a flank incision, but if the renal vein is occluded by tumor and if the tumor extends into the IVC, a midline incision often is used, which may be extended cephalad to create a sternotomy if necessary.[65]

Contrast-enhanced computed tomography is the preferred method of investigation for intravenous tumor extension, supplemented when necessary with magnetic resonance imaging or sonography. The latter modality has cost and convenience advantages over magnetic resonance imaging and can often answer directed questions, such as the superior extent of the tumor within the IVC. Duplex sonography is not as accurate as computed tomography or magnetic resonance imaging for de novo detection of tumor extension into the renal vein, particularly on the left side where the vein is frequently obscured by bowel gas.[66–72] If the renal vein and IVC are well visualized, sonographic accuracy is high (96% sensitivity, 100% specificity), but renal vein visualization is inadequate in 34% to 54% of patients, and the IVC is inadequately seen in 4% to 21% of cases.[67,70] Thus, the overall sensitivity of ultrasound for venous tumor extension may be as low as 18% for the renal veins and 33% for the IVC.[58]

As seen with ultrasound, renal vein tumor[53,54,68–72] is typically homogeneous and is low or intermediate in echogenicity. The tumor-containing renal vein is almost always distended to a distinctly abnormal size, and even the IVC may be distended when a tumor is present. Differentiation between intravenous tumor and thrombus is accomplished through color flow detection of small blood vessels within the tumor.

RENAL ALLOGRAFTS

The term *allograft* refers to any tissue transplanted from one human to another. The proper term for the transplanted kidney, therefore, is *renal allograft*. The allograft may be harvested (removed) from a living, related donor or from a brain-dead donor. The term *cadaveric renal allograft* is used in the latter circumstance, even though the donor's heart continues to function at the time the kidney is removed.

The renal allograft is almost always placed in the right or left iliac fossa of the recipient. Usually, the allograft is extraperitoneal (between the peritoneum and the iliacus muscle). In a child, the allograft may be placed intraperitoneally if it is too large for

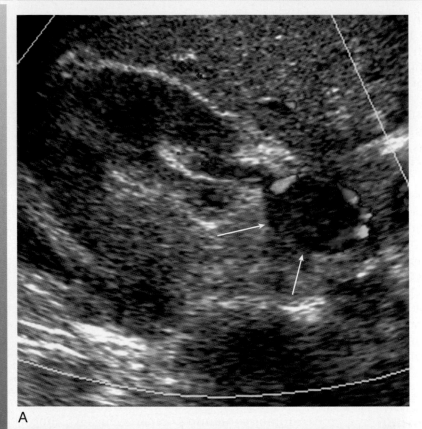

A

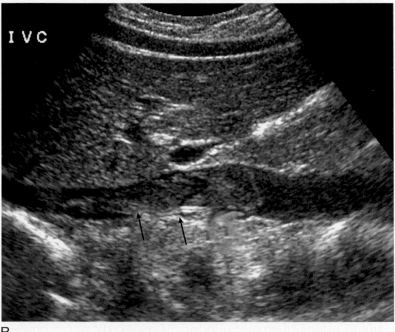

B

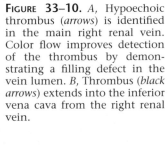

FIGURE 33–10. *A*, Hypoechoic thrombus (*arrows*) is identified in the main right renal vein. Color flow improves detection of the thrombus by demonstrating a filling defect in the vein lumen. *B*, Thrombus (*black arrows*) extends into the inferior vena cava from the right renal vein.

extraperitoneal transplantation. The allograft ureter is passed through an oblique tunnel in the muscular layer of the bladder, forming a nonrefluxing ureterovesical junction. The allograft artery is attached in one of three ways[73]: (1) The end of the allograft artery is attached to the side of the external iliac artery (end to side); (2) the end of the allograft artery is attached to the end of an internal iliac branch (end to end); or (3) for duplicated renal arteries or for a small renal artery from a child, a patch of the donor aorta containing the arterial orifice (Carrell's patch) is attached to an opening made in the external iliac artery. The renal vein anastomosis, in almost all cases, is end to side, with the cut end of the allograft vein attached to the side of the external iliac vein.

The native kidneys of the allograft recipient are usually left in place, but they are occasionally removed for a variety of reasons, including chronic or recurrent infection. Native kidneys are subject to the development of cysts and neoplasms in long-term dialysis patients, but these lesions do not result from renal transplantation per se.

Renal allografts are subject to a variety of complications including acute tubular necrosis (in the early postoperative period), acute rejection, chronic rejection, infection, ureteral obstruction, ureteral reflex, vascular obstruction, and extrarenal fluid collections.[73–129]

Technical Considerations

Renal allografts are usually quite superficial in location, which necessitates the use of high-frequency linear array or curved array transducers. These transducers provide a broad field of view and good near-field image quality. From an ultrasound perspective, a transplanted kidney looks like a native kidney, with several minor exceptions.[48,49] First, anatomic detail is often clearer than in native kidneys because of the superficial location of the allograft. Second, the cortex may appear more echogenic than that of a normotopic kidney because of the lack of ultrasound attenuation by overlying

structures. Third, the allograft usually enlarges over a period of several months following transplantation, and such enlargement should not be mistakenly attributed to rejection. In adults, the volume of the allograft typically increases up to 30%,[49,81] but this increase may be as great as 200% if a kidney from a young (and relatively small) donor is transplanted into a much larger recipient.[85] Finally, slight dilation of the allograft collecting system is a common finding, particularly in the postoperative period. In most instances, such dilation is not of urodynamic importance.

The sonographic diagnosis of allograft pathology is aided by a baseline scan conducted within the first 2 days after surgery. This scan represents an important standard against which later changes may be compared. Typically, a second scan is obtained at 1 to 2 weeks after transplantation, and a third scan is obtained at about 3 months.

Allograft Rejection and Acute Tubular Necrosis

Renal allograft rejection may produce a host of sonographic abnormalities, as listed in Table 33–1.[73,75–91] The most common and important manifestations of allograft rejection are (1) increased size of the graft (best appreciated through volume measurements), (2) increased cortical echogenicity, and (3) increased size or conspicuity of the renal pyramids.[79,84,88,91] Additional

---

Table 33–1. Sonographic Manifestations of Renal Allograft Rejection

Increased allograft size (volume)

Increased cortical echogenicity (cellular infiltration)

Increased prominence of the renal pyramids*

Focal cortical hypoechoic regions (edema, necrosis)

Decreased echogenicity of the renal sinus (edema)

Increased flow resistance in parenchymal arteries

*Due to increased pyramid size and increased contrast between the hypoechoic pyramids and the echogenic cortex.

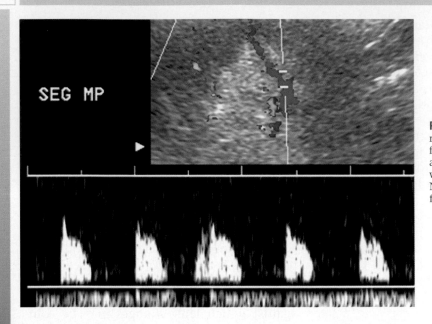

FIGURE 33–11. Abnormal high-resistance waveforms obtained from the midpole segmental artery (SEG MP) in this patient with renal transplant rejection. Note the absence of diastolic flow.

important features of acute rejection are peripheral hypoechoic zones and diminished sinus echogenicity, but these are seen only in cases of severe rejection.[75,77,79,82,84,91]

Doppler waveform abnormalities that indicate high peripheral arterial resistance (see Fig. 33–11) also occur in renal transplant rejection. These flow abnormalities are evident in the segmental, interlobar, or arcuate arteries of the allograft, in both acute and chronic rejection.[92–112] As summarized in Table 33–2, the waveform changes associated with rejection include (1) absence of flow throughout diastole, (2) flow reversal in diastole, (3) a resistivity index* that equals or exceeds 0.7, and (4) a pulsatility index[†] that equals or exceeds 1.8.[92–94,96–99,102–109] (Specificity for rejection is increased by using a resistivity index of 0.9 or greater.)

In contrast to allograft rejection, postsurgical acute tubular necrosis, resulting from ischemia, does not generally alter the B-mode appearance of the renal allografts or the Doppler flow characteristics. However, increased cortical echogenicity and increased arterial pulsatility result from severe post-transplant acute tubular necrosis.

*The RI is the peak systolic velocity minus the end-diastolic velocity, divided by the peak systolic velocity.
[†]The pulsatility index is the peak systolic velocity minus the lowest diastole velocity (including reversed flow), divided by the mean velocity.

Accuracy for Rejection and Acute Tubular Necrosis

Initially, it was hoped that sonography could be used to diagnose renal allograft rejection noninvasively and to differentiate between rejection and acute tubular necrosis in the postoperative period.[75–77,79,80,92,95,96] These hopes have faded with time, for experience has shown that sonography is neither sensitive nor specific for allograft rejection.[74,83,86–91,93,96–106,110,128] To optimize specificity (to avoid false-positive diagnosis), *rejection should not be diagnosed sonographically unless several rejection-related abnormalities are present.*[81,83,84,88,91] Unfortunately, this requirement reduces the sensitivity for rejection to 70% or less. To make matters worse, sonographic changes seen with cyclosporine toxicity mimic those seen with rejection.[87,97,101,112] (Cyclosporine is

---

Table 33–2. Doppler Features of Allograft Rejection

High-resistance waveform appearance
   Sharp, narrow systolic peaks
   Second systolic peak higher than first
   Minimal or absent diastolic flow
   Flow reversal early in diastole
Pulsatility index ≥1.8
Resistivity index ≥0.7

a commonly used immunosuppressant drug.)

In our opinion, ultrasound findings are most useful in cases of *severe* acute rejection. In such instances, the kidney is grossly enlarged, the pyramids are prominent, the renal sinus fat is hypoechoic, arterial flow resistance is elevated, and hypoechoic areas may be present in the renal cortex. Ultrasound findings may not be very helpful when rejection is mild or moderate in severity. Although sonography may play a limited role for the evaluation of renal transplant rejection, it is particularly useful for the detection of other complications—particularly hydronephrosis and fluid collections.

Allograft Hydronephrosis

As noted previously, mild allograft hydronephrosis may occur normally during the first or second week after renal transplantation and probably results from postoperative edema at the insertion site of the ureter into the bladder. In some cases, mild hydronephrosis persists indefinitely, for no apparent reason. This finding is insignificant as long as urine output is good, renal function is satisfactory, and the degree of dilation remains constant or regresses. The urodynamic significance of hydronephrosis may be evaluated with the Whitaker test,[101] scintigraphy, or pyelography in patients with abnormal renal function.

Moderate or severe hydronephrosis is a more disturbing finding, particularly if the degree of hydronephrosis increases over time. Functionally significant hydronephrosis in the immediate postoperative period usually results from edema at the ureterovesical junction or surgical complications. Hydronephrosis appearing later is generally due to one of the following problems: (1) scarring at the ureterovesical junction, (2) obstructing debris (blood clots or fungal mycelia) within the ureter, (3) ureteral compression by extrinsic fluid collections, (4) bladder-emptying disorders, and (5) vesicoureteral reflux. Sonographic findings cannot differentiate among many of these causes.

Perigraft Fluid

Fluid collections are quite common after renal transplantation.[114-117] In the immediate postoperative period, a small volume of serous fluid (seroma) commonly accumulates adjacent to the allograft or in the operative wound, and this fluid should not be viewed with alarm as long as it does not increase in volume over time. Moderate to large collections are generally pathologic, regardless of when they appear, and these usually require further investigation with percutaneous aspiration or other means. The differential possibilities for perigraft fluid collections include serous fluid (seroma), blood (hematoma), pus (abscess), urine (urinoma), and lymph (lymphocele). Ultrasound does not accurately differentiate among these collections in all cases, but an educated guess can be made by considering four factors: the time of appearance, symptoms, the location, and the sonographic appearance. These aspects of allograft-related fluid collections are outlined in Table 33–3.

Vascular Complications

The role of sonography in renal transplantation that is most germane to this text concerns the diagnosis of vascular problems.[115,118-129] We believe that color flow examination should be a routine component of renal allograft sonography, because such examination is relatively easy and yields valuable information. It is possible, in many cases, to trace the allograft vessels in their entirety, from the iliac anastomoses to the kidney,[128] and this should be the goal of the vascular examination, in addition to the assessment of arterial pulsatility, as discussed previously.

Vascular complications of renal allografts fall into four broad categories: arterial stenosis, vascular occlusion, arteriovenous fistula, and pseudoaneurysm.

Arterial Stenosis

The most common vascular complication of renal transplantation (about 10% of

Table 33–3. Diagnostic Features of Perigraft Fluid Collections

Collection	Clinical Features	Sonographic Features
Seroma and hematoma	Asymptomatic; immediate postoperative period	Anechoic or mixed echogenicity; adjacent to kidney or in wound; irregular shape; regresses in days or weeks
Abscess	Fever, leukocytosis, pain; may be relatively asymptomatic because of immunosuppression; often postoperative but may be later (weeks to months)	May be perinephric, in the parenchyma, or in the wound; usually well defined; contents anechoic to echogenic
Urinoma	Pain, decreased renal output, fever; virtually always in immediate postoperative period	Anechoic, often large, sometimes loculated; location variable; resembles lymphocele but too early; scintigraphy is diagnostic
Lymphocele	Asymptomatic or pain; may obstruct ureter by extrinsic compression; typically 1–2 mo or later after surgery, rarely earlier; attributed to interrupted allograft lymphatics	Classically multilocular with thin septae and anechoic fluid; may be unilocular; classically located medially between the allograft lower pole and the bladder

transplant patients) is arterial stenosis.[119] Typically, stenosis occurs within 3 years of transplantation and is heralded by hypertension.* Short-segment stenosis at the allograft artery origin that occurs early after transplantation is almost always a surgical complication. On occasion, however, such a stenosis results from allograft artery rejection. Long-segment, distal stenosis of the allograft artery is a later complication that usually results from intimal hyperplasia or scarring but may also result from rejection. In some cases, multiple distal stenoses are present. Stenosis of the recipient iliac artery is uncommon and almost invariably results from surgical injury.

The Doppler hallmark of renal artery stenosis is increased flow velocity in the stenotic segment, coupled with poststenotic disturbed flow (Fig. 33–12). Arterial waveforms may be damped distal to very severe stenoses, but distal waveforms alone cannot be relied on to diagnose or exclude renal artery stenosis.[128] The quantification of allograft stenosis has not been worked out in any detail, but a few diagnostic parameters are available, as listed in Table 33–4.[118–123,128]

*In approximately 80% of cases, post-transplantation hypertension is caused by conditions other than renal artery stenosis.[62]

Vascular Occlusion

Occlusion (thrombosis) of the allograft renal artery is an unusual complication (<1% of renal transplants)[119] that typically occurs acutely in the postoperative period and is related to either rejection or technical factors. Arterial occlusion is readily detected with color flow and Doppler ultrasound, because arterial and venous flow is absent in the allograft.[119,120]

Occlusion (thrombosis) of the allograft vein is also a rare complication (<1% of cases) that occurs primarily in the immediate post-transplant period.[107] The kidney

Table 33–4. Diagnostic Criteria of Allograft Renal Arteries

Normal flow parameters
1. Velocity: 80–118 cm/sec
2. Volume flow: 346–422 mL/min

Parameters for stenosis exceeding 50% or 60% decrease in diameter
1. Systolic velocity > 190 cm/sec (+ poststenotic disturbed flow)
2. Systolic velocity ≥ 250 cm/sec, highly specific
3. Systolic velocity ratio* > 3 (+ post-stenotic disturbed flow)

*Ratio of stenotic zone peak systolic velocity to external iliac artery peak systolic velocity.

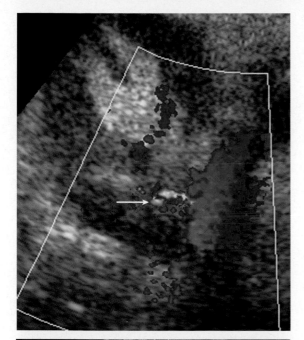

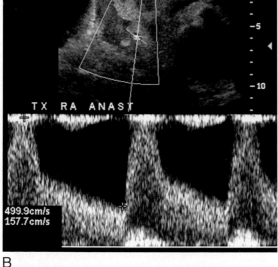

B

FIGURE 33-12. *A*, Color Doppler reveals focal aliasing (*arrow*) at the origin of the transplant renal artery, consistent with elevated velocities at the renal artery anastomosis with the external iliac artery. *B*, Pulsed Doppler interrogation of the transplant renal artery reveals a PSV = 500 cm/sec consistent with severe stenosis at the arterial anastomosis (TX RA ANAST).

is enlarged because of congestion, and the renal parenchyma typically has a non-homogeneous appearance. Flow is absent in the renal vein, which may be visibly distended with thrombus. A characteristic feature of renal vein thrombosis is a peculiar *renal artery* waveform pattern

consisting of sustained flow *reversal* in diastole.[119,124]

Arteriovenous Fistula

Fistula formation between an artery and a vein may occur within the renal allograft as a result of biopsy trauma.[119,125,126] Many such parenchymal fistulae are asymptomatic, but others are associated with sustained hypertension. Color flow sonography readily detects arteriovenous fistulae, because markedly disturbed flow within the fistula stands out like a beacon within the renal parenchyma. Additional findings are high-velocity flow in the artery that feeds the fistula, and a color flash artifact, called a *color bruit,* in the parenchyma adjacent to the fistula.

Pseudoaneurysm

Most pseudoaneurysms in renal allografts occur within the renal parenchyma and result from arterial laceration during renal biopsy.[119,126] These false aneurysms are represented on gray-scale images as well-defined, focal anechoic areas that are indistinguishable from renal cysts. Color flow sonography shows blood flow in the pseudoaneurysm, confirming the diagnosis. In some cases, a characteristic high-velocity jet or to-and-fro flow pattern is visible in the aneurysm neck. Pseudoaneurysms may also occur at the renal artery–iliac artery anastomosis, but these are uncommon.[119]

Acknowledgments. We would like to thank Saiedeh "Nanaz" Maghoul for her expertise and enthusiasm and James Cooper, MD, for his wonderful illustrations.

References

1. Dawson DL: Noninvasive assessment of renal artery stenosis. Semin Vasc Surg 9:172–181, 1996.
2. Baxter GM, Aitchison F, Sheppard D, et al: Colour Doppler ultrasound in renal artery stenosis: Intrarenal waveform analysis. Br J Radiol 69:810–815, 1996.

3. Miralles M, Cairols M, Cotillas J, et al: Value of Doppler parameters in the diagnosis of renal artery stenosis. J Vasc Surg 23:428–435, 1996.

4. Berland LL, Koslin DB, Routh WD, Keller FS: Renal artery stenosis: Prospective evaluation of diagnosis with color duplex US compared with angiography: Work in progress. Radiology 174:421–423, 1990.

5. Kliewer MA, Tupler RH, Hertzberg BS, et al: Doppler evaluation of renal artery stenosis: Interobserver agreement in the interpretation of waveform morphology. Am J Roentgenol 162:1371–1376, 1994.

6. Kliewer MA, Hertzberg BS, Keogan MT, et al: Early systole in the healthy kidney: Variability of Doppler US waveform parameters. Radiology 205:109–113, 1997.

7. Bakker J, Beek FJA, Beutler JJ, et al: Renal artery stenosis and accessory renal arteries: Accuracy of detection and visualization with gadolinium-enhanced breath-hold MR angiography. Radiology 207:487–504, 1998.

8. De Cobelli F, Vanzulli A, Sironi S, et al: Renal artery stenosis: Evaluation with breath-hold, three-dimensional, dynamic, gadolinium-enhanced versus three-dimensional, phase-contrast MR angiography. Radiology 205:689–695, 1997.

9. Strotzer M, Fellner CM, Geissler A, et al: Noninvasive assessment of renal artery stenosis: A comparison of MR angiography, color Doppler sonography, and intraarterial angiography. Acta Radiol 36:243–247, 1995.

10. Hoffmann U, Edwards JM, Carter S, et al: Role of duplex scanning for the detection of atherosclerotic renal artery disease. Kidney Int 39:1232–1239, 1991.

11. Hansen KJ, Tribble RW, Reavis S, et al: Renal duplex sonography: Evaluation of clinical utility. J Vasc Surg 12:227–236, 1990.

12. Kohler TR, Zierler RE, Martin RL, et al: Noninvasive diagnosis of renal artery stenosis by ultrasonic duplex scanning. J Vasc Surg 4:450–456, 1986.

13. Hélénon O, Rody FE, Correas JM, et al: Color Doppler US of renovascular disease in native kidneys. Radiographics 15:833–854, 1995.

14. Middleton WD: Doppler US evaluation of renal artery stenosis: Past, present, and future. Radiology 184:307–308, 1992.

15. Melany ML, Grant EG, Duerinckx AJ, et al: Ability of a phase shift US contrast agent to improve imaging of the main renal arteries. Radiology 205: 147–152, 1997.

16. Olin JW, Piedmonte MR, Young JR, et al: The utility of duplex ultrasound scanning of the renal arteries for diagnosing significant renal artery stenosis. Ann Intern Med 122:833–838, 1995.

17. Strandness DE Jr: Duplex scanning in diagnosis of renovascular hypertension. Surg Clin North Am 70:109–117, 1990.

18. Isikoff MB, Hill MC: Sonography of the renal arteries: Left lateral decubitus position. Am J Roentgenol 134:1177–1179, 1980.

19. Stavros AT, Parker SH, Yakes WF, et al: Segmental stenosis of the renal artery: Pattern recognition of tardus and parvus abnormalities with duplex sonography. Radiology 184:487–492, 1992.

20. Brun P, Kchouk H, Mouchet B, et al: Value of Doppler ultrasound for the diagnosis of renal artery stenosis in children. Pediatr Nephrol 11:27–30, 1997.

21. Aristizabal D, Frohlich ED: Hypertension due to renal arterial disease. Heart Dis Stroke 1:227–234, 1992.

22. Wilcox CS: Ischemic nephropathy: Noninvasive testing. Semin Nephrol 16:43–52, 1996.

23. Meyrier A: Renal vascular lesions in the elderly: Nephrosclerosis or atheromatous renal disease? Nephrol Dial Transplant 11(suppl 9):45–52, 1996.

24. Blaufox MD, Middleton ML, Bongiovanni J, et al: Cost efficacy of the diagnosis and therapy of renovascular hypertension. J Nucl Med 37:171–177, 1996.

25. Silverman JM, Friedman ML, Van Allan RJ: Detection of main renal artery stenosis using phase-contrast cine MR angiography. Am J Roentgenol 166:1131–1137, 1996.

26. Rubin GD, Walker PJ, Dake MD, et al: Three-dimensional spiral computed tomographic angiography: An alternative imaging modality for the abdominal aorta and its branches. J Vasc Surg 18:656–665, 1993.

27. Loubeyre P, Revel D, Garcia P, et al: Screening patients for renal artery stenosis: Value of three-dimensional time-of-flight MR angiography. Am J Roentgenol 162:847–852, 1994.

28. Nally JV, Black HR: State-of-the-art review: Captopril renography–pathophysiological considerations and clinical observations. Semin Nucl Med 22:85–97, 1992.

29. Postma CT, Bijlstra PJ, Rosenbusch G, Thien T: Pattern recognition of loss of early systolic peak by Doppler ultrasound has a low sensitivity for the detection of renal artery stenosis. J Hum Hypertens 10:181–184, 1996.

30. Pederson EB, Egeblad M, Jorgensen J, et al: Diagnosing renal artery stenosis: A comparison between conventional renography, captopril renography and ultrasound Doppler in a large consecutive series of patients with arterial hypertension. Blood Press 5:342–348, 1996.

31. Nazzal MM, Hoballah JJ, Miller EV, et al: Renal hilar Doppler analysis is of value in the management of patients with renovascular disease. Am J Surg 174:164–168, 1997.
32. Handa N, Fukanaga R, Ogawa S, et al: A new accurate and non-invasive screening method for renovascular hypertension: The renal artery Doppler technique. J Hypertens (Suppl) 6:458–460, 1988.
33. Kliewer MA, Tupler RH, Carroll BA, et al: Renal artery stenosis: Analysis of Doppler waveform parameters and tardus-parvus pattern. Radiology 189:779–787, 1993.
34. Patriquin HB, LaFortune M, Jéquier J-C, et al: Stenosis of the renal artery: Assessment of slowed systole in the downstream circulation with Doppler sonography. Radiology 184:470–485, 1992.
35. LaFortune M, Patriquin HB, Demeule E, et al: Renal arterial stenosis: Slowed systole in the downstream circulation—experimental study in dogs. Radiology 184:475–478, 1992.
36. Stanley JC: Renal vascular disease and renovascular hypertension in children. Urol Clin North Am 11:451–463, 1984.
37. Strandness DE Jr: Duplex Scanning in Vascular Disorders. New York, Lippincott-Raven, 1990, p 240.
38. Greene ER, Venters MD, Avasthi PS, et al: Non-invasive characterization of renal artery blood flow. Kidney Int 20:523–529, 1981.
39. Taylor DC, Kettler MD, Moneta GL, et al: Duplex ultrasound scanning in the diagnosis of renal artery stenosis: A prospective evaluation. J Vasc Surg 7:363–369, 1988.
40. Avasthi PS, Voyles WF, Greene ER: Noninvasive diagnosis of renal artery stenosis by echo-Doppler velocimetry. Kidney Int 25:824–829, 1984.
41. Dubbins PA: Renal artery stenosis: Duplex Doppler evaluation. Br J Radiol 59:225–229, 1986.
42. Reid JH, Mackay S, Lantz BMT: Noninvasive blood flow measurements by Doppler ultrasound with applications to renal artery flow determination. Invest Radiol 15:323–331, 1980.
43. Isaacson JA, Neumyer MM: Direct and indirect renal arterial duplex and Doppler color flow evaluations. J Vasc Technol 19:309–316, 1995.
44. Isaacson JA, Zierler RE, Spittell PC, Strandness DE: Noninvasive screening for renal artery stenosis: Comparison of renal artery and renal hilar duplex scanning. J Vasc Technol 19:105–110, 1995.
45. Norris CS, Pfeiffer JS, Rittgers SE, Barnes RW: Noninvasive evaluation of renal artery stenosis and renovascular resistance. J Vasc Surg 1:192–201, 1984.
46. Rittgers SE, Norris CS, Barnes RW: Detection of renal artery stenosis: Experimental and clinical analysis of velocity waveforms. Ultrasound Med Biol 11:523–531, 1985.
47. Fujitani RM, Murray SP: Surgical methods for renal revascularization. Semin Vasc Surg 9:198–217, 1996.
48. Handa N, Fukunaga R, Etani H, et al: Efficacy of echo-Doppler examination for the evaluation of renovascular disease. Ultrasound Med Biol 14:1–5, 1988.
49. Nichols BT, Rittgers SE, Norris CS, Barnes RW: Non-invasive detection of renal artery stenosis. Bruit 8:26–29, 1984.
50. van der Hulst VPM, van Baalen J, Kool LS, et al: Renal artery stenosis: Endovascular flow wire study for validation of Doppler US. Radiology 100:165–168, 1996.
51. Bude RO, Rubin JM, Platt JF, et al: Pulsus tardus: Its cause and potential limitations in detection of arterial stenosis. Radiology 190:779–784, 1994.
52. Radermacher J, Chavan A, Bleck J, et al: Use of Doppler ultrasonography to predict the outcome of therapy for renal artery stenosis. N Engl J Med 344:410–417, 2001.
53. Platt JF, Rubin JM, Ellis JH, DiPietro MA: Duplex Doppler US of the kidney: Differentiation of obstructive from nonobstructive dilatation. Radiology 171:515–517, 1989.
54. Platt JF, Ellis JH, Rubin JM, et al: Intrarenal arterial Doppler sonography in patients with nonobstructive renal disease: Correlation of resistive index with biopsy findings. Am J Roentgenol 154:1223–1227, 1990.
55. Keating MA, Althausen AF: The clinical spectrum of renal vein thrombosis. J Urol 133:938–945, 1985.
56. Clark RA, Wyatt GM, Colley D: Renal vein thrombosis: An underdiagnosed complication of multiple renal abnormalities. Radiology 132:43–50, 1979.
57. Llach F, Papper S, Massry SG: The clinical spectrum of renal vein thrombosis: Acute and chronic. Am J Med 69:819–827, 1980.
58. Rosenberg ER, Traught WS, Kirks DR, et al: Ultrasonic diagnosis of renal vein thrombosis in neonates. Am J Roentgenol 134:35–38, 1980.
59. Paling MR, Wakefield JA, Watson LR: Sonography of experimental acute renal vein occlusion. J Clin Ultrasound 13:647–653, 1985.
60. Metreweli C, Pearson R: Echographic diagnosis of neonatal renal venous thrombosis. Pediatr Radiol 14:105–108, 1984.
61. Lalmand B, Avni EF, Nasr A, et al: Perinatal renal vein thrombosis. J Ultrasound Med 9:437–442, 1990.
62. Rosenfield AT, Zeman RK, Cronan JJ, Taylor KJW: Ultrasound in experimental and clinical

renal vein thrombosis. Radiology 137:735–741, 1980.

63. Taylor KJW, Burns PN: Duplex Doppler scanning in the pelvis and abdomen. Ultrasound Med Biol 11:643–658, 1985.

64. Goncharenko V, Gerlock AJ Jr, Kadir S, Turner B: Incidence and distribution of venous extension in 70 hypernephromas. Am J Roentgenol 133:263–265, 1979.

65. Levine E: Malignant renal parenchymal tumors in adults. In Pollack HM (ed): Clinical Urography: An Atlas and Textbook of Urological Imaging. Philadelphia, WB Saunders, 1990, pp 1216–1291.

66. Goldstein HM, Green B, Weaver RM Jr: Ultrasonic detection of renal tumor extension into the inferior vena cava. Am J Roentgenol 130:1083–1085, 1978.

67. Schwerk WB, Schwerk WN, Rodeck G: Venous renal tumor extension: A prospective US evaluation. Radiology 156:491–495, 1985.

68. Didier D, Racle A, Etievent JP, Weill F: Tumor thrombus of the inferior vena cava secondary to malignant abdominal neoplasms: US and CT evaluation. Radiology 162:83–89, 1987.

69. Dubbins PA, Wells I: Renal carcinoma: Duplex Doppler evaluation. Br J Radiol 59:231–236, 1986.

70. London NJM, Messios N, Kinder RB, et al: A prospective study of the value of conventional CT, dynamic CT, ultrasonography and arteriography for staging renal carcinoma. Br J Urol 64:209–217, 1989.

71. Roubidoux MA, Dunnick NR, Sostman HD, Leder RA: Renal carcinoma: Detection of venous extension with gradient-echo MR imaging. Radiology 182:269–272, 1992.

72. Thomas JL, Bernardino ME: Neoplastic-induced renal vein enlargement: Sonographic detection. Am J Roentgenol 136:75–79, 1981.

73. Pozniak MA, Kelcz F, Dodd GD: Renal transplant ultrasound: Imaging and Doppler. Semin Ultrasound CT MR 12:319–334, 1991.

74. Lachance SL, Adamson D, Barry JM: Ultrasonically determined kidney transplant hypertrophy. J Urol 139:497–498, 1988.

75. Hillman BJ, Birnholz JC, Busch GJ: Correlation of echographic and histologic findings in suspected renal allograft rejection. Radiology 132:673–676, 1979.

76. Maklad NF, Wright CH, Rosenthal SJ: Gray scale ultrasonic appearances of renal transplant rejection. Radiology 131:711–717, 1979.

77. Hricak H, Toledo-Pereyra LH, Eyler WR, et al: The role of ultrasound in the diagnosis of kidney allograft rejection. Radiology 132:667–672, 1979.

78. Bricak H, Toledo-Pereyra LH, Eyler WR, et al: Evaluation of acute post-transplant renal failure by ultrasound. Radiology 133:443–447, 1979.

79. Singh A, Cohen WN: Renal allograft rejection: Sonography and scintigraphy. Am J Roentgenol 135:73–77, 1980.

80. Frick MP, Feinberg SB, Sibley R, Idstrom ME: Ultrasound in acute renal transplant rejection. Radiology 138:657–660, 1981.

81. Hricak H, Cruz C, Eyler WR, et al: Acute post-transplantation renal failure: Differential diagnosis by ultrasound. Radiology 139:441–449, 1981.

82. Hricak H, Romanski RN, Eyler WR: The renal sinus during allograft rejection: Sonographic and histopathologic findings. Radiology 142:693–699, 1982.

83. Fried AM, Woodring JH, Loh FK, et al: The medullary pyramid index: An objective assessment of prominence in renal transplant rejection. Radiology 149:787–791, 1983.

84. Slovis TL, Babcock DS, Hricak H, et al: Renal transplant rejection: Sonographic evaluation in children. Radiology 153:659–665, 1984.

85. Babcock DS, Slovis TL, Han BK, et al: Renal transplants in children: Long-term follow-up using sonography. Radiology 156:165–167, 1985.

86. Rosenfield AT, Zeman RK, Cicchetti DV, Siegel NJ: Experimental acute tubular necrosis: US appearance. Radiology 157:771–774, 1985.

87. Linkowski GD, Warvariv V, Filly RA, Vincenti F: Sonography in the diagnosis of acute renal allograft rejection and cyclosporine nephrotoxicity. Am J Roentgenol 148:291–295, 1987.

88. Swobodnik WL, Spohn BE, Wechsler JG, et al: Real-time ultrasound evaluation of renal transplant failure during the early postoperative period. Ultrasound Med Biol 12:97–105, 1986.

89. Hoddick W, Filly RA, Backman U, et al: Renal allograft rejection: US evaluation. Radiology 161:469–473, 1986.

90. Hricak H, Terrier F, Marotti M, et al: Post-transplant renal rejection: Comparison of quantitative scintigraphy, US, and MR imaging. Radiology 162:685–688, 1987.

91. Cochlin DL, Wake A, Salaman JR, Griffin PJA: Ultrasound changes in the transplant kidney. Clin Radiol 39:373–376, 1988.

92. Rifkin MD, Needleman L, Pasto ME, et al: Evaluation of renal transplant rejection by duplex Doppler examination: Value of the resistive index. Am J Roentgenol 148:759–762, 1987.

93. Taylor KJW, Morse SS, Rigsby CM, et al: Vascular complications in renal allografts: Detection with duplex Doppler US. Radiology 162:31–38, 1987.

94. Rigsby CM, Burns PN, Welton GG, et al: Doppler signal quantification in renal allografts: Comparison in normal and rejecting transplants with pathologic correlation. Radiology 162:39–42, 1987.

95. Sternberg HV, Nelson RC, Murphy FB, et al: Renal allograft rejection: Evaluation by Doppler US and MR imaging. Radiology 162:337–342, 1987.

96. Taylor KJW, Marks WH: Use of Doppler imaging for evaluation of dysfunction in renal allografts. Am J Roentgenol 155:536–537, 1990.

97. Grant EG, Perrella RR: Wishing won't make it so: Duplex sonography in the evaluation of renal transplant dysfunction. Am J Roentgenol 155:538–539, 1990.

98. Rigsby CM, Burns PN, Weltin GG, et al: Doppler signal quantification in renal allografts: Comparison in normal and rejecting transplants, with pathologic correlation. Radiology 162:39–42, 1987.

99. Genkins SM, Sanfilippo FP, Carroll BA: Duplex Doppler sonography of renal transplants: Lack of sensitivity and specificity in establishing pathologic diagnosis. Am J Roentgenol 152:535–539, 1989.

100. Waltzer WC, Shabtai M, Anaise D, Rapaport FT: Usefulness and limitations of Doppler ultrasonography in the evaluation of postoperative renal allograft dysfunction. Transplant Proc 21:1901–1902, 1989.

101. Ward RE, Bartlett ST, Koenig JO, et al: The use of duplex scanning in evaluation of the posttransplant kidney. Transplant Proc 21:1912–1916, 1989.

102. Allen KS, Jorkasky DK, Arger PH, et al: Renal allografts: Prospective analysis of Doppler sonography. Radiology 169:371–376, 1988.

103. Harris DCH, Allen AR, Gruenewald S, et al: Doppler assessment in renal transplantation. Transplant Proc 21:1895–1896, 1989.

104. Townsend RR, Tomlanovich SJ, Goldstein RB, Filly RA: Combined Doppler and morphologic sonographic evaluation of renal transplant rejection. J Ultrasound Med 9:199–206, 1990.

105. Drake DG, Day DL, Letourneau JG, et al: Doppler evaluation of renal transplants in children: A prospective analysis with histopathologic correlation. Am J Roentgenol 154:785–787, 1990.

106. Perchik JE, Baumgartner BR, Bernardino ME: Renal transplant rejection: Limited value of duplex Doppler sonography. Invest Radiol 26:422–426, 1991.

107. Kelcz F, Pozniak MA, Pirsch JD, Oberly TD: Pyramidal appearance and resistive index: Insensitive and nonspecific sonographic indicators of renal transplant rejection. Am J Roentgenol 155:531–535, 1990.

108. Schwaighofer B, Kainberger F, Fruehwald F, et al: Duplex sonography of normal renal allografts. Acta Radiol 30:53–56, 1989.

109. Don S, Kopechy KK, Filo RS, et al: Duplex Doppler US of renal allografts: Causes of elevated resistive index. Radiology 171:709–712, 1989.

110. Warshauer DM, Taylor KJW, Bia MJ, et al: Unusual causes of increased vascular impedance in renal transplants: Duplex Doppler evaluation. Radiology 169:367–370, 1988.

111. Pozniak MA, Kelcz F, Stratta RJ, Oberley TD: Extraneous factors affecting resistive index. Invest Radiol 23:899–904, 1988.

112. Pozniak MA, Kelcz F, D'Alessandro A, et al: Sonography of renal transplants in dogs: The effect of acute tubular necrosis, cyclosporine nephrotoxicity, and acute rejection on resistive index and renal length. Am J Roentgenol 158:791–797, 1992.

113. Jaffe RB, Middleton AW Jr: Whitaker test: Differentiation of obstructive from nonobstructive uropathy. Am J Roentgenol 134:9–15, 1980.

114. Siler TM, Campbell D, Wicks JD, et al: Peritransplant fluid collections. Radiology 138:145–151, 1981.

115. Coyne SS, Walsh JW, Tisnado WH, et al: Surgically correctable renal transplant complications: An integrated clinical and radiologic approach. Am J Roentgenol 136:1113–1119, 1981.

116. Hildell J, Aspelin P, Nyman U, et al: Ultrasonography in complications of renal transplantation. Acta Radiol Diag 25:299–304, 1984.

117. Surratt JT, Siegel MJ, Middleton WD: Sonography of complications in pediatric renal allografts. Radiographics 10:687–699, 1990.

118. McGee GS, Peterson-Kennedy L, Astleford P, Yao JST: Duplex assessment of the renal transplant. Surg Clin North Am 70:133–141, 1990.

119. Dodd GD, Tublin ME, Shah A, Zajko AB: Imaging of vascular complications associated with renal transplants. Am J Roentgenol 157:449–459, 1991.

120. Grenier N, Douws C, Morel D, et al: Detection of vascular complications in renal allografts with color Doppler flow imaging. Radiology 178:217–223, 1991.

121. Guzzo JA, Kupinski AM, Stone MP, et al: Evaluation of renal allograft blood flow rates by duplex ultrasonography. J Vasc Technol 14:232–234, 1990.

122. Snider JF, Hunter DW, Moradian GP, et al: Transplant renal artery stenosis: Evaluation with duplex sonography. Radiology 172:1027–1030, 1989.

123. Stringer DA, O'Halpin D, Daneman A, et al: Duplex Doppler sonography for renal artery

stenosis in the post-transplant pediatric patient. Pediatr Radiol 19:187–192, 1989.

124. Reuther G, Wanjura D, Bauer H: Acute renal vein thrombosis in renal allografts: Detection with duplex Doppler US. Radiology 170:557–558, 1989.

125. Middleton WD, Kellman GM, Melson GL, Madrazo BL: Postbiopsy renal transplant arteriovenous fistulas: Color Doppler US characteristics. Radiology 171:253–257, 1989.

126. Hübsch PJS, Mostbeck G, Barton PP, et al: Evaluation of arteriovenous fistulas and pseudoaneurysms in renal allografts following percutaneous needle biopsy: Color-coded Doppler sonography versus duplex Doppler sonography. J Ultrasound Med 9:95–100, 1990.

127. MacLennan AC, Baxter GM, Harden P, Rowe PA: Renal transplant vein occlusion: An early diagnostic sign? Clin Radiol 50:251–253, 1995.

128. Baxter GM, Ireland H, Moss JG, et al: Colour Doppler ultrasound in renal transplant artery stenosis: Which Doppler index? Clin Radiol 50:618–622, 1995.

129. Hilborn MD, Bude RO, Murphy KJ, et al: Renal transplant evaluation with power Doppler sonography. Br J Radiol 70:39–42, 1997.

Chapter 34

Duplex Ultrasound Evaluation of the Uterus and Ovaries

John S. Pellerito, MD

Duplex and color Doppler imaging have become a routine part of the ultrasound evaluation of the female pelvis.[1] These techniques are utilized for both the transabdominal and endovaginal examinations. The combination of Doppler ultrasound with endovaginal scanning is particularly valuable for gynecologic investigations because there is improved resolution and increased sensitivity to blood flow. I use the term *endovaginal color flow Doppler imaging* (EVCF) to describe this pairing of techniques.[2] In our department, we utilize Doppler ultrasound in a number of different applications, including:

1. Identification of the dominant follicle or corpus luteal cyst in patients with pelvic pain or suspected ectopic pregnancy
2. Detection of placental tissue in abnormal intrauterine pregnancy, ectopic pregnancy, and retained products of conception
3. Diagnosis of ovarian torsion
4. Characterization of ovarian and adnexal masses
5. Detection of a number of uterine abnormalities, including fibroids, polyps, and tumors, as well as vascular abnormalities such as arteriovenous malformation and the pelvic congestion syndrome

Endovaginal color flow Doppler imaging offers several advantages over endovaginal scans without Doppler. Integration of Doppler signal information into the sonographic analysis allows for tissue characterization and recognition of normal and abnormal flow patterns and may eliminate the need for computed tomographic or magnetic resonance imaging correlation in many cases. EVCF also improves the detection of flow compared with transabdominal scans with color Doppler. The endovaginal probe is closer to the areas of interest, so there is enhanced detection of vessel patency and tissue vascularity. This is extremely helpful in cases when the demonstration of blood flow is critical to the diagnosis (i.e., ovarian torsion).

TECHNICAL ISSUES

Because the technical aspects of color flow imaging are covered in Chapter 3, this chapter emphasizes just the key points relative to pelvic sonography. Similar to other color and pulsed Doppler examinations, Doppler evaluation of the uterus and ovaries should be considered a dynamic process, requiring adjustment of the color flow parameters according to the type of examination. Using the manufacturer's settings (presets) is a good starting point for any examination. They serve as a general guide and can be adjusted to improve visualization of blood flow. Presets are helpful to novice or beginner sonographers and sonologists, particularly when the demonstration of color flow is suboptimal but critical for diagnosis.

It is important to remember that color, power, and pulsed Doppler images are based on the same physical principles but display different information.[3] Color Doppler images are based on the mean velocity display of reflected frequency shifts. In other words, the frequencies reflected from the moving red blood cells are averaged over time and presented on the image. Color Doppler displays a range of velocities on the image but does not provide absolute or peak systolic velocity information. Pulsed Doppler is used to determine the peak velocity at a particular location.

Power (Amplitude) Doppler images are determined by the strength or amplitude of the returning Doppler shifts.[4] The frequency shifts are amplified and displayed along with the gray-scale information. Power Doppler provides three to five times increased sensitivity to blood flow, compared with color flow imaging. There is less dependence on the angle of insonation, so flow can be demonstrated at angles close to 90 degrees. Thus, very weak Doppler shifts are presented on the power Doppler image. Advantages of power Doppler include improved vascular detail, faster localization of blood flow for pulsed Doppler sampling, and assessment of global tissue perfusion.

Power Doppler images do not demonstrate color aliasing or direction of flow. This is not a significant limitation, as determination of flow direction or aliasing is achieved with color flow or pulsed Doppler sampling. Power Doppler is also susceptible to the same pitfalls associated with incorrect color flow settings as with color Doppler imaging. In general, there are three parameters that should always be checked to ensure optimal color and power Doppler imaging:

1. Color velocity range or pulse repetition frequency (PRF)
2. Color gain
3. Wall filter

These settings should be adjusted to improve the detection of color flow for each study, as they are fundamental to the detection of low-flow states.[3] To detect low-velocity flow, we decrease the PRF, increase the color gain, and/or decrease the wall filter settings. When flow velocities are high and we want to reduce the degree of color noise or aliasing in the image, we increase the PRF or color velocity scale, decrease color gain, and/or increase the wall filter. Experience and practice with different parameter settings will increase understanding of the interrelationships between these settings and lead to improved detection of flow. As always, the focal zone should be placed near the region of interest.

Most studies are performed with transducers in the 2.5- to 5-Mhz range for transabdominal studies. Endovaginal scans utilize probes in the 5- to 10-Mhz range. For pulsed Doppler evaluation, angle correction is performed when the direction of flow can be ascertained. We use no angle correction (0 degrees) for tiny or tortuous vessels when the direction of flow cannot be determined. A small sample volume is important for spectral analysis to avoid obtaining signals from multiple sources.

NORMAL ANATOMY AND HEMODYNAMICS

A thorough sonographic evaluation of the uterus and ovaries is usually performed prior to Doppler assessment of blood flow. We usually begin our evaluation with the uterus and then turn our attention to the adnexa and evaluation of the ovaries. The uterus is a pear-shaped, midline structure that is usually easy to identify (Fig. 34–1). Measurements of the length, width, and anteroposterior diameter of the uterus should be obtained. We also evaluate the thickness of the endometrium and the cervix and the presence and location of any uterine masses. The ovaries are variable in shape and location. Although the ovaries can be identified with either transabdominal or endovaginal scanning, a combination of techniques may be necessary for complete evaluation. The ovaries are also measured in three dimensions. The presence of cysts or masses is noted and correlated with the menstrual cycle.

Color and pulsed Doppler examination requires knowledge of the vascular anatomy and hemodynamic changes of the female pelvis. The vessels most frequently examined in the pelvis include the iliac, uterine, and ovarian arteries and veins (see Fig. 34–1).[5] These vessels may be identified with both transabdominal and endovaginal imaging. EVCF affords improved resolution and vascular detail compared with the transabdominal approach.

The uterine artery is a branch of the internal iliac artery and penetrates the uterus at the lower uterine segment (see Fig. 34–1B). Uterine artery branches course toward the uterine fundus and cervix as well as toward the ovaries in the broad ligament. Color and pulsed Doppler sampling of the uterine artery reveals high-impedance, low diastolic flow in the nongravid state.[5] A characteristic diastolic "notch" is usually noted (Fig. 34–2). Identification of the notch is helpful in characterizing waveforms found in the uterus and adnexa as originating from the uterine artery. There is a gradual decrease in resistance to flow in the spectral samples obtained from the uterine arteries during the second trimester of pregnancy. The decrease in resistance and resistive index is related to increased blood flow necessary for normal placental and fetal growth. Continuous low-resistance blood flow should be detected in the placenta and umbilical arteries supplying the fetus.

Each ovary receives a dual blood supply, as shown in Figure 34–1A. The ovarian artery originates from the abdominal aorta and descends to the pelvis. The ovary also receives branches from the uterine artery that course along the broad ligament. Flow patterns observed during color and pulsed Doppler sampling of the ovary vary depending on the phase of the ovulatory cycle. Low-velocity, high-impedance waveforms are usually noted early in menses into the follicular phase (Fig. 34–3). This is seen during the first menstrual week when the ovaries are dormant and before the formation of the dominant follicle and corpus luteal cyst.[6]

The luteal phase coincides with the extrusion of the mature egg or oocyte and formation of the corpus luteal cyst. Thickening of the cyst walls is seen with gray-scale imaging. Color Doppler demonstrates a ring of vascularity ("ring of fire" pattern) around the luteal cyst, related to formation of tiny vessels in the walls of the cyst.[7] Pulsed Doppler shows a marked increase in peak systolic and end-diastolic velocities (Fig. 34–4). The increased velocities are related to neovascularization of the corpus luteum, required for oocyte maturation and hormonal activity.[8]

We originally described the "ring of fire" color flow pattern to represent the increased vascularity noted around the periphery of an extrauterine gestational sac.[9] Subsequently, it became very clear that a similar pattern of peripheral blood flow occurs with the formation of a corpus luteal cyst. In fact, we look for the ring of increased vascularity in the ovary to locate and characterize luteal cysts. It should be clear that the "ring of fire" color flow pattern cannot distinguish between ectopic pregnancies and luteal cysts. Investigators have tried to identify

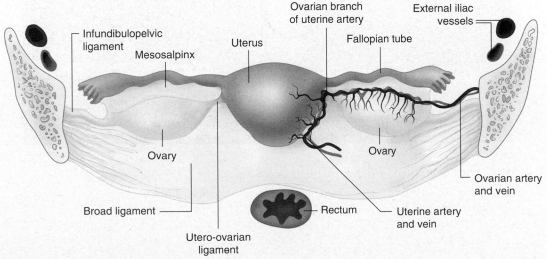

FIGURE 34–1. A, Normal pelvic anatomy.

Continued

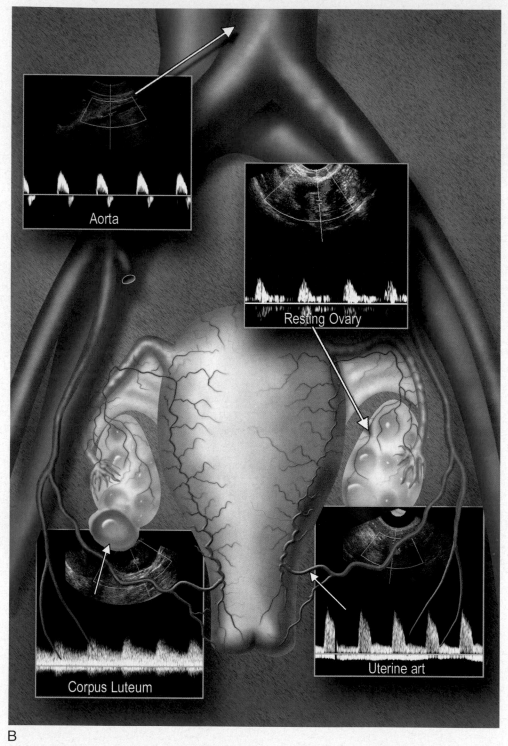

B

FIGURE 34–1—cont'd. *B*, Montage of normal pelvic Doppler waveforms.

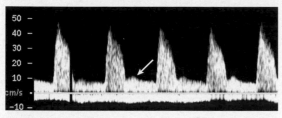

FIGURE 34–2. Normal uterine artery waveform. Pulsed Doppler evaluation reveals a high-resistance waveform with the early diastolic "notch" (*arrow*).

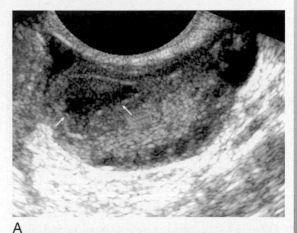

A

discriminating Doppler parameters to distinguish luteal from ectopic flow.[10,11] This is difficult due to overlap in peak systolic velocity and resistive index measurements between luteal cysts and ectopic pregnancies. The origin of the Doppler signal, from within the ovary or from an adnexal mass, allows more accurate characterization of a corpus luteal cyst or ectopic pregnancy than velocity or resistive index. Therefore, we do not use Doppler to distinguish luteal from ectopic flow but localize the site of origin of the signals to determine their significance.

Color and pulsed Doppler signals obtained from a postmenopausal ovary have low peak systolic velocities similar to ovaries in the follicular phase[7] (Fig. 34–5). This is typical of ovaries in the resting state. Because postmenopausal ovarian vessels carry low-velocity flow, they may be very difficult to visualize with conventional color Doppler flow settings. Low color velocity scale (PRF) and color wall filter adjustments may be necessary to detect postmenopausal ovarian blood flow. Power Doppler imaging improves the visualization of ovarian flow, particularly in

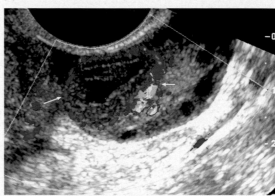

B

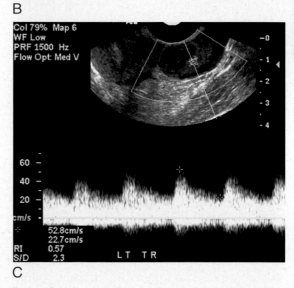

C

FIGURE 34–4. *A*, Corpus luteal cyst. Gray-scale image demonstrates a hypoechoic lesion with echogenic borders (*arrows*). *B*, Color Doppler shows a ring of increased color flow (*arrows*) around the periphery of the corpus luteal cyst. *C*, Pulsed Doppler demonstrates increased systolic and diastolic velocities associated with the vascular ring.

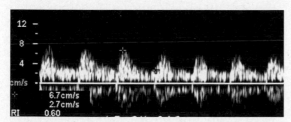

FIGURE 34–3. Normal follicular phase ovarian waveform. Pulsed Doppler evaluation of the ovary during the first week of the menstrual cycle reveals low-velocity, high-resistance flow.

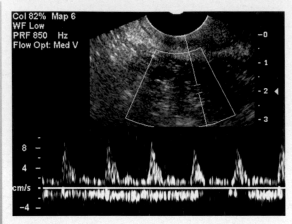

FIGURE 34-5. Normal postmenopausal ovarian waveform. Pulsed Doppler demonstrates typical low-velocity, high-resistance flow.

postmenopausal women. Because postmenopausal ovaries no longer ovulate, they remain relatively quiescent and are associated with little or no diastolic flow.

CURRENT APPLICATIONS

Current applications of transabdominal scanning and EVCF include identification of the corpus luteal cyst, detection of intrauterine placental flow, diagnosis of ectopic pregnancy and retained products of conception, evaluation of ovarian torsion, and the characterization of adnexal masses and uterine abnormalities.

Corpus Luteal Cyst

Identification of the dominant follicle or corpus luteal cyst has proven extremely helpful in patients who present with pelvic pain, adnexal mass, or ectopic pregnancy. Ovarian cysts are the most common cause of acute pelvic pain in premenopausal patients.[12] The pain is usually associated with enlargement of the cyst during the midportion of the menstrual cycle and precedes cyst rupture and the release of fluid.

Simple ovarian cysts are easily characterized by their lack of internal echoes; smooth, thin walls; and posterior sound enhancement. Complex ovarian cysts can be much harder to characterize as benign ovarian cysts. Hemorrhagic cysts may be filled with low-level echoes and are not easily recognized, as they become isoechoic to the ovarian parenchyma. These cysts may also contain solid regions and septations and may simulate ovarian neoplasms.

Color and pulsed Doppler are important tools in the characterization of complex ovarian cysts. Color Doppler can demonstrate the ring of increased vascularity in the wall of the corpus luteal cyst (Fig. 34–6). As mentioned earlier, the peripheral vascularity is related to neovascularization associated with the formation of the corpus luteal cyst.[8] The increased blood flow identified with color Doppler is associated with elevated peak systolic velocities and low-resistance flow. Dillon and colleagues[13] demonstrated a peak systolic velocity of 27 ± 10 cm/sec and a resistive index of 0.44 ± 0.09 for corpus luteal cysts. This color or power Doppler appearance makes the corpus luteal cyst conspicuous, even when it is filled with blood and is isoechoic to ovarian tissue on gray-scale images. The lack of vascularity within the central part of the lesion suggests it is a hemorrhagic cyst.[12] This is particularly helpful when gray-scale evaluation suggests the presence of wall thickening, nodules, or septations within the cyst cavity. The absence of flow within the cyst cavity suggests that any solid material within the cyst is likely related to hematoma or retracting clot and not tumor (Fig. 34–7). A follow-up study 6 to 8 weeks later, during the first week of a subsequent menstrual cycle, is recommended to assess for complete resolution of the complex cyst and to exclude the possibility of tumor.

The recognition of the corpus luteal cyst also aids in the diagnosis of ectopic pregnancy. Approximately 85% to 90% of ectopic pregnancies occur on the same side as the corpus luteal cyst.[9] Identification of the corpus luteum determines the side of ovulation and directs the examiner to the expected site of the ectopic pregnancy (Fig. 34–8). Color and pulsed Doppler also play a role in the identification and follow-up of ectopic pregnancy, which is our next topic of discussion.

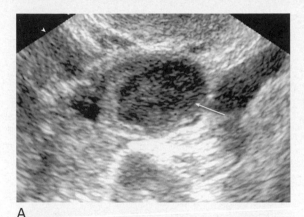

A

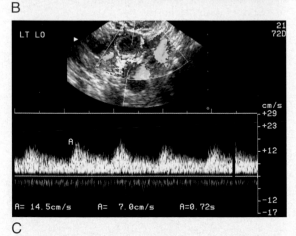

B

C

FIGURE 34–6. *A*, Hemorrhagic ovarian cyst. A hypoechoic lesion (*arrow*) is seen within the ovary, which contains low-level heterogeneous echoes consistent with hemorrhage. *B*, Color Doppler demonstrates a "ring of fire" (*arrowheads*) around the hemorrhagic cyst (*arrow*). Note that there is no color flow within the hemorrhagic component. *C*, Pulsed Doppler demonstrates low-resistance flow consistent with luteal flow.

ECTOPIC PREGNANCY

Ectopic pregnancy occurs in approximately 2% of pregnancies and is the leading cause of pregnancy-related deaths during the first trimester.[14] There is a rising incidence of ectopic pregnancy that is related to

An increased number of patients at risk
New techniques that allow earlier diagnosis
Improved treatment for salpingitis and ectopic pregnancy
Increased utilization of ovulation induction and assisted reproduction techniques

It is important to understand and solicit risk factors from patients with suspected ectopic pregnancy.[15] Any process that produces scarring or obstruction of the fallopian tube predisposes to ectopic pregnancy. The obstruction may be related to prior pelvic surgery or tubal ligation, prior ectopic pregnancy, or history of pelvic inflammatory disease or salpingitis. The use of an intrauterine contraceptive device may also increase the risk for ectopic pregnancy. In vitro fertilization also increases the rate of ectopic pregnancy due to multiple risk factors, including infertility, ovulation induction, and embryo transfer with retrograde migration of the embryo into the fallopian tube. Other important risk factors include in utero exposure to diethylstilbestrol and sterilization. (Infertility is associated with multiple anatomic and physiologic conditions that increase risk for ectopic pregnancy.)

The clinical presentation of ectopic pregnancy is variable; however, a positive pregnancy test, pelvic pain, an adnexal mass, and/or vaginal bleeding raise clinical suspicion for this condition. The classic triad of pelvic pain, adnexal mass, and vaginal bleeding occurs only in approximately 45% of patients.[16] Patients may be asymptomatic or have focal or generalized pelvic or abdominal pain.

Earlier diagnosis of ectopic pregnancy is possible due to improved sonographic techniques and increased awareness of the disease. Early detection reduces the risk of tubal rupture and significant hemorrhage. The evaluation of ectopic pregnancy usually includes a combination of endovaginal

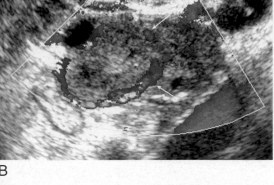
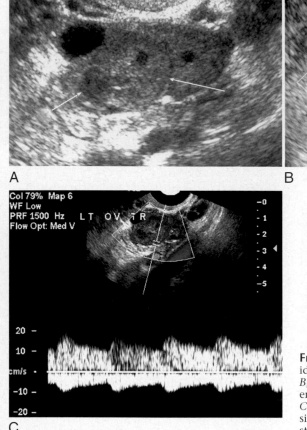

FIGURE 34–7. *A,* A heterogeneous solid lesion (*arrows*) is identified in the ovary, suspicious for neoplasm or mass. *B,* Color Doppler demonstrates flow around the periphery of the mass (*arrows*) but no central or internal flow. *C,* Pulsed Doppler evaluation reveals classic luteal flow signals. A follow-up examination after 8 weeks demonstrated resolution of the lesion.

sonography and serum human chorionic gonadotropin titers. Diagnostic laparoscopy is considered the gold standard and is usually reserved for difficult cases.

The sonographic findings associated with ectopic pregnancy include absence of a normal intrauterine pregnancy, a pseudo-gestational sac (described later), a live extrauterine embryo, pelvic fluid, and an adnexal mass.

A common sonographic feature is the extrauterine gestational sac. This appears as a ring-shaped adnexal mass with a thick wall, similar to a doughnut or life preserver. Occasionally, a complex or solid adnexal mass is identified, related to pelvic hematoma or hematosalpinx. The complex appearance of the mass is usually related to bleeding or rupture of the ectopic pregnancy. A live embryo is seen less commonly but provides the highest positive predictive value for the diagnosis of ectopic pregnancy.

Placental Flow

Color and pulsed Doppler imaging can also demonstrate placental flow features (described later) in the uterus or adnexa.[10]

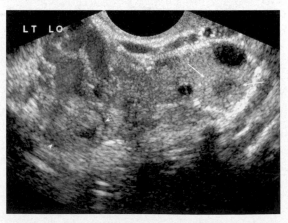

FIGURE 34–8. A well-defined extrauterine gestational sac (*arrowheads*) is identified on the same side as a hemorrhagic corpus luteal cyst (*arrows*) in the left ovary.

The presence or absence of placental flow in the uterus is an extremely valuable finding in the evaluation for suspected ectopic pregnancy, for when it is present, the focus of examination shifts toward an abnormal intrauterine pregnancy rather than an extrauterine gestation. Placental flow is related to invasion of the endometrium by growing trophoblastic tissue. As the trophoblast grows into the uterine tissue, the maternal spiral arteries will shunt arterial blood into the intervillous sinusoids. This results in relatively high-velocity, low-resistance blood flow that is readily detected with color Doppler imaging (Fig. 34–9). Pulsed Doppler examination of intrauterine placental flow reveals a peak systolic veloc-ity greater than 21 cm/sec, and the impedance decreases to a mean resistive index of 0.44 ± 0.09.[17] The increased vascularity related to trophoblastic implantation is detected 36–50 days after the last menstrual period.

Detection of the flow characteristics related to placentation is invaluable in the identification of gestational tissue in the uterus or in the adnexa. A peak systolic velocity cutoff at 21 cm/sec or more is uti-lized to characterize placental flow in the uterus. We utilize no (0-degree) angle cor-rection for the pulsed Doppler examination, as the vessels are too small to determine the direction of flow. Despite the lack of angle correction, Doppler is remarkably sensitive for the detection of placental flow. The detection of placental flow in the uterus confirms the presence of a normal or abnormal intrauterine pregnancy. In general, pulsed Doppler interrogation of a normal embryo is not performed due to potential bioeffects related to cavitation and heating.

PSEUDOGESTATION

Color and pulsed Doppler can also distin-guish between an abnormal intrauterine pregnancy and a pseudogestational sac related to ectopic pregnancy. The sono-graphic appearance of "pseudosacs" ranges from endometrial thickening to a fluid col-lection in the endometrial canal. Unlike normal intrauterine gestational sacs, pseu-dosacs tend to be oval and located centrally in the endometrial cavity rather than eccen-trically placed in the endometrium. They do not demonstrate a double decidual reaction, yolk sac, or embryo. They also do not exhibit placental flow, an important dis-criminatory factor (Fig. 34–10). Doppler sampling of the area surrounding the pseu-dosac will demonstrate velocities less than 21 cm/sec. Dillon and colleagues[17] showed that Doppler findings were 100% specific in the identification of pseudogestational sacs.

The diagnosis of ectopic pregnancy is based on the finding of a cystic, complex, or solid mass, separate from the uterus and ovaries, in a pregnant patient. Color

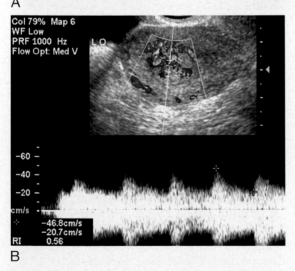

A

B

FIGURE 34–9. *A*, Endovaginal sonography reveals a ges-tational sac (*arrows*) within the endometrial canal. *B*, Color Doppler demonstrates increased flow around the gestational sac. Pulsed Doppler waveforms show char-acteristic high-velocity, low-resistance flow signals.

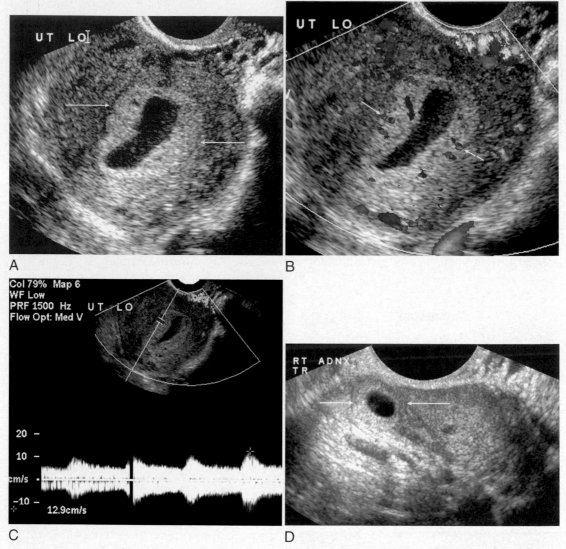

FIGURE 34–10. *A,* Endovaginal scan reveals a well-defined sac-like structure (*arrows*) within the endometrial canal in a patient with a positive human chorionic gonadotrophin titer and vaginal bleeding. This finding may be related to an abnormal intrauterine pregnancy or pseudogestational sac associated with an ectopic pregnancy. *B,* Color Doppler demonstrates flow in the myometrium and vessels associated with the intrauterine sac (*arrows*). *C,* Spectral analysis of the vessels around the sac demonstrates low-velocity signals (<21 cm/sec) consistent with a pseudogestational sac. *D,* Examination of the right adnexa demonstrates a ring-shaped mass (*arrows*) consistent with an ectopic sac.

Doppler is helpful in cases of ectopic pregnancy when the gray-scale findings are not diagnostic and increased vascularity is identified in the adnexa (Fig. 34–11). In a study of 155 patients with suspected ectopic pregnancy, my colleagues and I[9] found that placental flow was observed in 85% (55 of 65) of patients with ectopic pregnancy. Color and pulsed Doppler showed a sensitivity of 95% and specificity of 98% for the detection of ectopic pregnancy. We have been able to distinguish ectopic pregnancy from hematoma, bowel loops, and other adnexal masses on the basis of increased color flow (Fig. 34–12). Color and pulsed Doppler have also proven useful in cases of interstitial (cornual) and cervical ectopic pregnancies when no significant mass is identified but there is increased flow on color and power Doppler examination (Fig. 34–13).

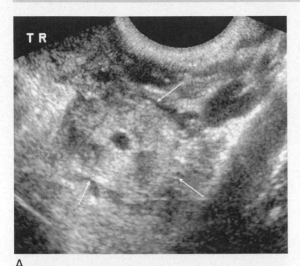

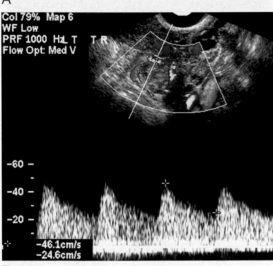

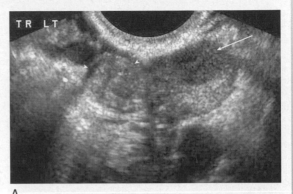

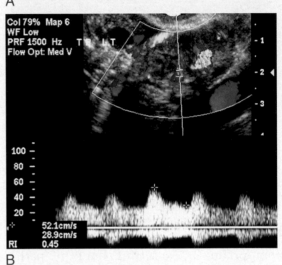

FIGURE 34–12. *A,* Endovaginal scan shows a round, solid region (*arrowheads*) adjacent to the left ovary in this pregnant patient with pain and vaginal bleeding. The differential diagnosis included hematoma, bowel, and ectopic pregnancy. Note that the left ovary contains a hemorrhagic luteal cyst (*arrow*). *B,* Color Doppler reveals increased flow within the tissue. Pulsed Doppler demonstrates high-velocity, low-resistance signals consistent with trophoblastic flow. Increased flow will not be seen in bowel or hematoma, and the findings are consistent with ectopic pregnancy.

FIGURE 34–11. *A,* A poorly defined hypoechoic region (*arrows*) is identified in the left adnexa, separate from the ovary, in this patient with positive human chorionic gonadotropin and pelvic pain. The finding is suspicious for an ectopic pregnancy. *B,* Color Doppler demonstrates increased flow within the mass. Pulsed Doppler shows high-velocity, low-impedance waveforms consistent with placental flow in this patient with proven ectopic pregnancy.

PITFALLS

As previously mentioned, one must use caution when interpreting color and pulsed Doppler images. There is significant overlap in the appearance of placental and luteal flow. Intrauterine and extrauterine gestational sacs, as well as corpus luteal cysts, exhibit the "ring of fire" appearance. Similarly, both placental and luteal wave-

forms demonstrate indistinguishable low-resistance arterial flow. The origin of the color Doppler signals must be considered for accurate diagnosis. Because intraovarian ectopic pregnancies are extremely rare (less than 1% of all ectopics),[18] increased flow obtained from within the ovary likely represents luteal flow.

Color and pulsed Doppler are also utilized to assess for persistent abnormal flow after ectopic pregnancy therapy. There is a trend toward nonsurgical treatment of small, uncomplicated ectopic pregnancies with methotrexate or careful clinical follow-up.

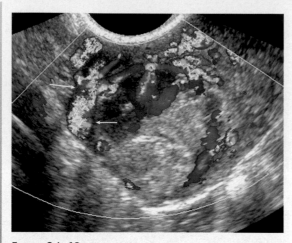

FIGURE 34–13. This cornual pregnancy was identified on the basis of increased color flow signals (*arrows*) in the absence of a sac or significant mass.

Doppler is used to assess for absence or persistence of placental flow after treatment or during follow-up. Ultrasound may show persistence or increase in size of the adnexal mass after methotrexate administration.[15] Serial sonograms demonstrate resolution of placental flow following methotrexate.

These techniques work very well in the appropriate clinical setting, but other pathologies may demonstrate high-velocity, low-resistance flow patterns that simulate placental flow. For example, fibroids or polyps can demonstrate similar low-resistance signals. The gray-scale features usually allow identification of the fibroid or polyp as the source of the signals. Other pathologies, such as endometritis, may demonstrate low-resistance signals similar to placental flow, but in this case, the clinical situation should clarify the diagnosis. Certain adnexal pathologies may also demonstrate signals that simulate placental flow. The keys to correct diagnosis relate to relevant clinical information and recognition of the source of the Doppler waveforms. Pitfalls can occur when the site of Doppler insonation is not clear. The most common pitfall is confusing a corpus luteal cyst with an ectopic pregnancy. Both the corpus luteal cyst and the ectopic pregnancy may present with a cystic, ring-shaped mass and low-resistance arterial signals. This situation is resolved by recognizing that the corpus luteal cyst is located

within the ovary and is not a separate adnexal mass. A mass that cannot be separated from the ovary is unlikely to represent an ectopic pregnancy for reasons mentioned previously. Other potential pitfalls include a tubo-ovarian abscess, pedunculated fibroid, ovarian malignancy, or other pelvic tumor or abscess. The location of Doppler flow and the clinical scenario should allow for correct diagnosis.

In summary, the value of color Doppler in the evaluation of ectopic pregnancy includes

Demonstration of an intrauterine pregnancy with identification of placental flow caused by spontaneous miscarriage or incomplete abortion

Absence of placental flow in a pseudogestational sac

Detection of placental flow in the adnexa when the gray-scale findings are not diagnostic or no mass is identified

Identification of retained products of conception following delivery or after therapeutic abortion

Assessment of therapeutic efficacy following methotrexate or laparoscopic surgery

Retained Gestational Tissue

Identification of placental flow is also useful in the diagnosis of incomplete abortion, retained products of conception, and gestational trophoblastic neoplasia. We use color and pulsed Doppler to assess for retained placental tissue after spontaneous miscarriage or therapeutic abortion and in patients following delivery (Fig. 34–14). Retained products may be suspected clinically due to persistent vaginal bleeding or elevated human chorionic gonadotropin titer. Color Doppler is able to demonstrate small foci of placental tissue, even in the absence of an appreciable endometrial mass or fluid collection (Fig. 34–15). Pulsed Doppler sampling in the region of increased color flow reveals peak systolic velocity measurements greater than 21 cm/sec, consistent with retained placental tissue. Conversely, the absence of placental flow in an endometrial mass suggests retained clot. Dillon and coworkers[13] reported that persistent high-

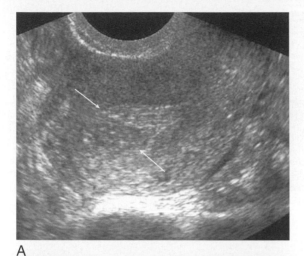

velocity, low-resistance flow was noted in half of patients studied after therapeutic abortion. This increased vascularity spontaneously resolved over the next few days. This is a pitfall for retained placental tissue, and treatment decisions in the first week after therapeutic abortion or dilation and curettage should be based on clinical factors and not Doppler findings.

Gestational Trophoblastic Disease

Gestational trophoblastic disease, or molar disease, is an uncommon complication of pregnancy. The clinical and sonographic presentations are variable. Typically, patients present in early pregnancy with symptoms and signs of threatened abortion, with elevated serum human chorionic gonadotropin levels, usually greater than 100,000 mIU/mL.[19] Sonographic examination of the uterus demonstrates an echogenic mass, which may appear complex. The molar tissue is usually extremely vascular and easily seen with color and power Doppler. Moles demonstrate multiple arteriovenous shunts with high-velocity, low-resistance blood flow. The detection of increased color flow is helpful when small amounts of tissue are noted on the grayscale image. Myometrial invasion of molar tissue can also be identified by the presence of abnormal color flow extending into the myometrium.

Ovarian Torsion

Ovarian torsion represents approximately 3% of gynecologic emergencies.[20] Although ovarian torsion occurs less commonly than other gynecologic problems, clinical symptoms may suggest other etiologies of acute pelvic pain, including ruptured ovarian cyst, pelvic inflammatory disease, appendicitis, renal colic, or bowel obstruction.[21] Duplex and color Doppler evaluation is the best noninvasive modality for the evaluation of ovarian torsion. Immediate diagnosis and surgical intervention is required to avoid irreversible ovarian injury.

FIGURE 34–14. *A,* Endovaginal scan reveals a thickened, heterogeneous endometrium (*arrows*) in this patient following incomplete abortion. *B,* Color Doppler shows markedly increased vascularity (*arrows*) in the region of endometrial thickening suggestive of retained products of conception. *C,* Pulsed Doppler demonstrates high-velocity (126 cm/sec), low-resistance (resistive index = 0.45) flow consistent with placental flow and retained products of conception.

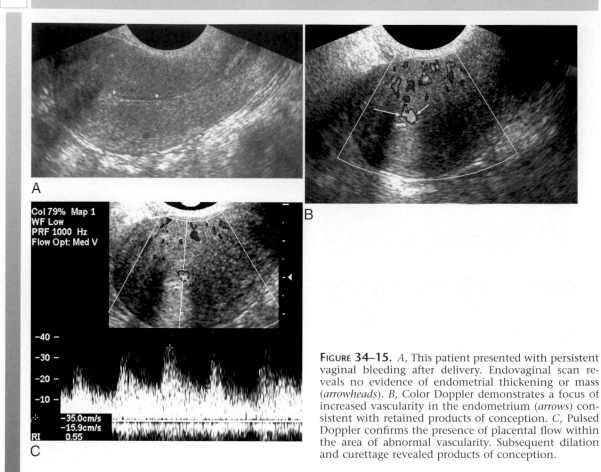

FIGURE 34–15. *A,* This patient presented with persistent vaginal bleeding after delivery. Endovaginal scan reveals no evidence of endometrial thickening or mass (*arrowheads*). *B,* Color Doppler demonstrates a focus of increased vascularity in the endometrium (*arrows*) consistent with retained products of conception. *C,* Pulsed Doppler confirms the presence of placental flow within the area of abnormal vascularity. Subsequent dilation and curettage revealed products of conception.

Torsion occurs more commonly in premenopausal patients and is related to partial or complete twisting of the vascular pedicle, usually due to ovarian or adnexal mass or swelling. The mass may be an ovarian or broad ligament cyst or neoplasm. The mass or broad ligament serves as the fulcrum for the torsion. Less commonly, torsion may be related to displacement or compression by a pelvic mass or enlarged uterus. Torsion occurs more commonly on the right side, which may be related to increased space and absence of the sigmoid colon. A hypermobile adnexa or abnormal attachment may also predispose to torsion. There is also increased incidence of torsion with pregnancy.[22,23]

Most patients with torsion present with a solid or cystic ovarian mass, which serves as the focal point for torsion. Typical sonographic findings include an enlarged ovary or adnexal mass, which may be cystic, complex, or solid.[24] The ovary may be edematous and associated with free fluid. An enlarged ovary in an unusual location, including the midline above the uterus, flank, or cul-de-sac, should raise suspicion for torsion.

The diagnosis of ovarian torsion relies on the failure to detect arterial flow within the ovarian parenchyma (Fig. 34–16).[21,22,25,26] The absence of flow within the torsed ovary during color flow, power, and pulsed Doppler is diagnostic.

Color Doppler may also demonstrate a coiling or twisting of the vascular pedicle (Fig. 34–17).[27] Absent or reversed diastolic flow in the ovarian vessels or within the ovarian parenchyma also suggests torsion. Other abnormal flow patterns are associated with ovarian torsion. Decreased arterial flow with no venous flow has been observed. A nonpulsatile, low-velocity venous-like pattern may occur that likely represents subtotal vascular occlusion with blunted,

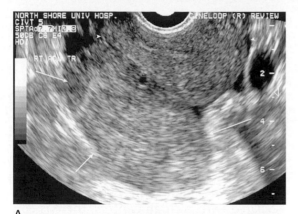

A

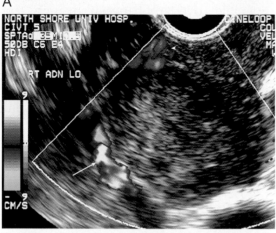

B

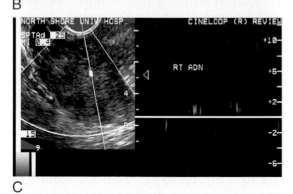

C

FIGURE 34–16. *A,* Endovaginal scan demonstrates a large right adnexal mass (*arrows*) behind the uterus (*arrowheads*) in this patient with acute pelvic pain. *B,* Color Doppler demonstrates flow in the adjacent right iliac artery (*arrow*) and parametrial vessels (*arrowhead*) but no flow in the right adnexal mass. *C,* Pulsed Doppler confirms the absence of flow in the right adnexal mass. Surgical exploration identified right ovarian torsion.

monophasic arterial flow signals (Fig. 34–18). Rarely, normal ovarian flow has also been detected in ovarian torsion.

There are important pitfalls to the diagnosis of ovarian torsion. Arterial signals may be detected from within the ovary when there is partial, or less than 360-degree, twisting of the vascular pedicle. This may be related in part to the dual arterial supply to the ovaries. Lack of intraovarian venous signals or damped arterial waveforms detected during pulsed Doppler interrogation should increase suspicion for partial or incomplete torsion. Patients with chronic torsion may present with absent internal vascularity and flow around the periphery of the ovary. The peripheral vascularity is related to reactive inflammation and scarring, similar to the "halo sign" associated with testicular torsion. Patients with intermittent torsion may present with episodic pain. Doppler examination may reveal increased hyperemic flow during periods of detorsion. Pain is typically relieved following detorsion. All color flow parameters must be optimized to ensure that the absence of flow is not related to technical factors, including high PRF, high wall filter, or low color gain settings. Power Doppler is very helpful to demonstrate low-velocity flow in the ovary when flow is not appreciated with color Doppler imaging.

Ovarian torsion remains a challenging diagnosis, and close correlation between clinical examination and Doppler findings is usually required.

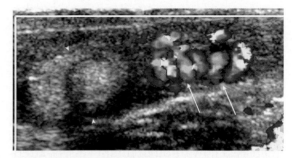

FIGURE 34–17. Color Doppler shows coiling or twisting of the vascular pedicle (*arrows*) in this patient with proven ovarian torsion. Note the absence of color flow in the ovary (*arrowheads*).

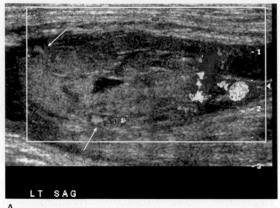

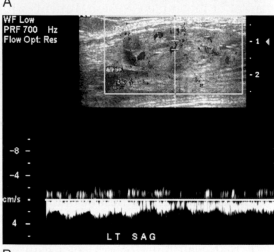

Figure 34–18. *A,* This patient presented with left adnexal pain. Endovaginal color flow Doppler imaging demonstrates an enlarged heterogeneous ovary with scattered internal blood vessels *(arrows). B,* Spectral Doppler reveals nonpulsatile low-velocity waveforms suggestive of partial ovarian torsion, proven at laparoscopy.

Characterization of Adnexal Masses

Ultrasound is utilized to detect neovascularity associated with malignant tumors.[28] Color Doppler demonstrates clusters of small abnormal tumor vessels within malignant masses and assists in placement of the sample volume for pulsed Doppler examination. Pulsed Doppler typically demonstrates high-velocity, low-resistance flow within cancers. These flow patterns are related to increased flow through tumor vessels, arteriovenous shunting, and absence of muscular media in the walls of tumor vessels. Power Doppler appears to improve visualization of malignant vascularity compared with conventional color flow imaging. Doppler techniques have proven valuable in the evaluation of cancers of the breast, kidney, liver, and prostate gland.

Color and pulsed Doppler is also used to characterize adnexal masses (Fig. 34–19).[29–34] Spectral tracings from ovarian cancer demonstrate high-velocity and/or low-impedance monophasic waveforms with no diastolic notch. Although color Doppler can demonstrate malignant neovascularity associated with ovarian cancers, there is considerable overlap between benign and malignant Doppler signals.[35,36] Apart from ovarian cancer, corpus luteal cysts, fibroids, endometriomas, abscesses, and other benign tumors can have similar low-impedance signals. The similarities in blood flow patterns between these entities limits the value of Doppler in their characterization.

Prior to Doppler evaluation, gray-scale morphologic findings were used to identify ovarian cancer. Thick cyst walls, complex masses, mural nodules, and septations more than 2 mm in thickness are associated with malignancy.[37] Like the Doppler findings, these features are nonspecific and overlap with benign lesions. Recent studies[38–41] have shown that a combination of morphologic and Doppler features increases specificity for the diagnosis of ovarian cancer. Scoring systems have been devised to assist in the recognition and characterization of ovarian cancer. In a study of 172 adnexal masses, my colleagues and I[40] showed that a scoring system consisting of elevated ovarian volume, abnormal morphologic features, and the detection of high-velocity, low-impedance flow in the abnormal solid components demonstrated a sensitivity of 95% and specificity of 92% for the detection of ovarian cancer. Brown and associates[39] reviewed 211 pelvic masses and demonstrated a sensitivity and specificity of 93% for a combination of gray-scale and Doppler parameters. Their scoring system included the presence of nonhyperechoic solid components, free fluid, absent or thick septations, and central location of blood flow. Both studies concluded that the identification of abnormal tumor vascularity within

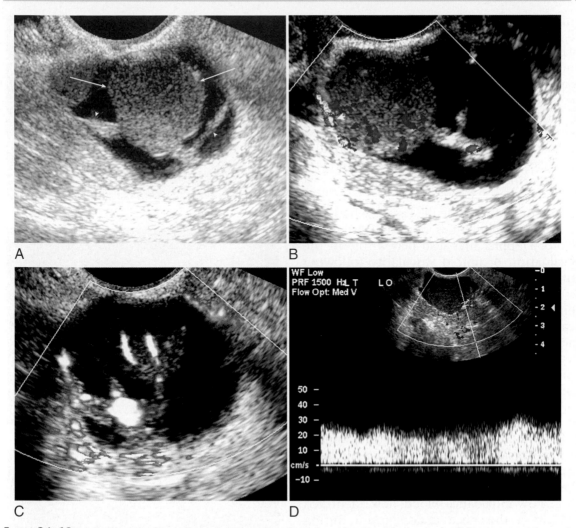

FIGURE 34–19. *A*, Endovaginal scan demonstrates a complex adnexal mass with a central solid component (*arrows*) and septations (*arrowheads*) in this postmenopausal patient. *B*, Color Doppler reveals flow in the central component (*arrowheads*) and septation (*arrow*), suggestive of malignancy. *C*, Power Doppler demonstrates increased flow (*arrows*) throughout all the solid components of the adnexal mass. *D*, Pulsed Doppler reveals high-velocity, low-resistance signals consistent with malignant vascularity in this ovarian cancer.

the complex and solid components of ovarian tumors has proven useful in the diagnosis of malignancy.

These findings are particularly useful in postmenopausal patients with adnexal masses. Normal postmenopausal ovaries are typically quiescent and small, with low-velocity (less than 20 cm/sec), high-resistance (resistive index ≥ 0.7) flow. Confusion with corpus luteal cysts, endometriosis, and pelvic inflammatory disease should not occur in this age group. The presence of an adnexal mass with high-velocity, low-impedance signals raises con-siderable suspicion for carcinoma in an elderly patient.

Uterine Abnormalites

Color Doppler also plays a role in the evaluation of uterine pathology. Through the demonstration of increased vascularity, color Doppler may improve the definition of fibroids and endometrial polyps. Fibroids may be highly vascular, and the vascularity is typically identified along the periphery of the mass. Spectral analysis may reveal high-velocity, low-resistance flow, similar to tumor signals seen in ovarian cancer. This is a significant pitfall for the misdiagnosis of ovarian cancer when the normal ispsilateral ovary is not identified with certainty.

Color Doppler is especially helpful for confirming that a solid adnexal mass is a subserosal fibroid. We look for the vascular pedicle attachment between the fibroid and the uterine body to confirm the nature of the mass (Fig. 34–20). Correlation with MRI is helpful for difficult cases, when the uterine attachment is not well visualized. Color Doppler may also play a role in the evaluation of fibroid vascularity following uterine artery embolization.

Uterine polyps may present as focal endometrial thickening or a mass. Identification of a feeding vessel assists in the characterization of focal endometrial lesions as polyps (Fig. 34–21). Sonohysterography improves the visualization of endometrial polyps and determines the size and number of endometrial lesions.

The value of color and pulsed Doppler in the evaluation of endometrial carcinoma is controversial.[42,43] Color Doppler imaging may be utilized to display abnormal vascularity associated with endometrial thickening. Low-impedance blood flow identified within a thickened endometrium during pulsed Doppler examination has been noted with endometrial carcinoma.[44] As is the case with adnexal masses, there is considerable overlap between the Doppler appearances of benign and malignant conditions. Low-resistance signals are also associated with endometrial hyperplasia, polyps, submucosal fibroids, adenomyosis, endometritis, molar disease, and placental tissue. Doppler studies may aid in the determination of the extent of tumor invasion and guide biopsy to regions of increased blood flow.[45]

We have had success with the identification of enlarged, tortuous parauterine vessels in patients with the pelvic congestion syndrome. Patients with this syndrome may present with complaints of nonspecific pelvic pain. Large venous varices are well visualized with endovaginal color Doppler imaging (Fig. 34–22). Mag-

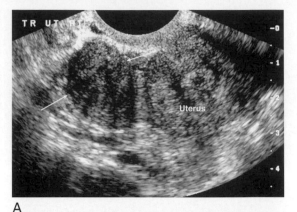

A

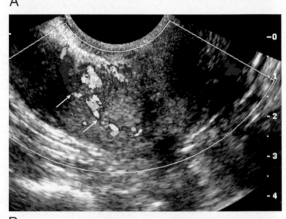

B

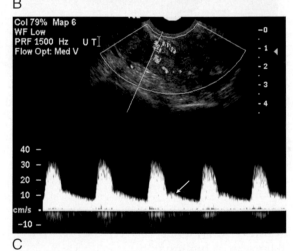

C

FIGURE 34–20. *A*, A solid hypoechoic mass (*arrows*) is identified adjacent to the uterus in this patient with pelvic pain. *B*, Color Doppler demonstrates the vascular pedicle (*arrows*) to this subserosal fibroid. *C*, Pulsed Doppler interrogation of the vascular pedicle reveals characteristic uterine artery waveforms with the diastolic notch (*arrow*).

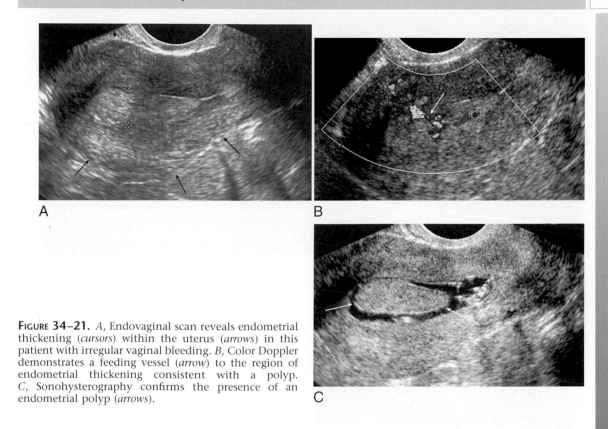

FIGURE 34–21. *A,* Endovaginal scan reveals endometrial thickening (*cursors*) within the uterus (*arrows*) in this patient with irregular vaginal bleeding. *B,* Color Doppler demonstrates a feeding vessel (*arrow*) to the region of endometrial thickening consistent with a polyp. *C,* Sonohysterography confirms the presence of an endometrial polyp (*arrows*).

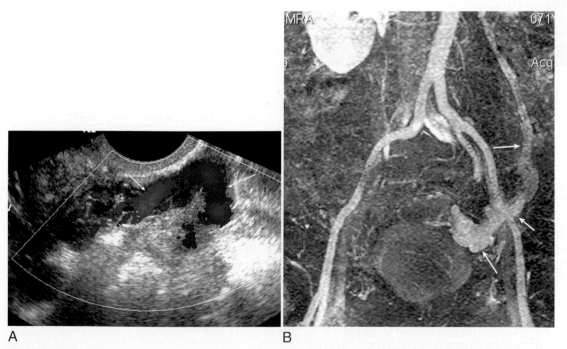

FIGURE 34–22. *A,* Color Doppler reveals large left parametrial venous varices (*arrows*) in this patient with chronic pelvic pain. *B,* Delayed three-dimensional magnetic resonance angiography reveals large left venous varices (*arrows*) consistent with pelvic congestion syndrome.

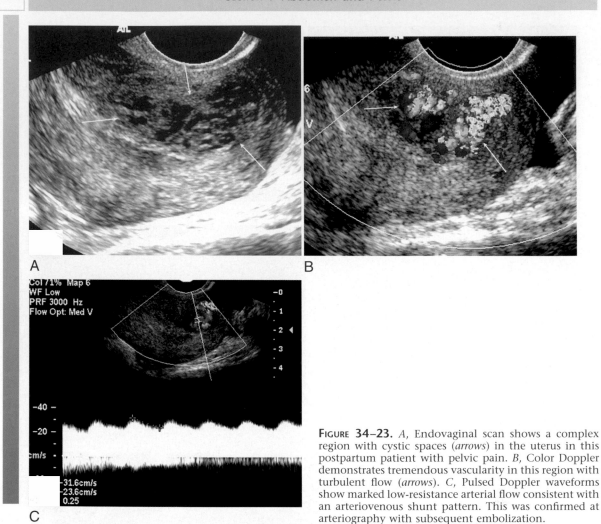

FIGURE 34–23. *A,* Endovaginal scan shows a complex region with cystic spaces (*arrows*) in the uterus in this postpartum patient with pelvic pain. *B,* Color Doppler demonstrates tremendous vascularity in this region with turbulent flow (*arrows*). *C,* Pulsed Doppler waveforms show marked low-resistance arterial flow consistent with an arteriovenous shunt pattern. This was confirmed at arteriography with subsequent embolization.

netic resonance imaging is also utilized to assess for evidence of enlarged vessels, abdominal or pelvic mass, or venous thrombosis.

Uncommon vascular lesions, including uterine vascular malformations, are also identified with color Doppler. Uterine arteriovenous malformations may appear as focal areas of uterine heterogeneity or a cystic, complex, or tubular mass, with or without prominent parametrial vessels on gray-scale imaging. Color Doppler will demonstrate increased vascularity in the region of the arteriovenous malformation. Pulsed Doppler will reveal high-velocity, low-resistance arterial signals consistent with arteriovenous shunting (Fig. 34–23).

CONCLUSIONS

Multiple applications of color Doppler have been defined clinically, and color Doppler is currently a routine component of gynecological sonography. Attention to technique and understanding of color flow parameters is key to maximum sensitivity. Integration of clinical and sonographic information, as well as recognition of diagnostic pitfalls, improves diagnostic accuracy and reduces misinterpretation.

Acknowledgments. I would like to recognize Dr. Kenneth J. W. Taylor for his dedication, innovations, and outstanding contributions to the field of pelvic Doppler.

References

1. Taylor KJ, Merritt CR, Hammers L, et al: Doppler color imaging. Obstetric and gynecologic applications. Clin Diagn Ultrasound 27:195–223, 1992.

2. Pellerito JS, Taylor KJW, Case CQ: Current applications of endovaginal color flow imaging. Radiology 193(P):395, 1994.

3. Pellerito JS, Troiano RN, Quedens-Case C, et al: Common pitfalls of endovaginal color flow imaging. Radiographics 15:37–47, 1995.

4. Rubin JM, Bude RO, Carson PL, et al: Power Doppler US: A potentially useful alternative to mean frequency-based color Doppler US. Radiology 190:853–856, 1994.

5. Taylor KJ, Burns PN, Wells PNT: Ultrasound Doppler flow studies of the ovarian and uterine arteries. Br J Obstet Gynaecol 92:240–246, 1985.

6. Hata K, Hata T, Senoh D, et al: Change in ovarian arterial compliance during the human menstrual cycle assessed by Doppler ultrasound. Br J Obstet Gynaecol 97:163, 1990.

7. D'Agostino, C, Pellerito JS: Color and pulsed Doppler imaging of the pelvic vasculature and pelvic organs. J Vasc Tech 19(5–6):331–335, 1995.

8. Parsons AK: Imaging the human corpus luteum. J Ultrasound Med 20:811–819, 2001.

9. Pellerito JS, Taylor KJ, Quedens-Case C, et al: Ectopic pregnancy: Evaluation with endovaginal color flow imaging. Radiology 183:407–411, 1992.

10. Taylor KJ, Ramos IM, Feyock AL, et al: Ectopic pregnancy: Duplex Doppler evaluation. Radiology 173:93–97, 1989.

11. Atri M: Ectopic pregnancy versus corpus luteal cyst revisited: Best Doppler predictors. J Ultrasound Med 22:1181–1184, 2003.

12. Pellerito JS: Acute pelvic pain. In Benson CB, Arger PH, Bluth EI (eds): Ultrasonography in Obstetric and Gynecology: A Practical Approach, 1st ed. New York, Thieme Publishers, 2000, pp 10–19.

13. Dillon EH, Quedens-Case C, Ramos IM, et al: Endovaginal pulsed and color flow Doppler in first trimester pregnancy. Ultrasound Med Biol 19:517–525, 1993.

14. NCHS: Advanced Report of Final Mortality Statistics, 1992. Report No. 43(Suppl). Hyattsville, MD, U.S. Department of Health and Human Services, Public Health Service, CDC, 1994.

15. Levine D: Ectopic pregnancy. In Callen PW (ed): Ultrasonography in Obstetrics and Gynecology, 4th ed. Philadelphia, W.B. Saunders, 2000, pp 912–934.

16. Schwartz R, Di Pietro DL: B-hCG as a diagnostic aid for suspected ectopic pregnancy. Obstet Gynecol 56:197, 1980.

17. Dillon EH, Feyock AL, Taylor KJW: Pseudogestational sacs: Doppler US differentiation from normal or abnormal intrauterine pregnancies. Radiology 176:359–364, 1990.

18. Chow TT, Lindahl S: Ectopic pregnancy. J Clin Ultrasound 7:217–218, 1979.

19. Taylor KJW, Schwartz PE, Kohorn EI: Gestational trophoblastic neoplasia: Diagnosis with Doppler US. Radiology 165:445–448, 1987.

20. Hibbard LT: Adnexal torsion. Am J Obstet Gynecol 152:456–461, 1985.

21. Albayram F, Hamper UM: Ovarian and adnexal torsion. Spectrum of sonographic findings with pathologic correlation. J Ultrasound Med 20:1083–1089, 2001.

22. Pena JE, Ufberg D, Cooney N, Denis AL: Usefulness of Doppler sonography in the diagnosis of ovarian torsion. Fertil Steril 73:1047–1050, 2000.

23. Bider D, Mashiach S, Dulitzky M, et al: Clinical, surgical and pathologic findings of adnexal torsion in pregnant and nonpregnant women [review]. Surg Gynecol Obstet 173:363–366, 1991.

24. Halvie MA, Silver TM: Ovarian torsion: Sonographic evaluation. J Clin Ultrasound 17: 327–332, 1989.

25. Rosado WM Jr, Trambert MA, Gosink BB, et al: Adnexal Torsion: Diagnosis by using Doppler sonography. AJR 159:1251–1253, 1992.

26. Fleischer AC, Stein SM, Cullinan JA, Warner MA: Color Doppler sonography of adnexal torsion. J Ultrasound Med 14:523–528, 1995.

27. Lee EJ, Kwon HC, Joo HJ, et al: Diagnosis of ovarian torsion with color Doppler sonography: Depiction of twisted vascular pedicle. J Ultrasound Med 17:83–89, 1998.

28. Taylor KJ, Ramos I, Carter D, et al: Correlation of Doppler US tumor signals with neovascular morphologic features. Radiology 166:57–62, 1988.

29. Fleischer AC, Rodgers WH, Rao BK, et al: Assessment of ovarian tumor vascularity with transvaginal color Doppler sonography. J Ultrasound Med 10:295–297, 1991.

30. Weiner Z, Thaler I, Beck D, et al: Differentiating malignant from benign ovarian tumors with transvaginal color flow imaging. Obstet Gynecol 79:159, 1992.

31. Fleischer AC, Rodgers WH, Kepple DM, et al: Color Doppler sonography of ovarian masses: A multiparameter analysis. J Ultrasound Med 12:41, 1993.

32. Brown DL, Frates MC, Laing FC, et al: Ovarian masses: Can benign and malignant lesions be

differentiated with color Doppler US? Radiology 190:333, 1994.

33. Pellerito JS, Taylor KJ, Schwartz PE, et al: Endovaginal color flow imaging of palpable adnexal masses. J Ultrasound Med 12:559, 1993.

34. Jain KA: Prospective evaluation of adnexal masses with endovaginal gray-scale and duplex and color Doppler US: Correlation with pathologic findings. Radiology 191:63, 1994.

35. Hamper UM, Sheth S, Abbas FM, et al: Transvaginal color Doppler sonography of adnexal masses: Differences in blood flow impedance in benign and malignant lesions. AJR 160:1225–1228, 1993.

36. Levine D, Feldstein VA, Babcock CJ, et al: Sonography of ovarian masses: Poor sensitivity of resistive index for identifying malignant lesions. AJR 162:1355,1994.

37. Lerner JP, Timor-Trisch IE, Federman A, Abramovich G: Transvaginal ultrasonographic characterization of ovarian masses with an improved, weighted scoring system. Am J Obstet Gynecol 170:81–85, 1994.

38. Kurjak A, Predanic M: New scoring system for prediction for ovarian malignancy based on transvaginal color Doppler sonography. J Ultrasound Med 11:631, 1992.

39. Brown DL, Doubilet PM, Miller FH, et al: Benign and malignant ovarian masses: Selection of the most discriminating gray-scale and Doppler sonographic features. Radiology 208:103–110, 1998.

40. Pellerito JS, Taylor KJ, Quedens-Case C, et al: Endovaginal color flow scoring system: A sensitive indicator of pelvic malignancy. Radiology 193(P):276, 1994.

41. Taylor KJW, Schwartz PE: Screening for early ovarian cancer. Radiology 192:1–10, 1994.

42. Bourne TH, Campbell S, Whitehead MI, et al: Detection of endometrial cancer in postmenopausal women by ultrasonography and color flow imaging. BMJ 301:369, 1990.

43. Nalaboff KM, Pellerito JS, Ben-Levi E: Imaging the endometrium: Disease and normal variants. RadioGraphics 21:1409–1424, 2001.

44. Bourne TH, Campbell S, Steer CV, et al: Detection of endometrial cancer by transvaginal ultrasonography with color flow imaging and blood flow analysis: A preliminary report. Gynecol Oncol 40:253–259, 1991.

45. Fleischer AC: Sonographic assessment of endometrial disorders. Semin Ultrasound CT MR 20:259–266, 1999.

Chapter 35

Duplex Ultrasound Evaluation of the Male Genitalia

WILLIAM J. ZWIEBEL, MD, CAROL B. BENSON, MD, AND PETER M. DOUBILET, MD, PhD

This chapter has two components; the first considers duplex ultrasound assessment of the scrotal contents, and the second describes the role that ultrasound plays in the diagnosis of erectile dysfunction. In both sections, emphasis is given to color flow and Doppler diagnosis, in keeping with the focus of the text. Because the treatment of scrotal pathology is fairly brief, some readers may wish to acquire additional information by referring to general ultrasound textbooks.

THE SCROTUM

Anatomy and Normal Sonograpic Features

The anatomy of the scrotum, testis, and epididymis is illustrated in Figures 35–1 and 35–2. As seen with ultrasound, each testis is homogeneous and medium in echogenicity (Fig. 35–3), with a smooth outer border but no visible capsule.[1-10] In adults, each testis measures 3 to 5 cm in long axis and 2 to 3 cm in short axis. The testes are relatively hypoechoic before the age of puberty and achieve adult echogenicity thereafter. In elderly individuals, they may also be relatively hypoechoic and somewhat heterogeneous in echotexture. The mediastinum testis is seen regularly as a strongly echogenic band running along the margin of the testis. The epididymis is slightly more echogenic and coarse in texture than the testis.

The arterial and venous anatomy of the testes is illustrated in Figures 35–4 and 35–5.

In postpubertal boys and adults, blood vessels[4-7,11,12] are normally visible in and about the testis with color flow sonography (Fig. 35–6). The capsular arteries, which course around the periphery, and the centripetal arteries, which penetrate the parenchyma, are seen most easily. Flow in the centripetal arteries is from the capsule inward. Testicular veins follow the same pattern as the arteries and generally are readily visualized. Differentiation between arteries and veins is possible only with spectral Doppler. In about 50% of normal individuals, one or more large artery/vein pair(s) may be seen to traverse the testis obliquely from the mediastinum to the opposite

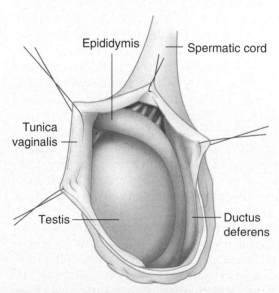

FIGURE 35–1. Scrotal anatomy. Each testis and epididymis is suspended in a sac lined by the tunica vaginalis.

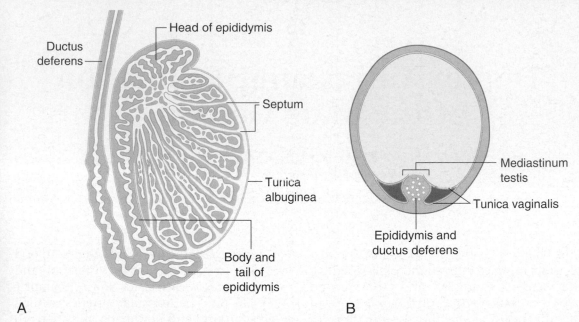

FIGURE 35–2. Testicular anatomy. *A,* The testis is encapsulated by a tough fibrous layer called the tunica albuginea and is divided into chambers by fibrous septae that are not visible with ultrasound. Myriad seminiferous tubules converge at the head of the epididymis, where they coalesce to form a single, but highly convoluted, tube that ultimately becomes the ductus deferens. For descriptive purposes, the epididymis is divided into the head (located superiorly), the body, and the tail (located inferiorly). *B,* The tunica vaginalis is a thin tissue layer that envelops the testis and epididymis and lines the scrotal sac, forming the mediastinum testis. The arrangement is analogous to the chest, where the pleura envelops the lungs, lines the chest cavity, and encloses the mediastinum of the thorax.

capsule.[4,5] These "transmediastinal" vessels may be visible on gray-scale images and should not be mistaken for pathology.

Arterial flow in the testis and epididymis characteristically exhibits a low-resistance pattern on spectral Doppler assessment, including continuous flow in diastole (Fig. 35–7). In contrast, a high-resistance flow pattern is seen in extragonadal arteries, which are part of the cremasteric system. These arteries are occasionally visualized along the course of the spermatic cord. It is important not to mistake extragonadal flow signals for testicular flow. Peak systolic velocity in testicular arteries ranges from 4 cm/sec to 19 cm/sec (mean 9.7 cm/sec), and end-diastolic velocity, from 1.6 cm/sec to 6.9 cm/sec (mean, 3.6 cm/sec).[11] These values permit quantitative assessment of arterial flow when a sufficiently long arterial segment is visualized with color flow, allowing for angle correction of the Doppler signal. When angle correction is not possible, spectral Doppler features are evaluated qualitatively.

Sonographic Technique

A linear array transducer with a frequency output of 7 MHz or higher is used to examine the testes, unless the scrotum is severely swollen and lower frequencies are required. A towel is draped over the penis for the sake of modesty and to keep it against the abdomen and out of the way. Several scanning approaches may be used. One method is to place towels between the patient's legs to support the scrotum, keeping both of the examiner's hands free. In another method, the examiner uses one hand to support to the scrotum and the other hand to maneuver the transducer. This method provides optimal control of the movable scrotal contents, but it requires a second individual to operate the ultrasound controls.

The first step in scanning the scrotal contents is to get oriented. The examiner then records a set of long- and short-axis images of each testis and epididymis, including

text continued on p. 663

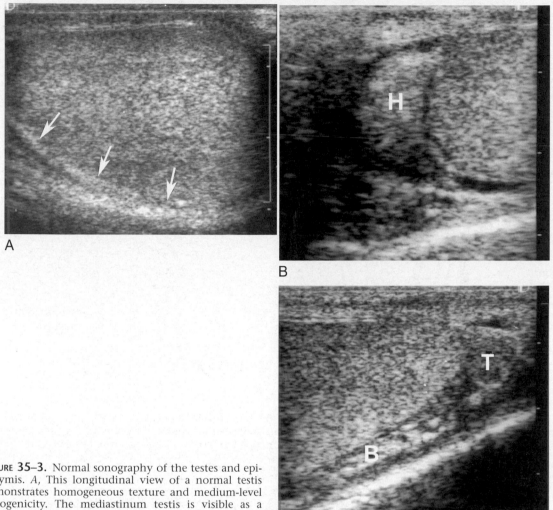

FIGURE 35–3. Normal sonography of the testes and epididymis. *A*, This longitudinal view of a normal testis demonstrates homogeneous texture and medium-level echogenicity. The mediastinum testis is visible as a slightly more echogenic region (*arrows*). *B* and *C*, Longitudinal views show the head (H), body (B), and tail (T) of the epididymis.

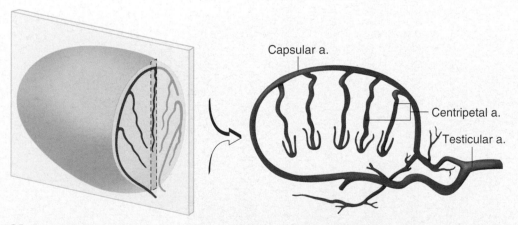

FIGURE 35–4. Vascular anatomy of the testis. The testicular (or spermatic) artery follows the course of the epididymal body through the mediastinum testis and gives off "capsular" branches that circle the periphery of the testis, beneath the tunica albuginea. The capsular arteries give off centripetal arteries that course through the testis toward the mediastinum and then loop back for a short distance as the recurrent rami. The venous drainage (not shown) parallels the arterial distribution.

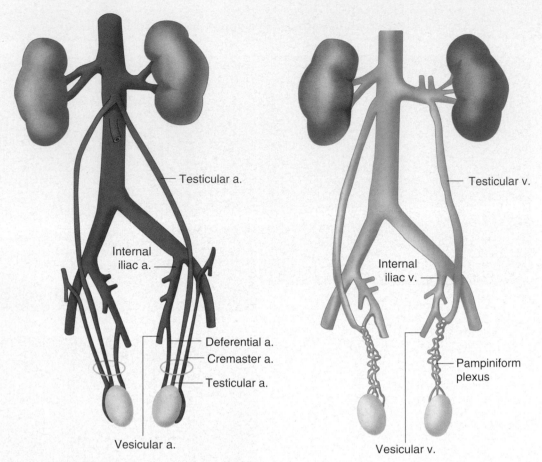

Testicular a.

Internal
iliac a.

Deferential a.
Cremaster a.
Testicular a.

Vesicular a.

Testicular v.

Internal
iliac v.

Pampiniform
plexus

Vesicular v.

FIGURE 35–5. Arterial supply and venous drainage of the scrotal contents. Each testicular artery arises from the aorta and extends directly to the testicle and epididymis, following the course of the spermatic cord and the body of the epididymis. Structures other than the testis and epididymis receive arterial flow via the cremasteric and deferential branches, which originate from the internal iliac arteries, as shown. Although the testicular arteries provide the principal arterial supply to the testis and epididymis, anastomotic channels exist among all of the scrotal arteries, permitting collateral flow. The venous drainage of each testis and epididymis is via a network of tiny veins called the pampiniform plexus. This network gradually coalesces to form two or three veins that follow the spermatic cord and unite as the spermatic vein. On the *left*, the spermatic vein drains into the ipsilateral renal vein, and on the *right*, the spermatic vein drains into the inferior vena cava.

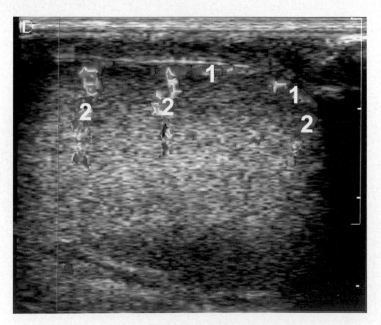

FIGURE 35–6. Normal testicular vessels. Longitudinal image shows capsular (1) and centripetal (2) arteries.

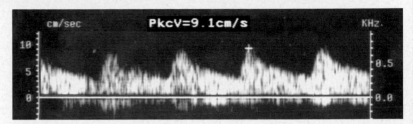

FIGURE   35–7. Low-resistance Doppler waveforms of normal testicular and epididymal flow. PckV, peak systolic velocity.

long- and short-axis testis dimensions. A composite transverse view showing both testicles simultaneously is also obtained, and this view is essential for comparing testicular echogenicity. If both testes cannot be viewed simultaneously on a transverse view, separate images should be recorded side by side, using identical ultrasound settings. When pathologic findings are present, they should be portrayed in whatever image plane best documents the abnormality, but long- and short-axis views should be used whenever possible as an aid to orientation.

The color flow examination may be conducted with color Doppler or power Doppler. In either case, the pulse repetition frequency must be set to detect very-low-velocity flow, and the wall filter must be low. Relatively high gain settings typically are needed, as the testicular vessels are quite small and produce weak Doppler signals. One method is to increase the gain until artifacts appear in the image and then back the gain down slightly. It is important to *make the spectral waveforms appear large on the images* by using an appropriate spectral display scale. If the waveforms are small, it is difficult to assess pulsatility patterns and compare testicular flow from one side to the other.

Scrotal Masses

Masses and masslike lesions of the scrotal contents may be caused by cysts, tumors, hematomas, inflammation, and abscesses. The location of the pathology, the gray-scale appearance, and the Doppler flow features are diagnostic in many cases.

Testicular Cysts

Cysts of the testis[1,2,6,7,10,13] are idiopathic and benign. They also are fairly common, being seen in 8% of adults examined sonographically. In most cases, a single testicular cyst is present, and it is uncommon to encounter more than three testicular cysts in a given individual. Most are 1 cm or less in diameter, but cysts as large as several centimeters are present occasionally. Cysts located on the testicular surface are called tunica cysts, since they are thought to arise in the tunica albuginea (fibrous layer that encapsulates the testis). These cysts may be palpable, leading to ultrasound investigation. More deeply located cysts are thought to arise from dilation of spermatic tubules called the rete testes. These may not be palpable.

The most important point about testicular cysts is distinguishing between these benign lesions and other pathology, including tumors and abscesses. Testicular cysts (Fig. 35–8) have the following sonographic features: (1) anechoic contents, (2) sharply defined borders and invisible wall, (3) enhanced through-transmission of ultrasound, and (4) no blood flow within or surrounding the cyst (other than normal testicular vessels). Cysts meeting these criteria are benign and inconsequential and require no follow-up.

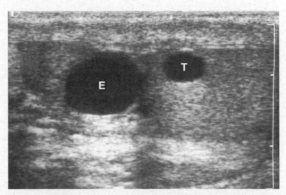

FIGURE 35–8. Testicular and epididymal cysts. This long-axis image shows both an epididymal (E) and a testicular (T) cyst.

Testicular Neoplasms

Testicular neoplasms are classified and described briefly in Table 35–1.[1,2,14] These neoplasms occur most frequently between the ages of 25 and 35 years and almost always are malignant. The prognosis generally is excellent, however, and 5-year survival is 90%, overall, assuming timely use of surgery, radiation therapy, or chemotherapy.[14] Testicular tumors usually present in one of two ways: as a palpable mass or with sudden pain and swelling due to hemorrhage. It is not uncommon for the latter presentation to follow minor trauma. A small number of patients present with signs and symptoms resulting from metastases.

Ultrasound can separate intratesticular and extratesticular pathology with about 98% accuracy.[1] Nevertheless, ultrasound generally cannot differentiate among histologic types of testicular tumors, nor can it generally differentiate between malignant and (uncommon) benign varieties. Most testicular tumors are well-defined hypoechoic lesions, but some may be poorly marginated or grossly infiltrating.[1,7,10,12,14–17] They may exhibit some degree of internal heterogeneity due to hemorrhage and/or necrosis, and calcification is occasionally present. Vascularity is evident within testicular neoplasms on color flow examination, which is a very important differential feature. Cysts, hematomas, and abscesses do not have internal vascularity. Testicular tumor vascularity (Fig. 35–9) is quite variable. Relative to the normal testis, some tumors are hypervascular, while in others, vascularity is similar to the normal testicle or even diminished.[4,10–12,14,16,17] In most tumors, focal dots or clumps of color are seen, with the occasional visualization of a linear vascular structure. The distribution of tumor blood vessels also is variable, with some lesions showing an orderly distribution of blood vessels and others, a chaotic distribution. In addition, large avascular areas may be present, due to necrosis and hemorrhage. Spectral Doppler generally shows low-pulsatility flow features in tumor vessels, which is typical of malignant neoplasms, regardless of location. Flow velocities are elevated substantially in hypervascular tumors but may be in the range of normal testicular vessels in less vascular lesions. Horstman and colleagues[12] found that testicular tumors larger than 1.6 cm were likely to be hypervascular, while smaller lesions tended to be hypovascular. Testicular microlithiasis, shown in Figure 35–9, has been associated with increased risk of testicular cancer in some series, but the level of risk and follow-up requirements remain controversial.[16]

Testicular Tumor Mimics

Lesions that can mimic the appearance of neoplasms include abscesses, inflamed areas (without frank abscess formation), contusions, hematomas, and infarcts.[1,7,10,14,18,19,20] The sonographic appearance of these lesions is nonspecific, as discussed later. Color and spectral Doppler features are of considerable importance in differentiating among these etiologies. No flow is present in abscesses, infarcts, and hematomas, but flow may be present in the periphery of abscesses.

Epididymal Cysts

Epididymal cysts[1,2,7,10,14] are much more common than testicular cysts, being found in about 40% of adult males examined

---

Table 35–1. Classification of Testicular Neoplasms

Seminoma: Most common (40%–50% primary testicular cancer). Least aggressive testicular cancer and exquisitely radiosensitive. Tends to occur in older age group.

Mixed Germ Cell Tumor: Accounts for 40% of primary testicular neoplasms. Mixture of different germ cell types. Teracarcinoma/teratoma/embryonal cell carcinoma is most common and is an aggressive tumor.

Embryonal Cell Carcinoma: Most aggressive primary germ cell tumor, as indicated by tunica invasion, testicular contour irregularity, and areas of hemorrhage or necrosis.

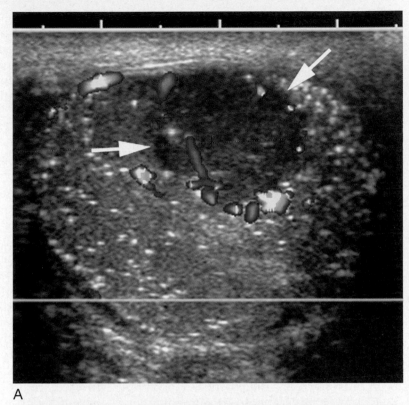

FIGURE 35–9. Seminoma. *A*, Color Doppler sonogram of small testicular seminoma (*arrows*) demonstrating a few blood vessels at the periphery and within the malignant testicular tumor. The punctate, strong reflections are caused by microlithiasis, which has been associated in some series with increased risk for testicular neoplasia. *B*, Color Doppler sonogram of a large testicular seminoma demonstrating disorganized blood vessels throughout the tumor.

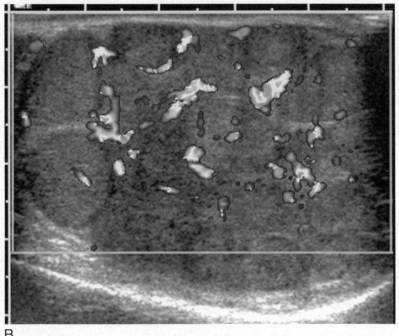

sonographically.[1] Most are located in the epididymal head, but cysts may occur anywhere in the epididymis. They may be single, multiple, unilateral, or bilateral. In some cases they are palpable, while in others they are found incidentally. Unlike testicular cysts, which usually are unilocular, epididymal cysts may be septated or even multilocular. Most are 2 to 3 mm in diameter, but larger cysts are common, and some may be several centimeters in size. The etiology of epididymal cysts is not entirely clear, and most are considered idiopathic. Some are spermatoceles, which are encapsulated collections of sperm.

The great majority of epididymal cysts have the same features as those described previously for testicular cysts, but there are other variations. Some may be septated or multilocular (see Fig. 35–8) and others may contain diffuse or dependent low-level echoes. It is hypothesized that the latter are spermatoceles, but this assumption has not been proven. From a diagnostic perspective, it is most important to document that benign epididymal cysts have no solid components, have exquisitely thin walls that are not visible sonographically, and show no visible blood flow on color flow examination (except for normal epididymal vessels).

Other Epididymal Masses

Other than cysts, the only common mass lesions of the epididymis are hematomas, abscesses, and inflammatory masses.[1,2,8,14,19,20] Tumors of the epididymis are uncommon, and their sonographic features are not well described in the medical literature. An important feature, however, is the presence of blood flow within the tumor, which is not present in some other lesions. Hematomas of the epididymis or spermatic cord usually occur in the context of recognized trauma but may occur spontaneously and in association with vigorous exercise. An epididymal hematoma usually presents as a hard, palpable (and possibly tender) mass that may mimic a neoplastic mass on physical examination. On ultrasound, a hematoma usually has a nonspe-

cific, hypoechoic, or heterogeneous appearance. Most importantly, blood flow is absent in and around the lesion (except for normal vessels) on color flow examination. Abscesses and inflammatory masses are differential considerations and are discussed later.

Epididymitis and Orchitis

Infection is the most common cause of acute scrotal pain and tenderness.[14] In the great majority of cases, the infection[2,6,7,10,12,13,17,18,21–23] is caused by sexually transmitted organisms (principally *Neisseria gonorrhoeae* and *Chlamydia trachomatis*) that "ascend" through the genital tract. The tail of the epididymis is infected first, and then the infection spreads throughout the epididymis (epididymitis). The infection may then extend to the testis (orchitis) and finally to the scrotal cavity, generating an infected hydrocele. Orchitis typically is present by the time patients seek medical care.[10]

Ultrasound is a very useful method for confirming the diagnosis of epididymitis or orchitis and for excluding other pathology that may cause acute scrotal pain or swelling. The key findings are enlargement and decreased echogenicity of the affected structures, accompanied by *increased blood flow* (hyperemia) on color or spectral Doppler examination[2,6,7,10,12,18,21–23] (Fig. 35–10). Because orchitis usually is present by the time the patient seeks care, involvement of both the testis and epididymis may be evident sonographically; however, in some patients, epididymal involvement may predominate. A hydrocele (excess scrotal fluid) often is present, and the scrotal wall may be edematous and/or inflamed. In some cases of epididymitis/orchitis, the ultrasound findings may be dramatic. In other instances, findings are less obvious and are based solely on side-to-side comparison of structure size, echogenicity, and blood flow. Obviously, side-by-side comparison is not helpful in cases of symmetrical, bilateral infection; nevertheless, hyperemia of the scrotal contents may still be evident in such cases. It is noteworthy that a focal,

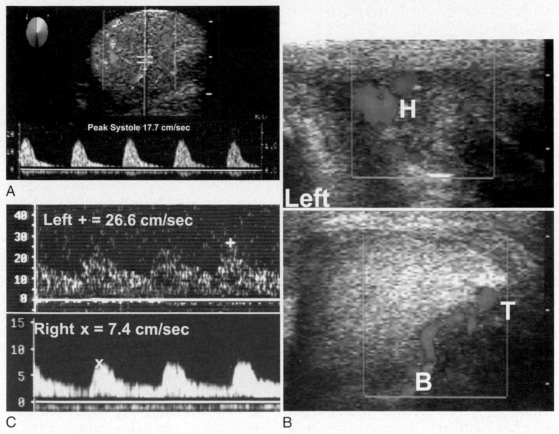

FIGURE 35–10. Epididymo-orchitis. *A*, Luxuriant blood flow is present in this infected testis. Peak systole is 17.1 cm/sec. *B*, In another patient, increased blood flow is present throughout the head (H), body (B), and tail (T) of the infected left epididymis. *C*, Doppler examination shows massively increased blood flow (peak systole, 26.6 cm/sec) in the left epididymis, as compared with the right (7.4 cm/sec).

hypoechoic area of inflammation may be seen in the periphery of the testis, adjacent to an infected epididymal head. This should not be mistaken for a testicular tumor but should be followed for resolution with antibiotic treatment.

The sonographic diagnosis of epididymo-orchitis generally is straightforward, but mimics occasionally may cause misdiagnoses; namely, hyperemia following detorsion of a testis (considered later) and diffusely infiltrating lymphoma or leukemia.[24] The epididymis and testis usually return to a normal sonographic appearance following an episode of infection, but in severe cases, testicular atrophy or infarction may occur. Atrophy is a noteworthy complication of mumps orchitis.

Abscesses may occur in the epididymis or testis in severe cases of epididymo-orchitis. These appear as heterogeneous masses or as fluid collections with irregular walls, possibly containing diffuse or dependent debris. Increased blood flow due to hyperemia may be apparent in the surrounding tissues, either focally or diffusely. In our experience, testicular abscesses are seen acutely rather than as chronic processes. Epididymal abscesses, however, may be chronic, and as a result, hyperemia may not be evident, causing a chronic abscess to be indistinguishable from other extratesticular masses.

In unusual cases of acute epididymo-orchitis, infection may spread to the scrotal sac, producing an infected hydrocele. The sonographic manifestation is echogenic debris within the hydrocele fluid, either diffusely or dependently, and possible loculation of the hydrocele. These findings are nonspecific, however, and may also be seen with chronic hydroceles in the absence of active infection. Therefore, infected hydrocele should be suggested only when there are concomitant findings of acute infection in the epididymis and/or testis.

Most cases of epididymo-orchitis are treated successfully and resolve, but untreated or incompletely treated cases may present with findings of chronic epididymitis, which may be manifested as diffuse thickening and heterogeneity of the epididymis or as a focal, heterogeneous epididymal mass. As noted previously, increased blood flow may not be a feature of chronic epididymitis. Hydrocele may also be present, and this may be loculated or may contain echogenic material.

Varicocele

Varicocele, or dilation of the pampiniform venous plexus, is a common cause of a palpable epididymal mass and scrotal discomfort.[1,2,7,10,13,25,26] In some individuals, a varicocele contributes to low sperm count, decreased sperm motility, and infertility. These problems have been attributed to persistent, hyperemia-induced elevation of testicular temperature, but the real cause may be more complex and is not known with certainty.

The veins of the pampiniform plexus, which drain the testis and epididymis, normally are quite small, but these may dilate due to valvular incompetence and/or elevated pressure, forming a tangle of enlarged veins along the course of the spermatic cord and epididymis. In unusual cases, dilated veins may even extend into the substance of the testis. Varicoceles are more common on the left side of the scrotum than the right, possibly due to elevated pressure in the left spermatic vein. The left spermatic vein inserts into the left renal vein, which drapes across the aorta and may be compressed between the aorta and superior mesenteric artery, raising venous pressure. The right renal vein drains into the inferior vena cava directly and is not subject to compressive effects. Because of the left side predominance of varicocele, the possibility of

neoplastic spermatic vein obstruction (due to intra-abdominal lymphadenopathy) should be considered when a varicocele is isolated to the right cord/epididymis. It is commonly suggested that an abdominal computed tomogram be obtained in such cases. In addition, the sonographer should examine the abdomen for evidence of retroperitoneal adenopathy in the vicinity of the aorta and inferior vena cava at the time of the scrotal examination.

Varicocele usually is a clinical diagnosis, as the tangle of veins is easily palpated and feels like a "bunch of worms." Ultrasound is required when the nature of the palpable mass is unclear or when pain or tenderness is present, as well as in men who experience infertility. Varicocele is diagnosed with color flow ultrasound when numerous veins of unusually large size are seen along the spermatic cord or epididymis, as shown in Figure 35–11. In all cases, the extent of the varicosities should be documented, and the largest veins should be measured, as discussed later. The presence of reflux within the veins should be investigated by having the patient perform the Valsalva maneuver during color flow observation. Normal pampiniform veins are barely detectable, so from one perspective, varicocele can be diagnosed whenever veins of unusual size and number are readily seen. More specific diagnosis may be important, however, in men with pain or infertility, in whom a decision must be made concerning the potential benefit of therapy. In this respect, veins 2 mm in diameter or less are generally regarded as not substantially dilated, while larger veins are considered varicose, especially those with a diameter of 3 mm or larger.[2,13,25,26] This definition includes veins reaching this size with the patient in positions not typically used during ultrasound examination (e.g., standing, squatting) and in any state of respiration, including straining or performing the Valsalva maneuver. The demonstration of reflux in the veins is further evidence of potential clinical significance. Although sonographic criteria such as these are used in an attempt to define the clinical significance of a varicocele, decisions concerning the need for veno-occlusive therapy are multifactoral and are

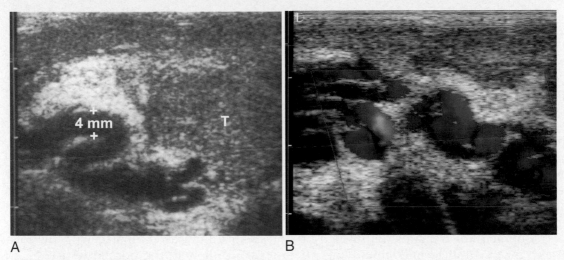

A   B

FIGURE 35–11. Varicocele. *A*, Gray-scale imaging shows a serpiginous vein measuring 4 mm in diameter in the head and body of the epididymis. T, testicle. *B*, Color Doppler confirms that the structure seen in *A* is a vein and shows additional dilated veins.

more a matter of clinical judgment than of specific ultrasound criteria.

Testicular Torsion

Torsion refers to twisting of the testis within the scrotal sac, such that the arteries and veins are compressed and blood flow is compromised.[2,10,12,13,17,18,21,22,27–36] Torsion results from abnormal mobility of the testis, due to narrow attachment of the testis to the scrotal wall by the reflection of the tunica vaginalis (see Fig. 35–2B). Normally, the parietal layer of the tunica vaginalis lines the inner wall of the scrotal sac until it reaches the edge of the testicle, where it reflects over the testicle, forming the visceral layer of the tunica vaginalis. The portion of the testicle that is not covered by the visceral layer of the tunica vaginalis is closely held against the scrotal wall and called the "bare area." Vessels and tubules from the spermatic cord enter and leave the testicle across the bare area. When the bare area is abnormally small (an abnormality called the "bell clapper deformity"), the attachment of the testicle to the scrotal wall is narrow and the testicle is at risk for torsion due to twisting at this attachment.

Torsion usually occurs in children or young adults, and two peaks of incidence have been noted: the neonatal period and puberty. Although scintigraphy continues to be utilized for testicular torsion diagnosis, color Doppler ultrasound has become the predominant diagnostic method. Ultrasound is reported to be 86% to 100% sensitive and virtually 100% specific for diagnosing testicular torsion.[27–32]

The pathologic sequence of events with torsion begins when the spermatic cord twists, with a rotation of at least 360 degrees, at the bare area. This causes venous obstruction, leading to swelling and increased pressure inside the testicle and within the spermatic cord. Subsequently, arterial flow becomes occluded and testicular ischemia results, progressing to infarction if detorsion does not occur surgically or spontaneously.

The pathologic process of torsion can be divided into *acute torsion*, during which the testicle suffers ischemia but can be saved if detorsion occurs, and *missed torsion*, the stage after which testicular infarction has occurred to the point that the testicle cannot be saved even if detorsed. The testicle is almost always salvageable during the first 6 to 10 hours of torsion and is progressively less likely to be salvageable thereafter. In virtually all cases of torsion lasting more than 24 hours, the testicle cannot be saved.[2,12,17,18,21,22]

Early on after the onset of torsion, the testicle may appear normal in echotexture. During this time, the only abnormal gray-scale sonographic findings may be in the spermatic cord and epididymis, which may appear as a thick echogenic structure with acoustic shadowing due to twisting.[33,34] On Doppler, blood flow will be diminished or absent in the testicle or the knotted cord and epididymis. As the torsion persists and blood flow remains occluded, the testicle becomes enlarged and mildly hypoechoic, due to swelling and edema. At this time, a small hydrocele is sometimes seen. With color Doppler, flow remains diminished or absent in the testicle and epididymis. If there is further progression to the development of testicular necrosis, the testicle becomes mottled and heterogeneous with hypoechoic areas, and the scrotal wall becomes thickened.

Gray-scale and Doppler findings are key to the diagnosis of testicular torsion. The examination should begin with gray-scale, including side-to-side comparison of testicular size and echogenicity and assessment of the epididymis to look for the knotted cord (Fig. 35–12). Color Doppler should then be performed for side-to-side assessment of blood flow. With testicular torsion, differences in perfusion, including absence or marked diminution of blood flow on the affected side, will be found. If blood flow is still present on the affected side, spectral waveforms typically demonstrate high-resistance flow, as compared with the low-resistance flow in the normal testicle.

Rarely, detorsion of the testicle occurs prior to the sonographic and Doppler assessment.[6,17,21,22] In such cases, the affected testicle may be hyperemic as compared with the normal testicle. In these cases, the knot

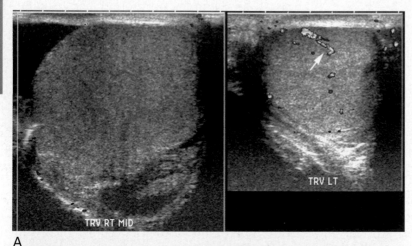

A

B

FIGURE 35–12. Testicular torsion. *A,* Transverse (TRV) views of right (RT) and left (LT) testicles demonstrate flow in several vessels on the left (*arrow*) and no flow in the right testicle due to acute torsion. The right testicle is markedly swollen and hypoechoic compared with the left. *B,* Transverse views of right and left testicles demonstrate flow in several vessels on the left (*arrow*) and no flow in the right testicle due to acute torsion. The knot of the twisted cord and epididymis (*arrowheads*) is seen adjacent to the testicle.

of the twisted cord and epididymis will not be present.

There are several pitfalls with respect to testicular torsion diagnosis.[2,17,18,21,22,27] First, blood flow is cut off completely only with fairly marked levels of torsion (360 degrees or greater). With lesser degrees of torsion, Doppler may be subtly abnormal or even normal. Second, appreciating side-to-side differences in blood flow may be problematic in young children, because the testicles may be small and blood flow may be difficult to detect even in a normal testicle.[35,36] Third, a torsed testis may undergo spontaneous detorsion, followed by a period of hyperemia. If the testis is examined during the hyperemic period, increased blood flow may be mistaken for orchitis, or torsion may be ascribed to the wrong testis.

Scrotal Trauma

Penetrating scrotal trauma usually requires surgical exploration and is not generally the subject of ultrasound examination. Ultrasound is useful, however, in concussion or crush injuries of the scrotum, which are difficult to evaluate clinically because of pain and scrotal swelling.[10,12,18,22,37–41] The primary role of ultrasound is to determine whether the testes are intact and to assess perfusion. Improved salvage of traumatized testes can be achieved if testicular rupture is recognized early and treated surgically. When testicular rupture is likely, based on the nature of the crush/contusion injury, then surgery is required and ultrasound may not have a role in patient management. Sonography is most useful when conservative (nonsurgical) management is anticipated. If the testes appear intact, conservative management is supported, but if there is evidence of rupture or if there are large nonperfused areas or a complete lack of perfusion (due to torsion), surgery is necessary.

A large hematocele (blood-filled scrotum) typically is present in trauma patients due to hemorrhage from the testis or other scrotal contents. The injured testis may be heterogeneous due to hematoma formation or infarction. Focal hematomas vary in echogenicity according to their age.

Acute hematomas tend to be moderately echogenic, and older hematomas, hypoechoic. Infarcted areas are isoechoic or hypoechoic. Color Doppler shows absent perfusion in both hematomas and infarcted areas; therefore, this does not differentiate one from the other. Fractures of the testicular tissue may be visualized as hypoechoic clefts that may or may not be associated with disruption of the tunica albuginea (testicular surface). If the testicular surface is clearly disrupted or tissue is extruded from the testis, the term *testicular rupture* is used, and this finding implies disruption of the tunica albuginea. This distinction is important, as fractures may not be surgical lesions, whereas rupture is generally treated surgically. The most useful signs of testicular rupture are distortion of the shape of the testicle, the detection of a frank cleft in the testicular surface, or the detection of extruded testicular tissue.[10,37,38,41] Heterogeneity is also associated with rupture due to intratesticular hemorrhage and contusion, but this finding may also be present without rupture.

The epididymis also may be injured, with or without associated testicular injury. Epididymal trauma is manifested by swelling and heterogeneity due to hemorrhage. Focal hematoma formation may also occur.

Color Doppler is used in blunt testicular injury to detect avascular areas representing infarction of testicular parenchyma or hematoma formation. Color Doppler may also detect the absence of venous or arterial flow due to post-traumatic torsion of the testis. Finally, large scrotal hematoceles may cause sufficient pressure to obstruct venous drainage, which is diagnosed through the absence of venous flow signals on Doppler examination.

The value of ultrasound in nonpenetrating scrotal trauma is well recognized, yet it appears that sonography is a less-than-perfect diagnostic method.[37–41] Statistics are limited because published series are small; however, it is clear that ultrasound cannot detect fractures reliably and even misses testicular rupture in some cases; furthermore, some testes that appear ruptured (even with apparent extrusion of testicular tissue) are found at surgery to be intact. In the latter cases, it appears that thrombus adherent to the testis may mimic tunica rupture and tissue extrusion. Epididymal injuries also may be difficult to detect due to absence of sonographic findings or obscuration by adherent thrombus.

ERECTILE DYSFUNCTION

Penile Anatomy

The normal penis comprises three columns of spongy tissue, each encased by a dense fibrous sheath. Two of the columns, the paired corpora cavernosa, lie in parallel on the dorsal side of the penis. The corpora cavernosa contain multiple sinusoidal spaces with smooth muscle in their walls, and it is this spongy tissue that expands and fills with blood during an erection. The tunica albuginea is the dense fibrous sheath that encapsulates the sinusoidal tissue, providing structure and support when the penis is erect.

Along the ventral side of the penis runs the corpus spongiosum. This column of spongiosal tissue surrounds the urethra, which remains in a collapsed state except during active urination. The corpus spongiosum is usually smaller than the corpora cavernosa, except at its distal end, where it broadens to form the glans penis. The spongiosal tissue of the corpus spongiosum expands somewhat with erection but not to the extent that the cavernosal tissues expand. The three columns of tissue are surrounded by a layer of subcutaneous tissue and skin.

Arterial blood supply to the penis is via bilateral penile arteries, each a branch of the internal pudendal artery. The penile artery has two main branches, the dorsal artery and the cavernosal artery. The dorsal artery travels along the dorsal side of the penis lateral to the midline dorsal vein and supplies blood to the glans penis and the corpus spongiosum. It has few or no branches before it reaches the glans penis. The cavernosal artery travels centrally within the corpus cavernosum and supplies blood to the cavernosal sinusoids via multiple branches called *helicine arteries* that extend radially from the cavernosal artery (Fig. 35–13). Most men have a single cavernosal artery on each side; however, anatomic variants of cavernosal blood supply are common. In some cases, the cavernosal artery arises from the dorsal artery. In other cases, more than one cavernosal artery is present. During the generation of an erection, flow in the cavernosal arteries and helicine branches is markedly increased.

The venous drainage from the corpora cavernosa is via small veins that perforate the tunica albuginea to drain into the deep dorsal vein. Toward the base of the penis are small crural veins that drain into the deep pelvic veins to the internal pudendal vein. When the penis is erect and the corpora cavernosa are expanded, the small draining

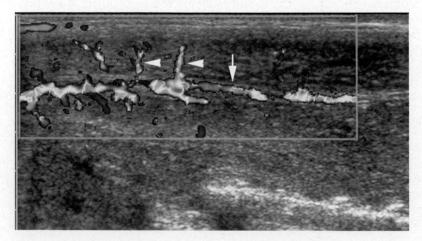

Figure 35–13. Cavernosal artery and helicine branches. Longitudinal color Doppler sonogram of corpus cavernosum demonstrating flow in the cavernosal artery (*arrow*) that courses through the middle of the corpus cavnernosum. Small helicine branches (*arrowheads*) extend radially from the cavernosal artery.

veins are occluded by stretching of the tunica albuginea.

Erectile Function

The physiologic process of a normal erection begins with increased parasympathetic motor nervous activity to the penis, involving sacral nerves two, three, and four. The parasympathetic motor activity causes the smooth muscle in the walls of the cavernosal sinusoids to relax, allowing the sinusoids to expand and decreasing the resistance to incoming blood flow. At the same time, the cavernosal arteries dilate and carry increased blood flow into the penis. The sinusoids fill with blood, and the corpora cavernosa expand and stretch to become rigid. With expansion of the corpora cavernosa, the draining veins are occluded, preventing blood from leaving the dilated sinusoids. Once the cavernosal sinusoids are filled, the cavernosal arterial blood flow decreases because of increased resistance within the corpora cavernosa. Continued parasympathetic nervous activity maintains the erection.[42]

Normal erectile function requires normal psychological health, normal endocrine balance, intact innervation to the penis, normal cavernosal sinusoids, adequate arterial blood supply, and normal venous occlusion with erection. Abnormalities of any of these systems may lead to erectile dysfunction. Impotence can be classified as organic, in which a physiologic abnormality is present, or psychogenic, in which impotence is due to psychological factors. Among men with previously normal erectile function who seek medical attention for impotence, an organic cause is found in 50% to 90%.[43-45]

The vast majority of patients with organic impotence have hemodynamic abnormalities: arterial insufficiency, venous incompetence, or both. Arteriogenic impotence occurs as a result of stenoses or occlusions that limit blood flow to the penis even in the presence of parasympathetic stimulation. If maximum flow is inadequate to fill the cavernosal sinusoids, tumescence and rigidity cannot occur. Without adequate filling of the corpora cavernosa, draining veins are not occluded but rather continue to carry blood away from the corpora cavernosa.[42,46] Arteriogenic impotence occurs most commonly in men with risk factors for atherosclerosis, including diabetes mellitus, hypertension, hypercholesterolemia, and smoking.[47,48]

Patients with mild to moderate arterial insufficiency in the absence of venous incompetence can often be successfully treated with self-injection therapy using prostaglandin E_1 or oral therapy with sildenafil citrate (Viagra). Patients with severe arterial insufficiency usually require a penile implant to restore sexual function.[42]

Venous incompetence results from failure of occlusion of the draining veins, despite adequate filling of the cavernosal sinusoids. Patients may experience partial erections, but rigidity cannot be fully achieved or maintained.

Other penile abnormalities, including scarring within the corpora cavernosa or involving the tunica albuginea, may also cause impotence. Scarring or fibrosis of sinusoidal tissue prevents that area of the corpora from expanding when an erection is developing. The sinusoidal tissue around the scar fills with blood and pulls on the abnormal area, causing penile curvature. If the scarring is severe, expansion of the surrounding sinusoids may also cause pain, leading to detumescence.

When scarring affects the tunica albuginea that surrounds the corpora cavernosa, the tunica becomes thickened and may even calcify. Calcified plaques of the tunica are called *Peyronie's disease*. Plaques involving the tunica albuginea most often cause painless curvature with erection. Sometimes, as with cavernosal plaques, there may be enough pain from the plaque with an erection that detumescence results.

Sonography

Sonographic evaluation of the penis is performed with high-frequency (7- to 15-MHz) linear transducers. The transducer is placed directly on the penis, and longitudinal and transverse images are obtained. The corpora

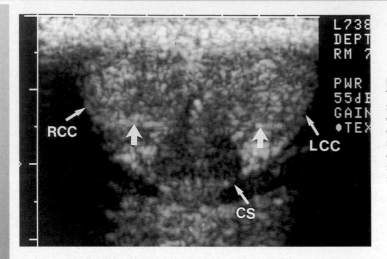

FIGURE 35–14. Normal nonerect penis. Transverse sonogram demonstrating two symmetric corpora cavernosa—right corpus cavernosum (RCC; *arrow*) and left corpus cavernosum (LCC; *arrow*)—dorsally and the corpus spongiosum (CS; *arrow*) ventrally. The tunica albuginea is seen as a thin line (*thick arrows*) encapsulating the corpora cavernosa.

of the normal penis have homogeneous echotexture. The two corpora cavernosa should be symmetric in size (Fig. 35–14). Within the corpora cavernosa, the bright walls of the cavernosal arteries may be seen in some areas (Fig. 35–15). The tunica albuginea surrounding the cavernosal tissue appears as a thin echogenic line encasing the corpora (see Fig. 35–14). The corpus spongiosum is usually smaller than the corpora cavernosa but has similar echogenicity to the flaccid corpora. The urethra cannot be seen when it is collapsed.

When the penis is erect, the corpora cavernosa are larger, and the spongiosal tissue has a speckled appearance with small anechoic areas representing dilated sinusoids, separated by the brightly echogenic sinusoidal septa (Fig. 35–16). The cavernosal arteries are dilated, and their walls are brightly echogenic (Fig. 35–17) because they are surrounded by blood-filled sinusoids.

Scarring of the corpora cavernosa or tunica albuginea can be diagnosed by ultrasound. Scars of the corpora cavernosa appear as irregular echogenic areas within the corpora (Fig. 35–18). With an erection and dilation of the surrounding sinusoids, the scars become more prominent and easier to delineate. Tunical plaques appear sonographically as focal areas of thickening of the tunica albuginea. Calcification in the plaque is brightly echogenic and casts an acoustic shadow (Fig. 35–19).

Doppler Evaluation

Color Doppler and pulsed Doppler assessments are used to evaluate the hemody-

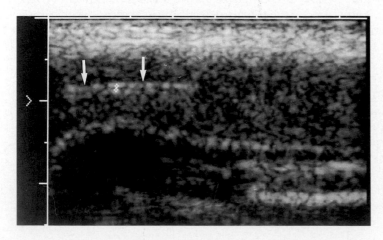

FIGURE 35–15. Cavernosal artery in nonerect penis. Longitudinal sonogram of the right corpus cavernosum demonstrating cavernosal artery (*calipers; arrows*) within sinusoidal tissue. The walls of the cavernosal artery are echogenic.

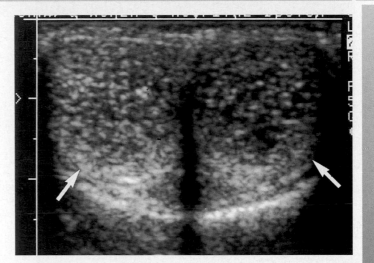

FIGURE 35–16. Erect penis. Transverse sonogram demonstrating the enlarged corpora cavernosa (*arrows*) with a speckled appearance because of blood-filled sinusoids.

namic function of the penis. Doppler assessment is performed after intracavernosal injection of a vasoactive pharmacologic agent to induce and maintain an erection. Either papaverine or prostaglandin E_1, both of which induce an erection by causing sinusoidal smooth muscle relaxation and dilation of the cavernosal arteries, can be used. The dose for papaverine is usually 30 to 60 mg, and that for prostaglandin E_1, 10 to 15 µg. The pharmacologic substance is injected directly into one corpus cavernosum using a small-gauge needle. A single injection acts on both corpora via multiple communications across the intercavernosal septum. Before injection, some examiners place a tourniquet at the base of the penis to prolong the local effect of the agent, leaving the tourni-

quet in place for 2 to 3 minutes until Doppler assessment is begun. Immediately after injection, some examiners use vibratory stimulation or ask the patient to manually stimulate the penis to promote the action of the drug.

Doppler assessment should begin 2 to 3 minutes after injection by obtaining Doppler waveforms from both cavernosal arteries and measuring the peak systolic velocity in each (Fig. 35–20). The waveforms are most easily obtained by scanning from the dorsal side of the penis, using color Doppler assessment, if necessary, to help localize the cavernosal artery (Fig. 35–21). Arterial waveforms should be obtained at 2- to 3-minute intervals until the peak systolic velocity is above 35 cm/sec or has plateaued. Once the penis has reached

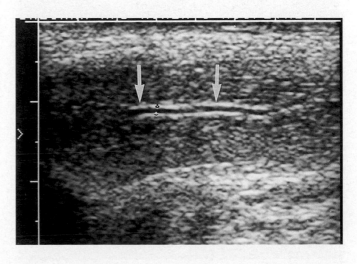

FIGURE 35–17. Cavernosal artery in erect penis. Longitudinal sonogram of the right corpus cavernosum demonstrating the cavernosal artery (*calipers; arrows*) with brightly echogenic walls running through blood-filled sinusoids.

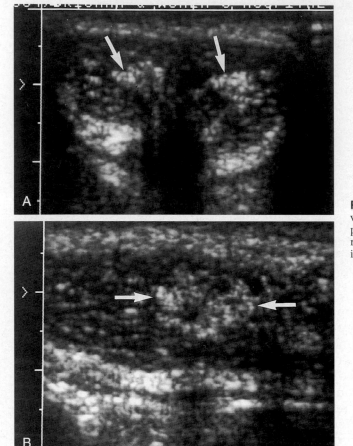

FIGURE 35–18. Sinusoidal scarring. *A,* Transverse sonogram demonstrating echogenic plaques (*arrows*) within both corpora cavernosa. *B,* Longitudinal sonogram demonstrating sinusoidal plaque (*arrows*).

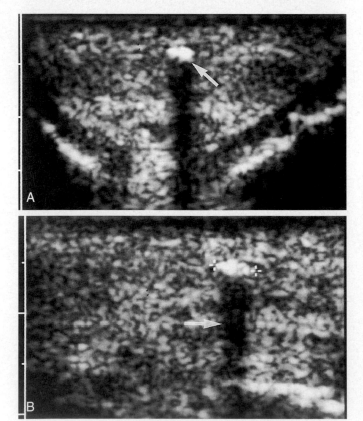

FIGURE 35–19. Peyronie's disease. *A,* Transverse sonogram demonstrating brightly echogenic calcified plaque (*arrow*) in midline, located dorsally between the corpora cavernosa. *B,* Longitudinal sonogram of calcified plaque (*calipers*) with acoustic shadowing behind calcification (*arrow*).

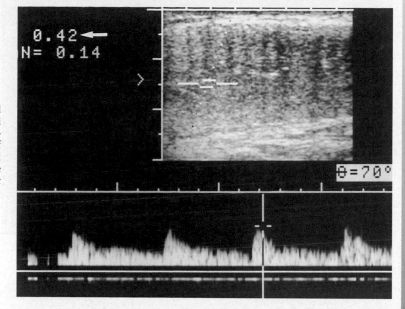

FIGURE 35–20. Normal cavernosal arterial waveform. Longitudinal sonogram with the Doppler waveform below, taken after injection of papaverine, demonstrating normal high velocities and low-resistance flow. Peak velocity is 42 cm/sec (0.42 m/sec; *arrow*).

maximal tumescence or the peak systolic velocity has plateaued, which usually occurs 8 to 10 minutes after injection but may be as long as 15 to 20 minutes in anxious patients,[49–52] the end-diastolic velocity is measured from the cavernosal arterial waveform. At this time, flow is also assessed in the deep dorsal vein by scanning the vein from the ventral side of the penis using color Doppler or pulsed Doppler assessments.[45,49–51,53–55]

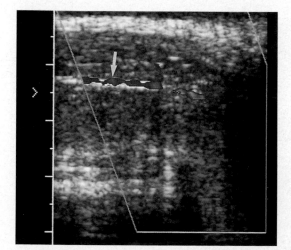

FIGURE 35–21. Color Doppler assessment of cavernosal artery. Longitudinal sonogram with the color Doppler image demonstrating flow in the cavernosal artery (*arrow*) located centrally within the corpus cavernosum.

The blood flow in men with normal hemodynamic function follows a predictable pattern during generation of an erection. Initially, in the flaccid state, Doppler waveforms of the cavernosal arteries demonstrate a high-resistance pattern, with low systolic peaks and absent or reverse diastolic flow (Fig. 35–22), and no flow is demonstrated in the deep dorsal vein. Two to three minutes after intracorporal injection of papaverine or prostaglandin E_1, the smooth muscles in the cavernosal sinusoids relax, leading to increased arterial inflow and a low-resistance arterial waveform, typified by high diastolic flow (Fig. 35–23). As the high flow continues in the cavernosal arteries and the sinusoids fill, the waveform changes to a higher-resistance pattern with sharp systolic waveforms and diminished or absent diastolic flow (Fig. 35–24). The peak systolic velocity increases over the first several minutes after injection, up to a maximum that exceeds 35 cm/sec in most normal men.[53,56–58] Because some men who achieve normal erections have peak systolic velocities between 30 and 35 cm/sec, some researchers classify patients with peak flows of 30 cm/sec or greater as normal.[48,50,55] With full tumescence, peak systolic velocities decline and there is absent or even reverse end-diastolic flow (Figs. 35–25 and

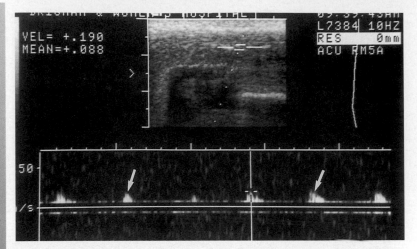

FIGURE 35–22. Cavernosal arterial waveform in the nonerect penis. Longitudinal sonogram with a Doppler waveform below demonstrating minimal arterial flow with short systolic peaks (*arrows*).

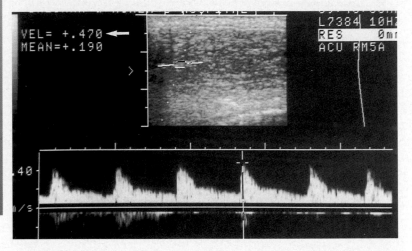

FIGURE 35–23. Cavernosal arterial waveform during the generation of erection. Longitudinal sonogram with a Doppler waveform below demonstrating low-resistance flow with normal systolic peak velocity of 47 cm/sec (0.47 m/sec; *arrow*).

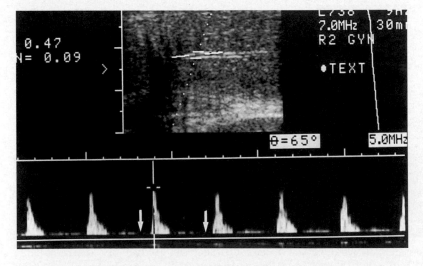

FIGURE 35–24. Cavernosal arterial waveform after full erection is achieved. Longitudinal sonogram with a Doppler waveform below demonstrating sharp systolic peaks with normal peak systolic velocity of 47 cm/sec and also absent end-diastolic flow (*arrows*).

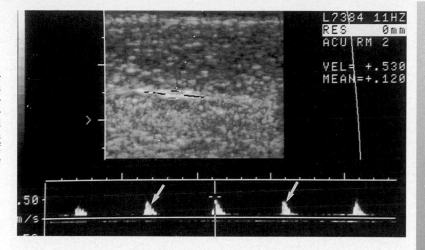

FIGURE 35–25. Cavernosal arterial waveform after full erection is achieved. Longitudinal sonogram with the Doppler waveform below demonstrating small systolic peaks (*arrows*) with normal peak systolic velocity of 53 cm/sec and also absent end-diastolic flow.

35–26). At this point, no flow should be seen in the deep dorsal vein with color Doppler examination.

Deviation from this normal pattern may be diagnostic of arterial or venous disease. Arterial insufficiency is best diagnosed using the maximum cavernosal arterial systolic velocity, as good correlation has been demonstrated between this measurement and the arteriographic findings at angiography.[46,59] The lower the peak systolic velocity, the greater the degree of severity of arterial disease. Patients with maximum systolic velocities somewhat below normal, in the range of 25 to 30 cm/sec, usually have mild to moderate arterial insufficiency. Patients with maximum velocities less than 25 cm/sec usually have severe arterial insuf-

ficiency[43,48,53,55,57,60] (Figs. 35–27 and 35–28). A discrepancy in maximum velocities of greater than 10 cm/sec between right and left sides is also usually indicative of some degree of arterial insufficiency.

Although the maximum systolic velocity correlates fairly well with arterial function of the penis, there are limitations to this diagnostic method. Patient anxiety can diminish the arterial response to the vasoactive pharmacologic agents to the point that maximum velocities fall below the normal range despite normal arterial function. A similar decrease may be found in some patients with psychogenic impotence.[61] In general, the maximum systolic velocity is lower in patients with psychogenic impotence and normal arterial function than

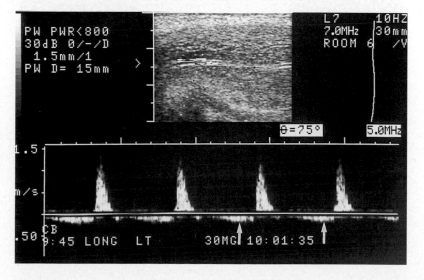

FIGURE 35–26. Cavernosal arterial waveform after full erection is achieved. Longitudinal sonogram with the Doppler waveform below demonstrating sharp systolic peaks and reverse end-diastolic flow (*arrows*).

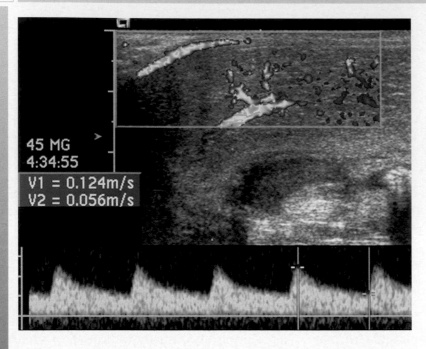

FIGURE 35–27. Arterial insufficiency. Cavernosal arterial waveform with arterial insufficiency. Longitudinal sonogram with color and spectral Doppler of cavernosal artery demonstrating an abnormally low peak systolic velocity of 12.4 cm/sec (V1 = 0.124 m/sec).

in patients without these conditions.[58] Patients with variants of cavernosal arterial anatomy, such as duplicated cavernosal arteries on one side, may have peak systolic velocities less than 30 cm/sec despite normal arterial flow. For this reason, when more than one artery is seen, conclusions about arterial function cannot be drawn if the maximum systolic velocity is less than 30 cm/sec.[62]

Doppler sonography can also be helpful for diagnosing venous incompetence, as a number of findings suggest this diagnosis when arterial function is normal. This diagnosis should be suspected in any patient who fails to generate an adequate erection despite normal cavernosal arterial Doppler waveforms.[45,53] The Doppler findings most suggestive of venous incompetence are flow in the dorsal vein or cavernosal arterial diastolic flow above 5 cm/sec (Fig. 35–29). Demonstration of dorsal vein flow, via either color Doppler or pulsed Doppler assessment (Fig. 35–30), is consistent with

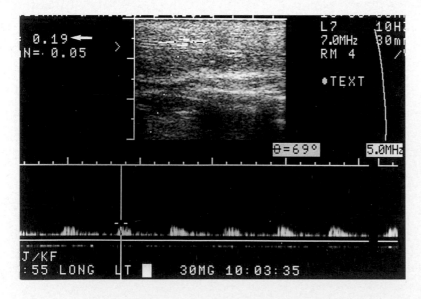

FIGURE 35–28. Cavernosal arterial waveform with arterial insufficiency. Longitudinal sonogram with the Doppler waveform below demonstrating an abnormally low peak systolic velocity of 19 cm/sec (0.19 m/sec; *arrow*).

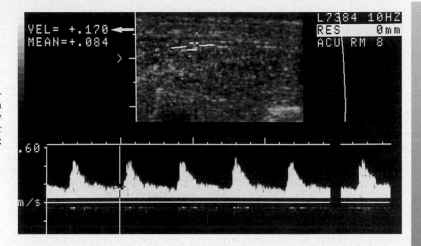

FIGURE 35–29. Venous incompetence. Longitudinal sonogram with the Doppler waveform below demonstrating persistent diastolic flow at 17 cm/sec (0.17 m/sec; *arrow*).

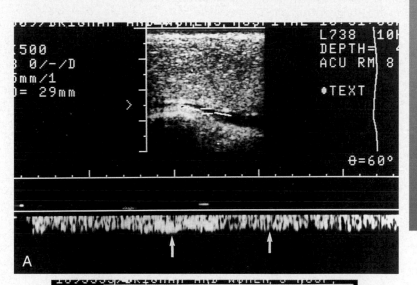

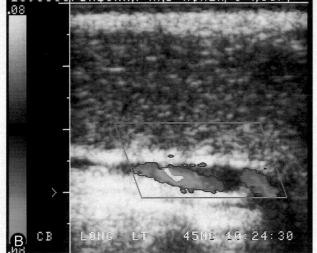

FIGURE 35–30. Venous incompetence. *A*, Longitudinal sonogram with the Doppler waveform below demonstrating flow in the dorsal vein (*arrows*). *B*, Longitudinal color Doppler sonogram demonstrating flow in the dorsal vein.

dorsal venous incompetence.[53,55,63] Persistently high diastolic flow without evident dorsal venous flow suggests venous leakage through the crural veins, as flow in these veins cannot be detected by Doppler sonography.

Although Doppler sonography can suggest the diagnosis of venous insufficiency, it is not the modality of choice for evaluating this disorder. Cavernosometry and cavernosography are preferable. Cavernosometry, performed with vasoactive pharmacologic agents, is the most accurate method for making the diagnosis. When venous incompetence is found, cavernosography provides anatomic delineation of the abnormal venous pathways.[63–66]

Venous competence can be assessed by Doppler only if arterial function is normal. Patients with arterial insufficiency may have too little arterial inflow to expand the sinusoids enough to occlude the draining veins, and hence, these patients may have venous flow regardless of whether the veins are intrinsically competent. For this reason, the results of the Doppler assessment of the cavernosal arteries should be kept in mind when evaluating for venous leakage. If the maximum systolic velocities in the cavernosal arteries are within the normal range, then further assessment for venous competence can be performed. If a diagnosis of arterial insufficiency is made based on abnormally low peak systolic velocities, conclusions about venous competence cannot be drawn from the arterial waveform or Doppler assessment of the dorsal vein.[45]

References

1. Doherty FJ: Ultrasound of the nonacute scrotum. Semin Ultrasound CT MRI 12:113–156, 1991.
2. Gerscovich EO: High-resolution ultrasonography in the diagnosis of scrotal pathology: I. Normal scrotum and benign disease. J Clin Ultrasound 21:355–373, 1993.
3. Hamm B, Fobbe F: Maturation of the testis: Ultrasound evaluation. Ultrasound Med Biol 21:143–147,1995.
4. Middleton WD, Bell MW: Analysis of intratesticular arterial anatomy with emphasis on transmediastinal arteries. Radiology 189:157–160, 1993.
5. Fakhry J, Khoury A, Barakat K: The hypoechoic band: A normal finding on testicular sonography. Am J Roentgenol 153:321–323, 1989.
6. Luker GD, Siegel MJ: Color Doppler sonography of the scrotum in children. Am J Roentgenol 163:649–655, 1994.
7. Ragheb D, Higgins JL: Ultrasonography of the scrotum, technique, anatomy and pathologic entities. J Ultrasound Med 21:171–185, 2002.
8. Black JAR, Patel A: Sonography of the normal extratesticular spaces. Am J Roentgenol 167:503–506, 1996.
9. Harris RD, Chouteau C, Patrick M, Schned A: Prevalence and significance of heterogeneous testes revealed on sonography: Ex vivo sonographic-pathologic correlation. Am J Roentgenol 175:347–352, 2000.
10. Winter T: Ultrasonography of the scrotum. Applied Radiology 31:9–18, 2002.
11. Middleton WD, Thorne DA, Melson GL: Color Doppler ultrasound of the normal testis. Am J Roentgenol 152:293–297, 1989.
12. Horstman WJ, Middleton WD, Melson GL, Siegel BA: Color Doppler US of the scrotum. RadioGraphics 11:941–957, 1991.
13. Watson LR, Abbitt PL, Woodard LL, Howard SS: Applied scrotal sonography. Applied Radiology 20:27–35, 1991.
14. Gerscovich EO: High-resolution ultrasonography in the diagnosis of scrotal pathology: II. Tumors. J Clin Ultrasound 21:375–386, 1993.
15. Lerner DM, Mevorach RA, Hulbert WC, Rabinowitz R: Color Doppler US in the evaluation of acute scrotal disease. Radiology 176:355–358, 1990.
16. Middleton WD, Teefey SA, Santillan CS: Testicular microlithiasis: Prospective analysis of prevalence and associated tumor. Radiology 224:425–428, 2002.
17. Luker GD, Siegel MJ: Pediatric testicular tumors: Evaluation with gray-scale and color Doppler US. Radiology 191:561–564, 1994.
18. Tumeh SS, Benson CB, Richie JP: Acute diseases of the scrotum. Semin Ultrasound CT MRI 12:115–130, 1991.
19. Oh C, Nisenbaum HL, Lanter J, et al: Sonographic demonstration, including color Doppler imaging, of recurrent sperm granuloma. J Ultrasound Med 19:333–335, 2000.
20. Frates MC, Benson CB, DiSalve DN, et al: Solid extratesticular masses evaluated with sonography: Pathologic correlation. Radiology 204:43–46, 1997.
21. Paltiel HJ, Connoly LP, Atala A, et al: Acute scrotal symptoms in boys with an indeterminate clinical presentation: Comparison of color Doppler sonography and scintigraphy. Radiology 207:223–231, 1998.

22. Paltiel HJ: Sonography of pediatric scrotal emergencies. Ultrasound Quarterly 16:53–71, 2000.

23. Gordon LM, Stein SM, Ralls PW: Traumatic epididymitis: Evaluation with color Doppler sonography. Am J Roentgenol 166:1323–1325, 1996.

24. Mazzu D, Greffrey RB, Ralls PW: Lymphoma and leukemia involving the testicles: Findings on gray-scale and color Doppler sonography. Am J Roentgenol 164:645–647, 1995.

25. Winkelbauer FW, Amman ME, Karnel F, Lammer J: Doppler sonography of varicocele: Long-term follow-up after venography and transcatheter sclerotherapy. J Ultrasound Med 13:953–958, 1994.

26. Graif M, Hauser R, Hirshebein A, et al: Varicocele and the testicular-renal venous route: Hemodynamic Doppler sonographic investigation. J Ultrasound Med 19:627–631, 2000.

27. Frush DP, Babcock DS, Lewis AG, et al: Comparison of color Doppler sonography and radionuclide imaging in different degrees of torsion in rabbit testes. Acad Radiol 2:945–951, 1995.

28. Weber DM, Rosslein R, Fliegel C: Color Doppler sonography in the diagnosis of acute scrotum in boys. Eur J Pediatr Surg 10:235–241, 2000.

29. Baker LA, Sigman D, Mathews RI, et al: An analysis of clinical outcomes using color Doppler testicular ultrasound for testicular torsion. Pediatrics 105:604–607, 2000.

30. Nussbaum-Blask AR, Bulas D, Shalaby-Rana E, et al: Color Doppler sonography and scintigraphy of the testis: A prospective, comparative analysis in children with acute scrotal pain. Pediatr Emerg Care 18:67–71, 2002.

31. Burks DD, Markey BJ, Burkhard TK, Balsara ZN, et al: Suspected testicular torsion and ischemia: Evaluation with color Doppler sonography. Radiology 175:815–821, 1990.

32. Kravchick S, Cytron S, Leibovici O, et al: Color Doppler sonography: Its real role in the evaluation of children with highly suspected testicular torsion. Eur Radiol 11:1000–1005, 2001.

33. Baud C, Veyrac C, Couture A, Ferran JL: Spiral twist of the spermatic cord: A reliable sign of testicular torsion. Pediatr Radiol 28:950–954, 1998.

34. Arce JD, Cortes M, Vargas JC: Sonographic diagnosis of acute spermatic cord torsion. Rotation of the cord: A key to the diagnosis. Pediatr Radiol 32:485–491, 2002.

35. Luker GD, Siegel MJ: Scrotal US in pediatric patients: Comparison of power and standard color Doppler US. Radiology 198:381–385, 1996.

36. Albrecht T, Lutzof K, Hussain JK, et al: Power Doppler US of the normal prepubertal testis: Does it live up to its promises? Radiology 203:227–231, 1997.

37. Lupetin AR, King W, Rich PJ, Lederman RB: The traumatized scrotum. Radiology 148:203–207, 1983.

38. Micallef M, Ahmad I, Hurley RN, McInerney D: Ultrasound features of blunt testicular injury. Injury 32:23–26, 2001.

39. Corrales JG, Corbel L, Cipolla B, et al: Accuracy of ultrasound diagnosis after blunt testicular trauma. J Urol 150:1834–1836, 1993.

40. Martinez-Pineiro L Jr, Cerezo E, Cozar JM, et al: Value of testicular ultrasound in the evaluation of blunt scrotal trauma without haematocele. Br J Urol 69:286–290, 1992.

41. Learch TJ, Hansch LP, Ralls PW: Sonography in patients with gunshot wounds of the scrotum: Imaging findings and their value. Am J Roentgenol 165:879–883, 1995.

42. Krane RJ, Goldstein I, Tejada IS: Impotence. N Engl J Med 321:1648–1659, 1989.

43. Krysiewicz S, Mellinger BC: The role of imaging in the diagnostic evaluation of impotence. Am J Roentgenol 153:1133–1139, 1989.

44. Paushter DM: Role of duplex sonography in the evaluation of sexual impotence. Am J Roentgenol 153:1161–1163, 1989.

45. Benson CB, Vickers MA Jr, Aruny J: Evaluation of impotence. Semin Ultrasound CT MR 12: 176–190, 1991.

46. Benson CB, Aruny JE, Vickers MA Jr: Correlation of duplex sonography with arteriography in patients with erectile dysfunction. Am J Roentgenol 160:71–73, 1993.

47. Kaufman JM, Borges FD, Fitch WP, et al: Evaluation of erectile dysfunction by dynamic infusion cavernosometry and cavernosography (DICC). Urology 41:445–451, 1993.

48. Kadioglu A, Erdogru T, Tellaloglu S: Evaluation of penile arteries in papaverine-induced erection with color Doppler ultrasonography. Arch Esp Urol 48:654–658, 1995.

49. Govier FE, Asase D, Hefty TR, et al: Timing of penile color flow duplex ultrasonography using a triple drug mixture. J Urol 153:1472–1475, 1995.

50. Schwartz AN, Wang KY, Mack LA, et al: Evaluation of normal erectile function with color flow Doppler sonography. Am J Roentgenol 153: 1155–1160, 1989.

51. Meuleman EJH, Bemelmans BLH, Doesburg WH, et al: Penile pharmacological duplex ultrasonography: A dose-effect study comparing papaverine, papaverine/phentolamine and prostaglandin E_1. J Urol 148:63–66, 1992.

52. Shabsigh R, Fishman IJ, Quesada ET, et al: Evaluation of vasculogenic erectile impotence using penile duplex ultrasonography. J Urol 142: 1469–1474, 1989.

53. Benson CB, Vickers MA: Sexual impotence caused by vascular disease: Diagnosis with

duplex sonography. Am J Roentgenol 153: 1149–1153, 1989.

54. Broderick GA, Arger P: Duplex Doppler ultrasonography: Noninvasive assessment of penile anatomy and function. Semin Roentgenol 28:43–56, 1993.

55. Quam JP, King BF, James EM, et al: Duplex and color Doppler sonographic evaluation of vasculogenic impotence. Am J Roentgenol 153: 1141–1147, 1989.

56. Hampson SJ, Cowie AGA, Rickards D, Lees WR: Independent evaluation of impotence by colour Doppler imaging and cavernosometry. Eur Urol 21:27–31, 1992.

57. Herbener TE, Seftel AD, Nehra A, Goldstein I: Penile ultrasound. Semin Urol 12:320–332, 1994.

58. Iacovo F, Barra S, Lotti T: Evaluation of penile deep arteries in psychogenic impotence by means of duplex ultrasonography. J Urol 149:1262–1264, 1993.

59. Mueller SC, Wallenberg-Pachaly H, Voges GE, Schild HH: Comparison of selective internal iliac pharmacoangiography, penile brachial index and duplex sonography with pulsed Doppler analysis for the evaluation of vasculogenic (arteriogenic) impotence. J Urol 143: 928–932, 1990.

60. Mueller SC, Lue TF: Evaluation of vasculogenic impotence. Urol Clin North Am 15:65–76, 1988.

61. Allen RP, Engel RME, Smolev JK, Brendler CB: Comparison of duplex ultrasonography and nocturnal penile tumescence in evaluation of impotence. J Urol 151:1525–1529, 1994.

62. Mancini M, Bartolini M, Maggi M, et al: The presence of arterial anatomical variations can affect the results of duplex sonographic evaluation of penile vessels in impotent patients. J Urol 155:1919–1923, 1996.

63. Vickers MA, Benson CB, Richie JR: High-resolution ultrasonography and pulsed-wave Doppler for detection of corporo-venous incompetence in erectile dysfunction. J Urol 43:1125–1127, 1990.

64. Gall H, Sparwasser DH, Stief CG, et al: Diagnosis of venous incompetence in erectile dysfunction. Urology 35:235–238, 1990.

65. Rudnick J, Bodecker R, Weidner W: Significance of intracavernosal pharmacological injection test, pharmacocavernosography, artificial erection and cavernosometry in the diagnosis of venous leakage. Urol Int 46:338–343, 1991.

66. Vickers MA, Benson CB, Dluhy R, Ball R: The current cavernosometric criteria for corporo-venous dysfunction are too strict. J Urol 147: 614–617, 1991.

Index

Note: Page numbers followed by f indicate figures; those followed by t indicate tables.